Handbook of Translational Medicine

Handbook of Translational Medicine

Editor: Kathlyn Rafferty

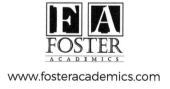

www.fosteracademics.com

www.fosteracademics.com

Cataloging-in-Publication Data

Handbook of translational medicine / edited by Kathlyn Rafferty.
   p. cm.
Includes bibliographical references and index.
ISBN 978-1-64646-625-2
1. Medicine. 2. Clinical medicine. 3. Medical sciences. 4. Medicine, Experimental.
5. Medical innovations. 6. Biomedical engineering. I. Rafferty, Kathlyn.
R852 .H36 2023
610.72--dc23

Foster Academics,
118-35 Queens Blvd., Suite 400,
Forest Hills, NY 11375, USA

ISBN 978-1-64646-625-2 (Hardback)

Contents

Preface

Translational medicine is an interdisciplinary branch of the biomedical field that aims to improve human health and longevity by determining the relevance of novel discoveries to human disease in the biological sciences. It is also referred to as translational science. This area of research is supported by three main pillars, namely, benchside, bedside and community. Translational medicine integrates disciplines, resources, expertise, and techniques within these pillars to promote enhancements in prevention, diagnosis, and therapies. It focuses on enhancing clinical medicine by incorporating the latest developments in research, reducing the gap between upcoming knowledge and its clinical application. Translational medicine plays an important role in shortening the duration of clinical trials and providing cost-effective solutions for healthcare delivery. This book provides comprehensive insights into the fundamentals of translational medicine. It is an essential guide for the graduate and postgraduate students, professionals and researchers engaged in this field.

Various studies have approached the subject by analyzing it with a single perspective, but the present book provides diverse methodologies and techniques to address this field. This book contains theories and applications needed for understanding the subject from different perspectives. The aim is to keep the readers informed about the progresses in the field; therefore, the contributions were carefully examined to compile novel researches by specialists from across the globe.

Indeed, the job of the editor is the most crucial and challenging in compiling all chapters into a single book. In the end, I would extend my sincere thanks to the chapter authors for their profound work. I am also thankful for the support provided by my family and colleagues during the compilation of this book.

Editor

1

Risk Factors, Pathogenesis and Strategies for Hepatocellular Carcinoma Prevention: Emphasis on Secondary Prevention and its Translational Challenges

Shen Li [1], Antonio Saviano [2], Derek J. Erstad [1], Yujin Hoshida [3]🆔, Bryan C. Fuchs [1]🆔, Thomas Baumert [2,*,†]🆔 and Kenneth K. Tanabe [1,*,†]

[1] Division of Surgical Oncology, Massachusetts General Hospital Cancer Center and Harvard Medical School, Boston, MA 02114, USA; sli8@bidmc.harvard.edu (S.L.); DERSTAD@partners.org (D.J.E.); Bryanfuchs1@gmail.com (B.C.F.)

[2] Inserm, U1110, Institut de Recherche sur les Maladies Virales et Hépatiques, Université de Strasbourg, 67000 Strasbourg, France; saviano@unistra.fr

[3] Simmons Comprehensive Cancer Center, UT Southwestern Medical Center, Department of Internal Medicine, Dallas, TX 75390, USA; Yujin.Hoshida@utsouthwestern.edu

* Correspondence: Thomas.Baumert@unistra.fr (T.B.); ktanabe@partners.org (K.K.T.)

† Indicates co-senior authorship.

Abstract: Hepatocellular carcinoma (HCC) is a leading cause of cancer-associated mortality globally. Given the limited therapeutic efficacy in advanced HCC, prevention of HCC carcinogenesis could serve as an effective strategy. Patients with chronic fibrosis due to viral or metabolic etiologies are at a high risk of developing HCC. Primary prevention seeks to eliminate cancer predisposing risk factors while tertiary prevention aims to prevent HCC recurrence. Secondary prevention targets patients with baseline chronic liver disease. Various epidemiological and experimental studies have identified candidates for secondary prevention—both etiology-specific and generic prevention strategies—including statins, aspirin, and anti-diabetic drugs. The introduction of multi-cell based omics analysis along with better characterization of the hepatic microenvironment will further facilitate the identification of targets for prevention. In this review, we will summarize HCC risk factors, pathogenesis, and discuss strategies of HCC prevention. We will focus on secondary prevention and also discuss current challenges in translating experimental work into clinical practice.

Keywords: hepatocellular carcinoma; hepatitis; NASH; chemoprevention

1. Introduction

Hepatocellular carcinoma (HCC) is the fifth most common malignancy and the fourth leading cause of cancer-associated mortality worldwide [1,2]. In 2015, there were 854,000 cases of HCC globally, with a male-to-female ratio of 2.4:1 [3]. Sub-Saharan Africa and East Asia have the highest incidence rate of HCC (more than 20 per 100,000 individuals), while North America and Europe have lower incidence levels (less than 5 per 100,000 individuals) [4–6]. Between 1996 and 2006, the HCC incidence rate in the US surveillance, epidemiology and end results (SEER) registries increased from 3.1 to 5.1 per 100,000 individuals, while the US liver cancer mortality rose from 3.3 to 4.0 per 100,000 individuals [7]. From 2006 to 2017, the rate of HCC has increased by 2–3% annually, largely due to the high prevalence of hepatitis C virus (HCV) cirrhosis and nonalcoholic steatohepatitis (NASH) [8,9].

Early HCC diagnosis occurs in 30–60% of cases, enabling curative treatments such as surgical resection and liver transplantation. Even with curative approaches, HCC recurrence is observed in up to 80% of patients within 5 years [10]. In advanced disease, surgical and systemic therapies have largely failed to yield survival benefits [11]. Until recently, Sorafenib was the only FDA-approved agent for advanced HCC. Since 2017, other multi-kinase inhibitors have been approved for second-line treatments, such as Cabozantinib and Ramucirumab [12–14]. Checkpoint inhibitors such as Nivolumab [15] and Pembrolizumab [16] have been either FDA approved or under investigation. Importantly, systemic therapies have substantial adverse effects that are difficult to manage in cirrhotic patients [17]. Finally, the high costs of approved therapies limit their use in low-resource countries [18]. Given the potential to identify high risk individuals and low survival rate once diagnosed, HCC prevention in at-risk patients can be a successful and alternative approach for HCC management. Here, we will review HCC risk factors, pathogenesis and current strategies for prevention, specifically secondary prevention and its clinical challenges.

2. Risk Factors and Carcinogenesis

2.1. Hepatitis B Virus (HBV)

Globally, 2 billion people have been exposed to HBV along with 250–350 million chronic carriers [19]. In high endemic areas, the HBV carrier rate is nearly 8% [20]. In areas of high incidence, 80% of patients with HCC are seropositive for the hepatitis B surface antigen (HBsAg) [21]. In East Asia, the HCC incidence rate in chronic HBV carriers ranges from 0.6 per 100 individuals without cirrhosis to 3.7 per 100 individuals with compensated cirrhosis. In Europe and the United states, the incidence rate ranges from 0.3 per 100 individuals without cirrhosis to 2.2 per 100 individuals in subjects with cirrhosis [22,23]. In addition, 10–20% of patients with HBV can develop HCC in the absence of cirrhosis [24]. Other factors that have been reported to increase the risk of HCC include duration of infection, viral load, environmental exposures (aflatoxin, alcohol, or tobacco), demographic features such as male sex, older age, family history of HCC, and co-infections with HCV, HDV, and HIV [25,26].

Two major mechanisms of HBV-induced HCC carcinogenesis have been proposed. First, chronic HBV can induce cirrhosis through the activation of HBV-specific T-cells, chemokine-mediated neutrophils, macrophages, and natural-killers [27,28]. These inflammatory cells promote carcinogenesis by stimulating hepatocyte regeneration, reactive oxygen species (ROSs) production, and DNA damage. Second, HBV DNA can be integrated into the host genome, prompting insertional activation of proto-oncogenes [29], induction of chromosomal instability [30], and the transcription of pro-carcinogenic HBV genes such as truncated envelope proteins [31], hepatitis B X gene (HBx) [32], and hepatitis B spliced proteins [33].

2.2. Hepatitis C Virus (HCV)

HCC induced by HCV has the highest HCC mortality rates per 100,000 individuals in the United States [34,35]. Chronic HCV is most prevalent in the "baby boomer" generation, defined as adults born between 1945 and 1965 who were exposed to blood transfusions, clotting factors, and hemodialysis prior to 1992 [36]. Moreover, the current opioid epidemic further contributes to the spread of HCV [37]. Between 2010 and 2017, a three-fold increase in acute HCV infections was reported by the CDC resulting from the opioid epidemic [38]. The annual incidence of HCV related HCC in patients with cirrhosis is extremely high, ranging from 1 to 12% per year [39,40]. In a large cohort of US patients with HCV, patients with genotype 3 are more likely to develop cirrhosis and HCC than other HCV genotypes [41].

HCC development in HCV is primarily associated with fibrosis and the viral copy number [42]. HCV associated HCC development occurs in a stepwise fashion, typically spanning over decades. All cases of HCV HCC arise from mutations in hepatocytes within a cirrhotic background. HCV proteins have also been shown to promote cellular proliferation, transformation, and tumor growth.

Over-expression of HCV core proteins, NS3 and NS5A, inhibit tumor suppressor genes *TP53*, *TP73*, and *RB1*, as well as negative cell cycle regulators such as CDKN1A. E2 and NS5B activate the RAF/mitogen-activated protein kinase (MAPK)/ERK kinase pathways [43]. NS5A activates the PI3K/AKT and beta-catenin/WNT pathways, and evades apoptosis by caspase-3 inhibition [44]. It is important to note that the interaction between nonstructural protein NS5A and HCV is dependent on Rab18-positive lipid droplets [45].

2.3. Nonalcoholic Fatty Liver Disease (NAFLD)/Nonalcoholic Steatohepatitis (NASH)

NAFLD/NASH has emerged as a leading cause of end-stage liver disease as well as HCC. Studies have demonstrated that the incidence of HCC in patients with NASH ranges from 2.4% over 7 years to 12.8% over 3 years [46]. Recent studies in the US have shown that NAFLD/NASH-related mortality has dramatically increased in the last 10 years together with NAFLD/NASH-related liver cirrhosis [47]. HCC in NAFLD/NASH is often diagnosed in patients without cirrhosis and is associated with late onset diagnosis and a higher tumor burden [48]. Moreover, patients with NASH receive sub-optimal HCC surveillance in comparison to patients with HCV cirrhosis [49].

The mechanism of HCC carcinogenesis as a result of NAFLD is not completely clear. Steatosis alone is not a driver of HCC as chronic inflammation is necessary for carcinogenesis [50]. Fat-tissue-derived free fatty acids (FFAs) lead to steatosis and lobular inflammation through the activation of intrahepatic lymphocytes and infiltrating macrophages. Hepatocyte cell death and compensatory proliferation together with increasing levels of tissue necrosis factor (TNF) superfamily members, transforming growth factor β (TGF-β), activation of hepatic stellate/liver sinusoidal endothelial cells, and hepatocyte chromosomal aberrations all contribute to HCC development [51]. The increased hepatocyte metabolism and oxidation of fatty acid induce overproduction of ROSs [52]. The excess of triglycerides and FFAs impair the initiation of autophagy through the activation of mammalian target of rapamycin (mTOR). When the antioxidant capacity of the hepatocytes is exceeded, DNA damage and oxidation occurs, eventually resulting in cell death [53,54].

It has also been suggested that the inflammatory responses seen in patients with NASH might be caused by an increase in gut permeability. Even though it is unclear whether a leaky gut is the consequence or the cause of NASH, it is evident that the translocation of lipopolysaccharide from gram-negative bacteria is an important aggravating factor for liver inflammation and fibrosis [55].

2.4. Lifestyle Risk Factors

Alcoholic liver disease (ALD) alters hepatic metabolism, causing progressive steatosis, fibrosis/cirrhosis, and HCC [56,57]. The risk of HCC increases with alcohol consumption as low as 10 g/day [58]. Perrsen et al. found that consuming more than three drinks daily was associated with an increase in HCC incidence and liver disease-related mortality [59]. There is a synergistic relationship between alcohol use of >60 g per day and viral hepatitis, with an approximately two-fold increase in the odds-ratio of developing HCC [60]. Alcohol use at least four times per week annually along with obesity (BMI > 30) increases the incidence of HCC [61]. Kimura et al. found that mild alcohol use (<20 g/day) in patients with NASH and advanced fibrosis was associated with a significant increase in the risk of HCC [62], while Ochiai et al. showed that ethanol intake ≥ 40 g was associated with a significant increase in multinodular HCCs [63].

The mechanism of ALD induced HCC is partially understood. Alcohol consumption can alter metabolic pathways including fatty acid oxidation and lipogenesis. Chronic alcohol consumption leads to an abnormal accumulation of acetaldehyde, which can exert carcinogenic effects through the formation of DNA-protein adduct [64]. Acetaldehyde has been shown in vitro to interfere with the transcriptional activities of peroxisome proliferator activated receptors (PPARs) and sterol regulatory element binding protein 1 (SREBP-1) [65,66]. Alcohol consumption can also reduce the level of 5′ AMP-activated protein kinase (AMPK), an important regulator of lipogenesis [67]. It is important to note that the severity of ALD is associated with genetic susceptibility. Genome-wide association studies (GWASs) have identified genetic risk loci for ALD, including *PNPLA3* [68] and *MBOAT7/TMC4* being related to a higher risk of cirrhosis in alcohol abusers [69].

Smoking is another important lifestyle risk factor for HCC. Tobacco smoking contributes to 13% of all HCC cases globally [70]. Current smokers have higher risks of HCC (hazard ratio 1.86, 95% CI: 1.57–2.20) [71], while those who quit for over 30 years have similar risks to non-smokers [72]. Tobacco contains multiple carcinogenic agents, including aromatic hydrocarbons [73], diethylnitrosamine (DEN) [74], and 4-aminobiphenyl [75]. Tobacco use is associated with an increase in inflammatory cytokines and ROS [76]. Tobacco also has been shown in rodent models to exacerbate the severity of NAFLD through the increasing of oxidative stress and hepatocellular apoptosis [77].

2.5. Environmental Carcinogens

A number of environmental chemicals have been implicated in HCC carcinogenesis. The best documented are aflatoxins. Other factors include vinyl chloride, arsenic compounds, polychlorinated biphenyls, and radioactive compounds [78]. Aflatoxins, mycotoxins produced by *Aspergillus flavus* and *Aspergillus parasiticus*, are frequently found in contaminated grain products such as maize and ground nuts in farming communities in sub-Saharan Africa, South America, and parts of Eastern Asia [79,80]. Aflatoxin B1 has been shown to form DNA adducts with hepatic DNA, leading to carcinogenesis in both humans and animal models [81]. In regions with high aflatoxin exposure, a 70-fold increase in the risk of HCC development has been observed [82].

2.6. Genetic Predisposition

Alpha 1-antitrypsin (AAT) deficiency is an autosomal recessive disease that results from mutations in the *SERPINA1* gene. This gene encodes a serine protease inhibitor, which functions to inhibit neutrophil elastase. A retrospective study in Sweden found an odds ratio of 20 for the development of HCC in patients with AAT deficiency [83]. Glycogen storage disease I, or Von Gierke's disease, leads to the impairment of glucose-6-phosphatase activity with excess glycogen storage in the liver [84]. Patients with glycogen storage disease I can develop hepatocellular adenomas by their second or third decade of life. A number of these patients go on to develop HCC [85]. The risk of HCC in patients with hemochromatosis is approximately 20 times higher than the general population [86]. Lastly, hereditary tyrosinemia type I is an autosomal recessive disease caused by an enzymatic deficiency in the catabolic pathway of tyrosine [87]. This disease can lead to acute hepatic failure or cirrhosis in infancy. In addition, 40% of patients who survive beyond the age of 2 develop HCCs [88].

GWAS have identified single-nucleotide polymorphisms (SNPs) that are associated with HCC carcinogenesis. A SNP in the epidermal growth factor (*EGF*) gene (rs4444903) was associated with an elevated risk of HCC in patients with cirrhosis [89]. A SNP (rs17401966) in Kinesin family member 1B (*KIF1B*) was associated with HBV-related HCC. Other SNPs in the Ubiquitination factor E4B (*UBE4B*) and Phosphogluconate dehydrogenase (*PDG*) genes were also shown to be associated with HCC amongst HBV positive patients [90]. Two SNPs (rs2596542 and rs1012068) discovered in a GWAS conducted in two large Japanese cohorts were significantly related with HCV-induced HCC [91,92].

2.7. Endocrine Risk Factors

Thyroid hormones are essential for lipid metabolism and have been shown to play a role in the pathogenesis of NAFLD/NASH [93]. Hypothyroidism has been demonstrated to be more common in patients with HCV, with a higher prevalence in those with cirrhosis [94]. Studies have also shown that patients with hypothyroidism have a two-fold higher risk of HCC than those with no prior history of thyroid cancer [95,96]. High thyroid stimulating hormone levels in HCC patients were found to be associated with larger tumor sizes [97]. Huang et al. demonstrated that 3,3'5-tri-iodo-L-thyronine (T_3) suppressed HCC cell proliferation through the inhibition of serine/threonine-protein kinase, PIM-1, via miRNA (miR-214-3p) [98]. T3 supplementation in rats resulted in fewer tumor nodules as well as a shift in global transcriptomic expression profile. T3 was shown to exert anti-carcinogenic effects through the maintaining of genes responsible for hepatocyte differentiation, such as *KLF9* and *HNF4a* [99].

Epidemiologically, HCC predominately occurs in males, with a male-to-female ratio ranging from 1.5:1 to 11:1. HCC prognosis, survival, and disease free survival after surgery are significantly better in females than males [100]. The predominance of HCC in males has been thought to be related to the effects of androgen/androgen receptors (ARs). ARs have been shown to promote HBV viral replication and HBV induced HCC [101], while AR knockout mice have fewer tumor nodules [102]. AR signaling has been demonstrated to promote key regulators of HCC carcinogenesis, including the MAPK/STAT/AKT pathway [103].

Estrogen/estrogen receptors (ERs) have been found to have protective effects against HCC while postmenopausal females have higher incidences of HCC [104,105]. Estrogen administration has been shown to reduce proinflammatory cytokines such as IL-6, a critical cytokine in HCC carcinogenesis [106]. Naugler et al. reported that estrogen treatment could reduce HCC carcinogenesis in DEN-injured rats by attenuating MyD88-dependent NF- κB signaling and inhibiting IL-6 signaling [107]. ER activation has also been shown to reduce STAT3 activation [108], a key regulator of the inflammatory tumor microenvironment [109].

3. Pathogenesis of HCC

A large body of research has been performed to address HCC pathogenesis. Large-scale genomic quantitative comparisons of HCC tumors have revealed the occurrence of chromosomal and microsatellite instability [110]. Loss of heterozygosity and SNP arrays have shown loss or mutations in tumor suppressor genes such as TP53 (*P53*) [111], retinoblastoma RB1 (*RB1*) [112], *CDKN2A* (*P16^{INK4A}*) [113], and insulin-like growth factor-2 receptor (*IGF-2R*) [114]. Gain of function mutations such as *CTNNBI* (β-catenin) can upregulate the transcription of MYC, cyclin D1, and COX2 [115]. There is a strong association between HBV encoded viral protein HBx and the suppression of *P53* induced apoptosis [116]. HCV core protein can also have direct carcinogenic effects by inducing ROSs [117].

Dysregulations of miRNAs, a class of small non-coding RNAs, can lead to HCC carcinogenesis [118]. Gene expression profiling has revealed that miR-181 upregulation is associated with the Wnt/B-catenin pathway [119]. MiR-26 downregulation has been shown to be associated with poor prognosis and a higher risk for metastasis [120]. Silencing of miR-122 was associated with increased cancer invasion, elevated alpha-fetoprotein expression, as well as higher HCC grades [121].

Genome-wide gene expression profiling has been used to capture dysregulated gene-expression signatures [122]. Numerous genome-wide expression studies have identified molecular sub-classes of HCC [123,124]. Aggressive HCC tumors are characterized by increased genetic instability, cellular proliferation, and impairment of tumor suppressor genes [125]. Hoshida et al. categorized HCC into three classes. S1 tumors are the most aggressive and are characterized by higher activation of *TGF-β*. S2 tumors overexpress EPCAM, AFP, and IGF-2 [126], while S3 tumors have matured hepatocyte-like phenotypes [127]. Zucman-Rossi et al. characterized proliferative vs. non-proliferative sub-classes of HCC. The main traits of the proliferative subclass are related to tumor proliferation and survival, while non-proliferative HCCs resemble normal hepatocytes [128].

It is also important to recognize that the hepatic microenvironment significantly promotes tumor progression [129] and concomitantly limits therapeutic interventions [130]. The normal liver stroma maintains tissue integrity and acts as a barrier against tumor formation [131]. During chronic inflammation, a modified stroma is formed, enriched in carcinoma-associated fibroblasts [132,133] and tumor-associated immune cells [134,135]. In such a pro-carcinogenic environment, cancer cells are potentiated to grow and proliferate such that responses to conventional treatments are altered (Figure 1).

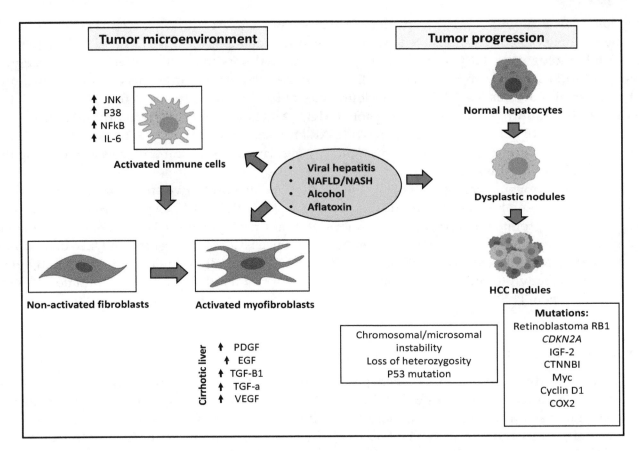

Figure 1. Mechanisms of hepatocellular carcinoma. Molecular pathways of HCC carcinogenesis are summarized. Risk factors include viral hepatitis, NAFLD, alcohol and toxins. HCC tumors develop as dysplastic nodules through the gaining of molecular aberrations and mutations. The cirrhotic microenvironment in the liver promotes HCC carcinogenesis through the activation of hepatic stellate cells into myofibroblasts. The cirrhotic background also promotes inflammation leading to the upregulation of pro-carcinogenic genes and pathways (text for details).

4. Molecular Biomarkers of HCC—The Prognostic Liver Signature

The major challenge in managing HCC is the complex and elusive mechanism of HCC carcinogenesis, leading to a scarcity of cancer biomarkers for targeted prevention trials. To circumvent this obstacle, a reverse engineering approach was developed to identify carcinogenic targets using long-term clinical follow-up patient cohorts, subsequently verified using in silico, in vitro, and in vivo models (Figure 2). It is hypothesized that cirrhosis leads to field cancerization, whereby cirrhotic liver tissue can harbor gene-expression signatures associated with carcinogenesis or recurrence after resection [136].

To verify this hypothesis, Hoshida et al. analyzed liver tissues surrounding resected HCV HCC tumors in 106 formalin-fixed, paraffin embedded blocks and identified a prognostic liver signature (PLS) containing 186 genes [137]. The poor-prognosis signature was found to be associated with an increase in liver-related deaths, progression of the Child–Pugh class, as well as HCC development. The 10-year HCC development rates were 42% and 18% for patients with poor and good prognostic signatures, respectively [138]. Though initially verified in HCV patients, the PLS also demonstrated significant concordance in liver tissues from HBV, alcohol, and NAFLD/NASH patients followed for 23 years [139]. This prognostic signature successfully verified the chemopreventive effect of erlotinib, a small molecule EGF pathway inhibitor, in multiple rodent models [140], and also led to the initiation of a cancer chemoprevention clinical trial (NCT02273362).

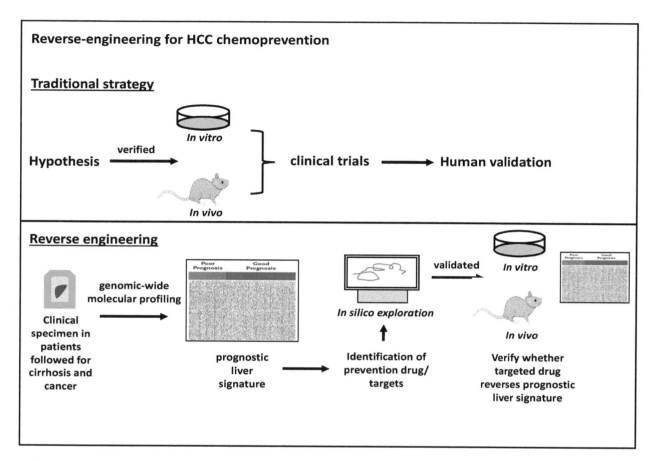

Figure 2. Reverse engineering for HCC chemoprevention. Traditionally, chemoprevention targets are verified in both in vitro and experimental animal models and then introduced into clinical trials (top panel). The reverse-engineering identifies targets for chemoprevention in human cohorts already followed for decades. Samples are genetically profiled into molecular signatures and then experimentally evaluated for mechanisms and therapeutic strategies (bottom panel).

Besides the EGF pathway, other inflammatory and fibrotic pathways have been identified as valuable cancer targets for prevention. Top enriched regulator genes were *AKT1, SLC35A1, DDX42, ILK,* and *LPAR1*. AKT-activated mTOR inhibitors, including everolimus and sirolimus, are currently being investigated for chemoprevention after transplantation [141]. Lysophosphatidic acid receptor 1 (LPAR1) is the receptor for the bioactive lipid lysophosphatidic acid (LPA) produced from lysophosphatidyl choline (LPC) through the actions of a secrete lysophospholipase D named autotaxin (ATX). LPAR1 overexpression has been shown to promote fibrosis [142], inflammation and HCC carcinogenesis via upregulation of its downstream effectors, including RhoA/ROCK, RAS/MAPK/ERK, and AKT/PI3K (Figure 3) [143]. In a DEN model of cirrhosis, LPAR1 upregulation coincided with the development of cirrhosis. Furthermore, LPAR1 inhibition with ATX inhibitors attenuated liver fibrosis, reduced the number of HCC nodules, and reversed the PLS risk gene signature [137,144].

The reverse-engineering technique along with the transcriptomic analysis of cancer-prone markers can be used to not only unearth key biomarkers of cancer prevention, but also be used for the proof-of-concept of other experimental compounds. Inhibition of chromatin reader Bromodomain 4—a target identified by reverse-engineering—by use of a small molecule, JQ1, reduced HCC carcinogenesis in experimental rodent models by reverting the epigenetic as well as the poor prognostic signature [145]. Villa et al. found a five-gene signature that predicted tumor doubling time as well as overall survival. In this study, ultrasound surveillance was used to identify newly diagnosed HCCs in cirrhotic patients. Patients then underwent two CT scans 6 weeks apart in order to determine tumor doubling time. In this study, five genes (*ANGPT2, NETO2, ESM1, NR4A1,* and *DLL4*) that regulated angiogenesis and endothelial cell migration were significantly upregulated and predicted tumor doubling time and survival [146].

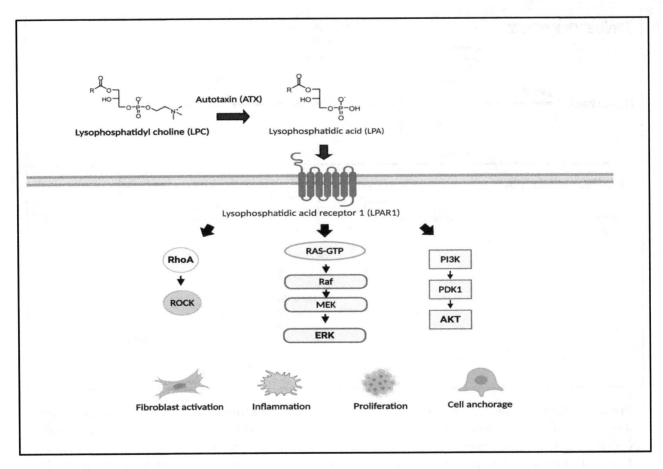

Figure 3. Lysophosphatidic acid (LPA) pathway as a novel chemoprevention target. Reverse engineering transcriptome analysis revealed the LPA pathway as a target for HCC prevention. LPA and its G protein-coupled receptors, lysophosphatidic acid receptors (LPARs), promote fibrosis, inflammation, and carcinogenesis through the activation of down-stream RhoA, Ras/mitogen-activated protein kinase (MAPK)/extracellular-signal-regulated kinase (ERK), and Akt/PI3K. LPA activation has been observed in human and rodent cirrhotic livers at risk for HCC.

5. Prevention Strategies

Understanding the risk factors and pathogenesis of HCC provides an opportunity for prevention strategies. Prevention can be sub-divided into primary, secondary, and tertiary prevention. Primary prevention focuses on eliminating cancer-predisposing factors through early vaccination, lifestyle modifications, as well as environmental interventions. Globally, a significant reduction in the incidence of HCC was observed after the implementation of hepatitis B vaccination [147–149]. Preventive actions against HCV can be taken through changes in social/cultural/medical practices such as the prevention of IV drug use and efficient screening of blood products and medical instruments [150]. In Australia, a substantial decline in the estimated intravenous drug use resulted in a decline in the number of new HCV infections from 14,000 per year in 2000 to 10,000 per year in 2005 [151]. Regulations of environmental carcinogens, such as Aflatoxin through information dissemination, have significantly reduced the Aflatoxin level in endemic areas [152].

Secondary prevention aims to delay the progression of chronic liver disease. This approach strives to eradicate the etiological agents (HBV and HCV) or inhibit the various steps in the carcinogenic progression. In general, chemoprevention agents should be inexpensive, well tolerated for long-term treatment, and available to the general population.

Tertiary prevention targets cancer recurrence or de-novo carcinogenesis within 1–2 years after curative treatment [153]. Ikeda et al. demonstrated in a randomized control trial that interferon-based immunotherapy after HCC resection resulted in a significant reduction in HCC recurrence [154]. Mazzaferro et al. demonstrated that adjuvant interferon therapy may reduce late recurrence of HCC [155]. Post-operative interferon-alpha is currently being investigated in patients with low miR-26 expression after HCC resection (NCT01681446). Immunosuppression with mTOR inhibitors has also been shown to reduce HCC recurrence [156,157] (Figure 4).

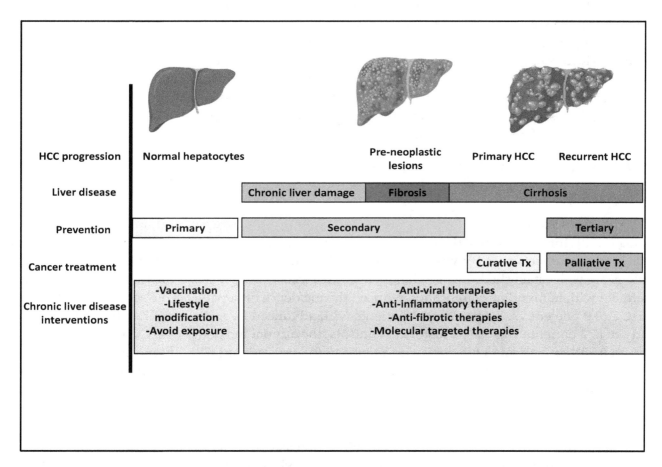

Figure 4. HCC-prevention strategies through the progression of HCC development. HCC prevention strategies, primary, secondary, and tertiary prevention, target various stages of liver disease progression (text for details).

6. Early Diagnosis and Surveillance

Compliance to HCC surveillance is associated with early diagnosis, allocation of curative treatment, and longer adjusted overall survival [158]. Practice guidelines from The American Association for the Study of Liver Diseases (AASLD) and The European Association for the Study of the Liver (EASL) recommend HCC surveillance for high risk patients by abdominal ultrasound performed by experienced personnel every 6 months [159,160]. Surveillance is indicated for all patients with cirrhosis. For patients with less advanced liver diseases, risk stratification using regression analysis is used to determine surveillance interval.

Models predicting the need for HCC surveillance in HCV patients use factors such as age, alcohol intake, platelet count, gamma-glutamyltransferase, and non-sustained virological response [161,162]. The ADRESS-HCC study, performed in 34,932 patients with decompensated cirrhosis from the US national liver transplant waiting list, identified six predictors of HCC (age, diabetes, race, etiology, sex, and severity of disease according to the Child–Turcotte–Pugh score) [163]. A retrospective analysis of the HALT-C trial demonstrated that the addition of the EGF SNP to clinical parameters (age, gender, smoking status, ALK-p level, and platelet count) could improve HCC risk stratification [164]. Furthermore, Ioannou et al. developed a risk stratification model for both NAFLD and ALD cirrhosis using seven predictors (age, gender, diabetes, BMI, platelet count, serum albumin, and AST/ALT ratio) [165].

HCC surveillance is often underutilized. Real-life worldwide retrospective cohorts reported screening adherence ranging from 5.7% to 78.8%, with higher rates occurring in countries with national screening programs [166]. A study from the US including 13,002 patients showed that only 42% of patients with HCV-cirrhosis received one or two surveillance tests during the first year and only 12% of them received surveillance two to four years after the diagnosis of cirrhosis [167].

Although ultrasound surveillance is currently the gold standard for HCC surveillance, there are downsides including sensitivities ranging from 47% to 84% depending on the operator's experience [168]. Magnetic resonance imaging (MRI) has high sensitivity and specificity for diagnosis of HCC and has the potential to improve HCC surveillance outcomes. In high-risk patients with cirrhosis, surveillance by MRI using liver-specific contrast increased early HCC detection compared to ultrasound but survival benefits and cost-effectiveness have not been demonstrated [169].

7. Etiology-Specific Secondary Chemoprevention

7.1. Hepatitis B

Antiviral treatments for HBV consist mainly of interferon therapies and nucleoside/nucleotide analogs [170]. Interferon alpha (IFN-α) therapy has shown inconsistent effects on HCC prevention due to its moderate effects on HBV viral replication [171]. The beneficial effects of nucleoside/nucleotide analogs are well established. In a randomized control trial, Liaw et al. demonstrated that continuous treatment with lamivudine significantly reduced the incidence of hepatic decompensation and the risk of HCC (3.9 percent vs. 7.4 percent) in patients with advanced liver disease [172]. In a retrospective study of 872 patients versus 699 historical controls, the annual incidence of HCC was reduced from 4.1% to 0.95% in patients with sustained response to lamivudine [173]. In one systemic review of 21 studies, the incidence of HCC was significantly lowered in HBV positive patients treated with lamivudine (2.8% vs. 6.4%; $p < 0.01$) [174].

7.2. Hepatitis C

Direct-acting anti-virals (DAAs) targeting viral protease, polymerase, and non-structural proteins have enabled improved sustained viral response compared to interferon-based therapies [175]. DAAs are better tolerated in cirrhotic patients in comparison to interferon-based therapies [176]. HCV-related cirrhosis mortality reached a plateau in 2014 and markedly declined from 2014 to 2016 after the introduction of DAAs [177]. After treatment, the sustained virologic response (SVR) is the best indication for successful HCV treatment [178]. Janjua et al. demonstrated that among DAA-treated patients, the HCC incidence rate was 6.9% in the SVR group vs. 38.2% in the non-SVR group [179]. Ioannou et al. found that DAA-induced SVR was associated with a 71% HCC risk reduction [180]. However, patients with pre-SVR fibrosis scores $\geq$ 3.25 have a higher annual incidence of HCC (3.66%/year) than those with <3.25 (1.16%/year) [181]. The persistence of HCC risk after HCV treatment can be partially explained by HCV-induced epigenetic modifications [182].

HCC surveillance should be continued in high-risk patients after DAA therapy. Despite the ongoing developments in HCV treatment options, the increasing rate of infection in young adults (age < 30) and the lack of screening are significant obstacles [183]. Barriers to HCV screening include lack of awareness, mental illness, lack of access to health care, and substance misuse [184]. The US Preventive Services Task Force recommends screening for adults at high risk, as well as one-time hepatitis C screening to all individuals born between 1945 and 1965. In high risk communities, the use of non-invasive fibroscanning can potentially identify individuals with chronic HCV [185].

Lifestyle intervention can be effective in patients with NAFLD and NASH. Weight loss > 10% has been shown to induce complete regression of NASH and partial regression of fibrosis [186]. Obese, sedentary individuals have increased risks of NAFLD in comparison to weight-matched physically active individuals [187]. EASL guidelines recommend moderate-intense aerobic physical activities in 3–5 sessions for a total of 150 min per week [188]. AASLD guidelines suggest the beneficial effects of physical activity but does not specify the exercise regimen [189]. There are currently no longitudinal studies demonstrating the effects of exercise on HCC risk reduction. Various pre-clinical rodent studies have demonstrated the efficacy of exercise in delaying HCC. In a hepatocyte-specific PTEN-deficient mouse model that developed steatohepatitis and spontaneous HCC, animals randomized to exercising developed fewer HCC nodules compared to sedentary animals (71% vs. 100%, respectively) [190].

Bariatric surgery is an effective option for weight loss in patients who are refractory to conservative treatment options. It has also been shown that bariatric surgery is a potential therapy for NASH. Lassailly et al. demonstrated that NASH resolved in 85% of patients after bariatric surgery while fibrosis was reduced in 33.8% of patients [191]. A meta-analysis demonstrated that bariatric surgery was associated with improvements in steatosis (91.6%), NASH (81.3%), as well as fibrosis (65.5%) [192]. Kwak et al. found that bariatric surgery was associated with a lower risk of HCC among matched cohorts of morbidly obese patients [193].

Diabetes mellitus (DM) has been shown to be an independent risk factor for HCC development [194]. Hyperinsulinemia can stimulate liver cell proliferation via the upregulation of IGF-1 [195] as well as hepatic stellate cell activation [196]. Insulin resistance is also an independent risk factor for liver fibrosis [197]. Given that NAFLD/NASH and DM commonly exist together, it is a reasonable hypothesis that anti-diabetic drugs have potential chemopreventive effects against NAFLD/NASH induced HCC. Metformin has been shown in several non-randomized studies to have HCC preventative effects in type-2 diabetic males [198]. In pre-clinical studies, the anti-carcinogenic effects of metformin have been shown to be mediated through the upregulation of AMPK, and the subsequent inactivation of mTOR via the upstream regulator of AMPK, LKB1 [199,200]. When exposed to DEN, male rats treated with metformin developed less fibrosis, cirrhosis, and overall fewer tumor nodules [201]. Metformin has been shown to improve liver histology and ALT levels in 30% of patients with NASH (NCT00063232). However, there are no completed clinical trials to date examining the effects of metformin administration on HCC prevention. The only trial to date (NCT02319200) was terminated early due to the lack of participants.

Long-term pioglitazone treatment can improve hepatic triglyceride content and fibrosis in patients with diabetes and NASH [202]. In a standard model, mice receiving a single injection of DEN, followed by the administration of a choline deficient L-amino acid diet, developed hepatic fibrosis and HCC nodules. In this model, pioglitazone administration at the initial onset of fibrosis resulted in a reduction in fibrosis and tumor nodules [203]. Pioglitazone targets downstream nuclear hormone PPARγ by binding to retinoid X receptor and subsequently regulating insulin sensitivity, glucose metabolism, and hepatic inflammation [204]. However, there are non-negligible side effects associated with pioglitazione, such as heart failure, weight gain, and bone loss.

Vitamin E is a lipid-soluble nutrient that acts as an antioxidant to prevent free radical damage in membranes and plasma lipoproteins [205]. Treatment with vitamin E has been shown to improve liver functions and fibrosis [206,207]. However, the effects of vitamin E on inflammation are controversial. A number of studies demonstrated no improvement in inflammation, while other studies concluded that vitamin E was associated with a significant improvement in steatosis, fibrosis, and inflammation [208–210]. No clinical data is available on vitamin E's HCC prevention effects.

7.3. Alcohol

Alcohol abstinence remains to be the most important treatment for alcohol-related hepatic disease. Alcohol cessation has been shown to decrease the risk of HCC by 6–10% per year. After two decades, the risk becomes equal to the general population [211]. Among former versus current drinkers, the odds-ratio of men developing HCC was significantly higher in those who stopped drinking for less than 10 years [212].

However, targeting sobriety is both complex and difficult to maintain. The current gold standard for alcohol use disorder is achieving total abstinence and preventing relapse [213]. Both inpatient and outpatient rehabilitation programs have shown efficacy in helping patients maintain abstinence [214]. It has also been shown that participation and communication with an alcohol addiction specialist in Alcoholic Anonymous can help to maintain abstinence [215]. Cognitive-behavioral coping skills therapy (CBT) is a psychotherapeutic approach that helps patients recognize risks for relapse and develop strategies to mitigate the risks. Patients are also encouraged to keep a diary to document the risk events [216].

Disulfiram, the most common and oldest pharmaceutical intervention for alcohol use disorder, works by inhibiting aldehyde dehydrogenase, resulting in an accumulation of aldehyde that usually results in a disulfiram–alcohol reaction, consisting primarily of tachycardia, flushing, nausea, and vomiting [217]. Studies have shown that disulfiram is effective in promoting short-term abstinence [218]. Naltrexone is an agent that blocks opioid receptors, which in turn leads to a reduction in dopamine levels and a reduction in alcohol intake [219]. The Combined Pharmacotherapies and Behavioral Interventions (COMBINE) study (NCT00006206) demonstrated that naltrexone, when given with medical counseling, resulted in an increase in the days of abstinence [220].

8. Etiology-Independent Secondary Chemoprevention Strategies

8.1. Statins

Statins, 3-hydroxy-3-methylgutaryl coenzyme A reductase inhibitors, are cholesterol-lowering agents that have cardiovascular protective effects [221]. Several randomized-controlled trials have demonstrated that statins have preventative effects in colorectal [222], breast [223], and prostate cancer [224]. Atorvastatin (10 mg/day) use in biopsy proven NASH patients demonstrated a 74% improvement in liver function tests as well as a rise in serum protein and adiponectin, a key regulator of lipid metabolism [225,226]. Statin use has been shown to correlate with a decreased risk of HCC carcinogenesis and recurrence after resection [227–229].

The anti-neoplastic effects of statins have been attributed to the inhibition of MYC [230], AKT [231,232], NF-κB, and IL6 production [233]. Statin use also reduces hepatic stellate cell activation via the induction of sterol regulatory element-binding protein 1 and PPAR [234], as well as reduction in portal hypertension via non-canonical hedgehog signaling [235]. Secondary prevention effects of simvastatin in patients with cirrhosis are being tested in a phase II clinical trial (NCT02968810). Currently, a multi-center double-blinded randomized clinical trial of tertiary prevention is being conducted with atorvastatin vs. placebo for HCC recurrence after completion ablation or hepatic resection (SHOT trial; NCT03024684).

8.2. Aspirin, COX2 Inhibitors and Anti-Platelet Agents

The major risk factor for HCC carcinogenesis is the non-resolving inflammation resulting in dysregulated production of cytokines, chemokines, growth factors, prostaglandins, and ROSs [236]. It is well established that TNF-α activated NF-κB is a critical mediator for HCC carcinogenesis [237]. In a large prospective study, the use of nonsteroidal anti-inflammatory drugs (NSAIDs) among men and women between the ages of 50 and 71 years was associated with a 37% reduced risk of HCC as well as a 51% reduced risk of mortality from chronic liver disease [238]. Cyclooxygenase-2 (COX2) controlled prostaglandins are upregulated in chronic liver disease [239]. Leng et al. demonstrated that COX2 overexpression in vitro resulted in cell growth and overexpression of AKT, while treatment with COX-2 inhibitor, celecoxib, resulted in a significant reduction in AKT activation and upregulation of apoptosis [240].

In two prospective cohorts of U.S. men and women, regular use of aspirin was associated with a significant reduction in the risk of developing HCC compared to non-regular use (2.1 vs. 5.2 cases per 100,000 person-years). However, prevention effects were not observed with other NSAIDs [241]. Aspirin has also been shown to inhibit platelet thromboxane, subsequently leading to the inhibition of spingosine-1-phosphate S1P, a lipid molecule that has been shown to promote HCC proliferation [242]. A study demonstrated that the combination of aspirin and clopidogrel reduced intrahepatic immune cell infiltration, NASH, and HCC [243]. However, increased risk of bleeding may limit the use of these drugs for long-term prevention, particularly in cirrhotic patients. Besides its anti-inflammatory properties, aspirin has also been shown to have anti-fibrotic properties. Wang et al. showed that aspirin targets P4HA2, an enzyme involved in collagen synthesis [244]. Aspirin administration to mice that were subcutaneously engrafted with HepG2 cells resulted in a reduction in collagen deposition and tumor growth [245]. Daily aspirin use was also shown to significantly lower the odds-ratio of NASH and fibrosis in 361 adults with biopsy-proven NAFLD [246].

8.3. Anti-Fibrosis Therapy

Fibrosis has been shown to be a key risk factor for HCC [247]. However, anti-fibrotic therapies for HCC prevention have not been established. Most clinical trials are designed to study the anti-fibrosis or anti-cancer effects of drugs, but rarely both. Though promising, therapies such as ASK-1 inhibitor, selonsertib (NCT02466516) and dual PPARα/δ agonist, elafibranor (NCT02704403), have demonstrated efficacy in reducing fibrosis but have not been tested for HCC prevention [248,249].

8.4. Nutritional Agents

Food-derived agents, nutritional supplements, and certain phytochemicals, plant-derived bioactive chemicals, have been recognized as potential prevention options for HCC. Glycyrrhizin, an extract of licorice root, has been shown to lower serum aminotransferases, improve liver histology, and delay HCC carcinogenesis in humans and animal models [250–253]. Sho-saiko-to, a Chinese herbal medicine that contains glycyrrhizin, was shown to increase survival in cirrhotic HBV patients as well as decrease the incidence of HCC [254]. Beta-carotene derived from fruits and vegetables reduced the number and size of hepatic nodules in rats injured by DEN and phenobarbital [255]. Epigallocatechin gallate (EGCG), the most abundant green tea catechin polyphenol, has been shown to inhibit tumor growth and induce apoptosis in vitro [256]. In a rodent HCC model of DEN and aflatoxin, EGCG treatment reduced the number of placental glutathione S-transferase positive pre-neoplastic nodules [257]. In a phase 2 clinical trial, consumption of green tea polyphenols led to a significant reduction in oxidative DNA damage in HBV positive patients exposed to aflatoxin [258]. EGCG was also shown to reverse the poor prognostic gene signature described by Hoshida et al. [137,259]. The mechanisms of HCC risk reduction with coffee consumption have yet to be determined. However, coffee has been shown to contain numerous anti-carcinogenic chemical compounds. Diterpenes have been shown to upregulate detoxifying enzymes and reduce the formation of aflatoxin–DNA adducts [260].

Higher vitamin D, 25(OH)D, levels have been associated with a reduced risk of HCC, while low levels are associated with increased risk of HBV-related HCC [261,262]. In DEN-injured mice, vitamin D3 up-regulated protein 1 (VDUP1) has been shown to suppress TNF and NF-κB activation [263]. Oral vitamin D3 is currently under investigation for the prevention of HCC in HBV patients (NCT02779465). Branched-chain amino acids (BCAA) have been shown to reduce hepatic fibrosis and HCC carcinogenesis in DEN-injured rats [264]. In an observational study of cirrhotic patients in Japan, BCAA supplementation was associated with a lower incidence of HCC development [265].

Fish is a rich source for n-3 polyunsaturated fatty acids and has been shown to reduce the risk of HCC by 35% [266] irrespective of the viral hepatitis status [267]. In a NAFLD HCC rodent model, mice fed with an n-3 polyunsaturated fatty acid supplemented diet have significant reductions in fibrosis and tumor nodules [268]. However, processed red meat has been shown to actually increase the risk of HCC [269] (Figure 5).

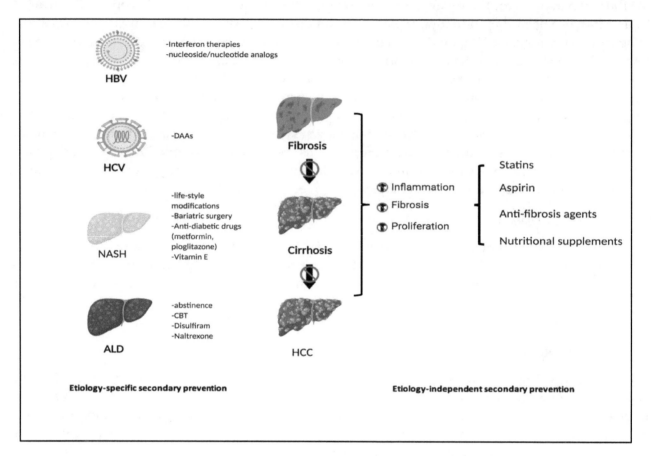

Figure 5. Etiology-specific and independent secondary HCC prevention. Etiology-specific secondary prevention targets the various risk factors of HCC development, including HBV, HCV, NAFLD/NASH, and ALD. Etiology independent prevention strategies include agents that have anti-fibrosis or anti-inflammatory activities.

9. Challenges and Obstacles in Prevention

A major obstacle in HCC chemoprevention is the lack of accurate pre-clinical models that closely mimic HCC carcinogenesis in humans. Many drugs that enter phase I clinical trials are able to progress to phase II [270]. However, 95% of drugs that enter clinical trials do not enter the market [271]. Many drugs are initially tested in the pre-clinical setting using in vitro systems. Cancer cell lines are invaluable in vitro models that are widely used for cancer research and novel drug discovery. The major concern is that they do not accurately reflect their tissues of origin due to genetic mutations and passage cycle-derived transcriptomic alterations. Many human HCC cell lines are strikingly different to their tumors of origin [272]. This is likely why compounds that show promise in in vitro models are ineffective clinically [273]. There lacks an in vitro system in cancer prevention research that captures cancer initiation, promotion, and progression. Most commonly established human HCC cell lines such as HepG3 and HuH7 can be used to investigate cancer treatment, but not prevention.

An ideal in vivo animal model should capture the key biological features of HCC and recapitulate the tumor microenvironment. Major etiologies for failure include the complex molecular heterogeneity as well as the limited understanding of HCC carcinogenesis. HCC genetically engineered mouse models (GEEMs) activate oncogenes such as *HRAS* or *MYC* [274] or disrupt tumor suppressor genes such as *PTEN* or *TP53* [275]. However, most GEMMs have failed in addressing the complex interaction between HCC and the representative microenvironment.

Chemical carcinogens such as carbon tetrachloride [276], DEN [277] and thioacetamide [278] induce fibrosis, cirrhosis and HCC sequentially. The repeated, low dose DEN cirrhosis-driven rat model [279] demonstrated an induction of the HCC prognostic gene signature similar to that of the human signature [139]. Chemical carcinogens such as DEN are an excellent model for chemoprevention research given the accurate recapitulation of all steps in the HCC carcinogenesis pathway.

Prior to the omics era, there were limited HCC prevention targets. Transcriptomic analysis of clinical specimens and reverse-engineering prevention targets may ultimately overcome this challenge. Cirrhotic patients expressing the poor prognostic signature would benefit the most from chemoprevention. HCC chemoprevention clinical trials are difficult to conduct and expensive given the requirement for a large sample size and long observation periods. Even if an agent demonstrates efficacy with a low toxicity profile, it still takes 5–10 years for a drug to move through phase III clinical trial [280]. Prevention trials focused on lifestyle modification, such as weight control, diet, and physical activity, can be challenging because these activities are typically clustered, thus identifying the change of a single behavior can be difficult if not impossible [281].

Another major challenge in HCC prevention is the lack of understanding of the long term tolerability and impact on quality of life of many drugs. To be acceptable for HCC prevention, a drug needs to be well tolerated for an extended period of time with minimal—if any—side effects. It is also important for physicians to be comfortable in prescribing these medications. Even minor side effects can be enough to affect quality of life and compliance with a cancer prevention medication, thus limiting its efficacy. This is especially of importance in HCC prevention, where a majority of this patient population have some form of chronic cirrhosis. Metformin is generally well tolerated with a good safety profile. However, lactic acidosis, one of its most notorious side effects, is more likely to occur in patients with hepatic insufficiency [282]. Aspirin is also commonly prescribed and well tolerated, but physicians may not be comfortable prescribing aspirin to cirrhotic patients who are at high risk of gastrointestinal bleeds.

10. Conclusions

Integration of HCC prevention research to the clinical setting is an extremely important strategy. Prevention clinical trials are very challenging to conduct because of the need for large sample sizes and long observation times. In addition, establishing the optimal dose and duration for chemopreventive drugs remains a challenge. Although there has been notable success in primary and secondary prevention for viral hepatitis such as the HBV vaccine or HCV cure by DAAs, similar successes for prevention of metabolic HCC are largely absent given the challenges associated with strategies of improved diet and regular exercise. Furthermore, there is no approved strategy to prevent HCC in advanced fibrosis or post HCC resection. Advances in the field of HCC chemoprevention will be aided by a more complete characterization of HCC carcinogenesis as well as a better understanding of the liver microenvironment. The main challenge in HCC prevention research will always be translating pre-clinical research into successful clinical trials but there is a promise for success as we develop more individualized therapies.

Author Contributions: S.L., A.S., B.C.F., T.B., and K.K.T. contributed to conceptualization; S.L., A.S., D.J.E. contributed to original draft preparation. S.L., A.S., D.J.E., Y.H., B.C.F., T.B., and K.K.T. contributed to reviewing and editing. S.L. contributed to visualization. K.K.T. contributed to supervision. All authors have read and agreed to the published version of the manuscript.

Abbreviations

AR	Androgen receptor
ALD	Alcoholic liver disease
AMPK	AMP-activated protein kinase

COX2	Cyclooxygenease-2
DAA	Direct-acting antivirals
DEN	N-diethylnitrosamine
DM	Diabetes mellitus
EGF	Epidermal growth factor
EGFR	Epidermal growth factor receptor
GWAS	Genome wide associated studies
HBV	Hepatitis B virus
HCV	Hepatitis C virus
HCC	Hepatocellular carcinoma
IFN-α	Interferon alpha
LAR	Lysophosphatidic acid receptor
LPAR1	Lysophosphatidic Acid Receptor 1
mTOR	Mammalian target of rapamycin
NAFLD	Nonalcoholic fatty liver disease
NF-κB	Nuclear factor κB
NASH	Nonalcoholic steatohepatitis
NSAIDS	Nonsteroidal anti-inflammatory drugs
PPAR	Peroxisome proliferator activated receptors
PLS	Prognostic liver signature
ROS	Reactive oxygen species
SNP	Single nucleotide polymorphism
SVR	Sustained virologic response
TNF-a	Tumor-Necrosis-Factor alpha

References

1. Yang, J.D.; Hainaut, P.; Gores, G.J.; Amadou, A.; Plymoth, A.; Roberts, L.R. A global view of hepatocellular carcinoma: Trends, risk, prevention and management. *Nat. Rev. Gastroenterol. Hepatol.* **2019**, *16*, 589–604. [CrossRef] [PubMed]

2. Bray, F.; Me, J.F.; Soerjomataram, I.; Siegel, R.L.; Torre, L.A.; Jemal, A. Global cancer statistics 2018: GLOBOCAN estimates of incidence and mortality worldwide for 36 cancers in 185 countries. *CA Cancer J. Clin.* **2018**, *68*, 394–424. [CrossRef] [PubMed]

3. Asrani, S.K.; Devarbhavi, H.; Eaton, J.; Kamath, P.S. Burden of liver diseases in the world. *J. Hepatol.* **2019**, *70*, 151–171. [CrossRef] [PubMed]

4. Siegel, R.L.; Miller, K.D.; Jemal, A. Colorectal cancer statistics, 2020. *CA Cancer J. Clin.* **2020**, *70*, 7–30. [CrossRef]

5. Beste, L.A.; Leipertz, S.L.; Green, P.K.; Dominitz, J.A.; Ross, D.; Ioannou, G.N. Trends in Burden of Cirrhosis and Hepatocellular Carcinoma by Underlying Liver Disease in US Veterans, 2001–2013. *Gastroenterology* **2015**, *149*, 1471–1482.e5. [CrossRef]

6. Mokdad, A.H.; Forouzanfar, M.H.; Daoud, F.; Mokdad, A.A.; El Bcheraoui, C.; Moradi-Lakeh, M.; Kyu, H.H.; Barber, R.M.; Wagner, J.; Cercy, K.; et al. Global burden of diseases, injuries, and risk factors for young people's health during 1990–2013: A systematic analysis for the Global Burden of Disease Study 2013. *Lancet* **2016**, *387*, 2383–2401. [CrossRef]

7. Kanwal, F.; Hoang, T.; Kramer, J.R.; Asch, S.M.; Goetz, M.B.; Zeringue, A.; Richardson, P.; El–Serag, H.B. Increasing Prevalence of HCC and Cirrhosis in Patients with Chronic Hepatitis C Virus Infection. *Gastroenterology* **2011**, *140*, 1182–1188.e1. [CrossRef]

8.   Howlader, N.; Noone, A.M.; Krapcho, M.; Miller, D.; Brest, A.; Yu, M.; Ruhl, J.; Tatalovich, Z.; Mariotto, A.; Lewis, D.R.; et al. *SEER Cancer Statistics Review, 1975-2016*; Based on November 2018 SEER Data Submission, Posted to the SEER Web Site; National Cancer Institute: Bethesda, MD, USA, 2019.

9.   Altekruse, S.F.; McGlynn, K.A.; Reichman, M.E. Hepatocellular Carcinoma Incidence, Mortality, and Survival Trends in the United States From 1975 to 2005. *J. Clin. Oncol.* **2009**, *27*, 1485–1491. [CrossRef]

10.   Lopez, P.M.; Villanueva, A.; Llovet, J.M. Systematic review: Evidence-based management of hepatocellular carcinoma—An updated analysis of randomized controlled trials. *Aliment. Pharmacol. Ther.* **2006**, *23*, 1535–1547. [CrossRef]

11.   Pompili, M.; Saviano, A.; De Matthaeis, N.; Cucchetti, A.; Ardito, F.; Federico, B.; Brunello, F.; Pinna, A.D.; Giorgio, A.; Giulini, S.M.; et al. Long-term effectiveness of resection and radiofrequency ablation for single hepatocellular carcinoma ≤ 3 cm. Results of a multicenter Italian survey. *J. Hepatol.* **2013**, *59*, 89–97. [CrossRef]

12.   Llovet, J.M.; Ricci, S.; Mazzaferro, V.; Hilgard, P.; Gane, E.; Blanc, J.-F.; De Oliveira, A.C.; Santoro, A.; Raoul, J.-L.; Forner, A.; et al. Sorafenib in Advanced Hepatocellular Carcinoma. *N. Engl. J. Med.* **2008**, *359*, 378–390. [CrossRef] [PubMed]

13.   Abou-Alfa, G.K.; Meyer, T.; Cheng, A.-L.; El-Khoueiry, A.B.; Rimassa, L.; Ryoo, B.-Y.; Cicin, I.; Merle, P.; Chen, Y.; Park, J.-W.; et al. Cabozantinib in Patients with Advanced and Progressing Hepatocellular Carcinoma. *N. Engl. J. Med.* **2018**, *379*, 54–63. [CrossRef] [PubMed]

14.   Zhu, A.X.; Galle, P.R.; Kudo, M.; Finn, R.S.; Qin, S.; Xu, Y.; Abada, P.; Llovet, J. A study of ramucirumab (LY3009806) versus placebo in patients with hepatocellular carcinoma and elevated baseline alpha-fetoprotein (REACH-2). *J. Clin. Oncol.* **2018**, *36*, TPS538. [CrossRef]

15.   El-Khoueiry, A.B.; Sangro, B.; Yau, T.; Crocenzi, T.S.; Kudo, M.; Hsu, C.; Kim, T.-Y.; Choo, S.-P.; Trojan, J.; Welling, T.H.; et al. Nivolumab in patients with advanced hepatocellular carcinoma (CheckMate 040): An open-label, non-comparative, phase 1/2 dose escalation and expansion trial. *Lancet* **2017**, *389*, 2492–2502. [CrossRef]

16.   Finn, R.S.; Ryoo, B.-Y.; Merle, P.; Kudo, M.; Bouattour, M.; Lim, H.-Y.; Breder, V.V.; Edeline, J.; Chao, Y.; Ogasawara, S.; et al. Results of KEYNOTE-240: Phase 3 study of pembrolizumab (Pembro) vs. best supportive care (BSC) for second line therapy in advanced hepatocellular carcinoma (HCC). *J. Clin. Oncol.* **2019**, *37*, 4004. [CrossRef]

17.   Pinter, M.; Jain, R.K.; Duda, D.G. The Current Landscape of Immune Checkpoint Blockade in Hepatocellular Carcinoma. *JAMA Oncol.* **2020**, *22*. [CrossRef]

18.   Zhang, P.; Yang, Y.; Wen, F.; He, X.; Tang, R.; Du, Z.; Zhou, J.; Zhang, J.; Li, Q. Cost-effectiveness of sorafenib as a first-line treatment for advanced hepatocellular carcinoma. *Eur. J. Gastroenterol. Hepatol.* **2015**, *27*, 853–859. [CrossRef]

19.   El-Serag, H.B.; Rudolph, K.L. Hepatocellular Carcinoma: Epidemiology and Molecular Carcinogenesis. *Gastroenterology* **2007**, *132*, 2557–2576. [CrossRef]

20.   Franco, E. Hepatitis B: Epidemiology and prevention in developing countries. *World J. Hepatol.* **2012**, *4*, 74–80. [CrossRef]

21.   Hsu, Y.-S.; Chien, R.-N.; Yeh, C.-T.; Sheen, I.-S.; Chiou, H.-Y.; Chu, C.-M.; Liaw, Y.-F. Long-term outcome after spontaneous HBeAg seroconversion in patients with chronic hepatitis B. *Hepatology* **2002**, *35*, 1522–1527. [CrossRef]

22.   Fattovich, G.; Olivari, N.; Pasino, M.; D'Onofrio, M.; Martone, E.; Donato, F. Long-term outcome of chronic hepatitis B in Caucasian patients: Mortality after 25 years. *Gut* **2007**, *57*, 84–90. [CrossRef] [PubMed]

23.   Fattovich, G. Natural History and Prognosis of Hepatitis B. *Semin. Liver Dis.* **2003**, *23*, 047–058. [CrossRef] [PubMed]

24.   Yang, J.D.; Kim, W.R.; Coelho, R.; Mettler, T.A.; Benson, J.T.; Sanderson, S.O.; Therneau, T.M.; Kim, B.; Roberts, L.R. Cirrhosis Is Present in Most Patients with Hepatitis B and Hepatocellular Carcinoma. *Clin. Gastroenterol. Hepatol.* **2011**, *9*, 64–70. [CrossRef] [PubMed]

25.   Osawa, M.; Akuta, N.; Suzuki, F.; Fujiyama, S.; Kawamura, Y.; Sezaki, H.; Hosaka, T.; Kobayashi, M.; Kobayashi, M.; Saitoh, S.; et al. Prognosis and predictors of hepatocellular carcinoma in elderly patients infected with hepatitis B virus. *J. Med. Virol.* **2017**, *89*, 2144–2148. [CrossRef] [PubMed]

26.   El-Serag, H.B. Epidemiology of Viral Hepatitis and Hepatocellular Carcinoma. *Gastroenterology* **2012**, *142*, 1264–1273.e1. [CrossRef]

27.   Soussan, P.; Garreau, F.; Zylberberg, H.; Ferray, C.; Brechot, C.; Kremsdorf, D. In vivo expression of a new hepatitis B virus protein encoded by a spliced RNA. *J. Clin. Investig.* **2000**, *105*, 55–60. [CrossRef]

28.   Edmunds, W.J.; Medley, G.F.; Nokes, D.J.; Hall, A.J.; Whittle, H.C. The influence of age on the development of the hepatitis B carrier state. *Proc. R. Soc. B Boil. Sci.* **1993**, *253*, 197–201. [CrossRef]

29.   Sung, W.-K.; Zheng, H.; Li, S.; Chen, R.; Liu, X.; Li, Y.; Lee, N.P.; Lee, W.H.; Ariyaratne, P.N.; Tennakoon, C.; et al. Genome-wide survey of recurrent HBV integration in hepatocellular carcinoma. *Nat. Genet.* **2012**, *44*, 765–769. [CrossRef]

30.   Yan, H.; Yang, Y.; Zhang, L.; Tang, G.; Wang, Y.; Xue, G.; Zhou, W.; Sun, S. Characterization of the genotype and integration patterns of hepatitis B virus in early- and late-onset hepatocellular carcinoma. *Hepatology* **2015**, *61*, 1821–1831. [CrossRef]

31.   Chemin, I.; Zoulim, F. Hepatitis B virus induced hepatocellular carcinoma. *Cancer Lett.* **2009**, *286*, 52–59. [CrossRef]

32.   Lucifora, J.; Arzberger, S.; Durantel, D.; Belloni, L.; Strubin, M.; Levrero, M.; Zoulim, F.; Hantz, O.; Protzer, U. Hepatitis B virus X protein is essential to initiate and maintain virus replication after infection. *J. Hepatol.* **2011**, *55*, 996–1003. [CrossRef] [PubMed]

33.   Bayliss, J.; Lim, L.; Thompson, A.J.; Desmond, P.; Angus, P.; Locarnini, S.; Revill, P.A. Hepatitis B virus splicing is enhanced prior to development of hepatocellular carcinoma. *J. Hepatol.* **2013**, *59*, 1022–1028. [CrossRef] [PubMed]

34.   Wong, R.J.; Cheung, R.; Ahmed, A. Nonalcoholic steatohepatitis is the most rapidly growing indication for liver transplantation in patients with hepatocellular carcinoma in the U.S. *Hepatology* **2014**, *59*, 2188–2195. [CrossRef] [PubMed]

35.   Galbraith, J.W.; Franco, R.A.; Donnelly, J.P.; Rodgers, J.B.; Morgan, J.M.; Viles, A.F.; Overton, E.T.; Saag, M.S.; Wang, H.E. Unrecognized chronic hepatitis C virus infection among baby boomers in the emergency department. *Hepatology* **2015**, *61*, 776–782. [CrossRef]

36.   Jacobson, I.M.; Davis, G.L.; El–Serag, H.; Negro, F.; Trepo, C. Prevalence and Challenges of Liver Diseases in Patients with Chronic Hepatitis C Virus Infection. *Clin. Gastroenterol. Hepatol.* **2010**, *8*, 924–933. [CrossRef]

37.   Liang, T.J.; Ward, J.W. Hepatitis C in Injection-Drug Users—A Hidden Danger of the Opioid Epidemic. *New Engl. J. Med.* **2018**, *378*, 1169–1171. [CrossRef]

38.   Khan, A.D.; Magee, E.; Grant, G. *National Center for HIV/AIDS, Viral Hepatitis, STD, and TB Prevention*; CDC Health Disparities Inequalities Report—United States; CDC: Atlanta, GA, USA, 2013; Volume 62, p. 149.

39.   Galbraith, J.W.; Donnelly, J.P.; Franco, R.A.; Overton, E.T.; Rodgers, J.B.; Wang, H.E. National Estimates of Healthcare Utilization by Individuals with Hepatitis C Virus Infection in the United States. *Clin. Infect. Dis.* **2014**, *59*, 755–764. [CrossRef]

40.   Yoshida, H.; Shiratori, Y.; Moriyama, M.; Arakawa, Y.; Ide, T.; Sata, M.; Inoue, O.; Yano, M.; Tanaka, M.; Fujiyama, S.; et al. Interferon Therapy Reduces the Risk for Hepatocellular Carcinoma: National Surveillance Program of Cirrhotic and Noncirrhotic Patients with Chronic Hepatitis C in Japan. *Ann. Intern. Med.* **1999**, *131*, 174–181. [CrossRef]

41.   Kanwal, F.; Kramer, J.R.; Ilyas, J.; Duan, Z.; El-Serag, H.B. HCV genotype 3 is associated with an increased risk of cirrhosis and hepatocellular cancer in a national sample of U.S. Veterans with HCV. *Hepatology* **2014**, *60*, 98–105. [CrossRef]

42.   Hoshida, Y.; Fuchs, B.C.; Bardeesy, N.; Baumert, T.F.; Chung, R.T. Pathogenesis and prevention of hepatitis C virus-induced hepatocellular carcinoma. *J. Hepatol.* **2014**, *61*, S79–S90. [CrossRef]

43.   Vescovo, T.; Refolo, G.; Vitagliano, G.; Fimia, G.; Piacentini, M. Molecular mechanisms of hepatitis C virus–induced hepatocellular carcinoma. *Clin. Microbiol. Infect.* **2016**, *22*, 853–861. [CrossRef] [PubMed]

44.   Street, A.; Macdonald, A.; McCormick, C.J.; Harris, M. Hepatitis C Virus NS5A-Mediated Activation of Phosphoinositide 3-Kinase Results in Stabilization of Cellular β-Catenin and Stimulation of β-Catenin-Responsive Transcription. *J. Virol.* **2005**, *79*, 5006–5016. [CrossRef]

45.   Salloum, S.; Wang, H.; Ferguson, C.; Parton, R.G.; Tai, A.W. Rab18 Binds to Hepatitis C Virus NS5A and Promotes Interaction between Sites of Viral Replication and Lipid Droplets. *PLoS Pathog.* **2013**, *9*, e1003513. [CrossRef]

46.   Yang, J.D.; Roberts, L.R. Hepatocellular carcinoma: A global view. *Nat. Rev. Gastroenterol. Hepatol.* **2010**, *7*, 448–458. [CrossRef] [PubMed]

47. Kim, D.; Li, A.A.; Gadiparthi, C.; Khan, M.A.; Cholankeril, G.; Glenn, J.S.; Ahmed, A. Changing Trends in Etiology-Based Annual Mortality From Chronic Liver Disease, From 2007 through 2016. *Gastroenterology* **2018**, *155*, 1154–1163.e3. [CrossRef] [PubMed]

48. Piscaglia, F.; Svegliati-Baroni, G.; Barchetti, A.; Pecorelli, A.; Marinelli, S.; Tiribelli, C.; Bellentani, S.; HCC-NAFLD Italian Study Group. Clinical patterns of hepatocellular carcinoma in nonalcoholic fatty liver disease: A multicenter prospective study. *Hepatology* **2016**, *63*, 827–838. [CrossRef]

49. White, D.L.; Kanwal, F.; El–Serag, H.B. Association Between Nonalcoholic Fatty Liver Disease and Risk for Hepatocellular Cancer, Based on Systematic Review. *Clin. Gastroenterol. Hepatol.* **2012**, *10*, 1342–1359.e2. [CrossRef]

50. McKeating, J.A.; Pfister, D.; O'Connor, T.; Pikarsky, E.; Heikenwalder, M. The immunology of hepatocellular carcinoma. *Nat. Immunol.* **2018**, *19*, 222–232. [CrossRef]

51. Younossi, Z.; Anstee, Q.M.; Marietti, M.; Hardy, T.; Henry, L.; Eslam, M.; George, J.; Bugianesi, E. Global burden of NAFLD and NASH: Trends, predictions, risk factors and prevention. *Nat. Rev. Gastroenterol. Hepatol.* **2018**, *15*, 11–20. [CrossRef]

52. Yuan, Y.; Liu, L.; Chen, H.; Wang, Y.; Xu, Y.; Mao, H.; Li, J.; Mills, G.B.; Shu, Y.; Li, L.; et al. Comprehensive Characterization of Molecular Differences in Cancer between Male and Female Patients. *Cancer Cell* **2016**, *29*, 711–722. [CrossRef]

53. Singh, R.; Kaushik, S.; Wang, Y.; Xiang, Y.; Novak, I.; Komatsu, M.; Tanaka, K.; Cuervo, A.M.; Czaja, M.J. Autophagy regulates lipid metabolism. *Nature* **2009**, *458*, 1131–1135. [CrossRef] [PubMed]

54. Tanaka, S.; Hikita, H.; Tatsumi, T.; Sakamori, R.; Nozaki, Y.; Sakane, S.; Shiode, Y.; Nakabori, T.; Saito, Y.; Hiramatsu, N.; et al. Rubicon inhibits autophagy and accelerates hepatocyte apoptosis and lipid accumulation in nonalcoholic fatty liver disease in mice. *Hepatology* **2016**, *64*, 1994–2014. [CrossRef] [PubMed]

55. Gäbele, E.; Dostert, K.; Hofmann, C.; Wiest, R.; Schölmerich, J.; Hellerbrand, C.; Obermeier, F. DSS induced colitis increases portal LPS levels and enhances hepatic inflammation and fibrogenesis in experimental NASH. *J. Hepatol.* **2011**, *55*, 1391–1399. [CrossRef] [PubMed]

56. European Association for the Study of the Liver (EASL). *Liver Int.* **2001**, *21*, 71. [CrossRef]

57. Ganne-Carrié, N.; Nahon, P. Hepatocellular carcinoma in the setting of alcohol-related liver disease. *J. Hepatol.* **2019**, *70*, 284–293. [CrossRef]

58. Meadows, G.G.; Zhang, H. Effects of Alcohol on Tumor Growth, Metastasis, Immune Response, and Host Survival. *Alcohol Res. Curr. Rev.* **2015**, *37*, 311–322.

59. Persson, E.C.; Schwartz, L.M.; Park, Y.; Trabert, B.; Hollenbeck, A.R.; Graubard, B.I.; Freedman, N.D.; McGlynn, K.A. Alcohol consumption, folate intake, hepatocellular carcinoma, and liver disease mortality. *Cancer Epidemiol. Biomark. Prev.* **2013**, *22*, 415–421. [CrossRef]

60. Donato, F.; Tagger, A.; Gelatti, U.; Parrinello, G.; Boffetta, P.; Albertini, A.; DeCarli, A.; Trevisi, P.; Ribero, M.L.; Martelli, C.; et al. Alcohol and hepatocellular carcinoma: The effect of lifetime intake and hepatitis virus infections in men and women. *Am. J. Epidemiol.* **2002**, *155*, 323–331. [CrossRef]

61. Loomba, R.; Yang, H.-I.; Su, J.; Brenner, D.A.; Iloeje, U.; Chen, C.-J. Obesity and Alcohol Synergize to Increase the Risk of Incident Hepatocellular Carcinoma in Men. *Clin. Gastroenterol. Hepatol.* **2010**, *8*, 891–898.e2. [CrossRef]

62. Kimura, T.; Tanaka, N.; Fujimori, N.; Sugiura, A.; Yamazaki, T.; Joshita, S.; Komatsu, M.; Umemura, T.; Matsumoto, A.; Tanaka, E. Mild drinking habit is a risk factor for hepatocarcinogenesis in non-alcoholic fatty liver disease with advanced fibrosis. *World J. Gastroenterol.* **2018**, *24*, 1440–1450. [CrossRef]

63. Ochiai, Y.; Kawamura, Y.; Kobayashi, M.; Shindoh, J.; Kobayashi, Y.; Okubo, S.; Muraishi, N.; Kajiwara, A.; Iritani, S.; Fujiyama, S.; et al. Effects of alcohol consumption on multiple hepatocarcinogenesis in patients with fatty liver disease. *Hepatol. Res.* **2020**. [CrossRef] [PubMed]

64. Setshedi, M.; Wands, J.R.; De La Monte, S.M. Acetaldehyde Adducts in Alcoholic Liver Disease. *Oxidative Med. Cell. Longev.* **2010**, *3*, 178–185. [CrossRef] [PubMed]

65. Fischer, M.; You, M.; Matsumoto, M.; Crabb, D.W. Peroxisome Proliferator-activated Receptor α (PPARα) Agonist Treatment Reverses PPARα Dysfunction and Abnormalities in Hepatic Lipid Metabolism in Ethanol-fed Mice. *J. Biol. Chem.* **2003**, *278*, 27997–28004. [CrossRef] [PubMed]

66. Li, C.; Yang, W.; Zhang, J.; Zheng, X.; Yao, Y.; Tu, K.; Liu, Q. SREBP-1 Has a Prognostic Role and Contributes to Invasion and Metastasis in Human Hepatocellular Carcinoma. *Int. J. Mol. Sci.* **2014**, *15*, 7124–7138. [CrossRef]

67. Hu, M.; Wang, F.; Li, X.; Rogers, C.Q.; Liang, X.; Finck, B.N.; Mitra, M.S.; Zhang, R.; Mitchell, D.A.; You, M. Regulation of hepatic lipin-1 by ethanol: Role of AMP-activated protein kinase/sterol regulatory element-binding protein 1 signaling in mice. *Hepatology* **2011**, *55*, 437–446. [CrossRef]

68. He, S.; McPhaul, C.; Li, J.Z.; Garuti, R.; Kinch, L.; Grishin, N.V.; Cohen, J.C.; Hobbs, H.H. A Sequence Variation (I148M) in PNPLA3 Associated with Nonalcoholic Fatty Liver Disease Disrupts Triglyceride Hydrolysis. *J. Biol. Chem.* **2010**, *285*, 6706–6715. [CrossRef]

69. Bucher, S.S.; Stickel, F.; Trépo, E.; Way, M.M.; Herrmann, A.; Nischalke, H.D.; Brosch, M.M.; Rosendahl, J.J.; Berg, T.; Ridinger, M.M.; et al. A genome-wide association study confirms PNPLA3 and identifies TM6SF2 and MBOAT7 as risk loci for alcohol-related cirrhosis. *Nat. Genet.* **2015**, *47*, 1443–1448. [CrossRef]

70. Baecker, A.; Liu, X.; La Vecchia, C.; Zhang, Z.-F. Worldwide incidence of hepatocellular carcinoma cases attributable to major risk factors. *Eur. J. Cancer Prev.* **2018**, *27*, 205–212. [CrossRef]

71. Petrick, J.L.; Campbell, P.T.; Koshiol, J.; Thistle, J.E.; Andreotti, G.; Freeman, L.E.B.; Buring, J.E.; Chan, A.T.; Chong, D.Q.; Doody, M.M.; et al. Tobacco, alcohol use and risk of hepatocellular carcinoma and intrahepatic cholangiocarcinoma: The Liver Cancer Pooling Project. *Br. J. Cancer* **2018**, *118*, 1005–1012. [CrossRef]

72. Kolly, P.; Knöpfli, M.; Dufour, J.-F.F. Effect of smoking on survival of patients with hepatocellular carcinoma. *Liver Int.* **2017**, *37*, 1682–1687. [CrossRef]

73. Staretz, M.E.; Murphy, S.E.; Patten, C.J.; Nunes, M.G.; Koehl, W.; Amin, S.; Koenig, L.A.; Guengerich, F.P.; Hecht, S.S. Comparative metabolism of the tobacco-related carcinogens benzo[a]pyrene, 4-(methylnitrosamino)-1-(3-pyridyl)-1-butanone, 4-(methylnitrosamino)-1-(3-pyridyl)-1-butanol, and N'-nitrosonornicotine in human hepatic microsomes. *Drug Metab. Dispos.* **1997**, *25*, 154–162. [PubMed]

74. Barbieri, S.S.; Zacchi, E.; Amadio, P.; Gianellini, S.; Mussoni, L.; Weksler, B.B.; Tremoli, E. Cytokines present in smokers' serum interact with smoke components to enhance endothelial dysfunction. *Cardiovasc. Res.* **2011**, *90*, 475–483. [CrossRef] [PubMed]

75. JM, D.P.; MJ, F.A.; MJ, L.A.; Álvarez, A. Tumor necrosis factor as an early marker of inflammation in healthy smokers. *Med. Clin.* **2012**, *139*, 47–53.

76. Dooley, K.; Von Tungeln, L.; Bucci, T.; Fu, P.; Kadlubar, F. Comparative carcinogenicity of 4-aminobiphenyl and the food pyrolysates, Glu-P-1, IQ, PhIP, and MeIQx in the neonatal B6C3F1 male mouse. *Cancer Lett.* **1992**, *62*, 205–209. [CrossRef]

77. Azzalini, L.; Ferrer, E.; Ramalho, L.N.; Moreno, M.; Domínguez, M.; Colmenero, J.; Peinado, V.I.; Barberà, J.A.; Arroyo, V.; Ginès, P.; et al. Cigarette smoking exacerbates nonalcoholic fatty liver disease in obese rats. *Hepatology* **2009**, *51*, 1567–1576. [CrossRef]

78. Kew, M. Aflatoxins as a cause of hepatocellular carcinoma. *J. Gastrointest. Liver Dis.* **2013**, *22*, 305–310.

79. Wu, H.-C.; Santella, R. The Role of Aflatoxins in Hepatocellular Carcinoma. *Zahedan J. Res. Med Sci.* **2012**, *12*. [CrossRef]

80. Woo, L.L.; Egner, P.A.; Belanger, C.L.; Wattanawaraporn, R.; Trudel, L.J.; Croy, R.G.; Groopman, J.D.; Essigmann, J.M.; Wogan, G.N.; Bouhenguel, J.T. Aflatoxin B1-DNA Adduct Formation and Mutagenicity in Livers of Neonatal Male and Female B6C3F1 Mice. *Toxicol. Sci.* **2011**, *122*, 38–44. [CrossRef]

81. Yu, M.-W.; Lien, J.-P.; Chiu, Y.-H.; Santella, R.M.; Liaw, Y.-F.; Chen, C.-J. Effect of aflatoxin metabolism and DNA adduct formation on hepatocellular carcinoma among chronic hepatitis B carriers in Taiwan. *J. Hepatol.* **1997**, *27*, 320–330. [CrossRef]

82. Yang, J.D.; A Mohamed, E.; Aziz, A.O.A.; I Shousha, H.; Hashem, M.B.; Nabeel, M.M.; Abdelmaksoud, A.H.; Elbaz, T.M.; Afihene, M.Y.; Duduyemi, B.M.; et al. Characteristics, management, and outcomes of patients with hepatocellular carcinoma in Africa: A multicountry observational study from the Africa Liver Cancer Consortium. *Lancet Gastroenterol. Hepatol.* **2017**, *2*, 103–111. [CrossRef]

83. Eriksson, S.G. Liver Disease in α 1 -Antitrypsin Deficiency: Aspects of Incidence and Prognosis. *Scand. J. Gastroenterol.* **1985**, *20*, 907–911. [CrossRef] [PubMed]

84. Janecke, A.R.; Mayatepek, E.; Utermann, G. Molecular Genetics of Type 1 Glycogen Storage Disease. *Mol. Genet. Metab.* **2001**, *73*, 117–125. [CrossRef] [PubMed]

85. Bianchi, L. Glycogen storage disease I and hepatocellular tumours. *Eur. J. Nucl. Med. Mol. Imaging* **1993**, *152*, 63–70. [CrossRef] [PubMed]

86. Elmberg, M.; Hultcrantz, R.; Ekbom, A.; Brandt, L.; Olsson, S.; Olsson, R.; Lindgren, S.; Lööf, L.; Stål, P.; Wallerstedt, S.; et al. Cancer risk in patients with hereditary hemochromatosis and in their first-degree relatives. *Gastroenterology* **2003**, *125*, 1733–1741. [CrossRef]

87. Scott, C.R. The genetic tyrosinemias. *Am. J. Med. Genet. Part C Semin. Med. Genet.* **2006**, *142*, 121–126. [CrossRef]

88. Weinberg, A.G.; Mize, C.E.; Worthen, H.G. The occurrence of hepatoma in the chronic form of hereditary tyrosinemia. *J. Pediatr.* **1976**, *88*, 434–438. [CrossRef]

89. Tanabe, K.K.; Lemoine, A.; Finkelstein, D.M.; Kawasaki, H.; Fujii, T.; Chung, R.T.; Lauwers, G.Y.; Kulu, Y.; Muzikansky, A.; Kuruppu, D.; et al. Epidermal Growth Factor Gene Functional Polymorphism and the Risk of Hepatocellular Carcinoma in Patients with Cirrhosis. *JAMA* **2008**, *299*, 53–60. [CrossRef]

90. Zhang, H.; Zhai, Y.; Hu, Z.; Wu, C.; Qian, J.; Jia, W.; Ma, F.; Huang, W.; Yu, L.; Yue, W.; et al. Genome-wide association study identifies 1p36.22 as a new susceptibility locus for hepatocellular carcinoma in chronic hepatitis B virus carriers. *Nat. Genet.* **2010**, *42*, 755–758. [CrossRef]

91. Kumar, V.; Kato, N.; Urabe, Y.; Takahashi, A.; Muroyama, R.; Hosono, N.; Otsuka, M.; Tateishi, R.; Omata, M.; Nakagawa, H.; et al. Genome-wide association study identifies a susceptibility locus for HCV-induced hepatocellular carcinoma. *Nat. Genet.* **2011**, *43*, 455–458. [CrossRef]

92. Miki, D.; Ochi, H.; Hayes, C.N.; Abe, H.; Yoshima, T.; Aikata, H.; Ikeda, K.; Kumada, H.; Toyota, J.; Morizono, T.; et al. Variation in the DEPDC5 locus is associated with progression to hepatocellular carcinoma in chronic hepatitis C virus carriers. *Nat. Genet.* **2011**, *43*, 797–800. [CrossRef]

93. Lonardo, A.; Mantovani, A.; Lugari, S.; Targher, G. NAFLD in Some Common Endocrine Diseases: Prevalence, Pathophysiology, and Principles of Diagnosis and Management. *Int. J. Mol. Sci.* **2019**, *20*, 2841. [CrossRef] [PubMed]

94. Antonelli, A.; Ferri, C.; Pampana, A.; Fallahi, P.; Nesti, C.; Pasquini, M.; Marchi, S.; Ferrannini, E. Thyroid disorders in chronic hepatitis C. *Am. J. Med.* **2004**, *117*, 10–13. [CrossRef] [PubMed]

95. Hassan, M.M.; Kaseb, A.; Li, D.; Patt, Y.Z.; Vauthey, J.-N.; Thomas, M.B.; Curley, S.A.; Spitz, M.R.; Sherman, S.I.; Abdalla, E.K.; et al. Association between hypothyroidism and hepatocellular carcinoma: A case-control study in the United States. *Hepatology* **2009**, *49*, 1563–1570. [CrossRef] [PubMed]

96. Lonardo, A.; Ballestri, S.; Mantovani, A.; Nascimbeni, F.; Lugari, S.; Targher, G. Pathogenesis of hypothyroidism-induced NAFLD: Evidence for a distinct disease entity? *Dig. Liver Dis.* **2019**, *51*, 462–470. [CrossRef]

97. Pinter, M.; Haupt, L.; Hucke, F.; Bota, S.; Bucsics, T.; Trauner, M.; Peck-Radosavljevic, M.; Sieghart, W. The impact of thyroid hormones on patients with hepatocellular carcinoma. *PLoS ONE* **2017**, *12*, e0181878. [CrossRef]

98. Huang, P.-S.; Lin, Y.-H.; Chi, H.-C.; Hsiang-Cheng, C.; Huang, Y.-H.; Yeh, C.-T.; Kwang-Huei, L.; Lin, K.-H. Thyroid hormone inhibits growth of hepatoma cells through induction of miR-214. *Sci. Rep.* **2017**, *7*, 1–11. [CrossRef] [PubMed]

99. Laurent–Puig, P.; Legoix, P.; Bluteau, O.; Belghiti, J.; Franco, D.; Binot, F.; Monges, G.; Thomas, G.; Bioulac–Sage, P.; Zucman-Rossi, J. Genetic alterations associated with hepatocellular carcinomas define distinct pathways of hepatocarcinogenesis. *Gastroenterology* **2001**, *120*, 1763–1773. [CrossRef]

100. Yeh, S.-H.; Chen, P.-J. Gender Disparity of Hepatocellular Carcinoma: The Roles of Sex Hormones. *Oncology* **2010**, *78*, 172–179. [CrossRef]

101. Wu, M.-H.; Ma, W.-L.; Hsu, C.-L.; Chen, Y.-L.; Ou, J.-H.J.; Ryan, C.K.; Hung, Y.-C.; Yeh, S.; Chang, C. Androgen Receptor Promotes Hepatitis B Virus-Induced Hepatocarcinogenesis Through Modulation of Hepatitis B Virus RNA Transcription. *Sci. Transl. Med.* **2010**, *2*, 32ra35. [CrossRef]

102. Ma, C.-L.; Hsu, C.; Wu, M.; Wu, C.; Wu, C.; Lai, J.; Jou, Y.; Cheng-Lung, H.; Yeh, S.; Chang, C. Androgen Receptor Is a New Potential Therapeutic Target for the Treatment of Hepatocellular Carcinoma. *Gastroenterology* **2008**, *135*, 947–955.e5. [CrossRef] [PubMed]

103. Kanda, T.; Yokosuka, O. The androgen receptor as an emerging target in hepatocellular carcinoma. *J. Hepatocell. Carcinoma* **2015**, *2*, 91–99. [CrossRef] [PubMed]

104. Shimizu, I. Impact of oestrogens on the progression of liver disease. *Liver Int.* **2003**, *23*, 63–69. [CrossRef] [PubMed]

105. McGlynn, K.A.; Sahasrabuddhe, V.V.; Campbell, P.T.; Graubard, B.I.; Chen, J.; Schwartz, L.M.; Petrick, J.L.; Alavanja, M.C.; Andreotti, G.; Boggs, D.A.; et al. Reproductive factors, exogenous hormone use and risk of hepatocellular carcinoma among US women: Results from the Liver Cancer Pooling Project. *Br. J. Cancer* **2015**, *112*, 1266–1272. [CrossRef] [PubMed]

106. Hsia, C.-Y.; Huo, T.-I.; Chiang, S.-Y.; Lu, M.-F.; Sun, C.-L.; Wu, J.-C.; Lee, P.-C.; Chi, C.-W.; Lui, W.-Y.; Lee, S.-D. Evaluation of interleukin-6, interleukin-10 and human hepatocyte growth factor as tumor markers for hepatocellular carcinoma. *Eur. J. Surg. Oncol.* **2007**, *33*, 208–212. [CrossRef]

107. Naugler, W.E.; Sakurai, T.; Kim, S.; Maeda, S.; Kim, K.; Elsharkawy, A.M.; Karin, M. Gender Disparity in Liver Cancer Due to Sex Differences in MyD88-Dependent IL-6 Production. *Science* **2007**, *317*, 121–124. [CrossRef]

108. He, G.; Yu, G.-Y.; Temkin, V.; Ogata, H.; Kuntzen, C.; Sakurai, T.; Sieghart, W.; Peck-Radosavljevic, M.; Leffert, H.L.; Karin, M. Hepatocyte IKKβ/NF-κB Inhibits Tumor Promotion and Progression by Preventing Oxidative Stress-Driven STAT3 Activation. *Cancer Cell* **2010**, *17*, 286–297. [CrossRef]

109. Calvisi, D.F. Dr. Jekyll and Mr. Hyde: A paradoxical oncogenic and tumor suppressive role of signal transducer and activator of transcription 3 in liver cancer. *Hepatology* **2011**, *54*, 9–12. [CrossRef]

110. Edamoto, Y.; Hara, A.; Biernat, W.; Terracciano, L.; Cathomas, G.; Riehle, H.-M.; Matsuda, M.; Fujii, H.; Scoazec, J.-Y.; Ohgaki, H. Alterations of RB1, p53 and Wnt pathways in hepatocellular carcinomas associated with hepatitis C, hepatitis B and alcoholic liver cirrhosis. *Int. J. Cancer* **2003**, *106*, 334–341. [CrossRef]

111. Murakami, Y.; Hayashi, K.; Hirohashi, S.; Sekiya, T. Aberrations of the tumor suppressor p53 and retinoblastoma genes in human hepatocellular carcinomas. *Cancer Res.* **1991**, *51*, 5520–5525.

112. Liew, C.T.; Li, H.-M.; Lo, K.-W.; Leow, C.K.; Chan, J.Y.; Hin, L.Y.; Lau, W.Y.; Lai, P.B.S.; Lim, B.K.; Huang, J.; et al. High frequency of p16INK4A gene alterations in hepatocellular carcinoma. *Oncogene* **1999**, *18*, 789–795. [CrossRef]

113. De Souza, A.T.; Hankins, G.R.; Washington, M.K.; Orton, T.C.; Jirtle, R.L. M6P/IGF2R gene is mutated in human hepatocellular carcinomas with loss of heterozygosity. *Nat. Genet.* **1995**, *11*, 447–449. [CrossRef] [PubMed]

114. Shang, S.; Hua, F.; Hu, Z.-W. The regulation of β-catenin activity and function in cancer: Therapeutic opportunities. *Oncotarget* **2017**, *8*, 33972–33989. [CrossRef] [PubMed]

115. Wong, C.M.; Fan, S.T.; Ng, I.O.L. β-catenin mutation and overexpression in hepatocellular carcinoma. *Cancer* **2001**, *92*, 136–145. [CrossRef]

116. Wang, X.W.; Forrester, K.; Yeh, H.; Feitelson, M.A.; Gu, J.R.; Harris, C.C. Hepatitis B virus X protein inhibits p53 sequence-specific DNA binding, transcriptional activity, and association with transcription factor ERCC3. *Proc. Natl. Acad. Sci. USA* **1994**, *91*, 2230–2234. [CrossRef]

117. Ji, J.; Wang, X.W. New kids on the block: Diagnostic and prognostic microRNAs in hepatocellular carcinoma. *Cancer Biol. Ther.* **2009**, *8*, 1683–1690. [CrossRef]

118. Ji, J.; Yamashita, T.; Budhu, A.; Forgues, M.; Jia, H.-L.; Li, C.; Deng, C.; Wauthier, E.; Reid, L.M.; Ye, Q.-H.; et al. Identification of microRNA-181 by genome-wide screening as a critical player in EpCAM-positive hepatic cancer stem cells. *Hepatology* **2009**, *50*, 472–480. [CrossRef] [PubMed]

119. Gong, J.; He, X.-X.; Tian, D.-A. Emerging role of microRNA in hepatocellular carcinoma (Review). *Oncol. Lett.* **2015**, *9*, 1027–1033. [CrossRef]

120. Kojima, K.; Takata, A.; Vadnais, C.; Otsuka, M.; Yoshikawa, T.; Akanuma, M.; Kondo, Y.; Kang, Y.J.; Kishikawa, T.; Kato, N.; et al. MicroRNA122 is a key regulator of α-fetoprotein expression and influences the aggressiveness of hepatocellular carcinoma. *Nat. Commun.* **2011**, *2*, 338. [CrossRef]

121. Lee, J.-S.; Chu, I.-S.; Heo, J.; Calvisi, D.F.; Sun, Z.; Roskams, T.; Durnez, A.; Demetris, A.J.; Thorgeirsson, S.S. Classification and prediction of survival in hepatocellular carcinoma by gene expression profiling. *Hepatology* **2004**, *40*, 667–676. [CrossRef]

122. Coulouarn, C.; Factor, V.M.; Thorgeirsson, S.S. Transforming growth factor-β gene expression signature in mouse hepatocytes predicts clinical outcome in human cancer. *Hepatology* **2008**, *47*, 2059–2067. [CrossRef]

123. Kaposi-Novak, P.; Lee, J.-S.; Gòmez-Quiroz, L.; Coulouarn, C.; Factor, V.M.; Thorgeirsson, S.S. Met-regulated expression signature defines a subset of human hepatocellular carcinomas with poor prognosis and aggressive phenotype. *J. Clin. Investig.* **2006**, *116*, 1582–1595. [CrossRef] [PubMed]

124. Goossens, N.; Sun, X.; Hoshida, Y. Molecular classification of hepatocellular carcinoma: Potential therapeutic implications. *Hepatic Oncol.* **2015**, *2*, 371–379. [CrossRef] [PubMed]

125. Liu, M.; Jiang, L.; Guan, X.-Y. The genetic and epigenetic alterations in human hepatocellular carcinoma: A recent update. *Protein Cell* **2014**, *5*, 673–691. [CrossRef] [PubMed]

126. Hoshida, Y.; Nijman, S.M.; Kobayashi, M.; Chan, J.A.; Brunet, J.-P.; Chiang, D.Y.; Villanueva, A.; Newell, P.; Ikeda, K.; Hashimoto, M.; et al. Integrative Transcriptome Analysis Reveals Common Molecular Subclasses of Human Hepatocellular Carcinoma. *Cancer Res.* **2009**, *69*, 7385–7392. [CrossRef]

127. Lachenmayer, A.; Alsinet, C.; Savic, R.; Cabellos, L.; Toffanin, S.; Hoshida, Y.; Villanueva, A.; Minguez, B.; Newell, P.; Tsai, H.W.; et al. Wnt-pathway activation in two molecular classes of hepatocellular carcinoma and experimental modulation by sorafenib. *Clin. Cancer Res.* **2012**, *18*, 4997–5007. [CrossRef]

128. Zucman-Rossi, J.; Villanueva, A.; Nault, J.-C.; Llovet, J.M. Genetic Landscape and Biomarkers of Hepatocellular Carcinoma. *Gastroenterology* **2015**, *149*, 1226–1239.e4. [CrossRef]

129. Castven, D.; Fischer, M.; Becker, D.; Heinrich, S.; Andersen, J.B.; Strand, D.; Sprinzl, M.F.; Strand, S.; Czauderna, C.; Heilmann-Heimbach, S.; et al. Adverse genomic alterations and stemness features are induced by field cancerization in the microenvironment of hepatocellular carcinomas. *Oncotarget* **2017**, *8*, 48688–48700. [CrossRef]

130. Elsharkawy, A.M.; Mann, D.A. Nuclear factor-κB and the hepatic inflammation-fibrosis-cancer axis. *Hepatology* **2007**, *46*, 590–597. [CrossRef]

131. Shimoda, M.; Mellody, K.T.; Orimo, A. Carcinoma-associated fibroblasts are a rate-limiting determinant for tumour progression. *Semin. Cell Dev. Biol.* **2010**, *21*, 19–25. [CrossRef]

132. Lau, E.Y.T.; Lo, J.; Cheng, B.Y.L.; Ma, M.K.F.; Lee, J.M.F.; Ng, J.K.Y.; Chai, S.; Lin, C.H.; Tsang, S.Y.; Ma, S.; et al. Cancer-associated fibroblasts regulate tumor-initiating cell plasticity in hepatocellular carcinoma through c-Met/FRA1/HEY1 signaling. *Cell Rep.* **2016**, *15*, 1175–1189. [CrossRef]

133. Faouzi, S.; Lepreux, S.; Bedin, C.; Dubuisson, L.; Balabaud, C.; Bioulac-Sage, P.; Desmoulière, A.; Rosenbaum, J. Activation of cultured rat hepatic stellate cells by tumoral hepatocytes. *Lab. Investig.* **1999**, *79*, 485–493. [PubMed]

134. Noy, R.; Pollard, J.W. Tumor-associated macrophages: From mechanisms to therapy. *Immunity* **2014**, *41*, 49–61. [CrossRef] [PubMed]

135. Mantovani, A.; Bottazzi, B.; Colotta, F.; Sozzani, S.; Ruco, L.P. The origin and function of tumor-associated macrophages. *Immunol. Today* **1992**, *13*, 265–270. [CrossRef]

136. Llovet, J.M.; Schwartz, M.; Mazzaferro, V. Resection and Liver Transplantation for Hepatocellular Carcinoma. *Semin. Liver Dis.* **2005**, *25*, 181–200. [CrossRef] [PubMed]

137. Hoshida, Y.; Villanueva, A.; Kobayashi, M.; Peix, J.; Chiang, D.Y.; Camargo, A.; Gupta, S.; Moore, J.; Wrobel, M.J.; Lerner, J.; et al. Gene Expression in Fixed Tissues and Outcome in Hepatocellular Carcinoma. *N. Engl. J. Med.* **2008**, *359*, 1995–2004. [CrossRef] [PubMed]

138. Hoshida, Y.; Villanueva, A.; SanGiovanni, A.; Sole, M.; Hur, C.; Andersson, K.L.; Chung, R.T.; Gould, J.; Kojima, K.; Gupta, S.; et al. Prognostic Gene Expression Signature for Patients with Hepatitis C–Related Early-Stage Cirrhosis. *Gastroenterology* **2013**, *144*, 1024–1030. [CrossRef]

139. Nakagawa, S.; Wei, L.; Song, W.M.; Higashi, T.; Ghoshal, S.; Kim, R.S.; Bian, C.B.; Yamada, S.; Sun, X.; Venkatesh, A.; et al. Molecular Liver Cancer Prevention in Cirrhosis by Organ Transcriptome Analysis and Lysophosphatidic Acid Pathway Inhibition. *Cancer Cell* **2016**, *30*, 879–890. [CrossRef]

140. Fuchs, B.C.; Hoshida, Y.; Fujii, T.; Wei, L.; Yamada, S.; Lauwers, G.Y.; McGinn, C.M.; Deperalta, D.K.; Chen, X.; Kuroda, T.; et al. Epidermal growth factor receptor inhibition attenuates liver fibrosis and development of hepatocellular carcinoma. *Hepatology* **2014**, *59*, 1577–1590. [CrossRef]

141. Burra, P.; Rodriguez-Castro, K.I. Neoplastic disease after liver transplantation: Focus onde novoneoplasms. *World J. Gastroenterol.* **2015**, *21*, 8753. [CrossRef]

142. Kihara, Y.; Mizuno, H.; Chun, J. Lysophospholipid receptors in drug discovery. *Exp. Cell Res.* **2015**, *333*, 171–177. [CrossRef]

143. Sakai, N.; Chun, J.; Duffield, J.S.; Wada, T.; Luster, A.D.; Tager, A.M. LPA 1 -induced cytoskeleton reorganization drives fibrosis through CTGF-dependent fibroblast proliferation. *FASEB J.* **2013**, *27*, 1830–1846. [CrossRef] [PubMed]

144. Hoshida, Y.; Toffanin, S.; Lachenmayer, A.; Villanueva, A.; Minguez, B.; Llovet, J.M. Molecular Classification and Novel Targets in Hepatocellular Carcinoma: Recent Advancements. *Semin. Liver Dis.* **2010**, *30*, 35–51. [CrossRef] [PubMed]

145. Jühling, F.; Hamdane, N.; Crouchet, E.; Li, S.; El Saghire, H.; Mukherji, A.; Fujiwara, N.; Oudot, M.A.; Thumann, C.; Saviano, A.; et al. Targeting clinical epigenetic reprogramming for chemoprevention of metabolic and viral hepatocellular carcinoma. *Gut* **2020**. [CrossRef] [PubMed]

146. Villa, E.; Critelli, R.; Lei, B.; Marzocchi, G.; Cammà, C.; Giannelli, G.; Pontisso, P.; Cabibbo, G.; Enea, M.; Colopi, S.; et al. Neoangiogenesis-related genes are hallmarks of fast-growing hepatocellular carcinomas and worst survival. Results from a prospective study. *Gut* **2015**, *65*, 861–869. [CrossRef] [PubMed]

147. Zanetti, A.R.; Van Damme, P.; Shouval, D. The global impact of vaccination against hepatitis B: A historical overview. *Vaccine* **2008**, *26*, 6266–6273. [CrossRef] [PubMed]

148. Ni, Y.-H.; Chang, M.-H.; Huang, L.-M.; Chen, H.-L.; Hsu, H.-Y.; Chiu, T.-Y.; Tsai, K.-S.; Chen, D.-S. Hepatitis B Virus Infection in Children and Adolescents in a Hyperendemic Area: 15 Years after Mass Hepatitis B Vaccination. *Ann. Intern. Med.* **2001**, *135*, 796–800. [CrossRef] [PubMed]

149. Chen, C.-H.; Yang, P.-M.; Huang, G.-T.; Lee, H.-S.; Sung, J.-L.; Sheu, J.-C. Estimation of Seroprevalence of Hepatitis B Virus and Hepatitis C Virus in Taiwan from a Large-scale Survey of Free Hepatitis Screening Participants. *J. Formos. Med. Assoc.* **2007**, *106*, 148–155. [CrossRef]

150. Aitken, C.; Lewis, J.; Hocking, J.; Bowden, D.; Hellard, M. Does information about IDUs' injecting networks predict exposure to the hepatitis C virus? *Hepat Monthly.* **2009**, *9*, 17–23.

151. Razali, K.; Thein, H.-H.; Bell, J.; Cooper-Stanbury, M.; Dolan, K.; Dore, G.; George, J.; Kaldor, J.; Karvelas, M.; Li, J.; et al. Modelling the hepatitis C virus epidemic in Australia. *Drug Alcohol Depend.* **2007**, *91*, 228–235. [CrossRef]

152. Azziz-Baumgartner, E.; Lindblade, K.; Gieseker, K.; Rogers, H.S.; Kieszak, S.; Njapau, H.; Schleicher, R.; McCoy, L.F.; Misore, A.; Decock, K.; et al. Case–Control Study of an Acute Aflatoxicosis Outbreak, Kenya, 2004. *Environ. Heal. Perspect.* **2005**, *113*, 1779–1783. [CrossRef]

153. Luedde, T.; Schwabe, R.F. NF-κB in the liver—Linking injury, fibrosis and hepatocellular carcinoma. *Nat. Rev. Gastroenterol. Hepatol.* **2011**, *8*, 108–118. [CrossRef] [PubMed]

154. Ikeda, K.; Arase, Y.; Saitoh, S.; Kobayashi, M.; Suzuki, Y.; Suzuki, F.; Tsubota, A.; Chayama, K.; Murashima, N.; Kumada, H. Interferon beta prevents recurrence of hepatocellular carcinoma after complete resection or ablation of the primary tumor—A prospective randomized study of hepatitis C virus–related liver cancer. *Hepatology* **2000**, *32*, 228–232. [CrossRef] [PubMed]

155. Mazzaferro, V.; Romito, R.; Schiavo, M.; Mariani, L.; Camerini, T.; Bhoori, S.; Capussotti, L.; Calise, F.; Pellicci, R.; Belli, G.; et al. Prevention of hepatocellular carcinoma recurrence with alpha-interferon after liver resection in HCV cirrhosis. *Hepatology* **2006**, *44*, 1543–1554. [CrossRef] [PubMed]

156. Chinnakotla, S.; Davis, G.L.; Vasani, S.; Kim, P.; Tomiyama, K.; Sanchez, E.; Onaca, N.; Goldstein, R.; Levy, M.; Klintmalm, G.B. Impact of sirolimus on the recurrence of hepatocellular carcinoma after liver transplantation. *Liver Transplant.* **2009**, *15*, 1834–1842. [CrossRef] [PubMed]

157. Toso, C.; Merani, S.; Bigam, D.L.; Shapiro, A.J.; Kneteman, N.M. Sirolimus-based immunosuppression is associated with increased survival after liver transplantation for hepatocellular carcinoma. *Hepatology* **2010**, *51*, 1237–1243. [CrossRef]

158. Costentin, C.; Layese, R.; Bourcier, V.; Cagnot, C.; Marcellin, P.; Guyader, D.; Pol, S.; Larrey, D.; De Lédinghen, V.; Ouzan, D.; et al. Compliance with Hepatocellular Carcinoma Surveillance Guidelines Associated With Increased Lead-Time Adjusted Survival of Patients With Compensated Viral Cirrhosis: A Multi-Center Cohort Study. *Gastroenterology* **2018**, *155*, 431–442.e10. [CrossRef]

159. Galle, P.R.; Forner, A.; Llovet, J.M.; Mazzaferro, V.; Piscaglia, F.; Raoul, J.-L.; Schirmacher, P.; Vilgrain, V. EASL Clinical Practice Guidelines: Management of hepatocellular carcinoma. *J. Hepatol.* **2018**, *69*, 182–236. [CrossRef]

160. Heimbach, J.K.; Kulik, L.M.; Finn, R.S.; Sirlin, C.B.; Abecassis, M.M.; Roberts, L.R.; Zhu, A.X.; Murad, M.H.; Marrero, J.A. AASLD guidelines for the treatment of hepatocellular carcinoma. *Hepatology* **2018**, *67*, 358–380. [CrossRef]

161. Ganne-Carrié, N.; Layese, R.; Bourcier, V.; Cagnot, C.; Marcellin, P.; Guyader, D.; Pol, S.; Larrey, D.; De Lédinghen, V.; Ouzan, D.; et al. Nomogram for individualized prediction of hepatocellular carcinoma occurrence in hepatitis C virus cirrhosis (ANRS CO12 CirVir). *Hepatology* **2016**, *64*, 1136–1147. [CrossRef]

162. Lok, A.S.; Seeff, L.B.; Morgan, T.R.; Di Bisceglie, A.M.; Sterling, R.K.; Curto, T.M.; Everson, G.T.; Lindsay, K.L.; Lee, W.M.; Bonkovsky, H.L.; et al. Incidence of Hepatocellular Carcinoma and Associated Risk Factors in Hepatitis C-Related Advanced Liver Disease. *Gastroenterology* **2009**, *136*, 138–148. [CrossRef]

163. Flemming, J.A.; Yang, J.D.; Vittinghoff, E.; Kim, W.R.; Terrault, N.A. Risk prediction of hepatocellular carcinoma in patients with cirrhosis: The ADRESS-HCC risk model. *Cancer* **2014**, *120*, 3485–3493. [CrossRef] [PubMed]

164. Abu Dayyeh, B.K.; Yang, M.; Fuchs, B.C.; Karl, D.L.; Yamada, S.; Sninsky, J.J.; O'Brien, T.R.; Dienstag, J.L.; Tanabe, K.K.; Chung, R.T. A Functional Polymorphism in the Epidermal Growth Factor Gene Is Associated with Risk for Hepatocellular Carcinoma. *Gastroenterology* **2011**, *141*, 141–149. [CrossRef] [PubMed]

165. Ioannou, G.N.; Green, P.; Kerr, K.F.; Berry, K. Models estimating risk of hepatocellular carcinoma in patients with alcohol or NAFLD-related cirrhosis for risk stratification. *J. Hepatol.* **2019**, *71*, 523–533. [CrossRef]

166. Mancebo, A.; González-Diéguez, M.L.; Navascués, C.A.; Cadahía, V.; Varela, M.; Pérez, R.; Rodrigo, L.; Rodríguez, M. Adherence to a Semiannual Surveillance Program for Hepatocellular Carcinoma in Patients With Liver Cirrhosis. *J. Clin. Gastroenterol.* **2017**, *51*, 557–563. [CrossRef]

167. Davila, J.A.; Henderson, L.; Kramer, J.R.; Kanwal, F.; Richardson, P.A.; Duan, Z.; El-Serag, H.B. Utilization of Surveillance for Hepatocellular Carcinoma Among Hepatitis C Virus–Infected Veterans in the United States. *Ann. Intern. Med.* **2011**, *154*, 85–93. [CrossRef]

168. Harris, P.S.; Hansen, R.M.; Gray, M.E.; Massoud, O.I.; McGuire, B.M.; Shoreibah, M.G. Hepatocellular carcinoma surveillance: An evidence-based approach. *World J. Gastroenterol.* **2019**, *25*, 1550–1559. [CrossRef]

169. Kim, S.Y.; Sang, L.Y.; Lim, Y.-S.; Han, S.; Lee, J.-Y.; Byun, J.H.; Won, H.J.; Lee, S.J.; Lee, H.C.; Lee, Y.S. MRI With Liver-Specific Contrast for Surveillance of Patients with Cirrhosis at High Risk of Hepatocellular Carcinoma. *JAMA Oncol.* **2017**, *3*, 456–463. [CrossRef] [PubMed]

170. Lin, S.-M.; Sheen, I.-S.; Chien, R.-N.; Chu, C.-M.; Liaw, Y.-F. Long-term beneficial effect of interferon therapy in patients with chronic hepatitis B virus infection. *Hepatology* **1999**, *29*, 971–975. [CrossRef] [PubMed]

171. Lin, S.-M.; Yu, M.-L.; Lee, C.-M.; Chien, R.-N.; Sheen, I.-S.; Chu, C.-M.; Liaw, Y.-F. Interferon therapy in HBeAg positive chronic hepatitis reduces progression to cirrhosis and hepatocellular carcinoma. *J. Hepatol.* **2007**, *46*, 45–52. [CrossRef] [PubMed]

172. Liaw, Y.-F.; Sung, J.J.; Chow, W.C.; Farrell, G.; Lee, C.-Z.; Yuen, H.; Tanwandee, T.; Tao, Q.-M.; Shue, K.; Keene, O.N.; et al. Lamivudine for Patients with Chronic Hepatitis B and Advanced Liver Disease. *N. Engl. J. Med.* **2004**, *351*, 1521–1531. [CrossRef]

173. Eun, J.R.; Lee, H.J.; Kim, T.N.; Lee, K.S. Risk assessment for the development of hepatocellular carcinoma: According to on-treatment viral response during long-term lamivudine therapy in hepatitis B virus-related liver disease. *J. Hepatol.* **2010**, *53*, 118–125. [CrossRef]

174. Papatheodoridis, G.V.; Lampertico, P.; Manolakopoulos, S.; Lok, A. Incidence of hepatocellular carcinoma in chronic hepatitis B patients receiving nucleos(t)ide therapy: A systematic review. *J. Hepatol.* **2010**, *53*, 348–356. [CrossRef]

175. Webster, D.P.; Klenerman, P.; Dusheiko, G.M. Hepatitis C. *Lancet* **2015**, *385*, 1124–1135. [CrossRef]

176. Morgan, R.L.; Baack, B.; Smith, B.D.; Yartel, A.; Pitasi, M.; Falck-Ytter, Y. Eradication of Hepatitis C Virus Infection and the Development of Hepatocellular Carcinoma. *Ann. Intern. Med.* **2013**, *158*, 329–337. [CrossRef]

177. Guarino, M.; Sessa, A.; Cossiga, V.; Morando, F.; Caporaso, N.; Morisco, F. Direct-acting antivirals and hepatocellular carcinoma in chronic hepatitis C: A few lights and many shadows. *World J. Gastroenterol.* **2018**, *24*, 2582–2595. [CrossRef]

178. Pearlman, B.L.; Traub, N. Sustained Virologic Response to Antiviral Therapy for Chronic Hepatitis C Virus Infection: A Cure and So Much More. *Clin. Infect. Dis.* **2011**, *52*, 889–900. [CrossRef]

179. Janjua, N.Z.; Wong, S.; Darvishian, M.; Butt, Z.A.; Yu, A.; Binka, M.; Alvarez, M.; Woods, R.; Yoshida, E.M.; Ramji, A.; et al. The impact of SVR from direct-acting antiviral- and interferon-based treatments for HCV on hepatocellular carcinoma risk. *J. Viral Hepat.* **2020**, *27*, 781–793. [CrossRef]

180. Ioannou, G.N.; Green, P.K.; Berry, K. HCV eradication induced by direct-acting antiviral agents reduces the risk of hepatocellular carcinoma. *J. Hepatol.* **2018**, *68*, 25–32. [CrossRef]

181. Ioannou, G.N.; Beste, L.A.; Green, P.K.; Singal, A.G.; Tapper, E.B.; Waljee, A.K.; Sterling, R.K.; Feld, J.J.; Kaplan, D.E.; Taddei, T.H.; et al. Increased Risk for Hepatocellular Carcinoma Persists Up to 10 Years after HCV Eradication in Patients with Baseline Cirrhosis or High FIB-4 Scores. *Gastroenterology* **2019**, *157*, 1264–1278.e4. [CrossRef]

182. Hamdane, N.; Jühling, F.; Crouchet, E.; El Saghire, H.; Thumann, C.; Oudot, M.A.; Bandiera, S.; Saviano, A.; Ponsolles, C.; Suarez, A.A.R.; et al. HCV-Induced Epigenetic Changes Associated with Liver Cancer Risk Persist After Sustained Virologic Response. *Gastroenterology* **2019**, *156*, 2313–2329.e7. [CrossRef]

183. Volk, M.L.; Tocco, R.; Saini, S.; Lok, A.S.-F. Public health impact of antiviral therapy for hepatitis C in the United States. *Hepatology* **2009**, *50*, 1750–1755. [CrossRef]

184. McGowan, C.E.; Fried, M.W. Barriers to hepatitis C treatment. *Liver Int.* **2012**, *32*, 151–156. [CrossRef]

185. Crowley, D.; Cullen, W.; Laird, E.; Lambert, J.S.; Mc Hugh, T.; Murphy, C.; Van Hout, M.C. Exploring patient characteristics and barriers to Hepatitis C treatment in patients on opioid substitution treatment attending a community based fibro-scanning clinic. *J. Transl. Intern. Med.* **2017**, *5*, 112–119. [CrossRef]

186. Romero-Gómez, M.; Zelber-Sagi, S.; Trenell, M. Treatment of NAFLD with diet, physical activity and exercise. *J. Hepatol.* **2017**, *67*, 829–846. [CrossRef]

187. Pälve, K.; Pahkala, K.; Suomela, E.; Aatola, H.; Hulkkonen, J.; Juonala, M.; Lehtimäki, T.; Rönnemaa, T.; Viikari, J.S.A.; Kähönen, M.; et al. Cardiorespiratory Fitness and Risk of Fatty Liver. *Med. Sci. Sports Exerc.* **2017**, *49*, 1834–1841. [CrossRef]

188. Byrne, C.D.; Targher, G. EASL–EASD–EASO Clinical Practice Guidelines for the management of non-alcoholic fatty liver disease: Is universal screening appropriate? *Diabetologia* **2016**, *59*, 1141–1144. [CrossRef] [PubMed]

189. Chalasani, N.; Younossi, Z.; LaVine, J.E.; Charlton, M.; Cusi, K.; Rinella, M.; Harrison, S.A.; Brunt, E.M.; Sanyal, A.J. The diagnosis and management of nonalcoholic fatty liver disease: Practice guidance from the American Association for the Study of Liver Diseases. *Hepatology* **2018**, *67*, 328–357. [CrossRef]

190. Piguet, A.-C.; Saran, U.; Simillion, C.A.M.; Keller, I.; Terracciano, L.; Reeves, H.L.; Dufour, J.-F.F. Regular exercise decreases liver tumors development in hepatocyte-specific PTEN-deficient mice independently of steatosis. *J. Hepatol.* **2015**, *62*, 1296–1303. [CrossRef]

191. Lassailly, G.; Caiazzo, R.; Buob, D.; Pigeyre, M.; Verkindt, H.; Labreuche, J.; Raverdy, V.; Leteurtre, E.; Dharancy, S.; Louvet, A.; et al. Bariatric Surgery Reduces Features of Nonalcoholic Steatohepatitis in Morbidly Obese Patients. *Gastroenterology* **2015**, *149*, 379–388. [CrossRef]

192. Mummadi, R.R.; Kasturi, K.S.; Chennareddygari, S.; Sood, G.K. Effect of Bariatric Surgery on Nonalcoholic Fatty Liver Disease: Systematic Review and Meta-Analysis. *Clin. Gastroenterol. Hepatol.* **2008**, *6*, 1396–1402. [CrossRef]

193. Kwak, M.; Mehaffey, J.H.; Hawkins, R.B.; Hsu, A.; Schirmer, B.; Hallowell, P.T. Bariatric surgery is associated with reduction in non-alcoholic steatohepatitis and hepatocellular carcinoma: A propensity matched analysis. *Am. J. Surg.* **2020**, *219*, 504–507. [CrossRef] [PubMed]

194. Singh, M.K.; Das, B.K.; Choudhary, S.; Gupta, D.; Patil, U.K. Diabetes and hepatocellular carcinoma: A pathophysiological link and pharmacological management. *Biomed. Pharmacother.* **2018**, *106*, 991–1002. [CrossRef]

195. Chou, C.K.; Ho, L.T.; Ting, L.P.; Hu, C.P.; Su, T.S.; Chang, W.C.; Suen, C.S.; Huang, M.Y.; Chang, C.M. Selective suppression of insulin-induced proliferation of cultured human hepatoma cells by somatostatin. *J. Clin. Investig.* **1987**, *79*, 175–178. [CrossRef]

196. Paradis, V.; Perlemuter, G.; Bonvoust, F.; Dargere, D.; Parfait, B.; Vidaud, M.; Conti, M.; Huet, S.; Bâ, N.; Buffet, C.; et al. High glucose and hyperinsulinemia stimulate connective tissue growth factor expression: A potential mechanism involved in progression to fibrosis in nonalcoholic steatohepatitis. *Hepatology* **2001**, *34*, 738–744. [CrossRef] [PubMed]

197. Evans, J.M.; Donnelly, L.A.; Emslie-Smith, A.M.; Alessi, D.R.; Morris, A.D. Metformin and reduced risk of cancer in diabetic patients. *BMJ* **2005**, *330*, 1304–1305. [CrossRef] [PubMed]

198. Tseng, C.-H. Metformin and risk of hepatocellular carcinoma in patients with type 2 diabetes. *Liver Int.* **2018**, *38*, 2018–2027. [CrossRef] [PubMed]

199. Zhou, G.; Myers, R.; Li, Y.; Chen, Y.; Shen, X.; Fenyk-Melody, J.; Wu, M.; Ventre, J.; Doebber, T.; Fujii, N.; et al. Role of AMP-activated protein kinase in mechanism of metformin action. *J. Clin. Investig.* **2001**, *108*, 1167–1174. [CrossRef]

200. Zheng, L.; Yang, W.; Wu, F.; Wang, C.; Yu, L.; Tang, L.; Qiu, B.; Li, Y.; Guo, L.; Wu, M.; et al. Prognostic Significance of AMPK Activation and Therapeutic Effects of Metformin in Hepatocellular Carcinoma. *Clin. Cancer Res.* **2013**, *19*, 5372–5380. [CrossRef]

201. Deperalta, D.K.; Wei, L.; Ghoshal, S.; Schmidt, B.; Lauwers, G.Y.; Lanuti, M.; Chung, R.T.; Tanabe, K.K.; Fuchs, B.C. Metformin prevents hepatocellular carcinoma development by suppressing hepatic progenitor cell activation in a rat model of cirrhosis. *Cancer* **2016**, *122*, 1216–1227. [CrossRef]

202. Cusi, K.; Orsak, B.; Bril, F.; Lomonaco, R.; Hecht, J.; Ortiz-Lopez, C.; Tio, F.; Hardies, J.; Darland, C.; Musi, N.; et al. Long-Term Pioglitazone Treatment for Patients with Nonalcoholic Steatohepatitis and Prediabetes or Type 2 Diabetes Mellitus. *Ann. Intern. Med.* **2016**, *165*, 305–315. [CrossRef]

203. Li, S.; Ghoshal, S.; Sojoodi, M.; Arora, G.; Masia, R.; Erstad, D.J.; Lanuti, M.; Hoshida, Y.; Baumert, T.F.; Tanabe, K.K.; et al. Pioglitazone Reduces Hepatocellular Carcinoma Development in Two Rodent Models of Cirrhosis. *J. Gastrointest. Surg.* **2018**, *23*, 101–111. [CrossRef] [PubMed]

204. Huang, M.-Y.; Chung, C.-H.; Chang, W.-K.; Lin, C.-S.; Chen, K.-W.; Hsieh, T.-Y.; Chien, W.-C.; Lin, H.-H. The role of thiazolidinediones in hepatocellular carcinoma risk reduction: A population-based cohort study in Taiwan. *Am. J. Cancer Res.* **2017**, *7*, 1606–1616. [PubMed]

205. Hasegawa, T.; Yoneda, M.; Nakamura, K.; Makino, I.; Terano, A. Plasma transforming growth factor-β1 level and efficacy of α-tocopherol in patients with non-alcoholic steatohepatitis: A pilot study. *Aliment. Pharmacol. Ther.* **2001**, *15*, 1667–1672. [CrossRef] [PubMed]

206. Kugelmas, M.; Hill, D.B.; Vivian, B.; Marsano, L.; McClain, C.J. Cytokines and NASH: A pilot study of the effects of lifestyle modification and vitamin E. *Hepatology* **2003**, *38*, 413–419. [CrossRef] [PubMed]

207. Vajro, P.; Mandato, C.; Franzese, A.; Ciccimarra, E.; Lucariello, S.; Savoia, M.; Capuano, G.; Migliaro, F. Vitamin E Treatment in Pediatric Obesity-Related Liver Disease: A Randomized Study. *J. Pediatr. Gastroenterol. Nutr.* **2004**, *38*, 48–55. [CrossRef]

208. Sanyal, A.J.; Chalasani, N.; Kowdley, K.V.; McCullough, A.; Diehl, A.M.; Bass, N.M.; Neuschwander-Tetri, B.A.; LaVine, J.E.; Tonascia, J.; Unalp, A.; et al. Pioglitazone, Vitamin E, or Placebo for Nonalcoholic Steatohepatitis. *N. Engl. J. Med.* **2010**, *362*, 1675–1685. [CrossRef]

209. Miller, E.R.; Pastor-Barriuso, R.; Dalal, D.; Riemersma, R.A.; Appel, L.J.; Guallar, E. Meta-analysis: High-dosage vitamin E supplementation may increase all-cause mortality. *Ann. Intern. Med.* **2005**, *142*, 37–46. [CrossRef]

210. Klein, E.A.; Thompson, I.M.; Tangen, C.M.; Crowley, J.J.; Lucia, M.S.; Goodman, P.J.; Minasian, L.M.; Ford, L.G.; Parnes, H.L.; Gaziano, J.M.; et al. Vitamin E and the Risk of Prostate Cancer: The selenium and vitamin e cancer prevention trial (SELECT). *JAMA* **2011**, *306*, 1549–1556. [CrossRef]

211. Testino, G.; Leone, S.; Borro, P. Alcohol and hepatocellular carcinoma: A review and a point of view. *World J. Gastroenterol.* **2014**, *20*, 15943–15954. [CrossRef]

212. Addolorato, G.; Mirijello, A.; Barrio, P.; Gual, A. Treatment of alcohol use disorders in patients with alcoholic liver disease. *J. Hepatol.* **2016**, *65*, 618–630. [CrossRef]

213. Miller, W.R.; Walters, S.T.; Bennett, M.E. How effective is alcoholism treatment in the United States? *J. Stud. Alcohol.* **2001**, *62*, 211–220. [CrossRef]

214. Menon, K.V.N.; Gores, G.J.; Shah, V.H. Pathogenesis, Diagnosis, and Treatment of Alcoholic Liver Disease. *Mayo Clin. Proc.* **2001**, *76*, 1021–1029. [CrossRef]

215. Humphreys, K.; Blodgett, J.C.; Wagner, T.H. Estimating the Efficacy of Alcoholics Anonymous without Self-Selection Bias: An Instrumental Variables Re-Analysis of Randomized Clinical Trials. *Alcohol. Clin. Exp. Res.* **2014**, *38*, 2688–2694. [CrossRef]

216. McHugh, R.K.; Hearon, B.A.; Otto, M.W. Cognitive Behavioral Therapy for Substance Use Disorders. *Psychiatr. Clin. N. Am.* **2010**, *33*, 511–525. [CrossRef]

217. Harrison, S.A.; Torgerson, S.; Hayashi, P.; Ward, J.; Schenker, S. Vitamin E and vitamin C treatment improves fibrosis in patients with nonalcoholic steatohepatitis. *Am. J. Gastroenterol.* **2003**, *98*, 2485–2490. [CrossRef]

218. Jørgensen, C.H.; Pedersen, B.; Tønnesen, H. The Efficacy of Disulfiram for the Treatment of Alcohol Use Disorder. *Alcohol. Clin. Exp. Res.* **2011**, *35*, 1749–1758. [CrossRef]

219. Benjamin, D.; Grant, E.R.; Pohorecky, L.A. Naltrexone reverses ethanol-induced dopamine release in the nucleus accumbens in awake, freely moving rats. *Brain Res.* **1993**, *621*, 137–140. [CrossRef]

220. Anton, R.F.; O'Malley, S.S.; Ciraulo, D.A.; Cisler, R.A.; Couper, D.; Donovan, D.M.; Gastfriend, D.R.; Hosking, J.D.; Johnson, B.A.; LoCastro, J.S.; et al. Combined Pharmacotherapies and Behavioral Interventions for Alcohol Dependence. *JAMA* **2006**, *295*, 2003–2017. [CrossRef]

221. Cholesterol Treatment Trialists' (CTT) Collaboration Efficacy and safety of more intensive lowering of LDL cholesterol: A meta-analysis of data from 170,000 participants in 26 randomised trials. *Lancet* **2010**, *376*, 1670–1681. [CrossRef]

222. Poynter, J.N.; Gruber, S.B.; Higgins, P.D.; Almog, R.; Bonner, J.D.; Rennert, H.S.; Low, M.; Greenson, J.K.; Rennert, G. Statins and the risk of colorectal cancer. *N. Engl. J. Med.* **2005**, *352*, 2184–2192. [CrossRef]

223. Campbell, M.J.; Esserman, L.J.; Zhou, Y.; Shoemaker, M.; Lobo, M.; Borman, E.; Baehner, F.; Kumar, A.S.; Adduci, K.; Marx, C.; et al. Breast Cancer Growth Prevention by Statins. *Cancer Res.* **2006**, *66*, 8707–8714. [CrossRef]

224. Shannon, J.; Tewoderos, S.; Garzotto, M.; Beer, T.M.; Derenick, R.; Palma, A.; Farris, P.E. Statins and Prostate Cancer Risk: A Case-Control Study. *Am. J. Epidemiol.* **2005**, *162*, 318–325. [CrossRef]

225. Hyogo, H.; Tazuma, S.; Arihiro, K.; Iwamoto, K.; Nabeshima, Y.; Inoue, M.; Ishitobi, T.; Nonaka, M.; Chayama, K. Efficacy of atorvastatin for the treatment of nonalcoholic steatohepatitis with dyslipidemia. *Metabolism* **2008**, *57*, 1711–1718. [CrossRef]

226. Athyros, V.; Alexandrides, T.K.; Bilianou, H.; Cholongitas, E.; Doumas, M.; Ganotakis, E.; Goudevenos, J.; Elisaf, M.S.; Germanidis, G.; Giouleme, O.; et al. The use of statins alone, or in combination with pioglitazone and other drugs, for the treatment of non-alcoholic fatty liver disease/non-alcoholic steatohepatitis and related cardiovascular risk. An Expert Panel Statement. *Metabolism* **2017**, *71*, 17–32. [CrossRef]

227. Tsan, Y.-T.; Lee, C.-H.; Wang, J.-D.; Chen, P.-C. Statins and the Risk of Hepatocellular Carcinoma in Patients with Hepatitis B Virus Infection. *J. Clin. Oncol.* **2012**, *30*, 623–630. [CrossRef]

228. Butt, A.A.; Yan, P.; Bonilla, H.; Abou-Samra, A.B.; Shaikh, O.S.; Simon, T.G.; Chung, R.T.; Rogal, S.S.; ERCHIVES (Electronically Retrieved Cohort of HCV Infected Veterans) Study Team. Effect of addition of statins to antiviral therapy in hepatitis C virus-infected persons: Results from ERCHIVES. *Hepatology* **2015**, *62*, 365–374. [CrossRef]

229. Kawaguchi, Y.; Sakamoto, Y.; Ito, D.; Ito, K.; Arita, J.; Akamatsu, N.; Kaneko, J.; Hasegawa, K.; Moriya, K.; Kokudo, N. Statin use is associated with a reduced risk of hepatocellular carcinoma recurrence after initial liver resection. *Biosci. Trends* **2017**, *11*, 574–580. [CrossRef]

230. Cao, Z.; Fan-Minogue, H.; Bellovin, D.I.; Yevtodiyenko, A.; Arzeno, J.; Yang, Q.; Gambhir, S.S.; Felsher, D.W. MYC phosphorylation, activation, and tumorigenic potential in hepatocellular carcinoma are regulated by HMG-CoA reductase. *Cancer Res.* **2011**, *71*, 2286–2297. [CrossRef]

231. Roudier, E.; Mistafa, O.; Stenius, U. Statins induce mammalian target of rapamycin (mTOR)-mediated inhibition of Akt signaling and sensitize p53-deficient cells to cytostatic drugs. *Mol. Cancer Ther.* **2006**, *5*, 2706–2715. [CrossRef]

232. Ghalali, A.; Martin-Renedo, J.; Högberg, J.; Stenius, U. Atorvastatin Decreases HBx-Induced Phospho-Akt in Hepatocytes via P2X Receptors. *Mol. Cancer Res.* **2017**, *15*, 714–722. [CrossRef]

233. Wang, J.; Tokoro, T.; Higa, S.; Kitajima, I. Anti-inflammatory Effect of Pitavastatin on NF-κB Activated by TNF-α in Hepatocellular Carcinoma Cells. *Biol. Pharm. Bull.* **2006**, *29*, 634–639. [CrossRef] [PubMed]

234. Marinho, T.D.S.; Kawasaki, A.; Bryntesson, M.; Souza-Mello, V.; Barbosa-Da-Silva, S.; Aguila, M.B.; Mandarim-De-Lacerda, C.A. Rosuvastatin limits the activation of hepatic stellate cells in diet-induced obese mice. *Hepatol. Res.* **2016**, *47*, 928–940. [CrossRef] [PubMed]

235. Uschner, F.E.; Ranabhat, G.; Choi, S.S.; Granzow, M.; Klein, S.; Schierwagen, R.; Raskopf, E.; Gautsch, S.; Van Der Ven, P.F.M.; Fürst, D.O.; et al. Statins activate the canonical hedgehog-signaling and aggravate non-cirrhotic portal hypertension, but inhibit the non-canonical hedgehog signaling and cirrhotic portal hypertension. *Sci. Rep.* **2015**, *5*, 14573. [CrossRef] [PubMed]

236. Pikarsky, E.; Porat, R.M.; Stein, I.; Abramovitch, R.; Amit, S.; Kasem, S.; Gutkovich-Pyest, E.; Urieli-Shoval, S.; Galun, E.; Ben-Neriah, Y. NF-κB functions as a tumour promoter in inflammation-associated cancer. *Nat. Cell Biol.* **2004**, *431*, 461–466. [CrossRef] [PubMed]

237. He, G.; Karin, M. NF-κB and STAT3—Key players in liver inflammation and cancer. *Cell Res.* **2011**, *21*, 159–168. [CrossRef] [PubMed]

238. Sahasrabuddhe, V.V.; Gunja, M.Z.; Graubard, B.I.; Trabert, B.; Schwartz, L.M.; Park, Y.; Hollenbeck, A.R.; Freedman, N.D.; McGlynn, K.A. Nonsteroidal Anti-inflammatory Drug Use, Chronic Liver Disease, and Hepatocellular Carcinoma. *J. Natl. Cancer Inst.* **2012**, *104*, 1808–1814. [CrossRef]

239. Chen, H.; Cai, W.; Chu, E.S.H.; Tang, J.; Wong, C.-C.; Wong, S.H.; Sun, W.; Liang, Q.; Fang, J.; Sun, Z.; et al. Hepatic cyclooxygenase-2 overexpression induced spontaneous hepatocellular carcinoma formation in mice. *Oncogene* **2017**, *36*, 4415–4426. [CrossRef]

240. Leng, J.; Han, C.; Demetris, A.J.; Michalopoulos, G.K.; Wu, T. Cyclooxygenase-2 promotes hepatocellular carcinoma cell growth through Akt activation: Evidence for Akt inhibition in celecoxib-induced apoptosis. *Hepatology* **2003**, *38*, 756–768. [CrossRef]

241. Simon, T.G.; Ma, Y.; Ludvigsson, J.F.; Chong, D.Q.; Giovannucci, E.L.; Fuchs, C.S.; Meyerhardt, J.A.; Corey, K.E.; Chung, R.T.; Zhang, X.; et al. Association Between Aspirin Use and Risk of Hepatocellular Carcinoma. *JAMA Oncol.* **2018**, *4*, 1683–1690. [CrossRef]

242. Funaki, M.; Kitabayashi, J.; Shimakami, T.; Nagata, N.; Kai, T.; Takegoshi, K.; Okada, H.; Murai, K.; Shirasaki, T.; Oyama, T.; et al. Peretinoin, an acyclic retinoid, inhibits hepatocarcinogenesis by suppressing sphingosine kinase 1 expression in vitro and in vivo. *Sci. Rep.* **2017**, *7*, 16978. [CrossRef]

243. Malehmir, M.; Pfister, D.; Gallage, S.; Szydlowska, M.; Inverso, D.; Kotsiliti, E.; Leone, V.; Peiseler, M.; Surewaard, B.G.J.; Rath, D.; et al. Platelet GPIbα is a mediator and potential interventional target for NASH and subsequent liver cancer. *Nat. Med.* **2019**, *25*, 641–655. [CrossRef] [PubMed]

244. Wang, T.; Fu, X.; Jin, T.; Zhang, L.; Liu, B.; Wu, Y.; Xu, F.; Wang, X.; Ye, K.; Zhang, W.; et al. Aspirin targets P4HA2 through inhibiting NF-κB and LMCD1-AS1/let-7g to inhibit tumour growth and collagen deposition in hepatocellular carcinoma. *EBioMedicine* **2019**, *45*, 168–180. [CrossRef] [PubMed]

245. Roehlen, N.; Baumert, T.F. Uncovering the mechanism of action of aspirin in HCC chemoprevention. *EBioMedicine* **2019**, *46*, 21–22. [CrossRef] [PubMed]

246. Simon, T.G.; Henson, J.; Osganian, S.; Masia, R.; Chan, A.T.; Chung, R.T.; Corey, K.E. Daily Aspirin Use Associated with Reduced Risk For Fibrosis Progression In Patients with Nonalcoholic Fatty Liver Disease. *Clin. Gastroenterol. Hepatol.* **2019**, *17*, 2776–2784.e4. [CrossRef] [PubMed]

247. Sakurai, T.; Kudo, M. Molecular Link between Liver Fibrosis and Hepatocellular Carcinoma. *Liver Cancer* **2013**, *2*, 365–366. [CrossRef] [PubMed]

248. Loomba, R.; Lawitz, E.; Mantry, P.S.; Jayakumar, S.; Caldwell, S.H.; Arnold, H.; Diehl, A.M.; Djedjos, C.S.; Han, L.; Myers, R.P.; et al. The ASK1 inhibitor selonsertib in patients with nonalcoholic steatohepatitis: A randomized, phase 2 trial. *Hepatology* **2018**, *67*, 549–559. [CrossRef]

249. Ratziu, V.; Harrison, S.A.; Francque, S.; Bedossa, P.; Lehert, P.; Serfaty, L.; Romero-Gomez, M.; Boursier, J.; Abdelmalek, M.; Caldwell, S.; et al. Elafibranor, an Agonist of the Peroxisome Proliferator−Activated Receptor−α and −δ, Induces Resolution of Nonalcoholic Steatohepatitis without Fibrosis Worsening. *Gastroenterol.* **2016**, *150*, 1147–1159.e5. [CrossRef]

250. Kumada, H. Long-term treatment of chronic hepatitis C with glycyrrhizin [stronger neo-minophagen C (SNMC)] for preventing liver cirrhosis and hepatocellular carcinoma. *Oncology* **2002**, *62*, 94–100. [CrossRef]

251. Arase, Y.; Ikeda, K.; Murashima, N.; Chayama, K.; Tsubota, A.; Koida, I.; Suzuki, Y.; Saitoh, S.; Kobayashi, M.; Kumada, H. The long term efficacy of glycyrrhizin in chronic hepatitis C patients. *Cancer* **1997**, *79*, 1494–1500. [CrossRef]

252. Van Rossum, T.G.J.; Vulto, A.G.; De Man, R.A.; Brouwer, J.T.; Schalm, S.W. glycyrrhizin as a potential treatment for chronic hepatitis C. *Aliment. Pharmacol. Ther.* **1998**, *12*, 199–205. [CrossRef]

253. Shiota, G.; Harada, K.-I.; Ishida, M.; Tomie, Y.; Okubo, M.; Katayama, S.; Ito, H.; Kawasaki, H. Inhibition of hepatocellular carcinoma by glycyrrhizin in diethylnitrosamine-treated mice. *Carcinogenesis* **1999**, *20*, 59–63. [CrossRef]

254. Oka, H.; Yamamoto, S.; Kuroki, T.; Harihara, S.; Marumo, T.; Kim, S.R.; Monna, T.; Kobayashi, K.; Tango, T. Prospective study of chemoprevention of hepatocellular carcinoma with sho-saiko-to (TJ-9). *Cancer* **1995**, *76*, 743–749. [CrossRef]

255. Bishayee, A.; Chatterjee, M.; Chatterjee, M. Further Evidence for Chemopreventive Potential of β-Carotene Against Experimental Carcinogenesis: Diethylnitrosamine-Initiated and Phenobarbital-Promoted Hepatocarcinogenesis Is Prevented More Effectively by β-Carotene Than by Retinoic Acid. *Nutr. Cancer* **2000**, *37*, 89–98. [CrossRef]

256. Mann, C.D.; Neal, C.P.; Garcea, G.; Manson, M.M.; Dennison, A.R.; Berry, D.P. Phytochemicals as potential chemopreventive and chemotherapeutic agents in hepatocarcinogenesis. *Eur. J. Cancer Prev.* **2009**, *18*, 13–25. [CrossRef]

257. Qin, G.; Ning, Y.; Lotlikar, P.D. Chemoprevention of Aflatoxin B1-Initiated and Carbon Tetrachloride-Promoted Hepatocarcinogenesis in the Rat by Green Tea. *Nutr. Cancer* **2000**, *38*, 215–222. [CrossRef]

258. Luo, H.; Tang, L.; Tang, M.; Billam, M.; Huang, T.; Yu, J.; Wei, Z.; Liang, Y.; Wang, K.; Zhang, Z.-Q.; et al. Phase IIa chemoprevention trial of green tea polyphenols in high-risk individuals of liver cancer: Modulation of urinary excretion of green tea polyphenols and 8-hydroxydeoxyguanosine. *Carcinogenesis* **2005**, *27*, 262–268. [CrossRef]

259. Sojoodi, M.; Wei, L.; Erstad, D.J.; Yamada, S.; Fujii, T.; Hirschfield, H.; Kim, R.S.; Lauwers, G.Y.; Lanuti, M.; Hoshida, Y.; et al. Epigallocatechin Gallate Induces Hepatic Stellate Cell Senescence and Attenuates Development of Hepatocellular Carcinoma. *Cancer Prev. Res.* **2020**, *13*, 497–508. [CrossRef]

260. Cavin, C.; Holzhäuser, D.; Constable, A.; Huggett, A.C.; Schilter, B. The coffee-specific diterpenes cafestol and kahweol protect against aflatoxin B1-induced genotoxicity through a dual mechanism. *Carcinogenesis* **1998**, *19*, 1369–1375. [CrossRef]

261. Wong, G.L.H.; Chan, H.L.-Y.; Chan, H.-Y.; Tse, C.-H.; Chim, A.M.-L.; Lo, A.O.-S.; Wong, V.W.-S. Adverse Effects of Vitamin D Deficiency on Outcomes of Patients with Chronic Hepatitis B. *Clin. Gastroenterol. Hepatol.* **2015**, *13*, 783–790.e1. [CrossRef]

262. Fedirko, V.; Duarte-Salles, T.; Bamia, C.; Trichopoulou, A.; Aleksandrova, K.; Trichopoulos, D.; Trepo, E.; Tjønneland, A.; Olsen, A.; Overvad, K.; et al. Prediagnostic circulating vitamin D levels and risk of hepatocellular carcinoma in European populations: A nested case-control study. *Hepatology* **2014**, *60*, 1222–1230. [CrossRef]

263. Kwon, H.-J.; Won, Y.-S.; Suh, H.-W.; Jeon, J.-H.; Shao, Y.; Yoon, S.-R.; Chung, J.-W.; Kim, T.-D.; Kim, H.-M.; Nam, K.-H.; et al. Vitamin D3 Upregulated Protein 1 Suppresses TNF-α–Induced NF-κB Activation in Hepatocarcinogenesis. *J. Immunol.* **2010**, *185*, 3980–3989. [CrossRef] [PubMed]

264. Cha, J.H.; Bae, S.H.; Kim, H.L.; Park, N.R.; Choi, E.S.; Jung, E.S.; Choi, J.Y.; Yoon, S.K. Branched-Chain Amino Acids Ameliorate Fibrosis and Suppress Tumor Growth in a Rat Model of Hepatocellular Carcinoma with Liver Cirrhosis. *PLoS ONE* **2013**, *8*, e77899. [CrossRef] [PubMed]

265. Kawaguchi, T.; Shiraishi, K.; Ito, T.; Suzuki, K.; Koreeda, C.; Ohtake, T.; Iwasa, M.; Tokumoto, Y.; Endo, R.; Kawamura, N.; et al. Branched-Chain Amino Acids Prevent Hepatocarcinogenesis and Prolong Survival of Patients with Cirrhosis. *Clin. Gastroenterol. Hepatol.* **2014**, *12*, 1012–1018.e1. [CrossRef] [PubMed]

266. Gao, M.; Sun, K.; Guo, M.; Gao, H.; Liu, K.; Yang, C.; Li, S.; Liu, N. Fish consumption and n-3 polyunsaturated fatty acids, and risk of hepatocellular carcinoma: Systematic review and meta-analysis. *Cancer Causes Control.* **2014**, *26*, 367–376. [CrossRef]

267. Sawada, N.; Inoue, M.; Iwasaki, M.; Sasazuki, S.; Shimazu, T.; Yamaji, T.; Takachi, R.; Tanaka, Y.; Mizokami, M.; Tsugane, S. Consumption of n-3 Fatty Acids and Fish Reduces Risk of Hepatocellular Carcinoma. *Gastroenterology* **2012**, *142*, 1468–1475. [CrossRef]

268. Liebig, M.; Dannenberger, D.; Vollmar, B.; Abshagen, K. n-3 PUFAs reduce tumor load and improve survival in a NASH-tumor mouse model. *Ther. Adv. Chronic Dis.* **2019**, *10*, 2040622319872118. [CrossRef]

269. Ma, Y.; Yang, W.; Li, T.; Liu, Y.; Simon, T.G.; Sui, J.; Wu, K.; Giovannucci, E.L.; Chan, A.T.; Zhang, X. Meat intake and risk of hepatocellular carcinoma in two large US prospective cohorts of women and men. *Int. J. Epidemiol.* **2019**, *48*, 1863–1871. [CrossRef]

270. Briske-Anderson, M.J.; Finley, J.W.; Newman, S.M. The Influence of Culture Time and Passage Number on the Morphological and Physiological Development of Caco-2 Cells. *Exp. Biol. Med.* **1997**, *214*, 248–257. [CrossRef]

271. Hartung, T. Food for thought look back in anger–What clinical studies tell us about preclinical work. *Altex* **2013**, *30*, 275. [CrossRef]

272. Chen, B.; Sirota, M.; Fan-Minogue, H.; Hadley, D.; Butte, A.J. Relating hepatocellular carcinoma tumor samples and cell lines using gene expression data in translational research. *BMC Med. Genom.* **2015**, *8*, S5. [CrossRef]

273. Gillet, J.-P.; Calcagno, A.M.; Varma, S.; Marino, M.; Green, L.J.; Vora, M.I.; Patel, C.; Orina, J.N.; Eliseeva, T.A.; Singal, V.; et al. Redefining the relevance of established cancer cell lines to the study of mechanisms of clinical anti-cancer drug resistance. *Proc. Natl. Acad. Sci. USA* **2011**, *108*, 18708–18713. [CrossRef] [PubMed]

274. Moon, H.; Ju, H.-L.; Chung, S.I.; Cho, K.J.; Eun, J.W.; Nam, S.W.; Han, K.-H.; Calvisi, D.F.; Ro, S.W. Transforming Growth Factor-β Promotes Liver Tumorigenesis in Mice via Up-regulation of Snail. *Gastroenterology* **2017**, *153*, 1378–1391.e6. [CrossRef] [PubMed]

275. Liu, Y.; Qi, X.; Zeng, Z.; Wang, L.; Wang, J.; Zhang, T.; Xu, Q.; Shen, C.; Zhou, G.; Yang, S.; et al. CRISPR/Cas9-mediated p53 and Pten dual mutation accelerates hepatocarcinogenesis in adult hepatitis B virus transgenic mice. *Sci. Rep.* **2017**, *7*, 2796. [CrossRef] [PubMed]

276. Recknagel, R.O.; Glende, E.A.; Dolak, J.A.; Waller, R.L. Mechanisms of carbon tetrachloride toxicity. *Pharmacol. Ther.* **1989**, *43*, 139–154. [CrossRef]

277. Hall, C.N.; Badawi, A.F.; O'Connor, P.J.; Saffhill, R. The detection of alkylation damage in the DNA of human gastrointestinal tissues. *Br. J. Cancer* **1991**, *64*, 59–63. [CrossRef]

278. Wallace, M.; Hamesch, K.; Lunova, M.; Kim, Y.; Weiskirchen, R.; Strnad, P.; Friedman, S.L. Standard Operating Procedures in Experimental Liver Research: Thioacetamide model in mice and rats. *Lab. Anim.* **2015**, *49*, 21–29. [CrossRef]

279. Kushida, M.; Kamendulis, L.M.; Peat, T.J.; Klaunig, J.E. Dose-Related Induction of Hepatic Preneoplastic Lesions by Diethylnitrosamine in C57BL/6 Mice. *Toxicol. Pathol.* **2011**, *39*, 776–786. [CrossRef]

280. Van Norman, G.A. Phase II Trials in Drug Development and Adaptive Trial Design. *JACC Basic Transl. Sci.* **2019**, *4*, 428–437. [CrossRef]

281. Rebholz, C.E.; Swiss Paediatric Oncology Group (SPOG); Rueegg, C.S.; Michel, G.; Ammann, R.A.; Von Der Weid, N.X.; Kuehni, C.E.; Spycher, B.D. Clustering of health behaviours in adult survivors of childhood cancer and the general population. *Br. J. Cancer* **2012**, *107*, 234–242. [CrossRef]

282. Perrone, J.; Phillips, C.; Gaieski, D. Occult Metformin Toxicity in Three Patients with Profound Lactic Acidosis. *J. Emerg. Med.* **2011**, *40*, 271–275. [CrossRef]

2

Frontline Management of Epithelial Ovarian Cancer—Combining Clinical Expertise with Community Practice Collaboration and Cutting-Edge Research

Edward Wenge Wang [1,*], Christina Hsiao Wei [2], Sariah Liu [1], Stephen Jae-Jin Lee [3], Susan Shehayeb [4], Scott Glaser [5], Richard Li [5], Siamak Saadat [1], James Shen [1], Thanh Dellinger [3], Ernest Soyoung Han [3], Daphne Stewart [1], Sharon Wilczynski [2], Mihaela Cristea [1] and Lorna Rodriguez-Rodriguez [3]

[1] Department of Medical Oncology and Therapeutics Research, City of Hope National Medical Center, Duarte, CA 91010, USA; sarliu@coh.org (S.L.); ssaadat@coh.org (S.S.); jashen@coh.org (J.S.); dapstewart@coh.org (D.S.); MCristea@coh.org (M.C.)
[2] Department of Pathology, City of Hope National Medical Center, Duarte, CA 91010, USA; cwei@coh.org (C.H.W.); swilczyn@coh.org (S.W.)
[3] Department of Surgical Oncology, City of Hope National Medical Center, Duarte, CA 91010, USA; stelee@coh.org (S.J.-J.L.); tdellinger@coh.org (T.D.); ehan@coh.org (E.S.H.); lorrodriguez@coh.org (L.R.-R.)
[4] Department of Population Sciences, City of Hope National Medical Center, Duarte, CA 91010, USA; sshehayeb@coh.org
[5] Department of Radiation Oncology, City of Hope National Medical Center, Duarte, CA 91010, USA; sglaser@coh.org (S.G.); rli@coh.org (R.L.)
*   Correspondence: edwang@coh.org

Abstract: Epithelial ovarian cancer (EOC) is the most common histology of ovarian cancer defined as epithelial cancer derived from the ovaries, fallopian tubes, or primary peritoneum. It is the fifth most common cause of cancer-related death in women in the United States. Because of a lack of effective screening and non-specific symptoms, EOC is typically diagnosed at an advanced stage (FIGO stage III or IV) and approximately one third of patients have malignant ascites at initial presentation. The treatment of ovarian cancer consists of a combination of cytoreductive surgery and systemic chemotherapy. Despite the advances with new cytotoxic and targeted therapies, the five-year survival rate for all-stage EOC in the United States is 48.6%. Delivery of up-to-date guideline care and multidisciplinary team efforts are important drivers of overall survival. In this paper, we review our frontline management of EOC that relies on a multi-disciplinary approach drawing on clinical expertise and collaboration combined with community practice and cutting edge clinical and translational research. By optimizing partnerships through team medicine and clinical research, we combine our cancer center clinical expertise, community practice partnership, and clinical and translational research to understand the biology of this deadly disease, advance therapy and connect our patients with the optimal treatment that offers the best possible outcomes.

Keywords: epithelial ovarian cancer; frontline treatment; surgical debulking; adjuvant chemotherapy; maintenance therapy; PARP inhibitor; genetics counseling; clinical research; team medicine

1. Introduction

Epithelial ovarian cancer (EOC) is the most common histology of ovarian cancer, defined as epithelial cancer derived from the ovaries, fallopian tubes, or primary peritoneum [1]. It is the fifth most common cause of cancer-related death in women in the United States, with an estimated 21,750 new cases and 13,940 deaths in 2020 [2]. Because of a lack of effective screening [3] and non-specific symptoms, EOC is typically diagnosed at an advanced stage (FIGO stage III or IV) and approximately one third of patients have malignant ascites at initial presentation. The treatment of ovarian cancer is primarily limited to cytoreductive surgery and systemic chemotherapy. Despite the advances with new cytotoxic and targeted therapies, the five-year survival rate for all-stage EOC in the United States is 48.6% [4]. The delivery of up-to-date guideline care and multidisciplinary team efforts are important drivers of overall survival [5].

The City of Hope National Medical Center (COH) is an NCI-designated Comprehensive Cancer Center based in Duarte, California. Its service area includes Los Angeles, San Bernadino, Riverside, and Orange Counties. Together, these four counties are home to 46% of California's total population. COH delivers high quality cancer care to this sizable demographic through its large network of community oncology practice clinics in the area. In this paper, we review the frontline management of EOC and how we combine our cancer center clinical expertise, community practice partnership, and clinical and translational research to understand the biology of this deadly disease and advance therapy.

2. Surgical Management

Cytoreductive surgery (debulking) plays a fundamental role in managing EOC. Studies show that survival is inversely correlated with the volume of residual disease after cytoreductive surgery [6–13]. Thus, the goal of surgery is to remove all visible disease [6,9,12,14–18]. In a 2011 meta-analysis of 11 retrospective studies of primary cytoreduction for advanced EOC, there was improved survival with optimal (residual disease ≤ 1 cm in maximum tumor diameter) versus suboptimal (residual disease > 1 cm in maximum tumor diameter) cytoreduction (hazard ratio (HR) 1.36, 95% CI 1.10–1.68), and further improved survival with no gross residual disease (HR 2.20, 95% CI 1.90–2.54) [19]. In a 2013 meta-analysis of 18 studies (retrospective and prospective) of women with stage IIB or higher EOC who underwent cytoreduction and platinum/taxane chemotherapy, each 10% increase in the proportion of patients undergoing complete cytoreduction was associated with a 2.3 month increase in median survival compared with a 1.8 month increase for optimal cytoreduction [14].

Furthermore, improved outcomes in advanced EOC have been shown in high volume hospitals (≥20 cases/year) and high-volume surgeons (≥10 cases/year) [20]. Given the importance of the extent of cytoreduction and volume of cases on outcome and the potential morbidity with an extensive major abdominal surgery, predicting which patients will be able to have at least an optimal cytoreduction is valuable. This is primarily performed through physical examination and computed tomography (CT) of the chest, abdomen, and pelvis. Diagnostic laparoscopy can also be utilized to help triage patients with primary debulking or neoadjuvant chemotherapy [21–23]. It is of utmost importance that a gynecologic oncologist experienced in extensive cytoreductive surgeries evaluates the patient to determine resectability, as achieving no gross residual disease or optimal cytoreduction largely depends on the judgment, experience, skill, and aggressiveness of the surgeon. Additionally, patient factors, such as age, performance status, medical comorbidities, and preoperative nutritional status, are important considerations, as some patients may not be able to tolerate an extensive cytoreduction. The commonly accepted criteria for unresectability include mesenteric root involvement, diffuse involvement of the stomach and/or large parts of the small or large bowel, extra-abdominal disease, infiltration of the duodenum and/or parts of the pancreas (not limited to the pancreatic tail), or involvement of the large vessels of the hepatoduodenal ligament, celiac trunk, or behind the porta hepatis [24].

Our strong partnership with community practices provides a large number of patients in Los Angeles and the Greater Los Angeles area with access to a high volume, high complexity cancer center. In addition to hysterectomy, bilateral salpingo-oophorectomy, and omentectomy, additional procedures can include small bowel resection, large bowel resection, stoma formation, diaphragm peritonectomy plus/minus segmental full-thickness diaphragm resection, splenectomy plus/minus distal pancreatectomy, segmental liver resection, cholecystectomy, partial stomach resection, and partial bladder/ureteral resection. We advocate against routine lymphadenectomy (pelvic, para-aortic) in patients undergoing cytoreduction for stage III or IV disease as it has not been shown to improve overall survival and results in increased postoperative morbidity [25]. However, we do resect suspicious or enlarged lymph nodes to achieve a complete or optimal cytoreduction. An intraperitoneal (IP) catheter for IP delivery of adjuvant chemotherapy may be placed in select patients who have obtained optimal primary cytoreduction, as combination treatment with intravenous (IV) and IP chemotherapy has been shown to prolong overall survival [26–28]; although newer trials have advocated for IV delivery of chemotherapeutics that may have similar outcomes but less morbidity than IP chemotherapy [29].

Patients referred to COH from our community clinics for the surgical management of EOC are assessed by our gynecologic surgical oncologist team and we perform primary cytoreduction for EOC in selected patients (those medically fit to undergo an extensive surgery and in whom it is deemed a resection to no gross residual disease or at least in whom an optimal debulking can be achieved) followed by adjuvant chemotherapy. Other patients deemed unresectable may undergo neoadjuvant chemotherapy and then re-evaluation for possible interval cytoreduction. We perform heated intraperitoneal chemotherapy (HIPEC) in a clinical trial setting for translational purpose toward personalized medicine. We collect biospecimens including peritoneal samples with and without tumor cells, blood samples before and after HIPEC. Paired tumor/normal whole exome sequencing (WES) and whole transcriptome sequencing (RNAseq) is performed for analyses of germline and somatic genomic landscapes, as well as gene expression phenotypes before and after treatment, including the assessment of driver mutations, mutation signatures, tumor mutation burden, and immune signatures. Hyperthermia increases the penetration of chemotherapy and increases the chemosensitivity of the cancer by impairing DNA repair. Additionally, hyperthermia induces apoptosis and activates heat-shock proteins that serve as receptors for natural killer cells, inhibits angiogenesis, and has a direct cytotoxic effect by promoting the denaturation of proteins. In a 2018 randomized trial, van Driel et al. reported a nearly 12-month survival benefit in those receiving HIPEC versus no HIPEC after undergoing at least an optimal interval cytoreduction with a similar rate of grade 3 or 4 adverse events between the two groups [30]. It is unclear if the IP administration, the heat, or the additional dose of chemotherapy is responsible for the benefit as all three interventions were utilized. These results are encouraging; however, further studies are needed before there is widespread adoption of this technique, which requires additional technical expertise [31,32].

Pressurized intraperitoneal aerosol chemotherapy (PIPAC) is another approach we are evaluating in the clinical trial setting. PIPAC is a novel minimally-invasive drug delivery system in which normothermic chemotherapy is administered into the abdominal cavity as an aerosol under pressure [33,34]. This approach uses the advantage of the physical properties of gas and pressure by generating an artificial pressure gradient and enhancing tissue uptake of the aerosolized chemotherapy. Due to high local bioavailability during PIPAC, lower concentrations of chemotherapy can be utilized, thus minimizing side effects and toxicity.

3. Gynecologic Pathology: Diagnostic Evaluation

Accurate pathologic diagnosis is the cornerstone of our treatment approach. When patients come to COH with a diagnosis of EOC made in the community, their surgical pathology is reviewed by our gynecologic pathology team. There are four major histologic types of ovarian epithelial tumors—serous, mucinous, endometrioid, and clear cell. High grade serous carcinoma (HGSC) is the most common, and lethal histologic subtypes of all ovarian epithelial malignancies are diagnosed, often presenting at an advanced stage. A subset of these patients carry germline mutations in double-strand DNA repair genes, such as BRCA1, BRCA2, RAD51c, and PALB2. Therefore, diagnosis of HGSC carries specific prognostic, therapeutic, and genetic implications. The ovarian cancer TCGA study showed that HGSC is characterized by a near universal p53 mutation [35]. Most of the p53 mutations lead to the overexpression or deletion of the protein, and these can be detected using immunohistochemistry.

In morphologically ambiguous cases, performing a p53 mutation analysis may be helpful, and p53 mutation status can be used to temporally track patients' tumors over time. Knowledge about the clinical and functional consequences of various p53 mutations is emerging. We perform whole-exome and RNA sequencing using the next generation sequencing platform for HGSC tumors. This allows us to define the p53 mutation profile in tumors and helps us to better understand clinical and treatment significance.

HGSC also displays genomic instability with high copy-number variations across the genome [36]. This unstable genomic landscape is a collective reflection of high tumor replication rate and the tumor cells' underlying defective DNA repair mechanisms, specifically homologous recombination repair (HRR) [37]. In HGSC, which displays homologous recombination deficiency (HRD), tumors rely on alternative but error-prone pathways, including non-homologous end-joining and single-strand annealing repair pathways [38]. Women with germline BRCA1/2 mutations are enriched for the HRD phenotype [39]. The underlying HRD phenotype explains why some HGSC patients are sensitive to platinum-based chemotherapy (carboplatin, paclitaxel, or docetaxel) or poly-(ADP-ribose)-polymerase 1 (PARP1) inhibitors (such as olaparib and niraparib). Platinum-based chemotherapy induces synthetic lethality by covalent binding with DNA, forming DNA-platinum adducts that eventually trigger double strand break. PARP1 inhibitors impede the PARP1-mediated repair of DNA single strand breaks, a component of the HRR pathway. In HGSC with underlying HRD, double strand breaks cannot be repaired efficiently and their accumulation in the genome result in cell death [38].

HGSC is diagnosed using the MD Anderson histologic 2-tier system [40,41]. Corroborating with the molecular event of p53 mutation, the diagnosis of HGSC can be further supported by performing immunohistochemical staining for p53. HGSC is staged using the current American Joint Committee on Cancer/College of American Pathologists Cancer Staging Form and the FIGO Staging System. The molecular diagnosis of ovarian cancer subtypes that correlate with prognosis may also be adopted as standard procedure in the future. Verhaak et al. analyzed the TCGA database and revealed four ovarian tumor subtypes, each associated with a different prognosis [42].

4. Molecular Studies Available for Diagnostic or Therapeutic Decision Support and Emerging Translational Research

We perform extensive molecular testing, including whole exome sequencing, transcriptomic sequencing, copy number information, mismatch repair (MMR) deficiency, microsatellite instability (MSI) status, tumor mutation burden (TMB), HRD, and PD-L1 protein expression levels, using paired formalin-fixed paraffin-embedded tumor tissue and patient saliva or peripheral blood. This comprehensive approach allows us to detect somatic and germline mutations, clinically actionable mutations, potential therapeutic targets, and markers to help guide checkpoint inhibitor therapy. The genomic analysis makes tailored therapy possible and informs clinical trial options that best match with patient tumor genotype.

Germline and somatic BRCA1 and BRCA2 mutations are assessed in specific clinical contexts to inform genetic counseling and therapy selection. Younger age at presentation and family history of tubo-ovarian and breast cancer malignancies are risk factors suggestive of the presence of germline cancer predisposition syndrome. Referral to a genetic counselor and establishing germline mutation information is crucial for informing patients about BRCA-related cancer risks for themselves and their family members. Most importantly, this allows patients the opportunity to access BRCA-related cancer risk reduction surgeries (e.g., risk-reducing salpingo-oophorectomy, mastectomy), where the timing of surgery can be crucial to successful risk reduction.

Germline and somatic BRCA1/2 mutation information is also important for informing PARP inhibitor eligibility in Stage II, III, and IV HGSC patients post primary treatment. The NCCN guidelines recommend screening for BRCA mutations early in the treatment course to avoid the possibility of delay in instituting PARP inhibitor therapy [43].

HRD positivity is determined by BRCA mutation status (deleterious or suspected deleterious) or HRD/genomic instability score (mathematically derived from genomic assessment of loss of heterozygosity, telomeric allelic imbalance, and large-scale state transitions). Due to the inherent biocomputational complexity with HRD score derivation and inter-laboratory analytic variability, most large medical centers perform HRD testing on a research basis and not for routine clinical diagnostic use.

Circulating miRNAs in blood and urine are being explored as potential early detection markers. However, the evidence on this approach is currently limited, and no consistent miRNA signatures have emerged [44–46]. The lack of reproducibility may be attributable, in part, to technical issues, such as different statistical modeling and approaches, the utilization of different miRNA detection platforms, and patient and tumor heterogeneity [46]. Besides early detection, liquid biopsy-based circulating tumor cells have been leveraged in a recent small pilot preclinical study to provide chemosensitivity information and therapy response prediction in patients presenting with recurrent ovarian cancer [47]. The quest for providing precision oncology to patients using minimally invasive liquid biopsies is expanding, and hopefully it will become a reality in the not so distant future.

With numerous genomic alterations present in HGSC, an integrative analytical approach is necessary to characterize the dominant biologic drivers of carcinogenesis, cancer progression, and prognosis. The TCGA (Cancer Genome Atlas Research Network) and CPTAC (Clinical Proteomic Tumor Analysis Consortium) investigators have paved the way for combining multiple omics in ovarian HGSC—including genomics, proteomics, and phosphoproteomics. Using transcriptomic data, TCGA has built a HGSC molecular taxonomy comprised of four subtypes: differentiated, mesenchymal, immunoreactive, and proliferative [35]. This framework was recapitulated using the proteomic data [36]. However, this molecular taxonomy does not correlate with patient survival [36]. Instead, proteomic signatures (cytoskeleton involved in invasion and migration, apoptosis, and epithelial junction/adhesion) showed more robust correlation with survival [36]. However, this proteomic signature is currently research-based only, awaiting further validation in larger independent cohorts, and is not currently used in clinical setting.

5. Adjuvant Chemotherapy

With the exception of patients with early-stage disease and low-grade cancers with a high cure rate, such as stage 1A and 1B grade 1 endometrioid ovarian cancer, mucinous carcinoma, and low grade serous carcinoma [48–50], patients with EOC who have undergone surgical debulking usually require adjuvant platinum- and taxane-based chemotherapy to reduce the risk of recurrence or prolong disease-free survival. Optimal time from surgery to initiate adjuvant chemotherapy has been shown to be 4–6 weeks [49,51]. Table 1 summarizes the main clinical studies of frontline treatment and maintenance of EOC. The standard adjuvant chemotherapy regimen includes: IV paclitaxel 175 mg/m^2 and carboplatin AUC 5–6 every 3 weeks. Alternatively, dose dense weekly paclitaxel 80 mg/m^2 and carboplatin AUC 5–6 every 3 weeks may be applied [52–55]—although this regimen has shown differing outcomes in different studies—the JGOG3016 study [52,56] showed a favorable outcome over every 3-week standard regimen, while the ICON-8 [55], and GOG-262 studies [53] failed to showed a significant improvement. The MITO-7 study used weekly paclitaxel 60 mg/m^2 and carboplatin AUC 2 for up to 18 weeks—this regimen has a high tolerance and is effective for elderly patients or those with poor performance status [54]. Single agent carboplatin is also acceptable if patients cannot tolerate the combination treatment. Docetaxel is an acceptable taxane alternative to paclitaxel with equivalent efficacy [57]. Carboplatin plus liposomal doxorubicin is also an acceptable combination for adjuvant chemotherapy when patients cannot tolerate taxanes [58,59]. Recently, bevacizumab was incorporated into the adjuvant chemotherapeutic regimen, showing improved progression-free survival and also overall survival in the high risk of progression subgroup, including those with stage IV disease and inoperable or sub-optimally debulked stage III disease (ICON-7, GOG-218) [60,61], especially in patients with ascites [60,62,63].

In patients with EOC, the peritoneal cavity is usually the primary site of recurrence. Thus, the administration of adjuvant IV/IP chemotherapy to treat residual cancer cells with highly concentrated chemotherapeutics is an attractive approach. The GOG-172 study showed that IV paclitaxel 135 mg/m^2 on day 1 plus IP cisplatin 75–100 mg/m^2 on day 2 and IP paclitaxel 60 mg/m^2 on day 8, every 3 weeks for up to six cycles, improved survival by 16 months in patients with optimally debulked stage III EOC compared with IV delivery of paclitaxel and cisplatin [27]; IP carboplatin is a suitable substitute for IP cisplatin in the GOG-252 study, as the median progression-free survival and overall survival were similar in the IP carboplatin and IP cisplatin arms [28]. However, the IV/IP chemotherapy regimen resulted in more side effects [64], including abdominal pain, catheter-related infection and blockage, and myelosuppression, all of which may delay treatment and compromise efficacy. We routinely use IV/IP adjuvant chemotherapy based on the favorable survival outcomes [27,65]. A recent publication showed that, when bevacizumab was added to IV/IV carboplatin and paclitaxel, IV/IP carboplatin and paclitaxel, or IV/IP cisplatin and paclitaxel, there was no significant difference in progression-free survival in all of these groups of patients [28]. Therefore, there is debate as to whether or not IP chemotherapy is still an acceptable option in primary adjuvant chemotherapy for patients with advanced EOC, given its higher toxicity, inconvenience, catheter complications, and uncertain long-term benefits [29]. At City of Hope, we have been treating patients with the IV/IP protocol. Due to recent advances in maintenance therapy, we are reconsidering if it is still necessary to perform the IP delivery of chemotherapeutics.

6. Maintenance Therapy

EOC patients who undergo surgical debulking and adjuvant chemotherapy still experience a high rate of disease recurrence. Thus, there is a need for effective maintenance therapy after adjuvant chemotherapy for patients with EOC to help prevent recurrence or prolong disease-free survival. In the past, patients who completed adjuvant chemotherapy usually underwent active surveillance with regular follow-up, labs, and imaging as needed. However, this practice was changed after the ICON-7 and GOG-218 studies showed clinical benefit by adding bevacizumab to the adjuvant chemotherapy regimen [59–62]. The ICON-7 study added bevacizumab (7.5 mg/kg) to IV paclitaxel and carboplatin on day 1, repeated every 3 weeks for 5–6 cycles, continuing bevacizumab for up to 12 additional cycles and showed a modest prolongation of progression-free survival by 2.4 months. Overall, survival was also increased in patients with a poor prognosis [61,66]. The GOG-218 study added bevacizumab to IV paclitaxel and carboplatin on day 1 of cycle 2 (15 mg/kg), every 3 weeks for up to 22 cycles. This regimen showed a significant benefit to progression-free survival (14.1 months vs. 10.3 months, $p < 0.001$). Patients with ascites who received bevacizumab in addition to paclitaxel and carboplatin had significantly improved progression-free survival and overall survival compared to those who received paclitaxel and carboplatin alone [63]. However, maintenance with PARP inhibitors may be favored over bevacizumab due to improved survival.

Following success in treating recurrent EOC, PARP inhibitors have also recently become an attractive choice for maintenance after adjuvant chemotherapy in newly diagnosed EOC patients. Olaparib was FDA-approved (2018) for the maintenance treatment of adult patients with deleterious or suspected deleterious germline or somatic BRCA-mutated advanced EOC who are experiencing a complete or partial response to first-line platinum-based chemotherapy. This is based on the SOLO-1 study [67], a randomized, double-blind, placebo-controlled, multi-center trial that compared the efficacy of olaparib with placebo in patients with BRCA-mutated advanced ovarian, fallopian tube, or primary peritoneal cancer following first-line platinum-based chemotherapy. After a median follow-up of 41 months, the risk of disease progression or death was 70% lower with olaparib than with placebo. In May 2020, the FDA expanded the indication of olaparib to include its combination with bevacizumab for first-line maintenance treatment of adult patients with advanced EOC who have complete or partial response to first-line platinum-based chemotherapy and whose cancers are HRD-positive, defined by either a deleterious or suspected deleterious BRCA mutation and/or genomic instability score. This recommendation was based on the study by Ray-Coquard et al. [68], which showed that, in patients with advanced EOC receiving first-line standard therapy bevacizumab, the addition of maintenance olaparib provided a significant progression-free survival benefit, which was substantial in patients with HRD-positive tumors (37.2 vs. 17.7 months). Patients with HRD-positivity but without a BRCA mutation also had significantly improved progression-free survival (28.1 vs. 16.6 months).

Niraparib, another PARP inhibitor, was granted approval by the FDA in April 2020 as a first-line maintenance treatment of adult patients with advanced EOC who experienced a complete or partial response to first-line platinum-based chemotherapy, regardless of biomarker status. This recommendation is based on the PRIMA study [69] (Table 1) which showed that patients with newly diagnosed advanced EOC who had a response to platinum-based chemotherapy and received niraparib had significantly longer progression-free survival than those who received placebo (13.8 vs. 8.2 months), regardless of the presence or absence of HRD. We use niraparib for patients without BRCA mutation or HRD, or patients with unknown BCRA/HRD status.

Additional maintenance options are being studied in clinical trials, including new PARP inhibitors, anti-angiogenesis agents, immune checkpoint inhibitors, agents targeting other signal transduction pathways, and new rational combinations. We expect to have improved maintenance options in the future to further reduce recurrence and prolong disease-free survival. Choosing the right maintenance therapy for each patient is highly complex and benefits from multi-disciplinary discussion. At COH, the community oncologists have access to the COH Gynecologic Cancer Tumor Board (discussed further below) to present their challenging cases for in-depth discussion.

Table 1. Major clinical trials on frontline treatment of epithelial ovarian cancer.

Study	Patients	Experimental	Control	Progression Free Survival	Overall Survival
JGOG 3016 [52,56]	Stage II-IV EOC	three-weekly carboplatin (AUC 6) and weekly paclitaxel (80 mg/m²) for six cycles	three-weekly carboplatin (AUC 6) and paclitaxel (180 mg/m²) for six cycles	28.0 vs. 17.2 months; HR 0.71, 95% CI 0.58–0.88; p = 0.0015	100.5 vs. 62.2 months (HR 0.79, 95% CI 0.63–0.99; p = 0.039
MITO-7 [54]	FIGO stage IC-IV EOC	Weekly carboplatin (AUC 2) and paclitaxel (60 mg/m²) for 18 weeks	three-weekly carboplatin (AUC 6) and paclitaxel (175 mg/m²) for six cycles	18.3 vs. 17.3 months; HR 0.96, 95% CI 0.80–1.16; p = .66	-
ICON-8 [55]	FIGO stage IC-IV EOC	Group 2: three-weekly carboplatin (AUC 5/6) and weekly paclitaxel (80 mg/m²) for six cycles Group 3: Weekly carboplatin (AUC 6) and paclitaxel (60 mg/m²) for 18 weeks	Group 1: three-weekly carboplatin (AUC 5/6) and paclitaxel (175 mg/m²) for six cycles	Group 1 vs. Group 2 vs. Group 3: 17.7 vs. 20.8 vs. 21.0 Group 2 vs. Group 1: p = 0.35 Group 3 vs. Group 1: p = 0.51	-
GOG-172 [27,65]	FIGO stage III with optimal debulking	paclitaxel 135 mg/m² continuous IV infusion over 24 h on day 1, cisplatin 100 mg/m² IP on day 2, paclitaxel 60 mg/m² IP on day 8 for six cycles	paclitaxel 135 mg/m² continuous IV infusion over 24 h on day 1, cisplatin 75 mg/m² IV on day 2 for six cycles	23.8 vs. 18.3 months; HR 0.80, 95% CI 0.64–1.00; p = 0.05	65.6 vs. 49.7 months; HR 0.75, 95% CI, 0.58–0.97; p = 0.03 61.8 vs. 51.4 months; Adjusted HR 0.77; 95% CI, 0.65–0.90; p = 0.002
GOG-252 [28]	FIGO stage II-IV EOC	paclitaxel 80 mg/m² IV on days 1, 8, and 15 plus carboplatin AUC 6 IP on day 1 every 21 days for cycles 1-6 plus bevacizumab 15 mg/kg IV every 21 days for cycles 2-22 paclitaxel 135 mg/m² IV on day 1 plus cisplatin 75 mg/m² IP on day 2 plus paclitaxel 60 mg/m² IV on day 8 every 21 days for cycles 1-6 plus bevacizumab 15 mg/kg IV every 21 days for cycles 2-22	paclitaxel 80 mg/m² IV on days 1, 8, and 15 plus carboplatin AUC 6 IV on day 1 every 21 days for cycles 1-6 plus bevacizumab 15 mg/kg IV every 21 days for cycles 2-22	IV vs. IP-carboplatin vs. IP-cisplatin: 24.9 vs. 27.4 vs. 26.2 months IP-carboplatin: HR 0.93, 95% CI 0.80–1.07 IP-cisplatin: HR 0.98, 95% CI 0.84–1.13	IV vs. IP-carboplatin vs. IP-cisplatin: 75.5 vs. 78.9 vs. 72.9 months IP-carboplatin: HR 0.95, 95% CI 0.80–1.13 IP-cisplatin: HR 1.05, 95% CI; 0.88–1.24;
GOG-262 [53]	FIGO stage III-IV EOC	three-weekly carboplatin (AUC 6) and weekly paclitaxel (80 mg/m²), plus/minus three-weekly bevacizumab 15 mg/kg for six cycles	three-weekly carboplatin (AUC 6) and paclitaxel (175 mg/m²), plus/minus three-weekly bevacizumab 15 mg/kg for six cycles	With bevacizumab: 14.9 vs. 14.7 months; HR 0.99, 95% CI 0.83–1.20; p = 0.60 Without bevacizumab: 14.2 vs. 10.3 months; HR 0.62, 95% CI 0.40–0.95; p = 0.03	With and without bevacizumab: 40.2 vs. 39.0 months; HR 0.94; 95% CI, 0.72–1.2
SOLO-1 [67]	FIGO stage III or IV high-grade serous or endometrioid EOC patients with a deleterious or suspected deleterious germline or somatic BRCA1/2 mutation, completed frontline platinum-based chemotherapy	olaparib	placebo	Not reached vs. 13.8 months; HR 0.30, 95% CI 0.23–0.41); p < 0.0001 3-year: 60% vs. 27%; 4-year: 53% vs. 11%	-
PAOLA-1 [68]	FIGO stage III or IV high-grade EOC patients after first-line treatment with platinum–taxane chemotherapy plus bevacizumab	olaparib plus bevacizumab	placebo plus bevacizumab	22.1 vs. 16.6 months; HR 0.59; 95% CI 0.49–0.72; p < 0.001 HRD plus BRCA mutation: 37.2 vs. 17.7 months; HR 0.33, 95% CI 0.25–0.45 HRD minus BRCA mutation: 28.1 vs. 16.6 months; HR 0.43, 95% CI 0.28–0.66	-
PRIMA [69]	FIGO stage III or IV high-grade serous or endometrioid EOC patients after first-line treatment with platinum-based chemotherapy	niraparib	placebo	Overall: 13.8 vs. 8.2 months; HR .62, 95% CI 0.50–0.76; p < 0.001 HRD-positive: 21.9 vs. 10.4 months; HR 0.43, 95% CI 0.31–0.59; p < 0.001	-

7. Genetic Counseling

HGSC is a single case indicator for germline genetic testing [70]. Germline genetic testing should be considered both due to the relatively high percentage of hereditary ovarian cancer with some studies estimating that more than 20% is hereditary in etiology [71–73], and due to the potential for treatment implications [74]. Generally, it is preferable for an individual to undergo germline testing as soon as diagnosis occurs [75,76]. This allows ample time to obtain and disclose results, especially in the setting of a patient who may have a guarded prognosis. Urgent testing of BRCA1/2 and other breast cancer genes with high or moderate penetrance by multi-gene panel can currently be performed. While this strategy is often used for women with breast cancer undergoing surgical decision-making, it can also be employed in the gynecologic oncology setting to provide results that may affect eligibility for PARP inhibitors or other therapies in a timely manner.

Germline testing in an affected individual is the most informative strategy and can help clarify risk for relatives. Close female relatives may have increased empiric risk to develop EOC, although older studies may include some families with risk alleles that would be identified by current technology [77,78]. The ascertainment of a multi-generational pedigree allows both for appropriate test selection as well as for proper assessment of family structure and identification of at-risk relatives [79]. Pedigree assessment in the setting of genetic counseling can also facilitate understanding of social relationships between relatives to help develop appropriate strategies to encourage familial communication about risk.

Germline testing for women with EOC at our center typically includes evaluation via a multi-gene panel to include EOC risk genes beyond BRCA1/2, such as the mismatch repair (Lynch syndrome) genes, BRIP1, RAD51C, and RAD51D [71,80]. Beyond informing therapeutic strategy, germline testing in the setting of appropriate counseling can have significant implications for patients and family members. Germline testing can help stratify the risk of developing other cancers and guide the development of appropriate management strategies, especially as the prognosis for EOC improves with better treatment options. For example, patients with Lynch syndrome are at significantly elevated risk to develop colorectal cancer [81] and patients with pathogenic alterations in the BRCA genes are at significantly elevated risk to develop breast cancer [82]. Understanding a patient's risk may help prevent a second primary cancer, especially in the setting of well-controlled ovarian disease or in the setting where the development of a new cancer may interfere with the patient's current treatment.

Germline testing may be even more impactful in terms of implications for relatives. Identifying an ovarian cancer risk allele can allow relatives with the same allele to undergo preventative measures, such as risk-reducing salpingo-oopherectomy, which is especially relevant when screening is not effective. Moreover, in some cases, over-treatment may be avoided in relatives who do not carry the risk allele but who may have otherwise chosen to move forward with preventative measures or screening due to concerns over risk, based on family history. Many genes implicated in EOC in the setting of a monoallelic pathogenic variant also have implications for typically childhood-onset syndromes in the setting of biallelic pathogenic variants. For example, biallelic variants in BRCA1/2, BRIP1, and RAD51C [83–86] are associated with Fanconi anemia and biallelic variants in the mismatch repair genes are associated with Constitutional Mismatch Repair Deficiency syndrome [81]. Thus, individuals contemplating childbearing may also wish to learn their germline status to inform reproductive decisions.

Importantly, negative somatic testing does not obviate the need for germline testing. Reasons for this can include the loss of a germline mutation in the tumor, limited analysis of the tumor genome, and differences in variant calling between somatic and germline laboratories. Conversely, somatic testing may identify variants that are germline in origin [87,88]. Therefore, patients should be counseled about this possibility, and if somatic results are available, they should be reviewed to help inform germline test selection. Other genes may also be included based on clinical suspicion and the evaluation of additional personal and family history. Reevaluation should be considered over time as changes to the family history, as well as advances in the field of cancer genetics, occur [79].

8. Team Medicine: Optimizing Partnerships and Clinical Research

We have a number of initiatives to ensure the inclusion of our community partners in research, education, and the integration of research-based advances into novel therapeutics by clinical trials. We aim to personalize therapy for patients so our community physicians can recommend improved therapy considerations, including clinical trials beyond the standard of care. One way we achieve this is via comprehensive molecular testing. All EOC patients at COH undergo GEM ExTra® testing (facilitated by TGen, a COH affiliate). This test reports clinically actionable mutations, copy number alterations, transcript variants, and fusions, detected in any gene in patient DNA or RNA. The goal is to uncover true tumor-specific (somatic) alterations by comparing the sequence of the tumor against the paired normal DNA from each patient. The test also includes whole-transcriptome RNA profiling, interrogating the patient's tumor transcriptome for fusions and transcriptional variants known to be relevant to cancer (e.g., EGFR vIII). Each tumor's cancer-specific alterations are then queried against a proprietary knowledge base algorithm to identify potential therapeutic associations. The final report provides the physician with a list of FDA-approved agents that are associated with tumor-specific DNA alterations, as well as biomarker summaries on the variants found and tumor-specific evidence for drug matches, including matches with investigational agents, as available on clinicaltrials.gov. The results are reviewed by our multidisciplinary gynecologic cancer research team to aid in treatment decision-making, highlight on-going studies and identify study candidates.

Our current clinical research portfolio in the frontline management of EOC focuses on developing superior treatment options for patients that reduce recurrence and prolong disease-free survival. We are exploring the use of HIPEC and PIPAC in the clinical trial setting as well as novel drug combinations that help to tailor and personalize treatment for superior results. Our HIPEC trial includes studying the molecular changes triggered by HIPEC to identify molecular signatures of response. Our PIPAC trial is the first in the United States to study aerosolized, pressurized chemotherapy for patients with peritoneal carcinomatosis, including ovarian cancer. Our community oncologists play an important role in these studies by referring patients, thereby allowing us to complete accrual expeditiously.

9. Summary

Management of EOC requires a multi-disciplinary approach, drawing on clinical expertise and collaboration combined with community practice and cutting edge clinical and translational research. Our goal is to understand the biology of this disease, advance therapy and connect our patients with the optimal treatment that offers the best possible outcomes.

Author Contributions: Conceptualization, E.W.W., C.H.W., S.L., S.J.-J.L., S.S. (Susan Shehayeb), S.G., R.L., S.S. (Siamak Saadat), J.S.; validation, E.W.W., M.C. and L.R.-R.; writing—original draft preparation, E.W.W., C.H.W., S.L., S.J.-J.L., S.S. (Susan Shehayeb), S.G., R.L., S.S. (Siamak Saadat), J.S.; writing—review and editing, E.W.W., C.H.W., S.L., S.J.-J.L., S.S. (Susan Shehayeb), T.D., E.S.H., D.S., S.W., M.C. and L.R.-R.; supervision, E.W.W. and L.R.-R.; project administration, E.W.W.; funding acquisition, E.W.W. All authors have read and agreed to the published version of the manuscript.

Acknowledgments: The authors thank Nicola Welch, CMPP for assistance with writing and editing the manuscript. This work was supported by the National Cancer Institute of the National Institutes of Health under award number K12CA001727. The content is solely the responsibility of the authors and does not necessarily represent the official views of the National Institutes of Health.

References

1.   Board PDQATE. *Ovarian Epithelial, Fallopian Tube, and Primary Peritoneal Cancer Treatment (PDQ(R)): Health Professional Version*; PDQ Cancer Information Summaries; National Cancer Institute: Bethesda, MD, USA, 2002.
2.   Siegel, R.L.; Miller, K.D.; Jemal, A. Cancer statistics, 2020. *CA A Cancer J. Clin.* **2020**, *70*, 145–164. [CrossRef]
3.   Nebgen, D.R.; Lu, K.H.; Bast, R.C., Jr. Novel Approaches to Ovarian Cancer Screening. *Curr. Oncol. Rep.* **2019**, *21*, 75. [CrossRef]
4.   Howlader, N.N.A.; Krapcho, M.; Miller, D.; Brest, A.; Yu, M.; Ruhl, J.; Tatalovich, Z.; Mariotto, A.; Lewis, D.R.; Chen, H.S.; et al. *SEER Cancer Statistics Review, 1975–2017*; National Cancer Institute: Bethesda, MD, USA; Available online: https://seer.cancer.gov/csr/1975_2017/ (accessed on 25 August 2020).

5.   Cliby, W.A.; Powell, M.A.; Al-Hammadi, N.; Chen, L.; Miller, J.P.; Roland, P.Y.; Mutch, D.G.; Bristow, R.E. Ovarian cancer in the United States: Contemporary patterns of care associated with improved survival. *Gynecol. Oncol.* **2015**, *136*, 11–17. [CrossRef] [PubMed]

6.   Hoskins, W.J.; McGuire, W.P.; Brady, M.; Homesley, H.D.; Creasman, W.T.; Berman, M.; Ball, H.; Berek, J.S. The effect of diameter of largest residual disease on survival after primary cytoreductive surgery in patients with suboptimal residual epithelial ovarian carcinoma. *Am. J. Obs. Gynecol.* **1994**, *170*, 974–979. [CrossRef]

7.   Eisenkop, S.M.; Friedman, R.L.; Wang, H.J. Complete cytoreductive surgery is feasible and maximizes survival in patients with advanced epithelial ovarian cancer: A prospective study. *Gynecol. Oncol.* **1998**, *69*, 103–108. [CrossRef] [PubMed]

8.   Allen, D.G.; Heintz, A.P.; Touw, F.W. A meta-analysis of residual disease and survival in stage III and IV carcinoma of the ovary. *Eur. J. Gynaecol. Oncol.* **1995**, *16*, 349–356. [PubMed]

9.   Chi, D.S.; Eisenhauer, E.L.; Lang, J.; Huh, J.; Haddad, L.; Abu-Rustum, N.R.; Sonoda, Y.; Levine, D.; Hensley, M.; Barakat, R. What is the optimal goal of primary cytoreductive surgery for bulky stage IIIC epithelial ovarian carcinoma (EOC)? *Gynecol. Oncol.* **2006**, *103*, 559–564. [CrossRef]

10. Winter, W.E., 3rd; Maxwell, G.L.; Tian, C.; Carlson, J.W.; Ozols, R.F.; Rose, P.G.; Markman, M.; Armstrong, D.K.; Muggia, F.; McGuire, W.P. Prognostic factors for stage III epithelial ovarian cancer: A Gynecologic Oncology Group Study. *J. Clin. Oncol. Off. J. Am. Soc. Clin. Oncol.* **2007**, *25*, 3621–3627. [CrossRef]

11. Wimberger, P.; Lehmann, N.; Kimmig, R.; Burges, A.; Meier, W.; Du Bois, A. Prognostic factors for complete debulking in advanced ovarian cancer and its impact on survival. An exploratory analysis of a prospectively randomized phase III study of the Arbeitsgemeinschaft Gynaekologische Onkologie Ovarian Cancer Study Group (AGO-OVAR). *Gynecol. Oncol.* **2007**, *106*, 69–74.

12. Bristow, R.E.; Tomacruz, R.S.; Armstrong, D.K.; Trimble, E.L.; Montz, F.J. Survival effect of maximal cytoreductive surgery for advanced ovarian carcinoma during the platinum era: A meta-analysis. *J. Clin. Oncol. Off. J. Am. Soc. Clin. Oncol.* **2002**, *20*, 1248–1259. [CrossRef]

13. Teramukai, S.; Ochiai, K.; Tada, H.; Fukushima, M. Japan Multinational Trial Organization OC. PIEPOC: A new prognostic index for advanced epithelial ovarian cancer–Japan Multinational Trial Organization OC01–01. *J. Clin. Oncol. Off. J. Am. Soc. Clin. Oncol.* **2007**, *25*, 3302–3306. [CrossRef] [PubMed]

14. Chang, S.J.; Hodeib, M.; Chang, J.; Bristow, R.E. Survival impact of complete cytoreduction to no gross residual disease for advanced-stage ovarian cancer: A meta-analysis. *Gynecol. Oncol.* **2013**, *130*, 493–498. [CrossRef] [PubMed]

15. Eisenkop, S.M.; Spirtos, N.M.; Lin, W.C. "Optimal" cytoreduction for advanced epithelial ovarian cancer: A commentary. *Gynecol. Oncol.* **2006**, *103*, 329–335. [CrossRef] [PubMed]

16. Winter, W.E., 3rd; Maxwell, G.L.; Tian, C.; Sundborg, M.J.; Rose, G.S.; Rose, P.G.; Rubin, S.C.; Muggia, F.; McGuire, W.P. Tumor residual after surgical cytoreduction in prediction of clinical outcome in stage IV epithelial ovarian cancer: A Gynecologic Oncology Group Study. *J. Clin. Oncol. Off. J. Am. Soc. Clin. Oncol.* **2008**, *26*, 83–89. [CrossRef] [PubMed]

17. Eisenhauer, E.L.; Abu-Rustum, N.R.; Sonoda, Y.; Aghajanian, C.; Barakat, R.R.; Chi, D.S. The effect of maximal surgical cytoreduction on sensitivity to platinum-taxane chemotherapy and subsequent survival in patients with advanced ovarian cancer. *Gynecol. Oncol.* **2008**, *108*, 276–281. [CrossRef] [PubMed]

18. Hoskins, W.J. Epithelial ovarian carcinoma: Principles of primary surgery. *Gynecologic Oncol.* **1994**, *55* (3 Pt 2), S91–S96. [CrossRef]

19. Elattar, A.; Bryant, A.; Winter-Roach, B.A.; Hatem, M.; Naik, R. Optimal primary surgical treatment for advanced epithelial ovarian cancer. *Cochrane Database Syst. Rev.* **2011**, *2011*, Cd007565. [CrossRef]

20. Wright, J.D.; Chen, L.; Hou, J.Y.; Burke, W.M.; Tergas, A.I.; Ananth, C.V.; Neugut, A.I.; Hershman, D.L. Association of Hospital Volume and Quality of Care With Survival for Ovarian Cancer. *Obstet. Gynecol.* **2017**, *130*, 545–553. [CrossRef]

21. Rutten, M.J.; Gaarenstroom, K.N.; Van Gorp, T.; van Meurs, H.S.; Arts, H.J.; Bossuyt, P.M.; Ter Brugge, H.G.; Hermans, R.H.; Opmeer, B.C.; Pijnenborg, J.M.; et al. Laparoscopy to predict the result of primary cytoreductive surgery in advanced ovarian cancer patients (LapOvCa-trial): A multicentre randomized controlled study. *BMC Cancer* **2012**, *12*, 31. [CrossRef]

22. Rutten, M.J.; van Meurs, H.S.; van de Vrie, R.; Gaarenstroom, K.N.; Naaktgeboren, C.A.; van Gorp, T.; Ter Brugge, H.G.; Hofhuis, W.; Schreuder, H.W.; Arts, H.J.; et al. Laparoscopy to Predict the Result of Primary Cytoreductive Surgery in Patients With Advanced Ovarian Cancer: A Randomized Controlled Trial. *J. Clin. Oncol. Off. J. Am. Soc. Clin. Oncol.* **2017**, *35*, 613–621. [CrossRef]

23. Fagotti, A.; Ferrandina, G.; Fanfani, F.; Ercoli, A.; Lorusso, D.; Rossi, M.; Scambia, G. A laparoscopy-based score to predict surgical outcome in patients with advanced ovarian carcinoma: A pilot study. *Ann. Surg. Oncol.* **2006**, *13*, 1156–1161. [CrossRef] [PubMed]

24. Wright, A.A.; Bohlke, K.; Armstrong, D.K.; Bookman, M.A.; Cliby, W.A.; Coleman, R.L.; Dizon, D.S.; Kash, J.J.; Meyer, L.A.; Moore, K.N.; et al. Neoadjuvant Chemotherapy for Newly Diagnosed, Advanced Ovarian Cancer: Society of Gynecologic Oncology and American Society of Clinical Oncology Clinical Practice Guideline. *J. Clin. Oncol. Off. J. Am. Soc. Clin. Oncol.* **2016**, *34*, 3460–3473. [CrossRef] [PubMed]

25. Harter, P.; Sehouli, J.; Lorusso, D.; Reuss, A.; Vergote, I.; Marth, C.; Kim, J.-W.; Raspagliesi, F.; Lampe, B.; Aletti, G.; et al. A Randomized Trial of Lymphadenectomy in Patients with Advanced Ovarian Neoplasms. *N. Engl. J. Med.* **2019**, *380*, 822–832. [CrossRef] [PubMed]

26. Walker, J.L.; Armstrong, D.K.; Huang, H.Q.; Fowler, J.; Webster, K.; Burger, R.A.; Clarke-Pearson, D. Intraperitoneal catheter outcomes in a phase III trial of intravenous versus intraperitoneal chemotherapy in optimal stage III ovarian and primary peritoneal cancer: A Gynecologic Oncology Group Study. *Gynecol. Oncol.* **2006**, *100*, 27–32. [CrossRef] [PubMed]

27. Armstrong, D.K.; Bundy, B.; Wenzel, L.; Huang, H.Q.; Baergen, R.; Lele, S.; Copeland, L.J.; Walker, J.; Burger, R.A. Intraperitoneal cisplatin and paclitaxel in ovarian cancer. *N. Engl. J. Med.* **2006**, *354*, 34–43. [CrossRef] [PubMed]

28. Walker, J.L.; Brady, M.F.; Wenzel, L.; Fleming, G.F.; Huang, H.Q.; DiSilvestro, P.A.; Fujiwara, K.; Alberts, D.S.; Zheng, W.; Tewari, K.S.; et al. Randomized Trial of Intravenous Versus Intraperitoneal Chemotherapy Plus Bevacizumab in Advanced Ovarian Carcinoma: An NRG Oncology/Gynecologic Oncology Group Study. *J. Clin. Oncol. Off. J. Am. Soc. Clin. Oncol.* **2019**, *37*, 1380–1390. [CrossRef] [PubMed]

29. Monk, B.J.; Chan, J.K. Is intraperitoneal chemotherapy still an acceptable option in primary adjuvant chemotherapy for advanced ovarian cancer? *Ann. Oncol. Off. J. Eur. Soc. Med. Oncol.* **2017**, *28* (Suppl. 8), viii40–viii45. [CrossRef]

30. van Driel, W.J.; Koole, S.N.; Sikorska, K.; Schagen van Leeuwen, J.H.; Schreuder, H.W.R.; Hermans, R.H.M.; De Hingh, I.H.; Van Der Velden, J.; Arts, H.J.; Massuger, L.F.; et al. Hyperthermic Intraperitoneal Chemotherapy in Ovarian Cancer. *N. Engl. J. Med.* **2018**, *378*, 230–240. [CrossRef]

31. Bouchard-Fortier, G.; Cusimano, M.C.; Fazelzad, R.; Sajewycz, K.; Lu, L.; Espin-Garcia, O.; May, T.; Bouchard-Fortier, A.; Ferguson, S.E. Oncologic outcomes and morbidity following heated intraperitoneal chemotherapy at cytoreductive surgery for primary epithelial ovarian cancer: A systematic review and meta-analysis. *Gynecol. Oncol.* **2020**, *158*, 218–228. [CrossRef]

32. Pletcher, E.; Gleeson, E.; Labow, D. Peritoneal Cancers and Hyperthermic Intraperitoneal Chemotherapy. *Surg. Clin. N. Am.* **2020**, *100*, 589–613. [CrossRef]

33. Nadiradze, G.; Horvath, P.; Sautkin, Y.; Archid, R.; Weinreich, F.J.; Königsrainer, A.; Reymond, M.A. Overcoming Drug Resistance by Taking Advantage of Physical Principles: Pressurized Intraperitoneal Aerosol Chemotherapy (PIPAC). *Cancers* **2019**, *12*, 34. [CrossRef]

34. Tate, S.J.; Torkington, J. Pressurized intraperitoneal aerosol chemotherapy: A review of the introduction of a new surgical technology using the IDEAL framework. *BJS Open* **2020**, *4*, 206–215. [CrossRef] [PubMed]

35. Cancer Genome Atlas Research Network. Integrated genomic analyses of ovarian carcinoma. *Nature* **2011**, *474*, 609–615. [CrossRef] [PubMed]

36. Zhang, H.; Liu, T.; Zhang, Z.; Payne, S.H.; Zhang, B.; McDermott, J.E.; Zhou, J.-Y.; Petyuk, V.A.; Chen, L.; Ray, D.; et al. Integrated Proteogenomic Characterization of Human High-Grade Serous Ovarian Cancer. *Cell* **2016**, *166*, 755–765. [CrossRef] [PubMed]

37. Gee, M.E.; Faraahi, Z.; McCormick, A.; Edmondson, R.J. DNA damage repair in ovarian cancer: Unlocking the heterogeneity. *J. Ovarian Res.* **2018**, *11*, 50. [CrossRef] [PubMed]

38. Milanesio, M.C.; Giordano, S.; Valabrega, G. Clinical Implications of DNA Repair Defects in High-Grade Serous Ovarian Carcinomas. *Cancers* **2020**, *12*, 1315. [CrossRef]

39. Takaya, H.; Nakai, H.; Takamatsu, S.; Mandai, M.; Matsumura, N. Homologous recombination deficiency status-based classification of high-grade serous ovarian carcinoma. *Sci. Rep.* **2020**, *10*, 2757. [CrossRef]

40. Bodurka, D.C.; Deavers, M.T.; Tian, C.; Sun, C.C.; Malpica, A.; Coleman, R.L.; Lu, K.H.; Sood, A.K.; Birrer, M.J.; Ozols, R.; et al. Reclassification of serous ovarian carcinoma by a 2-tier system: A Gynecologic Oncology Group Study. *Cancer* **2012**, *118*, 3087–3094. [CrossRef]

41. Malpica, A.; Deavers, M.T.; Lu, K.; Bodurka, D.C.; Atkinson, E.N.; Gershenson, D.M.; Silva, E.G. Grading ovarian serous carcinoma using a two-tier system. *Am. J. Surg. Pathol.* **2004**, *28*, 496–504. [CrossRef]

42. Verhaak, R.G.; Tamayo, P.; Yang, J.Y.; Hubbard, D.; Zhang, H.; Creighton, C.J.; Fereday, S.; Lawrence, M.; Carter, S.L.; Mermel, C.; et al. Prognostically relevant gene signatures of high-grade serous ovarian carcinoma. *J. Clin. Investig.* **2013**, *123*, 517–525. [CrossRef]

43. Armstrong, D.K.; Alvarez, R.D.; Bakkum-Gamez, J.N.; Barroilhet, L.; Behbakht, K.; Berchuck, A.; Berek, J.S.; Chen, L.-M.; Cristea, M.; DeRosa, M.; et al. NCCN Guidelines Insights: Ovarian Cancer, Version 1.2019. *J. Natl. Compr. Cancer Netw.* **2019**, *17*, 896–909. [CrossRef] [PubMed]

44. Yokoi, A.; Yoshioka, Y.; Hirakawa, A.; Yamamoto, Y.; Ishikawa, M.; Ikeda, S.I.; Kato, T.; Niimi, K.; Kajiyama, H.; Kikkawa, F.; et al. A combination of circulating miRNAs for the early detection of ovarian cancer. *Oncotarget* **2017**, *8*, 89811–89823. [CrossRef] [PubMed]

45. Otsuka, I.; Matsuura, T. Screening and Prevention for High-Grade Serous Carcinoma of the Ovary Based on Carcinogenesis-Fallopian Tube- and Ovarian-Derived Tumors and Incessant Retrograde Bleeding. *Diagnostics* **2020**, *10*, 120. [CrossRef] [PubMed]

46. Elias, K.M.; Fendler, W.; Stawiski, K.; Fiascone, S.J.; Vitonis, A.F.; Berkowitz, R.S.; Frendl, G.; Konstantinopoulos, P.A.; Crum, C.P.; Kedzierska, M.; et al. Diagnostic potential for a serum miRNA neural network for detection of ovarian cancer. *eLife* **2017**, *6*, e28932. [CrossRef] [PubMed]

47. Guadagni, S.; Clementi, M.; Masedu, F.; Fiorentini, G.; Sarti, D.; Deraco, M.; Kusamura, S.; Papasotiriou, I.; Apostolou, P.; Aigner, K.R.; et al. A Pilot Study of the Predictive Potential of Chemosensitivity and Gene Expression Assays Using Circulating Tumour Cells from Patients with Recurrent Ovarian Cancer. *Int. J. Mol. Sci.* **2020**, *21*, 4813. [CrossRef]

48. Young, R.C.; Walton, L.A.; Ellenberg, S.S.; Homesley, H.D.; Wilbanks, G.D.; Decker, D.G.; Miller, A.; Park, R.; Major, F. Adjuvant therapy in stage I and stage II epithelial ovarian cancer. Results of two prospective randomized trials. *N. Eng. J. Med.* **1990**, *322*, 1021–1027. [CrossRef]

49. Winter-Roach, B.A.; Kitchener, H.C.; Lawrie, T.A. Adjuvant (post-surgery) chemotherapy for early stage epithelial ovarian cancer. *Cochrane Database Syst. Rev.* **2012**, *3*, Cd004706.

50. Hogberg, T.; Glimelius, B.; Nygren, P. A systematic overview of chemotherapy effects in ovarian cancer. *Acta Oncolog.* **2001**, *40*, 340–360. [CrossRef]

51. Chan, J.K.; Java, J.J.; Fuh, K.; Monk, B.J.; Kapp, D.S.; Herzog, T.; Bell, J.; Young, R. The association between timing of initiation of adjuvant therapy and the survival of early stage ovarian cancer patients—An analysis of NRG Oncology/Gynecologic Oncology Group trials. *Gynecol. Oncol.* **2016**, *143*, 490–495. [CrossRef]

52. Harano, K.; Terauchi, F.; Katsumata, N.; Takahashi, F.; Yasuda, M.; Takakura, S.; Takano, M.; Yamamoto, Y.; Sugiyama, T. Quality-of-life outcomes from a randomized phase III trial of dose-dense weekly paclitaxel and carboplatin compared with conventional paclitaxel and carboplatin as a first-line treatment for stage II-IV ovarian cancer: Japanese Gynecologic Oncology Group Trial (JGOG3016). *Ann. Oncol. Off. J. Eur. Soc. Med.Oncol.* **2014**, *25*, 251–257.

53. Chan, J.K.; Brady, M.F.; Penson, R.T.; Huang, H.; Birrer, M.J.; Walker, J.L.; DiSilvestro, P.A.; Rubin, S.C.; Martin, L.P.; Davidson, S.A.; et al. Weekly vs. Every-3-Week Paclitaxel and Carboplatin for Ovarian Cancer. *N. Eng. J. Med.* **2016**, *374*, 738–748. [CrossRef] [PubMed]

54. Pignata, S.; Scambia, G.; Katsaros, D.; Gallo, C.; Pujade-Lauraine, E.; De Placido, S.; Bologna, A.; Weber, B.; Raspagliesi, F.; Panici, P.B.; et al. Carboplatin plus paclitaxel once a week versus every 3 weeks in patients with advanced ovarian cancer (MITO-7): A randomised, multicentre, open-label, phase 3 trial. *Lancet Oncol.* **2014**, *15*, 396–405. [CrossRef]

55. Clamp, A.R.; James, E.C.; McNeish, I.A.; Dean, A.; Kim, J.W.; O'Donnell, D.M.; Hook, J.; Coyle, C.; Blagden, S.; Brenton, J.D.; et al. Weekly dose-dense chemotherapy in first-line epithelial ovarian, fallopian tube, or primary peritoneal carcinoma treatment (ICON8): Primary progression free survival analysis results from a GCIG phase 3 randomised controlled trial. *Lancet* **2019**, *394*, 2084–2095. [CrossRef]

56. Katsumata, N.; Yasuda, M.; Isonishi, S.; Takahashi, F.; Michimae, H.; Kimura, E.; Aoki, D.; Jobo, T.; Kodama, S.; Terauchi, F.; et al. Long-term results of dose-dense paclitaxel and carboplatin versus conventional paclitaxel and carboplatin for treatment of advanced epithelial ovarian, fallopian tube, or primary peritoneal cancer (JGOG 3016): A randomised, controlled, open-label trial. *Lancet Oncol.* **2013**, *14*, 1020–1026. [CrossRef]

57. Hsu, Y.; Sood, A.K.; Sorosky, J.I. Docetaxel versus paclitaxel for adjuvant treatment of ovarian cancer: Case-control analysis of toxicity. *Am. J. Clin. Oncol.* **2004**, *27*, 14–18. [CrossRef]

58.   Nguyen, J.; Solimando, D.A., Jr.; Waddell, J.A. Carboplatin and Liposomal Doxorubicin for Ovarian Cancer. *Hosp. Pharm.* **2016**, *51*, 442–449. [CrossRef]

59.   Pignata, S.; Scambia, G.; Ferrandina, G.; Savarese, A.; Sorio, R.; Breda, E.; Gebbia, V.; Musso, P.; Frigerio, L.; Del Medico, P.; et al. Carboplatin plus paclitaxel versus carboplatin plus pegylated liposomal doxorubicin as first-line treatment for patients with ovarian cancer: The MITO-2 randomized phase III trial. *J. Clin. Oncol. Off. J. Am. Soc. Clin. Oncol.* **2011**, *29*, 3628–3635. [CrossRef]

60.   Burger, R.A.; Brady, M.F.; Rhee, J.; Sovak, M.A.; Kong, G.; Nguyen, H.P.; Bookman, M.A. Independent radiologic review of the Gynecologic Oncology Group Study 0218, a phase III trial of bevacizumab in the primary treatment of advanced epithelial ovarian, primary peritoneal, or fallopian tube cancer. *Gynecol. Oncol.* **2013**, *131*, 21–26. [CrossRef]

61.   Perren, T.J.; Swart, A.M.; Pfisterer, J.; Ledermann, J.A.; Pujade-Lauraine, E.; Kristensen, G.; Carey, M.S.; Beale, P.; Cervantes, A.; Kurzeder, C.; et al. A phase 3 trial of bevacizumab in ovarian cancer. *N. Eng. J. Med.* **2011**, *365*, 2484–2496. [CrossRef]

62.   Burger, R.A.; Brady, M.; Bookman, M.A.; Fleming, G.F.; Monk, B.J.; Huang, H.; Mannel, R.S.; Homesley, H.D.; Fowler, J.; Greer, B.E.; et al. Incorporation of bevacizumab in the primary treatment of ovarian cancer. *N. Eng. J. Med.* **2011**, *365*, 2473–2483. [CrossRef]

63.   Ferriss, J.S.; Java, J.J.; Bookman, M.A.; Fleming, G.F.; Monk, B.J.; Walker, J.L.; Homesley, H.D.; Fowler, J.; Greer, B.E.; Boente, M.P.; et al. Ascites predicts treatment benefit of bevacizumab in front-line therapy of advanced epithelial ovarian, fallopian tube and peritoneal cancers: An NRG Oncology/GOG study. *Gynecol. Oncol.* **2015**, *139*, 17–22. [CrossRef]

64.   Wenzel, L.B.; Huang, H.Q.; Armstrong, D.K.; Walker, J.L.; Cella, D. Health-related quality of life during and after intraperitoneal versus intravenous chemotherapy for optimally debulked ovarian cancer: A Gynecologic Oncology Group Study. *J. Clin. Oncol. Off. J. Am. Soc. Clin. Oncol.* **2007**, *25*, 437–443. [CrossRef] [PubMed]

65.   Tewari, D.; Java, J.J.; Salani, R.; Armstrong, D.K.; Markman, M.; Herzog, T.; Monk, B.J.; Chan, J.K. Long-term survival advantage and prognostic factors associated with intraperitoneal chemotherapy treatment in advanced ovarian cancer: A gynecologic oncology group study. *J. Clin. Oncol. Off. J. Am. Soc. Clin. Oncol.* **2015**, *33*, 1460–1466. [CrossRef]

66.   Oza, A.M.; Cook, A.D.; Pfisterer, J.; Embleton, A.; Ledermann, J.A.; Pujade-Lauraine, E.; Kristensen, G.; Carey, M.S.; Beale, P.; Cervantes, A.; et al. Standard chemotherapy with or without bevacizumab for women with newly diagnosed ovarian cancer (ICON7): Overall survival results of a phase 3 randomised trial. *Lancet Oncol.* **2015**, *16*, 928–936. [CrossRef]

67.   Moore, K.N.; Colombo, N.; Scambia, G.; Kim, B.-G.; Oaknin, A.; Friedlander, M.; Lisyanskaya, A.; Floquet, A.; Leary, A.; Sonke, G.S.; et al. Maintenance Olaparib in Patients with Newly Diagnosed Advanced Ovarian Cancer. *N. Eng. J. Med.* **2018**, *379*, 2495–2505. [CrossRef] [PubMed]

68.   Ray-Coquard, I.; Pautier, P.; Pignata, S.; Pérol, D.; González-Martín, A.; Berger, R.; Fujiwara, K.; Vergote, I.; Colombo, N.; Mäenpää, J.; et al. Olaparib plus Bevacizumab as First-Line Maintenance in Ovarian Cancer. *N. Eng. J. Med.* **2019**, *381*, 2416–2428. [CrossRef] [PubMed]

69.   González-Martín, A.; Pothuri, B.; Vergote, I.; Christensen, R.D.; Graybill, W.; Mirza, M.R.; McCormick, C.; Lorusso, D.; Hoskins, P.; Freyer, G.; et al. Niraparib in Patients with Newly Diagnosed Advanced Ovarian Cancer. *N. Engl. J. Med.* **2019**, *381*, 2391–2402. [CrossRef]

70.   Daly, M.B.; Pilarski, R.; Yurgelun, M.B.; Berry, M.P.; Buys, S.S.; Dickson, P.; Domchek, S.M.; Elkhanany, A.; Friedman, S.; Garber, J.E.; et al. NCCN Guidelines Insights: Genetic/Familial High-Risk Assessment: Breast, Ovarian, and Pancreatic, Version 1.2020. *J. Natl. Compr. Cancer Netw.* **2020**, *18*, 380–391. [CrossRef]

71.   Walsh, T.; Casadei, S.; Lee, M.K.; Pennil, C.C.; Nord, A.S.; Thornton, A.M.; Roeb, W.; Agnew, K.J.; Stray, S.M.; Wickramanayake, A.; et al. Mutations in 12 genes for inherited ovarian, fallopian tube, and peritoneal carcinoma identified by massively parallel sequencing. *Proc. Natl. Acad. Sci. USA* **2011**, *108*, 18032–18037. [CrossRef]

72.   Zhang, S.; Royer, R.; Li, S.; McLaughlin, J.R.; Rosen, B.; Risch, H.A.; Fan, I.; Bradley, L.; Shaw, P.A.; Narod, S.A. Frequencies of BRCA1 and BRCA2 mutations among 1,342 unselected patients with invasive ovarian cancer. *Gynecol. Oncol.* **2011**, *121*, 353–357. [CrossRef]

73.   Pal, T.; Permuth-Wey, J.; Betts, J.A.; Krischer, J.P.; Fiorica, J.; Arango, H.; Lapolla, J.; Hoffman, M.; Martino, M.A.; Wakeley, K.; et al. BRCA1 and BRCA2 mutations account for a large proportion of ovarian carcinoma cases. *Cancer* **2005**, *104*, 2807–2816. [CrossRef] [PubMed]

74. Fong, P.C.; Boss, D.S.; Yap, T.A.; Tutt, A.; Wu, P.; Mergui-Roelvink, M.; Mortimer, P.; Swaisland, H.; Lau, A.; O'Connor, M.J.; et al. Inhibition of poly(ADP-ribose) polymerase in tumors from BRCA mutation carriers. *N. Engl. J. Med.* **2009**, *361*, 123–134. [CrossRef] [PubMed]

75. Novetsky, A.; Smith, K.; Babb, S.A.; Jeffe, N.B.; Hagemann, A.R.; Thaker, P.H.; Powell, M.A.; Mutch, D.G.; Massad, L.S.; Zighelboim, I. Timing of referral for genetic counseling and genetic testing in patients with ovarian, fallopian tube, or primary peritoneal carcinoma. *Int. J. Gynecol. Cancer* **2013**, *23*, 1016–1021. [CrossRef] [PubMed]

76. Neviere, Z.; De La Motte Rouge, T.; Floquet, A.; Johnson, A.; Berthet, P.; Joly, F. How and when to refer patients for oncogenetic counseling in the era of PARP inhibitors. *Adv. Med. Oncol.* **2020**, *12*, 1758835919897530. [CrossRef]

77. Stratton, J.F.; Pharoah, P.; Smith, S.K.; Easton, D.; Ponder, B.A. A systematic review and meta-analysis of family history and risk of ovarian cancer. *Br. J. Obstet. Gynaecol.* **1998**, *105*, 493–499. [CrossRef] [PubMed]

78. Jervis, S.; Song, H.; Lee, A.; Dicks, E.; Harrington, P.; Baynes, C.; Manchanda, R.; Easton, U.F.; Jacobs, I.; Pharoah, P.P.D.; et al. A risk prediction algorithm for ovarian cancer incorporating BRCA1, BRCA2, common alleles and other familial effects. *J. Med. Genet.* **2015**, *52*, 465–475. [CrossRef]

79. Lu, K.H.; Wood, M.E.; Daniels, M.S.; Burke, C.; Ford, J.; Kauff, N.D.; Kohlmann, W.; Lindor, N.M.; Mulvey, T.M.; Robinson, L.; et al. American Society of Clinical Oncology Expert Statement: Collection and use of a cancer family history for oncology providers. *J. Clin. Oncol. Off. J. Am. Soc. Clin. Oncol.* **2014**, *32*, 833–840. [CrossRef]

80. Desmond, A.; Kurian, A.W.; Gabree, M.; Mills, M.A.; Anderson, M.J.; Kobayashi, Y.; Horick, N.; Yang, S.; Shannon, K.M.; Tung, N.; et al. Clinical Actionability of Multigene Panel Testing for Hereditary Breast and Ovarian Cancer Risk Assessment. *JAMA Oncol.* **2015**, *1*, 943–951. [CrossRef]

81. Wimmer, K.; Kratz, C.P. Constitutional mismatch repair-deficiency syndrome. *Haematologica* **2010**, *95*, 699–701. [CrossRef]

82. Ford, D.; Easton, D.; Stratton, M.; Narod, S.; Goldgar, D.; Devilee, P.; Bishop, D.T.; Weber, B.; Lenoir, G.; Chang-Claude, J.; et al. Genetic heterogeneity and penetrance analysis of the BRCA1 and BRCA2 genes in breast cancer families. The Breast Cancer Linkage Consortium. *Am. J. Hum. Genet.* **1998**, *62*, 676–689. [CrossRef]

83. Rafnar, T.; Gudbjartsson, D.F.; Sulem, P.; Jonasdottir, A.; Sigurdsson, A.; Jonasdottir, A.; Besenbacher, S.; Lundin, P.; Stacey, S.N.; Gudmundsson, J.; et al. Mutations in BRIP1 confer high risk of ovarian cancer. *Nat. Genet.* **2011**, *43*, 1104–1107. [CrossRef] [PubMed]

84. Vaz, F.; Hanenberg, H.; Schuster, B.; Barker, K.; Wiek, C.; Erven, V.; Neveling, K.; Endt, D.; Kesterton, I.; Autore, F.; et al. Mutation of the RAD51C gene in a Fanconi anemia-like disorder. *Nat. Genet.* **2010**, *42*, 406–409. [CrossRef] [PubMed]

85. Sawyer, S.L.; Tian, L.; Kähkönen, M.; Schwartzentruber, J.; Kircher, M.; Majewski, J.; Dyment, D.A.; Innes, A.M.; Boycott, K.M.; Moreau, L.A.; et al. Biallelic mutations in BRCA1 cause a new Fanconi anemia subtype. *Cancer Discov.* **2015**, *5*, 135–142. [CrossRef] [PubMed]

86. Wagner, J.E.; Tolar, J.; Levran, O.; Scholl, T.; Deffenbaugh, A.; Satagopan, J.; Ben-Porat, L.; Mah, K.; Batish, S.D.; Kutler, D.I.; et al. Germline mutations in BRCA2: Shared genetic susceptibility to breast cancer, early onset leukemia, and Fanconi anemia. *Blood* **2004**, *103*, 3226–3229. [CrossRef] [PubMed]

87. Ngeow, J.; Eng, C. Precision medicine in heritable cancer: When somatic tumour testing and germline mutations meet. *NPJ Genomic Med.* **2016**, *1*, 15006. [CrossRef]

88. Slavin, T.P.; Banks, K.C.; Chudova, D.; Oxnard, G.R.; Odegaard, J.I.; Nagy, R.J.; Tsang, K.W.; Neuhausen, S.L.; Gray, S.W.; Cristofanilli, M.; et al. Identification of Incidental Germline Mutations in Patients With Advanced Solid Tumors Who Underwent Cell-Free Circulating Tumor DNA Sequencing. *J. Clin. Oncol. Off. J. Am. Soc. Clin. Oncol.* **2018**, *36*, JCO1800328.

3D Bioprinted Human Cortical Neural Constructs Derived from Induced Pluripotent Stem Cells

Federico Salaris [1,2], Cristina Colosi [1], Carlo Brighi [1], Alessandro Soloperto [1], Valeria de Turris [1], Maria Cristina Benedetti [2], Silvia Ghirga [1], Maria Rosito [1], Silvia Di Angelantonio [1,3,*] and Alessandro Rosa [1,2,*]

[1]   Center for Life Nano Science, Istituto Italiano di Tecnologia, Viale Regina Elena 291, 00161 Rome, Italy; federico.salaris@uniroma1.it (F.S.); cristinacolosi@gmail.com (C.C.); carlo.brighi@uniroma1.it (C.B.); alessandro.soloperto@iit.it (A.S.); valeria.deturris@iit.it (V.d.T.); silvia.ghirga@uniroma1.it (S.G.); maria.rosito@iit.it (M.R.)

[2]   Department of Biology and Biotechnology Charles Darwin, Sapienza University of Rome, P.le A. Moro 5, 00185 Rome, Italy; benedetti.1690350@studenti.uniroma1.it

[3]   Department of Physiology and Pharmacology, Sapienza University of Rome, P.le A. Moro 5, 00185 Rome, Italy

*   Correspondence: silvia.diangelantonio@uniroma1.it (S.D.A.); alessandro.rosa@uniroma1.it (A.R.)

Abstract: Bioprinting techniques use bioinks made of biocompatible non-living materials and cells to build 3D constructs in a controlled manner and with micrometric resolution. 3D bioprinted structures representative of several human tissues have been recently produced using cells derived by differentiation of induced pluripotent stem cells (iPSCs). Human iPSCs can be differentiated in a wide range of neurons and glia, providing an ideal tool for modeling the human nervous system. Here we report a neural construct generated by 3D bioprinting of cortical neurons and glial precursors derived from human iPSCs. We show that the extrusion-based printing process does not impair cell viability in the short and long term. Bioprinted cells can be further differentiated within the construct and properly express neuronal and astrocytic markers. Functional analysis of 3D bioprinted cells highlights an early stage of maturation and the establishment of early network activity behaviors. This work lays the basis for generating more complex and faithful 3D models of the human nervous systems by bioprinting neural cells derived from iPSCs.

Keywords: 3D bioprinting; biofabrication; 3D cultures; iPSCs; cortical neurons; calcium imaging; patch clamp

1. Introduction

In three-dimensional (3D) bioprinting, cells and biocompatible materials are used as a biological ink (bioink) that can be organized in the 3D space with the goal of generating constructs mimicking organs and tissues. Recent advancements in biofabrication techniques have opened the possibility to apply 3D bioprinting methodologies to human pluripotent stem cells (hPSCs), including embryonic stem cells (ESCs) and induced pluripotent stem cells (iPSCs). The interest in using hPSCs as building blocks in 3D bioprinting comes from their ability to generate ideally any cell type of interest by in vitro differentiation. Laser-assisted [1] and extrusion-based [2] bioprinting are two layer-by-layer deposition methods recently applied to undifferentiated hPSCs [3–6]. Once embedded in a 3D construct, hPSCs maintain their plurilineage potential [3–5] and could be converted by directed differentiation into neural [4], cartilage [6] or cardiac cells [3]. An alternative approach relies on prior differentiation of hPSCs into cell types of interest, which are then printed to generate tissue-like 3D constructs. Examples of liver [7–9], cardiac [9,10], vascular [11], cornea [12] and spinal cord [13,14] cells, all derived from hPSCs by conventional differentiation and subsequently used for bioprinting, have been recently reported. Notably, to the best of our knowledge, cortical neurons and glial cells derived from hPSCs have never been successfully used for bioprinting. Obtaining cells that cannot be isolated from primary human tissues is one of the major purposes of hPSCs, which have been successfully used to generate a wide variety of derivatives of the nervous system, including neuron subtypes of interest for translational or basic science applications [15].

In this work we took advantage of a custom-made extrusion-based bioprinter, implemented with co-axial wet-spinning microfluidic devices [16], to build 3D constructs made of iPSC-derived cortical neurons and glial cells. Optimization of the printing process and bioink composition resulted in high survival of human neural cells. Bioprinting did not impair further differentiation of the cells within the 3D construct. We also report long term maintenance and acquisition of mature functional properties.

2. Experimental Section

2.1. Cell Culture and Differentiation

Generation and maintenance of iPSCs (WT I line) is described in Lenzi et al. (2015) [17]. In brief, cells were cultured in Nutristem-XF (Biological Industries, Cromwell, CT, USA) supplemented with 0.1% Penicillin-Streptomycin (Thermo Fisher Scientific, Waltham, MA, USA) in hESC-qualified Matrigel (CORNING, New York, NY, USA) coated plates. Medium was changed every day and cells were passaged every 4–5 days using 1 mg/mL Dispase (Gibco, Waltham, MA, USA). The cortical neurons differentiation protocol has been adapted and modified from Shi et al. (2012) [18]. iPSCs were treated with Accutase (Thermo Fisher Scientific) promoting single cell dissociation and plated in Matrigel coated dishes in Nutristem-XF supplemented with 10 μM Rock Inhibitor (Enzo Life Sciences, Farmingdale, NY, USA) and 0.1% Penicillin-Streptomycin with a seeding density of 65,000 cells per cm^2. After three days, medium was changed to N2B27 medium (DMEM-F12, Dulbecco's Modified Eagle's Medium/Nutrient Mixture F-12 Ham, Sigma Aldrich; Neurobasal Medium, Gibco; 1X N2 supplement, Thermo Fisher Scientific; 1X Glutamax, Thermo Fisher Scientific; 1X NEAA, Thermo Fisher Scientific; 1X B27, Miltenyi Biotech; 1X Penicillin-Streptomycin) supplemented with SMAD inhibitors, 10 μM SB431542 and 500 nM LDN-193189 (both from Cayman Chemical, Ann Arbor, MI, USA). This was considered day 0 (D0). Medium was changed every day. After 10 days, cells were passaged with 1 mg/mL Dispase and re-plated into poly-L-ornithine/laminin (Sigma Aldrich, St. Louis, MO, USA) coated dishes in N2B27 medium. Starting from day 10, medium was changed every other day. At day 20, cells were dissociated using Accutase and plated into poly-L-ornithine/laminin coated dishes with a seeding density of 65,000 cells per cm^2 in N2B27 medium supplemented with 10 μM Rock Inhibitor for 24 h. Medium was changed twice a week and 2 μM Cyclopamine (Merck, Kenilworth, NJ, USA) was supplemented to N2B27 medium at day 27 for 4 d. Around day 30, cells were dissociated again with Accutase and re-plated into poly-L-ornithine/laminin coated dishes with a seeding density of 65,000 cells/cm^2 in N2B27 medium supplemented with 10 μM Rock Inhibitor for 24 h. From day 40, N2B27 medium was supplemented with 20 ng/mL BDNF (Sigma Aldrich, St. Louis, MO, USA), 20 ng/mL GDNF (Peprotech, London, UK), 200 ng/mL Ascorbic Acid (Sigma Aldrich), 1 mM cyclic AMP (Sigma Aldrich, St. Louis, MO, USA) and 5 μM DAPT (Adipogen Life Sciences, San Diego, CA, USA).

2.2. Preparation of Gel-Adhesive Glass Substrates and Bioink for 3D Bioprinting

Standard microscopy glass slides were functionalized following a published protocol [19] with minor changes. Briefly, standard glass slides were exposed to air plasma (3 min, 27 W, 600 mTorr) and quickly soaked in a 5% v/v solution of 3-aminopropyl triethoxysilane (Aptes, Sigma Aldrich, St. Louis, MO, USA) in deionized water for 2 h, washed with deionized water and ethanol and then air dried. Afterwards, slides were soaked in 0.2 M solution of 4-morpholineethanesulfonic acid (MES, PH4.5,

Sigma Aldrich, St. Louis, MO, USA) containing 1% w/v alginate (Fmc Biopolymers, Philadelphia, PA, USA), EDC (0.4% w/v; Sigma Aldrich, St. Louis, MO, USA) and NHS (0.3% w/v; Sigma Aldrich, St. Louis, MO, USA) overnight at room temperature. Finally, slides were washed with water and ethanol, air dried, cut into 5 mm × 5 mm squares using a glass cutting pen, UV-sterilized and stored for later use. Alginate solution was prepared by dissolving alginate powder (GP1740, Fmc Biopolymers, Philadelphia, PA, USA) in 25 mM HEPES buffered saline (HBS). A stock solution of alginate was prepared at a concentration of 4% w/v, sterile-filtered, divided in working aliquots and stored at +4 °C for later use. The day of the bioprinting experiment, Matrigel precursor solution was thawed in ice for 2 h and mixed with alginate stock solution at a ratio of 1:1 v/v. Typically, 300 µL of Matrigel/alginate mixture was prepared for each experiment. All solutions were manipulated and kept in ice baths. Differentiating cells were collected from cell culture plates by single cell dissociation mediated by Accutase treatment. Cells were resuspended in the Matrigel/alginate mixture at a 1:1 ratio to obtain the bioink with 2% alginate as final concentration.

2.3. 3D Cell Printing and Post-Processing of Printed Samples

The bioink was loaded in a reservoir consisting of a micro-tube coil of known internal volume, as schematized in Figure 1A. The reservoir was placed in a poly(methyl methacrylate) cylindrical tank (3 cm radius, 15 cm height) covered with a thermal isolating tape (Armaflex L414, Armacell, Munster, DE) and filled with ice in order to prevent the gelation of Matrigel in the reservoir. The total dimension of the system, shown in Figure S1, was rationalized in order to limit the encumbrance of the extruder while ensuring the maintenance of a temperature around 0 °C for the total duration of the printing step (~1 h). The reservoir was connected with the internal needle of a coaxial wet-spinning extruder, while the outer needle was fed with a calcium chloride solution (225 mM $CaCl_2$ in HBS). Two independent microfluidic pumps (Cetoni, Korbussen, DE) controlled the flow of the bioink (5 µL/min) and the crosslinking solution (3.5 µL/min) through the coaxial extruder. The extruder and the ice-bath tank were mounted on a three-axis motorized system (PI-miCos, Eschbach, DE) with a computer-numerical-control (CNC) interface (Twintec, Auburn, WA, USA). Printing instructions were expressed in g-code language, and printing codes were generated using a custom MATLAB algorithm. The geometry described in these codes consisted of two alternating perpendicular layers of microfibers with theoretical diameter of 100 µm, separated by gaps of 200 µm, a layer thickness of 100 µm, deposited at a speed of 240 mm/min, forming a squared fiber mesh of 5 mm × 5 mm × 200 µm. Typically, printing time for generated codes was around 40–50 s, and each sample was constituted of 3 to 5 µL of solution depending on the desired dimension of the construct. Printed samples were collected, washed with sterile saline solution and placed in cell culture incubator for 10 min to trigger the gelation process of Matrigel. Samples were then transferred in 12-well cell culture plates, soaked with cell culture media and incubated for additional 2 h to terminate Matrigel gelation. Afterwards, samples were exposed to alginate-lyase enzyme (Sigma Aldrich, 0.2 µg/mL in cell culture media) overnight, washed with fresh media and maintained in culture for characterization and maturation.

2.4. RNA Analysis

Total RNA was extracted with the Quick RNA MiniPrep (Zymo Research, Freiburg, DE) and retrotranscribed with iScript Reverse Transcription Supermix for RT-qPCR (Bio-Rad, Hercules, CA, USA). Targets were analyzed by PCR with the enzyme MyTaq DNA Polymerase (Bioline, Boston, MA, USA). Thirty cycles of amplification were used for PAX6 and GAPDH, while FOXG1, TBR1, TBR2 and GFAP were amplified for 34 reaction cycles. The internal control used was the housekeeping gene GAPDH. Primer sequences are reported in Table S1.

2.5. Live/Dead Cell Analysis

Cell viability was assessed with the LIVE/DEAD Viability/Cytotoxicity Kit (Thermo Fisher Scientific), which uses green-fluorescent calcein AM and red-fluorescent ethidium homodimer-1 to identify live and dead cells, respectively, according to the manufacturer's instructions. Briefly, bioprinted constructs were incubated with calcein-AM and ethidium homodimer-1 at 37 °C for 30 min, followed by a PBS wash, and a further media change before acquisition. Image acquisition was performed with a custom fluorescent integrated system (Crisel Instruments, Rome, IT) based on an IX73 Olympus inverted microscope equipped with the x-light spinning disk module (Crestoptics, Rome, IT) for confocal acquisition, Lumencor Spectra X LED illumination and a CoolSNAP MYO CCD camera (Photometrics, Tucson, AZ, USA). The widefield images were acquired using Metamorph software version 7.10.2 (Molecular Device, San Jose, CA, USA) with 10×, 20× and 40× air objectives. The construct was sectioned in z with a step size of 5 μm to obtain at least five optical planes per construct to capture the whole structure. For the live/dead cells quantification, the entire image stacks were analyzed in 3D and cells were counted using Spots in Imaris 8.1.2 (Bitplane, Belfast, UK); nine fields were analyzed for each time point. Percentage of viability is reported as the mean value ± standard deviation of the mean, from three independent bioprinted constructs at DPP1 and DPP7 and one bioprinted construct at DPP50.

2.6. Immunostaining

Cells were fixed in 4% paraformaldehyde for 15 min at room temperature and washed twice with PBS. Fixed cells were then permeabilized with PBS containing 0.2% Triton X-100 for 10 min at room temperature and incubated overnight with primary antibodies at 4 °C. The primary antibodies used were anti-PAX6 (1:50, sc-81649, Santa Cruz Biotechnology, Dallas, TX, USA), anti-NCAD (1:100, ab18203, Abcam, Cambridge, UK), anti-TUJ1 (1:1000, T2200, Sigma-Aldrich), anti-MAP2 (1:2000, ab5392, Abcam), anti-NeuN (1:50, MAB377, Merck Millipore), anti-GFAP (1:500, MAB360, Merck Millipore) and anti-TBR1 (1:150, 20932-1-AP, Proteintech, Rosemont, IL, USA). The secondary antibodies used were goat anti-mouse Alexa Fluor 488 (1:250, Immunological Sciences, Rome, IT), goat anti-chicken Alexa Fluor 488 (1:500, Thermo Fisher Scientific), goat anti-rabbit Alexa Fluor 488 (1:250, Immunological Sciences), goat anti-mouse Alexa Fluor 594 (1:500, Thermo Fisher Scientific), goat anti-rabbit Alexa Fluor 594 (1:500, Thermo Fisher Scientific) and goat anti-rabbit Alexa Fluor 647 (1:500, Thermo Fisher Scientific). DAPI (Sigma-Aldrich) was used to label nuclei.

2.7. Microscopy Imaging

Confocal images of panels 1D, 2D and 2D' were acquired at the Olympus iX83 FluoView1200 laser scanning confocal microscope using an air 10× NA0.4 or a silicon oil 30× NA1.05 objective (Olympus, Shinjuku, JP) and 405, 473, 559 and 635 nm lasers. Filter setting for DAPI, Alexa Fluor 488, Alexa Fluor 594 and Alexa Fluor 647 were used when needed. Each stack consisted of individual images with a z-step of 0.5, 5 and 1 μm respectively. Stack images of 1024 × 1024 pixels were stitched together in a mosaic view with the Multi Area Viewer tool of Fluoview 4.2 image software (Olympus). The 3D rendering shown was performed using the Imaris image analysis software v.8.1.2 (Bitplane). Widefield images of panels 2C were acquired with the same system described above with a 20× air objective.

2.8. Patch Clamp Recordings

Whole-cell patch-clamp recordings were used for the functional characterization of 3D bioprinted constructs. Cells in the 3D bioprinted structures were visualized with a BX51WI microscope (OLYMPUS), in a recording chamber continuously perfused with an external solution containing 140 mM NaCl, 2.8 mM KCl, 2 mM $CaCl_2$, 2 mM $MgCl_2$, 10 mM HEPES and 10 mM D-glucose (pH 7.3 with NaOH; 290 mOsm) at room temperature. Borosilicate pipettes were filled with a solution containing 140 mM K-gluconate, 5 mM BAPTA, 2 mM $MgCl_2$, 10 mM HEPES, 2 mM Mg-ATP and 0.3 mM Na-GTP (pH 7.3 with KOH; 280 mOsm). Voltage- and current-clamp recordings were performed using Axon DigiData 1550 (MOLECULAR DEVICES). Signals were filtered at 10 KHz, digitized (25 kHz) and collected using Clampex 10 (MOLECULAR DEVICES). Whole-cell capacitance (Cm), cell membrane resistance (Rm) and resting membrane potential (RMP) were measured on-line by Clampex. Cells were clamped at −70 and 0 mV to measure spontaneous activity. An on-line P4 leak subtraction protocol was used for all recordings of voltage-activated currents. Voltage steps (50 ms duration) from −80 to +40 mV (10 mV increment; holding potential −70 mV) were applied to study voltage-activated sodium currents. Voltage-activated potassium currents were evoked by voltage steps (50 ms duration) from −80 to +40 mV (10 mV increment; holding potential −70 mV). Firing properties were investigated in current-clamp mode, injecting current pulses (1 s duration) of increasing amplitude (from 10 to 80 pA; 10 pA increment), after imposing a membrane potential of −70 mV to each cell (injection of −79 ± 20 pA). Data were analyzed off-line with Clampfit 10 and Origin 7 software.

2.9. Calcium Imaging Recordings

Fluorescence images were acquired at room temperature using a customized digital imaging microscope. Between 5–8 field of views (FOVs) per bioprinted construct were recorded in each experiment session. Excitation of calcium dye was achieved using a 1-nm-bandwidth monocromator (Cairn Optoscan, Faversham, UK) equipped with a 150 W xenon lamp. Fluorescence was visualized using the upright microscope Olympus BX51WI equipped with a 40× water immersion objective and a CoolSnap Myo camera. Image acquisition and processing were obtained using MetaFluor software (Molecular Devices). Changes in the intracellular Ca^{2+} level were monitored using the high-affinity Ca^{2+}-sensitive indicator Fluo4-AM (Invitrogen). 3D bioprinted constructs were loaded by incubating for 30 min at 37 °C in external solution containing the following: 140 mM NaCl, 2.8 mM KCl, 2 mM $CaCl_2$, 2 mM $MgCl_2$, 10 mM HEPES, 10 mM D-glucose (pH 7.3 with NaOH; 290 mOsm) plus 5 μM Fluo4-AM. A custom-made MATLAB guided user interface (GUI) was used to perform calcium imaging data analysis. Fluorescence data collected as a series of images were converted to three-dimensional MATLAB files and the neurons were manually selected from the time-averaged fluorescence recording before running the trace extraction and analysis. Tens of neurons were identified for each field scanned, depending on the confluence and seeding density of the cultures. The calcium traces were acquired with a sampling frequency of 2 Hz and signals were normalized as a function of $\Delta F/F_0 = (F − F_0)/F_0$, where F is the current fluorescence intensity at any time point and F_0 is the basal fluorescence intensity. Single calcium events were detected on the basis of a previously published method [20]. Threshold for peak amplitude, initially set to 3% of the baseline value, was manually adjustable to improve the detection depending on the recording conditions (signal-to-noise ratio, acquisition rate, etc.). Results were visualized, and eventual false or missing detections were manually corrected. Raster plots were created to visualize asynchronous (appearing as sparse vertical lines) and synchronous (appearing as a series of vertically aligned lines) results and the linear dependence between each pair of neurons was calculated by means of Pearson correlation coefficient from binary traces. Neuron firing rate, amplitude of the events and synchrony of the network (evaluated as the relative number of simultaneous events) were exported in Microsoft Excel to perform statistics. Statistical analysis was performed in GraphPad Prism 7 or OriginPro 6.0.

3. Results

3.1. 3D Bioprinting of Differentiating Human iPSC-Derived Neurons and Glia

An outline of the 3D bioprinting method developed in this work is shown in Figure 1A. We used a customized extrusion bioprinter developed in-house (Figure S1). This platform consists of a custom extrusion 3D bioprinter integrating a microfluidic printing head constituted of two independent needles arranged in a coaxial configuration. The deposition strategy is based on the use of calcium-alginate gel as templating agent for the printing of blended extracellular matrices and cells. This provides a precise control on the relative position of cells within the 3D construct, down to the micrometer scale with high reproducibility [16], independently on the 3D embedding matrix of election. Reportedly, bioink composition is crucial to ensure long-term iPSCs viability and maintenance of 3D structures [3,6]. Pilot experiments revealed that Matrigel is the best candidate for in vitro differentiation of neuronal cells in 3D, when compared with transglutaminase/gelatin or photo-crosslinked gelatin methacryloyl gels. For

3D printing experiments, different ratios of Matrigel/alginate and post-printing treatments have been tested. We obtained the best results using a solution containing 2% w/v alginate and 0.5× Matrigel (~50% dilution from stock), printed using 0.33 mM $CaCl_2$ crosslinking solution, and subsequently exposing the printed construct to alginate-lyase enzyme at a concentration of 0.2 μg/mL in cell culture media for 12 h, starting the exposure 3 h after the printing protocol.

The cellular components of the bioink, neuronal and glial precursors, were derived by differentiation of human iPSCs by a multistep protocol in conventional bidimensional (2D) culture conditions (Figure 1B). Efficient induction of a neural cortical fate was obtained by initial dual SMAD inhibition and subsequent block of Hedgehog signaling with cyclopamine [16]. Representative images of differentiating cells are shown in Figure S2. During this standard differentiation process, human iPSCs exited from pluripotency (loss of *NANOG* expression) and gradually acquired a neural character, as shown by the progressive expression of neural progenitor cells (NPCs; *PAX6, NCAD*), neuronal precursors (*TBR2, FOXG1*) and neurons (*TBR1, TUJ1, NeuN, MAP2*) markers (Figure S2A). Further characterization by immunostaining analysis showed progressive acquisition of a neuronal morphology and expression of neurofilament proteins (Figure S2B,C). The astrocyte marker *GFAP* was also expressed at late time points (Figure S2B,C).

3.2. Characterization of 3D Bioprinted Neural Constructs

Neural cells differentiated for about 4 weeks were dissociated, resuspended in the Matrigel/alginate solution and printed. We have performed several experiments in which cells were dissociated in the window of time between day 25 and day 35 of differentiation (indicated in red in the diagram of Figure 1B). During the printing process, the bioink and the crosslinking solution met at the ending tip of the coaxial extruder. Here, Ca^{2+} ions triggered the gelation of alginate in the bioink. This gel adhered to the functionalized glass substrate so that, by moving the extruder, a micrometric cell-embedding gel fiber was spun out and deposited in pre-determined positions. In this work we printed the cells as a reticulum (Figure 1C; Movies S1 and S2). Such architecture was chosen as it allows optimal perfusion of culture medium, which can reach all the cells in the construct. Moreover, areas with lower and higher cell densities are formed along the fibers and at the crossing points, respectively, providing useful information on the behavior of the cells in the 3D construct under different density conditions. Alginate removal by enzymatic treatment 3 h after the printing process promoted the acquisition of neuronal morphology by the first day post printing (Figure S3). Notably, such mild enzymatic treatment did not affect the shape of the printed construct, which was stabilized by Matrigel polymerization. Immunostaining of neurofilaments showed that the structure of the reticulum was maintained over time and that neuronal cells projected their axons and dendrites both within and across the fibers (Figure 1D). Printed cells were then analyzed in terms of viability at different days post printing (DPP). Results shown in Figure 1E indicated that the great majority of the cells were viable at DPP1 (78 ± 3.8% live cells; average ± standard deviation; three constructs, nine fields each) and DPP7 (71 ± 3.5% live cells; average ± standard deviation; three constructs, nine fields each), suggesting that both physical parameters and bioink formulation did not harm neural cells during and immediately after the printing process. Moreover, viability was consistently maintained over time as assessed by live/dead staining up to DPP50 (68 ± 8% live cells; average ± standard deviation; one construct, nine fields). We noticed that the reticulum structure was to some extent maintained at this late time point.

We then assessed possible alterations in neuronal cell fate acquisition caused by either the printing process and/or subsequent cell differentiation within the 3D bioprinted construct. Bioprinted cells were compared with cells maintained in conventional 2D conditions for the same time and cells that were encapsulated in bioink droplets not subjected to printing process (3D bulk). Neuronal morphology was maintained intact in both 3D bulk and 3D bioprinted cells at DPP7 and DPP40 (Figure 2A). In the same samples, marker analysis by RT-PCR showed proper expression of: *PAX6, FOXG1* and *TBR2* as neuronal progenitor markers; *TBR1*, which reveals the presence of mature cortical neurons; and *GFAP*, a common astrocyte marker (Figure 2B and Figure S4). These results were further supported by immunostaining analyses of TBR1 and MAP2 at DPP7 (Figure 2C). Bioprinted neural cells were maintained in neuronal differentiation medium up to DPP70. At this late time point the reticulum structure was, to some extent, maintained and cells properly expressed neuronal and astroglial markers (Figure 2D,D').

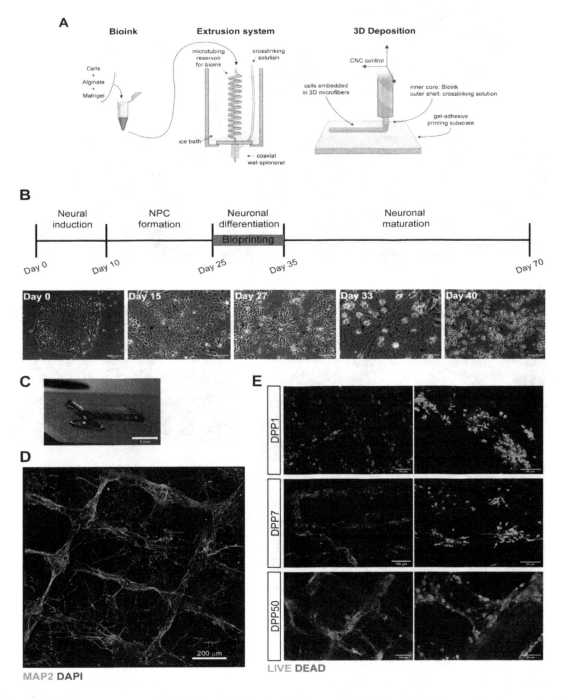

Figure 1. 3D bioprinting method and analysis of viability post printing. (**A**) Schematic representation of the outline of the bioprinting method. (**B**) Outline of the human induced pluripotent stem cell (iPSC) neural differentiation protocol in conventional 2D culture and representative images of differentiating cells in these conditions at the indicated time points. The window of time in which cells have been dissociated for bioprinting experiments in this work is indicated in red. (**C**) Image of the printed 3D construct. Scalebar: 2 mm. (**D**) Mosaic reconstruction of confocal images of bioprinted neural cells at DPP7, stained with a MAP2 antibody (green) and DAPI (blue). Scalebar: 200 μm. (**E**) Live (green) and dead (red) cell staining in the bioprinted construct at the indicated days post printing (DPP). Scalebar: 150 μm (left panels); 50 μm (right panels).

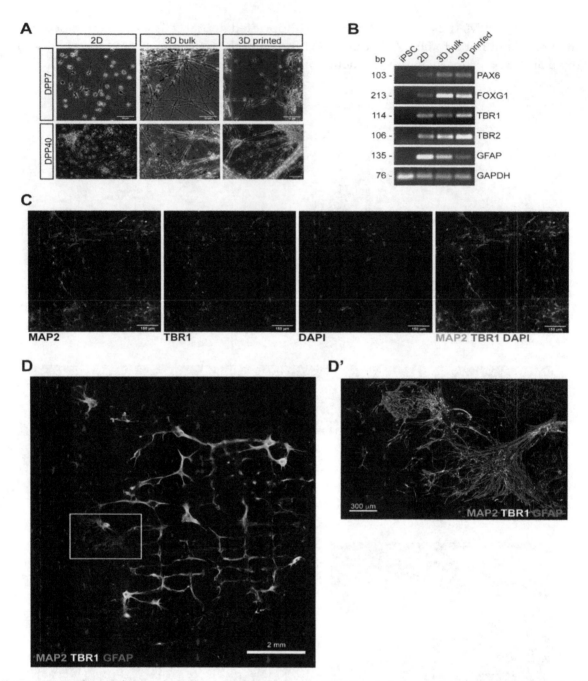

Figure 2. Analysis of neural marker expression in the 3D bioprinted construct. (**A**) Phase contrast images of cells within the 3D bioprinted construct ("3D printed" panels), at the indicated days post printing, and cells in conventional monolayer conditions ("2D" panels) or resuspended in the bioink ("3D bulk" panels) and maintained for the same time of differentiation. (**B**) RT-PCR analysis of neuronal progenitor markers (*PAX6, FOXG1, TBR2*), a cortical neuron marker (*TBR1*) and an astrocyte marker (*GFAP*). GAPDH was used as a housekeeping control. (**C**) Immunostaining analysis of bioprinted cells at DPP7. MAP2 (green), TBR1 (red) and DAPI (blue) signals are shown. Scalebar: 150 μm. (**D**) Mosaic reconstruction of confocal images of bioprinted neural cells at DPP70, showing the entire sample, stained with MAP2 (green), TBR1 (white) and GFAP (red) antibodies. Scalebar: 2 mm. (**D′**) Mosaic reconstruction of confocal images of the region inside the white box in panel D, acquired at higher resolution. Scalebar: 300 μm.

Collectively, these results demonstrate that iPSC-derived cortical neuronal cells can be bioprinted and further cultured in 3D constructs without causing major survival and differentiation issues.

3.3. Functional Analysis

Single-cell patch-clamp and time-lapse calcium imaging recordings were then performed to assess the degree of maturation achieved by the 3D bioprinted construct. Even though the 3D construct was 300 μm thick, the selected bioink displayed sufficient transparency to visible light and softness to patch pipette insertion (Figure 3A). Using patch clamp recordings, we investigated the expression of the passive and active membrane properties on 3D bioprinted cortical neurons at day 7 after printing. As expected at this experimental point, resting membrane potential (-17.7 ± 1.5 mV; $n = 36$), cell capacitance (14.8 ± 0.89 pF; $n = 45$) and membrane resistance values (1.97 ± 0.23 MΩ; $n = 44$) were typical of neuronal progenitors [21] and similar to those observed in parallel 2D cultures (Figure S5), indicating that the printing process did not impair neuronal viability. We then characterized the ability of cortical neurons to generate action potentials. Neurons in the 3D construct displayed large inward voltage-dependent Na^+ currents (-777.31 ± 73.16 pA at 0 mV; $n = 43$; Figure 3B,C and Figure S5) which activated near -40 mV and peaked at 0 mV, and voltage-dependent K+ currents (865.75 ± 63.28 pA at $+40$ mV; $n = 43$; Figure 3B,D and Figure S5). Current pulses were able to induce action potentials in almost all tested cells. The mean threshold for first action potential generation was -32.85 ± 2.86 mV ($n = 15$; 20 pA of current injection). However, the minimum current required to elicit firing in some of the tested cells was 10 pA (Figure 3E,F). As expected, no synaptic activity was recorded at 7 days post printing (data not shown).

Given the optical transparency of the 3D bioprinted constructs at DPP7, fluorescence time-lapse recordings lasting 5 min each were performed, thus preserving a good signal-to-noise ratio (Figure 3G). Fluorescence time-lapse analysis of spontaneous calcium oscillation in Fluo4-AM loaded 3D neuronal network indicated the presence of individual calcium activity (mean firing frequency = 0.015 ± 0.001 Hz; FOVs = 38; mean firing amplitude = 0.083 ± 0.002 A.U.) with little synchronized firing (syncro index = 0.223 ± 0.020; FOVs = 38). The small degree of synchronous activity was confirmed by the low correlation coefficient value between each pair of neurons in the field as displayed by the heatmap in Figure 3G (average correlation coefficient value = 0.006; max correlation coefficient value = 0.046 ± 0.005; FOV = 38), thus indicating the establishment of early and immature neuronal networks.

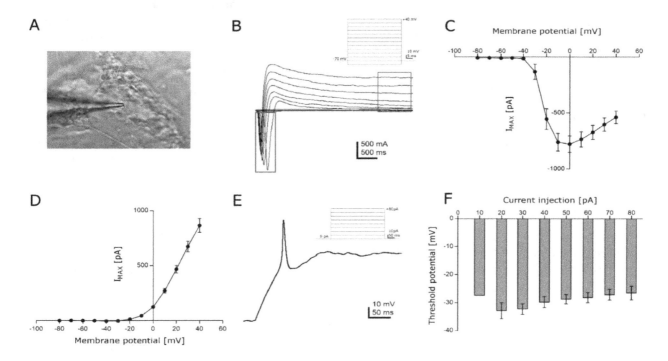

Figure 3. *Cont.*

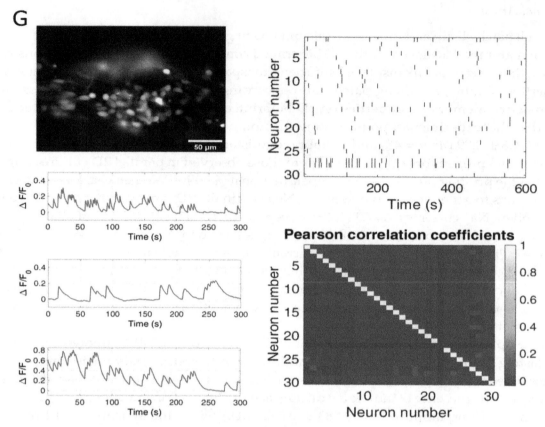

Figure 3. Functional analysis of the 3D bioprinted construct. (**A**) Single-cell patch-clamp recording of an iPSC-derived neuronal cell encapsulated in the 3D bioprinted construct at DPP7. (**B**) Representative scheme of the recording protocol is shown. The inward sodium currents are highlighted in the purple box and the permanent outward potassium currents are highlighted in the green box. (**C**) Average trace of the large inward voltage-dependent Na^+ currents. (**D**) Average trace of the outward voltage-dependent K^+ currents. (**E**) A single action potential evoked in current clamp recording is shown. The minimum current required to elicit firing was 10 pA, however more of the 50% of tested cells ($n = 9$ out of 15) responded to 20 pA (**F**). (**G**) Calcium traces as a function of $\Delta F/F_0$ of cortical neurons isolated within the 3D network shown on the left at DPP7. On the right, a representation of the firing pattern and a relative heatmap of the Pearson correlation coefficients within the cells of the same network are shown.

4. Discussion

In this paper we describe a method to obtain 3D cortical constructs in which human cortical neurons and glial cells survive in the long term, holding their cellular characteristics and functional properties. Moving from conventional neuronal cultures, in 2D, to more realistic 3D models is considered a crucial advancement in neurobiology [22]. The recent discovery that differentiating hPSCs have the ability to self-assemble into brain organoids, which recapitulate to some extent the brain structure in 3D [23], has given a twist in the way neurodevelopmental and neurodegenerative diseases are modeled and approached [24]. 3D bioprinting could provide important advantages, in terms of automation and reproducibility, over self-assembled brain organoids [25]. Recent reports showed that undifferentiated human iPSCs and ESCs can be bioprinted and then converted, post-printing, into cell types of interest [4]. This approach will not likely generate useful artificial tissues, as it does not allow control on the position of individual cell types, generated during differentiation, within the construct. The complementary approach, used in this work and in [13,14], and consisting in bioprinting specific cell types obtained by pre-printing hPSCs differentiation, would be more advantageous, allowing better control of the resulting bioprinted construct.

Bioprinting neurons and glial cells represents a challenge. Neurons are vulnerable cells in vitro and environmental stress due to the printing process may affect neural cell viability and influence further differentiation and maturation. Our work is the result of an extensive effort in the optimization of the bioprinting process and bioink composition, with the goal to define proper conditions for generating human artificial 3D cortical neural tissues from hiPSCs. The generation of a bioprinted constructs, by combining hiPSC-derived spinal neuronal progenitor cells and mouse oligodendrocyte progenitor cells, has been recently reported by Joung et al. [13]. Moreover, spinal cord neural progenitors from hiPSCs have been successfully bioprinted by using a commercial lab-on-a-printer platform [14,26]. Here, for the first time, we describe the generation of constructs made of cortical neurons and glial cells by a custom extrusion bioprinter. In this work, we have obtained the best results with a bioink made of Matrigel and alginate. The selection of the bioink most suitable for the viability of the 3D construct remains a controversial issue. Indeed, both fibrin-based and Matrigel-based bioinks have been previously used for bioprinting hiPSC-derived spinal neural cells [13,14]. Matrigel, which is a matrix preparation extracted from the Engelbreth-Holm-Swarm mouse sarcoma, had been successfully used as a bioink component for the generation of hiPSC-derived cardiac and spinal cord bioprinted constructs [3,13]. However, its composition is rather undefined. This could represent an important limitation for basic and translational applications of bioprinted models, including those of the nervous system. Future studies are necessary for identifying more physiological, standardized and defined alternatives to Matrigel. To this direction, promising results have been recently obtained with decellularized extracellular matrix, used for the bioprinting of liver and hearth constructs [9].

Due to the vulnerability of neurons, their viability post printing is a major concern. In this regard, our results (70–80% of live cells) are comparable to previous works using hiPSC-derived neural progenitors [13,14] or an immortalized human neural stem cell line [27]. Moreover, our method allows long term survival of human neurons, up to 70 days post printing. To the best of our knowledge, this is the longest time of maintenance of hiPSC-derived neurons in 3D bioprinted constructs (14 days in [13], 30 days in [14], 40 days in [4] and 41 days in [26]). Further, this work suggests a possible approach to overcome some practical challenges associated with the bioprinting of 3D in vitro models containing cells of limited availability. In order to be able to produce constructs with arbitrary, high cellular density, without affecting the number of samples obtainable from each experiment, we adjusted the amount of bioink necessary for each construct to a few microliters (3 to 5 µL per sample). The dimension, visibility and weight of these samples are very limited, and their handling and maintenance in floating culture condition can be very challenging. To overcome this, we used functionalized micro-slides as receiving substrate during the printing step that guaranteed a prolonged adhesion of the samples to a flat, clear glass surface.

We here report that cortical 3D bioprinted constructs, as well as parallel 2D cultures, display functional properties typical of immature neuronal networks. Indeed, calcium imaging experiments showed sustained calcium spontaneous activity already at DPP7, in line with that reported for 3D bioprinted iPSCs [4,27], and spinal neural progenitors [13], thus suggesting that the printing process does not prevent the development of a functional network. However, passive and active neuronal properties, analyzed at single cell level by means of patch clamp recordings, were typical of immature neurons, and the absence of spontaneous synaptic activity indicated that network activity was mainly not dependent on action potential firing. This result is in line with data on 2D culture at the same time point.

This study opens the possibility for generating more complex human neural 3D constructs, for instance by printing mixed populations with precise ratios of neuronal and glial cells and/or printing iPSCs carrying pathogenic mutations associated to neurological diseases. Notably, the bioprinting approach used herein can be further implemented with more sophisticated microfluidic platforms that might allow the deposition of multiple materials and/or multicellular bioink within a single scaffold, by simultaneously extruding different bioinks or by rapidly switching between one bioink and another, as previously described [16], with the aim of controlling the localization of individual cell types in predetermined positions of the 3D construct. Different specific neuronal subtypes, which can be obtained by iPSC differentiation, might be used as the cellular components of 3D constructs for disease models and drug screening. In the case of complex diseases with clear non-cell autonomous contribution, neural and non-neural cells could be printed together. In the long term, further development of this technology could provide bioprinted cortical neural constructs that can be exploited as customized, standardized and scalable pre-clinical models for drug safety and toxicity studies.

5. Conclusions

In this paper we report the generation of a novel type of bioprinted 3D neuronal construct, based on cortical neurons and glial cells derived from hiPSCs. The cortical construct develops molecular, morphological and functional properties of neuronal networks and can be used for future disease modeling studies as well as for drug screening.

Author Contributions: Conceptualization, F.S., C.C., S.D.A. and A.R.; Formal analysis, A.S., V.d.T., S.G. and M.R.; Investigation, F.S., C.C., C.B., A.S., V.d.T. and M.C.B.; Methodology, F.S., C.C. and C.B.; Project administration, S.D.A. and A.R.; Supervision, S.D.A. and A.R.; Writing – original draft, S.D.A. and A.R.

Acknowledgments: The authors wish to thank the Imaging Facility at Center for Life Nano Science (CLNS), Istituto Italiano di Tecnologia, for support and technical advice. We are grateful to Giorgia Belloni for technical help in the qRT-PCR experiments of Figure S2 and Chiara Scognamiglio for advice on 3D bioprinting. We thank Giancarlo Ruocco and the other colleagues of CLNS for helpful discussion.

References

1. Koch, L.; Gruene, M.; Unger, C.; Chichkov, B. Laser assisted cell printing. *Curr. Pharm. Biotechnol.* **2013**, *14*, 91–97. [PubMed]
2. Jiang, T.; Munguia-Lopez, J.G.; Flores-Torres, S.; Kort-Mascort, J.; Kinsella, J.M. Extrusion bioprinting of soft materials: An emerging technique for biological model fabrication. *Appl. Phys. Rev.* **2019**, *6*, 011310. [CrossRef]
3. Koch, L.; Deiwick, A.; Franke, A.; Schwanke, K.; Haverich, A.; Zweigerdt, R.; Chichkov, B. Laser bioprinting of human induced pluripotent stem cells-the effect of printing and biomaterials on cell survival, pluripotency, and differentiation. *Biofabrication* **2018**, *10*, 035005. [CrossRef] [PubMed]
4. Gu, Q.; Tomaskovic-Crook, E.; Wallace, G.G.; Crook, J.M. 3D Bioprinting Human Induced Pluripotent Stem Cell Constructs for In Situ Cell Proliferation and Successive Multilineage Differentiation. *Adv. Healthc. Mater.* **2017**, *6*. [CrossRef]
5. Reid, J.A.; Mollica, P.A.; Johnson, G.D.; Ogle, R.C.; Bruno, R.D.; Sachs, P.C. Accessible bioprinting: Adaptation of a low-cost 3D-printer for precise cell placement and stem cell differentiation. *Biofabrication* **2016**, *8*, 025017. [CrossRef] [PubMed]
6. Nguyen, D.; Hägg, D.A.; Forsman, A.; Ekholm, J.; Nimkingratana, P.; Brantsing, C.; Kalogeropoulos, T.; Zaunz, S.; Concaro, S.; Brittberg, M.; et al. Cartilage Tissue Engineering by the 3D Bioprinting of iPS Cells in a Nanocellulose/Alginate Bioink. *Sci Rep.* **2017**, *7*, 658. [CrossRef]
7. Faulkner-Jones, A.; Fyfe, C.; Cornelissen, D.-J.; Gardner, J.; King, J.; Courtney, A.; Shu, W. Bioprinting of human pluripotent stem cells and their directed differentiation into hepatocyte-like cells for the generation of mini-livers in 3D. *Biofabrication* **2015**, *7*, 044102. [CrossRef]
8. Ma, X.; Qu, X.; Zhu, W.; Li, Y.-S.; Yuan, S.; Zhang, H.; Liu, J.; Wang, P.; Lai, C.S.E.; Zanella, F.; et al. Deterministically patterned biomimetic human iPSC-derived hepatic model via rapid 3D bioprinting. *Proc. Natl. Acad. Sci. USA* **2016**, *113*, 2206–2211. [CrossRef]
9. Yu, C.; Ma, X.; Zhu, W.; Wang, P.; Miller, K.L.; Stupin, J.; Koroleva-Maharajh, A.; Hairabedian, A.; Chen, S. Scanningless and continuous 3D bioprinting of human tissues with decellularized extracellular matrix. *Biomaterials* **2019**, *194*, 1–13. [CrossRef]
10. Ong, C.S.; Fukunishi, T.; Zhang, H.; Huang, C.Y.; Nashed, A.; Blazeski, A.; Di Silvestre, D.; Vricella, L.; Conte, J.; Tung, L.; et al. Biomaterial-Free Three-Dimensional Bioprinting of Cardiac Tissue using Human Induced Pluripotent Stem Cell Derived Cardiomyocytes. *Sci. Rep.* **2017**, *7*, 4566. [CrossRef]

11. Moldovan, L.; Barnard, A.; Gil, C.-H.; Lin, Y.; Grant, M.B.; Yoder, M.C.; Prasain, N.; Moldovan, N.I. iPSC-Derived Vascular Cell Spheroids as Building Blocks for Scaffold-Free Biofabrication. *Biotechnol. J.* **2017**, *12*. [CrossRef] [PubMed]

12. Sorkio, A.; Koch, L.; Koivusalo, L.; Deiwick, A.; Miettinen, S.; Chichkov, B.; Skottman, H. Human stem cell based corneal tissue mimicking structures using laser-assisted 3D bioprinting and functional bioinks. *Biomaterials* **2018**, *171*, 57–71. [CrossRef] [PubMed]

13. Joung, D.; Truong, V.; Neitzke, C.C.; Guo, S.-Z.; Walsh, P.J.; Monat, J.R.; Meng, F.; Park, S.H.; Dutton, J.R.; Parr, A.M.; et al. 3D Printed Stem-Cell Derived Neural Progenitors Generate Spinal Cord Scaffolds. *Adv. Funct. Mater.* **2018**, *28*, 1801850. [CrossRef]

14. De la Vega, L.; Rosas Gómez, A.D.; Abelseth, E.; Abelseth, L.; Allisson da Silva, V.; Willerth, S. 3D Bioprinting Human Induced Pluripotent Stem Cell-Derived Neural Tissues Using a Novel Lab-on-a-Printer Technology. *Appl. Sci.* **2018**, *8*, 2414. [CrossRef]

15. Bellin, M.; Marchetto, M.C.; Gage, F.H.; Mummery, C.L. Induced pluripotent stem cells: The new patient? *Nat. Rev. Mol. Cell Biol.* **2012**, *13*, 713–726. [CrossRef]

16. Colosi, C.; Costantini, M.; Barbetta, A.; Dentini, M. Microfluidic Bioprinting of Heterogeneous 3D Tissue Constructs. *Methods Mol. Biol.* **2017**, *1612*, 369–380.

17. Lenzi, J.; De Santis, R.; de Turris, V.; Morlando, M.; Laneve, P.; Calvo, A.; Caliendo, V.; Chiò, A.; Rosa, A.; Bozzoni, I. ALS mutant FUS proteins are recruited into stress granules in induced Pluripotent Stem Cells (iPSCs) derived motoneurons. *Dis. Model. Mech.* **2015**, *8*, 755–766. [CrossRef]

18. Shi, Y.; Kirwan, P.; Livesey, F.J. Directed differentiation of human pluripotent stem cells to cerebral cortex neurons and neural networks. *Nat. Protoc.* **2012**, *7*, 1836–1846. [CrossRef]

19. Yuk, H.; Zhang, T.; Lin, S.; Parada, G.A.; Zhao, X. Tough bonding of hydrogels to diverse non-porous surfaces. *Nat. Mater.* **2016**, *15*, 190–196. [CrossRef]

20. Palazzolo, G.; Moroni, M.; Soloperto, A.; Aletti, G.; Naldi, G.; Vassalli, M.; Nieus, T.; Difato, F. Fast wide-volume functional imaging of engineered in vitro brain tissues. *Sci Rep.* **2017**, *7*, 8499. [CrossRef]

21. Vitali, I.; Fièvre, S.; Telley, L.; Oberst, P.; Bariselli, S.; Frangeul, L.; Baumann, N.; McMahon, J.J.; Klingler, E.; Bocchi, R.; et al. Progenitor Hyperpolarization Regulates the Sequential Generation of Neuronal Subtypes in the Developing Neocortex. *Cell* **2018**, *174*, 1264–1276. [CrossRef] [PubMed]

22. Centeno, E.G.Z.; Cimarosti, H.; Bithell, A. 2D versus 3D human induced pluripotent stem cell-derived cultures for neurodegenerative disease modelling. *Mol. Neurodegener.* **2018**, *13*, 27. [CrossRef] [PubMed]

23. Lancaster, M.A.; Renner, M.; Martin, C.-A.; Wenzel, D.; Bicknell, L.S.; Hurles, M.E.; Homfray, T.; Penninger, J.M.; Jackson, A.P.; Knoblich, J.A. Cerebral organoids model human brain development and microcephaly. *Nature* **2013**, *501*, 373–379. [CrossRef] [PubMed]

24. Kelava, I.; Lancaster, M.A. Dishing out mini-brains: Current progress and future prospects in brain organoid research. *Dev. Biol.* **2016**, *420*, 199–209. [CrossRef] [PubMed]

25. Salaris, F.; Rosa, A. Construction of 3D in vitro models by bioprinting human pluripotent stem cells: Challenges and opportunities. *Brain Res.* **2019**, *1723*, 146393. [CrossRef] [PubMed]

26. Abelseth, E.; Abelseth, L.; De la Vega, L.; Beyer, S.T.; Wadsworth, S.J.; Willerth, S.M. 3D Printing of Neural Tissues Derived from Human Induced Pluripotent Stem Cells Using a Fibrin-Based Bioink. *ACS Biomater. Sci. Eng.* **2019**, *5*, 234–243. [CrossRef]

27. Gu, Q.; Tomaskovic-Crook, E.; Lozano, R.; Chen, Y.; Kapsa, R.M.; Zhou, Q.; Wallace, G.G.; Crook, J.M. Functional 3D Neural Mini-Tissues from Printed Gel-Based Bioink and Human Neural Stem Cells. *Adv. Healthc. Mater.* **2016**, *5*, 1429–1438. [CrossRef] [PubMed]

4

Non-Small Cell Lung Cancer from Genomics to Therapeutics: A Framework for Community Practice Integration to Arrive at Personalized Therapy Strategies

Swapnil Rajurkar [†], Isa Mambetsariev [†], Rebecca Pharaon, Benjamin Leach, TingTing Tan, Prakash Kulkarni and Ravi Salgia *

Department of Medical Oncology and Therapeutics Research, City of Hope, Duarte, CA 91010, USA; srajurkar@coh.org (S.R.); Imambetsariev@coh.org (I.M.); rpharaon@coh.org (R.P.); bleach@coh.org (B.L.); titan@coh.org (T.T.); pkulkarni@coh.org (P.K.)
* Correspondence: rsalgia@coh.org
† These authors contributed equally to this work and should be considered co-first authors.

Abstract: Non-small cell lung cancer (NSCLC) is a heterogeneous disease, and therapeutic management has advanced with the identification of various key oncogenic mutations that promote lung cancer tumorigenesis. Subsequent studies have developed targeted therapies against these oncogenes in the hope of personalizing therapy based on the molecular genomics of the tumor. This review presents approved treatments against actionable mutations in NSCLC as well as promising targets and therapies. We also discuss the current status of molecular testing practices in community oncology sites that would help to direct oncologists in lung cancer decision-making. We propose a collaborative framework between community practice and academic sites that can help improve the utilization of personalized strategies in the community, through incorporation of increased testing rates, virtual molecular tumor boards, vendor-based oncology clinical pathways, and an academic-type singular electronic health record system.

Keywords: non-small cell lung cancer; driver mutations; testing rates; receptor tyrosine kinases; team medicine

1. Introduction

Lung cancer remains the leading cause of cancer deaths in the United States and, in 2020, it will be responsible for an estimated 230,000 cases and 135,000 deaths in the US alone [1]. Non-small cell lung cancer (NSCLC) is the major histological subtype that accounts for approximately 85% of all lung cancer cases and encompasses several subtypes, including adenocarcinoma, squamous cell carcinoma, and large cell carcinoma [2]. Despite advances in screening and diagnosis, most patients still present with metastatic disease, at which point surgical intervention is no longer an option [3]. The advent of targeted therapy and immunotherapy has altered the course of treatment for the majority of patients—with molecular testing now a standard recommendation for late-stage lung adenocarcinoma patients. Tyrosine kinase inhibitors (TKIs) that target abnormalities in several genes, such as *ALK* and *EGFR*, have shown better progression-free survival (PFS) as compared with standard chemotherapy in a number of NSCLC trials [4–6]. More recently, other molecular markers, including ROS1, RET, NTRK, BRAF, and MET, have delivered similar clinical benefits to patients with late-stage NSCLC [7–12]. Furthermore, mature outcome data from second-generation TKIs is showing durable overall survival benefit for patients [13,14], a factor that was previously disputed with earlier TKIs [15].

Several molecular targets that were previously considered "unactionable", such as KRAS, now have several targeted therapies under consideration with promising early results [16,17]. Nevertheless, for patients without an actionable target or progression of disease, immune checkpoint inhibitors (ICIs) have resulted in durable outcomes and clinical benefit across several NSCLC trials in various lines of therapy [18–24]. Protein expression testing of programmed death-ligand 1 (PD-L1) has been identified as a potential, though not definitive, biomarker of predicting response to immunotherapy [21,25–27]. Beyond tumor response, recent results from KEYNOTE-001 showed that pembrolizumab monotherapy was associated with a 23.2% 5-year overall survival as compared to 15.5% for previously treated patients [28]. However, therapeutic advancements and outcome improvements have not been uniformly applied in practice, with the majority of trials and novel therapies being more prevalent in academic sites as compared to community practice. We previously showed in a retrospective study that in a cohort of 253 patients from nine community practice centers, the molecular testing rate for first-line treatment decisions was 81.75%, with testing for PD-L1 at only 56% [29]. This suggests that while community sites are on pace to improving their testing rates, the current results are inadequate and require more education and understanding of novel upcoming personalized therapies. The purpose of the current review is to shed light on the available and upcoming therapies in lung cancer, to report the gaps in community practice testing rates, and to identify the available tools that can assist in complex lung cancer management and decision-making.

2. Advances in Genomic Testing and Personalized Therapy

In the last 20 years, therapeutic management of lung cancer has progressed from cytotoxic chemotherapies to personalized targeted therapies that act upon specific genomic alterations. Prior to this, while cytotoxic therapies showed a benefit for early-stage disease [30,31], there was no reported outcome benefit in patients with late-stage lung cancer [32]. Following the completion of the multi-billion dollar endeavor of the Human Genome Project in 2003 [33], the development of next-generation sequencing with high-throughput has enabled large-scale parallel sequencing of the lung cancer genome revealing a plethora of genomic targets including EGFR (10–50%), KRAS (25%), ALK (2–7%), ROS1 (1–2%), RET (1%), BRAF (4%), and others [34,35]. Initially, EGFR tyrosine kinase inhibitors were evaluated in unselected populations with mixed responses due to inadequate selection of patients with EGFR alterations [36,37]. However, the results from randomized Phase III trials for EGFR and ALK tyrosine kinase inhibitors [5] led to the acceptance of genomic testing for ALK and EGFR alterations in routine clinical practice, and in turn, led to the development of faster and more efficient next-generation sequencing platforms that were Clinical Laboratory Improvement Amendments (CLIA)-certified and became widely accepted commercially and at academic sites [38]. While first-generation EGFR TKIs, including gefitinib and erlotinib, showed improved progression-free survival, retrospective studies and outcomes data failed to show improvements in overall survival outcomes [13,39–42]. In contrast to these results, the FLAURA trial for second-generation TKI, osimertinib, showed significant progression-free survival benefit (median PFS 18.9 vs. 10.2 months) and a considerable overall survival benefit of 35.8 months as compared to 27.0 months in the control [43]. The durable survival benefit of targeted therapies had previously been disputed, but recent results from the long-term survival of advanced ALK-rearranged patients treated with crizotinib showed an undisputable benefit of median OS of 6.8 years and a 5-year OS rate of 36% as compared to the historical 2% [44]. Moreover, advances in immunotherapy have yielded similar improvements and KEYNOTE-189 showed that patients who received immunotherapy resulted in a 20% improvement in the overall survival [45].

The promise of precision medicine and the arrival of personalized therapy has transformed lung cancer care with a number of genetic alterations that have come to fruition or are quickly rising with promising trial results, including EGFR, ALK, ROS1, MET, RET, NTRK, BRAF, KRAS, and immunotherapies (Table 1). However, the rapid and dynamic nature of emerging trial results has made lung cancer management difficult and while academic sites are familiar with trial results and the latest available therapies, a community oncologist, who may see a variety of solid tumors, may have difficulty grasping the complexity of these genomic alterations. In our experience at the academic site, actionable alterations were identified in 53.5% of patients with lung cancer, and the use of genomic-informed therapy was associated with improved survival benefit as compared to patients with no actionable alterations [46]. The use of genomic-informed therapy and selective immunotherapy must be standardized within community practice to ensure improved outcomes.

Table 1. Actionable targets in lung cancer and available therapeutics.

Biomarker Strategy	Approved and Investigational Therapies	Toxicities	Preferred Frontline Therapy	Incidence Rates in NSCLC
EGFR	Osimertinib, Erlotinib, Gefitinib, Afatinib, Dacomitinib	Cutaneous (acneiform rash), gastrointestinal (diarrhea)	Osimertinib	10–50%
ALK	Crizotinib, Ceritinib, Alectinib, Brigatinib, Lorlatinib	Gastrointestinal (nausea, diarrhea), transaminitis, visual changes, pneumonitis	Alectinib	1–7%
ROS1	Crizotinib, Ceritinib, Entrectinib, Lorlatinib	Gastrointestinal (nausea, diarrhea), transaminitis, visual changes, pneumonitis	Crizotinib or Entrectinib	1–2%
MET	Crizotinib, Capmatinib, Tepotinib, Telisotuzumab vedotin	Gastrointestinal, transaminitis	Crizotinib or Capmatinib	3–6%
RET	Cabozantinib, Vandetanib, Sunitinib, Selpercatinib, Pralsetnib(BLU-667) Selpercatinib (LOXO-292)	Fatigue, transaminitis, hypertension, diarrhea	Selpercatinib	1–2%
NTRK	Larotrectinib, Entrectinib, Loxo-195	Fatigue, edema, dizziness, constipation, diarrhea, liver abnormalities	Larotrectinib or Entrectinib	3–4%
BRAF	Dabrafenib, Trametinib, Vemurafenib	Rash, fever, headache, diarrhea	Dabrafenib+Trametinib	7%
PD-L1 expression	Pembrolizumab, Nivolumab, Ipilimumab, Atezolizumab, Durvalumab	Immune-mediated toxicities, including pulmonary and gastrointestinal	Various combination options of chemotherapy and immunotherapy or single-agent immunotherapy	~22–47% [47]

2.1. EGFR

The epidermal growth factor receptor is a transmembrane cell-surface receptor that is activated in 10–50% of patients with NSCLC, which varies based on populations and is more common in Asians and nonsmokers [34,48]. The receptors in the EGFR family exist as inactive monomers, but the binding of extracellular growth factors, such as epidermal growth factor (EGF), has been shown to cause receptor dimerization and induced autophosphorylation of the tyrosine kinase domain, with downstream and intercellular signaling cascades that in turn affect cell motility, invasion, proliferation, and angiogenesis [49]. Initial mutations in EGFR were first described in 2004 and activating mutations in EGFR occurring in exons 18–21 of the kinase domain were associated with sensitivity and response to gefitinib and erlotinib [50–52]. This led to the selection of patients with adenocarcinoma histology and EGFR alterations and, in 2009, a landmark Phase III Iressa Pan-Asia Study (IPASS) identified clinical responsiveness and increased progression-free survival in EGFR mutant patients who received gefitinib as compared to standard chemotherapy [50]. The landmark Phase III trial, EURTAC, evaluating erlotinib, an EGFR TKI, as a first-line therapy for patients with EGFR mutations, showed an increased median PFS of 9.7 months as compared to 5.2 months with standard chemotherapy [53]. Two other Phase III trials, the OPTIMAL and ENSURE trials, showed a similar improvement with erlotinib and the US Food and Drug Administration (FDA) approved erlotinib as a first-line cancer therapy for EGFR mutation-positive patients [4,53,54]. Similarly, afatinib, a second-generation TKI, received FDA approval in 2013 following two Phase III trials, Lux-Lung 3 and Lux-Lung 6, that both showed improved PFS of 11.1 months and 11 months respectively, as compared to standard chemotherapy in the first-line setting [55,56].

In 2015, efficacy results for patients with exon 19 deletions or exon 21 (L858R) mutations treated with gefitinib showed a 50% objective response rate (ORR) and led to the FDA approval of gefitinib as a first-line therapy for EGFR mutation-positive patients [57]. However, at that time erlotinib became the standard choice of therapy for many EGFR mutated patients, and mechanisms of primary and secondary resistance to TKI therapy began to emerge. The most commonly identified acquired resistance to early-generation TKIs was the T790M substitution, a secondary EGFR mutation in exon 20, that accounted for approximately 60% of cases [53,55,58,59]. The development of mutant selective pyrimidine-based third-generation TKIs that could block the T790M substitution led to the AURA3 trial evaluating osimertinib, a third-generation TKI, as second-line therapy following T790M EGFR TKI resistance [6]. In 2017, the results of the AURA3 trial showed a significantly improved PFS of 10.1 months and a response rate of 71% as compared to standard chemotherapy [6], and this led to the issuance of FDA approval for osimertinib in the second-line setting for EGFR T790M mutation-positive patients treated with first-line EGFR TKI. Compounding results also exhibited higher CNS response rates with osimertinib (40% vs. 17%) and a longer CNS PFS of 11.7 months vs. 5.6 months [60]. Brain metastases occur in approximately 20–40% of EGFR patients at presentation [61,62] and CNS activity of osimertinib hinted at its potential as a first-line therapy. Unsurprisingly, in 2018, the results of the FLAURA trial showed osimertinib as superior in the first-line setting as compared to first-generation TKIs, with a median PFS of 18.9 months (vs. 10.2 months), ORR of 77% (vs. 69%), and a median duration of response (DOR) at 17.6 months (vs. 9.6 months) [13]. This led to the issuance of FDA approval for osimertinib as the first-line therapy option for EGFR mutant lung cancer. Furthermore, mature data from the FLAURA trial also showed a medial overall survival benefit of 38.6 months over 31.8 months in the control and there was a significant improvement in quality of life, a clinical factor that was never previously achieved in first-generation TKIs [43].

However, despite advances in therapy, acquired resistance inevitably occurs, including EGFR-dependent resistance (6–10%), MET and HER2 amplifications (8–17%), small cell lung cancer (SCLC), and squamous cell carcinoma (SCC) transformation (15%), and others [63]. EGFR-dependent resistance includes S768I, L861Q, G719X, and other alterations that are resistant to most first-generation TKIs except for afatinib that was approved for first-line therapy for patients with rare EGFR alterations [64]. Additional TKIs such as poziotinib are currently under consideration for such alterations and Phase II preliminary data showed a response rate of 43% and a median PFS of 5.5 months in previously treated EGFR-mutant patients [65]. Additionally, other TKIs including TAK-788 (NCT03807778), TAS6417 (NCT04036682), and tarloxotinib (TH-4000) (NCT03805841) are currently under investigation in this setting. There are other trials available for less-frequent mutations of EGFR, such as exon 18 or exon 20 EGFR insertions. The availability of numerous EGFR TKIs in the first and refractory setting is strictly contingent upon appropriate assignment to therapy following reflex molecular testing. The improvements in survival are dependent on early identification of molecular markers and appropriate sequence of TKI therapy. In one retrospective study of rates of molecular testing in a community-based academic center, EGFR testing following the approval of reflex testing was only 62% [66]. In another larger cohort of 814 community practice patients, testing rates were similarly low, with only 69% of patients who were tested for EGFR mutations, and approximately 70% of patients who tested positive received appropriate targeted therapy [67]. In a retrospective evaluation of 1,203 advanced NSCLC patients from five community oncology practices, the testing rates of EGFR were at 54% [68]. A comprehensive retrospective cohort of 191 community oncology practices with 5688 patients performed by Flatiron Health, selected patients who were tested for EGFR alterations with either broad genomic sequencing or routine-testing and identified 154 EGFR-mutated patients in the broad-based sequencing group, but reported that only 25% of these patients received appropriate EGFR-targeted therapy [69]. The findings of the study concluded that there was no survival difference between broad-based and routine genomic sequencing, but this misrepresented the utility of broad-based genomic sequencing in the community, as better outcomes cannot be achieved without appropriate assignment to targeted therapy. Meanwhile, in our own community practice experience of 253 patients, we reported testing rates of 94% for EGFR and 96.2% of patients with an EGFR sensitizing mutation received a TKI therapy [29]. The translation of outcomes reported in clinical trials to real-world outcomes requires cooperation and acceptance of molecular testing within community practice and the integration of targeted therapies in community decision-making.

2.2. ALK

ALK, a receptor tyrosine kinase, was originally identified in lung cancer in 2007 with the detection of an echinoderm microtubule-associated protein-like 4 (EML4) gene and anaplastic lymphoma kinase (ALK) gene fusion from a surgically resected lung adenocarcinoma patient [70]. This gene rearrangement is largely independent of EGFR alterations and has been described as an actionable oncogene with incidence in 1–7% of lung cancer patients [71]. ALK-rearranged patients tend to be younger and—similar to EGFR—have a limited history of smoking. Crizotinib, while originally developed as a MET therapeutic, showed a preclinical efficacy for ALK [72]. The Phase I trial lead to the FDA approval of crizotinib in ALK-positive NSCLC [5]. In 2013, the results of the Phase III trial evaluating crizotinib compared to standard chemotherapy showed PFS of 7.7 months (vs. 3.0 months) and ORR of 65% (vs. 20%) [5], resulting in FDA approval of crizotinib for first-line therapy as a standard of care. As with other TKIs, while patients initially respond to ALK inhibitors, resistance invariably develops and one of the most common resistance mechanisms is an acquired ALK mutation (1151Tins, L1152R, C1156Y, F1174V/L, G1269A, and others) [73]. Other resistance mechanisms include EGFR activation, KIT activation, KRAS mutation, and IGF1R activation [74–79]. It was estimated that 25% of ALK-mutated patients do not respond to crizotinib in the first-line setting and, in response to these resistance mechanisms [77], other ALK TKIs have been developed. In 2014, the results from the Phase I trial evaluating ceritinib as a potential therapy in ALK-rearranged NSCLC patients with disease progression on crizotinib showed a median progression-free survival of 7.0 months and a response rate of 56% [80]. Based on only the Phase I trial results, the FDA approved ceritinib in patients who have progressed on crizotinib, and in 2017, it expanded its approval for first-line use. Alectinib received similar approval in 2015 in the refractory setting that was later expanded to first-line in 2017 [81–83]. In the first-line, alectinib showed a median PFS of 34.8 months with an OS rate of 62.5% as compared to crizotinib with 11 months and 52% [81–83]. Brigatinib, a second-generation ALK TKI, was initially identified to have preclinical efficacy and grater potency against all 17 ALK mutants as compared with crizotinib [84,85]. Initial results for brigatinib from a Phase II trial in the refractory setting showed promising responses and yielded FDA approval in 2017 [86]. While alectinib has been shown to be effective against L1196M, C1156Y, and F1174L ALK gatekeeper mutations [87], brigatinib has shown efficacy against ROS1, FLT3, and IGF-1 secondary mutations [88]. The results of the Phase III trial for brigatinib vs. crizotinib in the first-line showed an estimated PFS of 12 months as compared to 11 months with crizotinib, and two-year follow-up data showed brigatinib reduced the risk of progression or death by 76% [14,89]. Several other new generation ALK TKIs including lorlatinib and ensartinib demonstrated 73% and 72% ORR, respectively, following crizotinib and we are awaiting first-line results [90,91].

The availability of a number of ALK inhibitors has complicated management of ALK patients, but in a long-term assessment of 110 patients with an ALK inhibitor, a remarkable OS for advanced ALK NSCLC patients of 6.8 years was reported with 78.4% of patients receiving another ALK inhibitor after first-line progression [44]. Therefore, many studies are reporting that the success of ALK inhibition therapy may lie in the sequence of administrating ALK inhibitors based on metastatic progression and resistance profiles [92,93]. In a retrospective analysis of 31,483 patients with advanced NSCLC at community practices, ALK overall testing rates were 53.1% and rose to 62.1% in 2016, with 21.5% of patients who were initiated into non-targeted therapy before receiving test results [94]. Gierman et al. in 2019 evaluated 1,203 advanced NSCLC patients from five community practices and results showed that only 51% of patients were tested for ALK rearrangement, with approximately 45% of actionable patients receiving targeted therapy [68]. A concurrent study of 814 community practice patients showed that only 65% were tested for ALK alterations [67]. A retrospective study of advanced NSCLC across over 70 community sites in the US showed that only ~50% of patients were tested for ALK alterations during their cancer care [95], suggesting that advancements in liquid biopsies and testing are not translating to real-world practice. The use of liquid biopsies in a large cfDNA study showed that genomic results were concordant with tissue and utilizing cfDNA liquid biopsies increased detection and rates of testing by 48% [96]. The integration of liquid biopsy testing and further controls on tissue biopsy testing may improve the rates of ALK testing and translate the 6.8-year median survival benefit from academic site-wide studies into real-world efficacy.

2.3. ROS1

ROS1 has been identified as an oncogene in lung cancer and rearrangements have been reported in 1 to 2% of patients with NSCLC [34]. The fusion mutations lead to the dysregulation of the tyrosine-kinase dependent multi-use intracellular signaling pathway, which in turn accelerates growth, proliferation, and progression [97]. Similar to EGFR and ALK alterations, ROS1 fusions and rearrangements are mutually exclusive and independent of other oncogenes such as KRAS or MET [98]. Following the discovery of ROS1 fusions in 2007 and in part due to the high degree of homology between ALK and ROS1, the tyrosine kinase inhibitor crizotinib was explored as a therapeutic option [99,100]. Crizotinib was approved by the FDA in 2016 contingent upon clinical benefit from a PROFILE 1001 Phase I study, where patients had a median PFS of 19.2 months and an ORR of 72% [101]. A Phase II study of ceritinib with 32 patients showed an ORR response rate of 62% and a PFS of 19.3 months for crizotinib-naïve patients, but FDA approval is pending and ceritinib was ineffective against resistance mutations but had activity against CNS disease, as intracranial ORR was 25% and intracranial DCR was 63% [102]. Unlike ceritinib, entrectinib has been shown to be effective against some resistance mutations and had similar CNS activity with a median PFS of 13.6 months and ORR of 55% for patients with CNS disease [103]. This led to the FDA's approval of entrectinib in the management of ROS1-positive NSCLC. However, lorlatinib is currently the only inhibitor under consideration for ROS1 that is effective against most resistance mutations and in a Phase II trial it induced an ORR of 26.5% with a PFS of 8.5, with considerable CNS activity inducing an ORR of 52.6% [104]. Other agents such as DS6051b (NCT02279433) and repotrectinib (NCT03093116) are also currently under investigation with results awaiting. A 2018 study by Friends of Cancer Research and Deerfield Institute announced the response of a survey of 157 oncologists and showed that ROS1 testing in the community centers was 32% [105]. However, a comprehensive study of 14,461 patients treated in the community showed testing rates for ROS1 were incrementally lower at 5.7% with 35.5% and 32.9% for EGFR and ALK respectively [106]. Of the three major approved alterations, ROS1 has the lowest testing rates in several studies [67,105,106]. While tissue biopsies remain the gold standard in detecting ROS1 fusions and rearrangements, advances in liquid biopsy have shown that it is a viable option for ROS1 and implementation of this practice may increase the testing rates within the community practice [29,107].

2.4. MET

MET oncogenic mutations and amplification has been noted in various solid tumor malignancies, including NSCLC, breast cancer, and head and neck cancer [108–112]. MET alterations or its ligand activation (hepatocyte growth factor) causes the activation of the tyrosine kinase which subsequently activates downstream signaling pathways related to cell growth, apoptosis, motility, and invasiveness [113]. Initially discovered in familial and sporadic papillary renal carcinomas [114], subsequent studies revealed the incidence of *MET* alterations in SCLC and NSCLC, especially MET exon 14 skipping as identified initially by our laboratory [115,116]. *MET* alterations have an incidence rate of 6% in lung adenocarcinoma and 3% of lung squamous cell carcinoma [117,118]. The most frequent alteration is the *MET* exon 14 skipping mutation, which has been identified in 4% of lung cancers. A 2015 study was the first to demonstrate clinical efficacy of crizotinib or cabozantinib in NSCLC patients with *MET* exon 14 skipping mutations [119]. A recent study enrolled 69 NSCLC patients harboring *MET* exon 14 alterations that were treated with crizotinib and reported an ORR of 32% and a median PFS of 7.3 months, suggesting antitumor activity with crizotinib treatment [120]. Several clinical trials, such as the GEOMETRY mono-1 trial and the VISION trial, are evaluating other TKIs like capmatinib and tepotinib in MET exon 14-mutated NSCLC and have shown promising results [12,121]. Interim results of the Phase II GEOMETRY mono-1 trial with 97 enrolled patients reported good ORR and a median PFS of 9.13 months in the treatment-naïve cohort [12]. Recently, capmantinib was granted accelerated FDA approval in metastatic NSCLC patients with *MET* exon 14 skipping mutation, the first TKI approved for MET NSCLC patients. MET amplification, which accounts for 1–4% of NSCLC patients who have not been treated with EGFR TKIs, is associated with a poor prognosis [122,123]. A Phase I trial investigated telisotuzumab vedotin, an antibody-drug conjugate, in NSCLC patients with MET overexpression and demonstrated safety and tolerability of the drug with promising antitumor efficacy [124]. In a study of NGS testing rates of genomic biomarkers in NSCLC patients treated at community sites, only 15% of the 814 patients underwent NGS testing for MET, a sharp decline compared to EGFR (69%) or ALK (65%) testing rates [67]. This testing rate was recapitulated in another community analysis [69], however, MET testing rates were reported as low as 6% in an analysis of NGS screening rates between private clinics, academic centers, and community sites [105].

2.5. RET

Activation of RET results in downstream pathway signaling including MAPK, JAK/STAT, and PI3K/AKT, leading to cell proliferation and migration. Alterations in *RET* are most frequently found in medullary thyroid carcinoma and NSCLC. In NSCLC, RET rearrangements are found in approximately 1–2% of cases [117]. These patients tend to be non- or former light smokers with adenocarcinoma histology and present with advanced disease [125]. Since its discovery, several targeted therapies have been investigated including multikinase inhibitors and selective RET inhibitors. A Phase II trial of RET fusion-positive NSCLC patients were treated with cabozantinib, a TKI targeting RET, VEGFR, and MET. The results demonstrated good clinical efficacy with an ORR of 28% and a median PFS of 5.5 months [126]. The most promising selective RET inhibitors currently under investigation are BLU-677 and selpercatinib (LOXO-292). Interim results from a Phase I clinical trial of 79 RET fusion-positive NSCLC patients treated with BLU-677 demonstrated an ORR of 56% among the 57 evaluable patients and encouraging central nervous system (CNS) activity against brain metastases [127]. The Phase I/II LIBRETTO-001 trial evaluating selpercatinib in a cohort of previously treated NSCLC patients with RET rearrangements (N = 105) also demonstrated marked antitumor efficacy with an ORR of 68%, a remarkable CNS response of 91%, and a median PFS of 18.4 months [8]. In the treatment-naïve cohort (N = 34) of the trial, the ORR was 85%, resulting in the FDA approval of selpercatinib for patients with RET-positive NSCLC. Like MET testing rates, RET demonstrated a 14–15% testing rate in community NSCLC patients [67,69]. Also similar to MET, RET testing rates were reported as low as 8% [105]. This is a staggeringly low rate considering the recent FDA approval and great antitumor activity of selective RET inhibitors.

2.6. NTRK

NTRK genes (*NTRK1, NTRK2,* and *NTRK3)* encode three TRK proteins (TRKA, TRKB, and TRKC), which play an important role in the cell growth, differentiation, and apoptosis of peripheral and CNS neurons [128]. *NTRK1* and *NTRK2* rearrangements account for 3–4% of NSCLC cases [129]. Several clinical trials have shown the efficacy of TRK inhibitor treatment in *TRK*-positive tumors. Larotrectinib (LOXO-101), a highly selective pan-TRK inhibitor, was first evaluated in a study of 55 pediatric and adult patients with various *TRK* fusion-positive malignancies, four of whom had lung cancer, and reported an ORR of 75% [10]. Remarkably, responses were shown to be durable with a response rate of 71% while 51% of patients stayed progression-free at one year. A multicenter analysis of three major Phase I/II clinical trials—STARTRK-1, STARTRK-2, and ALKA-372-001—investigating entrectinib in 54 patients diagnosed with advanced or metastatic *NTRK*-positive tumors demonstrated an ORR of 57%, a median PFS of 11.2 months, and a median OS of 20.9 months [130]. Larotrectinib and entrectinib are currently FDA-approved for the treatment of advanced *NTRK* fusion-positive NSCLC. Although these clinical trials have shown strong and durable responses to first-generation TRK TKIs, acquired resistance mutations have been identified in colorectal and mammary analogue secretory carcinomas, requiring the development of second-generation TKIs [131,132]. LOXO-195, a second-generation TRK-selective inhibitor, has shown preclinical efficacy and clinical activity in a Phase I trial of *NTRK* fusion-positive cancers previously treated with larotrectinib, demonstrating an ORR of 45% [133,134]. Despite the great clinical response elicited by NTRK-targeted therapies, NTRK testing rates were shown to range from 0–15% in several community site analyses [69,105].

2.7. BRAF

BRAF mutations represent 7% of NSCLC cases and are more commonly found in current or former smokers and female patients [117]. The most frequent *BRAF* activating mutation, V600E, carries a poorer prognosis and a shorter disease-free survival [135]. A Phase II trial investigated combination treatments of dabrafenib and trametinib in chemotherapy-pretreated patients diagnosed with *BRAF* V600E-mutated NSCLC and reported an ORR of 63% and a median PFS of 9.7 months in 52 evaluable patients [11]. In a Phase II trial of treatment-naïve patients with *BRAF* V600E-mutated NSCLC, treatment with dabrafenib and trametinib resulted in an ORR of 64% and a median PFS of 10.9 months, although 69% of patients experienced at least one grade 3/4 adverse event [136]. Currently, the combination of dabrafenib and trametinib is FDA approved for the treatment of advanced NSCLC harboring the *BRAF* V600E mutation regardless of the previous therapy. In an analysis by Gutierrez et al., BRAF NGS testing rates in 814 community site patients were reported to be 18%, similar to MET and RET NGS testing rates [67]. Other analyses demonstrated consistent rates of 12–29% [68,69,105]. Interestingly, rates of BRAF testing were shown to be as low as 0.1% in a larger analysis of 14,461 NSCLC patients treated in the community [106].

2.8. KRAS

Alterations in *KRAS*, one of the most frequent oncogenes in solid tumor malignancies, represent up to 32% of lung adenocarcinoma cases [117]. They are generally found in smokers [137] and are associated with a poor prognosis [138], although recent data have reported that it has a minimal effect on overall survival in early-stage NSCLC [139]. Therapeutic targeting of *KRAS* has been notoriously difficult, thus dubbing the molecular marker as an "undruggable" target. However, research into KRAS small molecule inhibitors targeting mutational variants of *KRAS* has shown preclinical and clinical efficacy. AMG-510, an inhibitor targeting KRAS G12C, which accounts for 13% of *KRAS* mutant NSCLC [140], is currently under investigation in a Phase I/II clinical trial of advanced *KRAS* mutant solid tumors. Interim results were recently presented and showed that out of the 29 patients, 10 were diagnosed with NSCLC, of which 90% ($N = 9$) of patients exhibited either a partial response or stable disease [16]. Although there are currently no FDA-approved drugs targeting *KRAS*, small molecule inhibitors like AMG-510 and JNJ-74699157 continue to demonstrate good clinical activity. Another drug, MRTX849, has also shown potent efficacy in vitro and in vivo for G12C positive lung cancer, with pronounced tumor regression in 17 of 26 (65%) KRAS G12C positive cell lines [141]. Preliminary data from the Phase I trial also showed a ~30% decrease in target lesions in heavily pre-treated lung cancer patients [141]. NGS testing of KRAS, although still important now, will become necessary once targeted therapies become approved. In several studies of molecular testing rates in community sites, KRAS testing has widely varied, ranging from 0–43% [66,67,69,105]. As more and more targets such as KRAS become clinically actionable, the landscape of lung cancer therapeutic management will continue to change. However, a number of actionable alterations are currently FDA approved and have distinct therapeutic strategies currently available (Figure 1).

The testing rates reported in the community have been rising over the years, and the main driver of this transformation has been education and dissemination of novel therapeutics available for the different oncogenes. However, more effort is required as the primary challenge remains that many newly approved targets face an astronomical hurdle in being implemented in daily community practice (Table 2). The most distinct example of this is the testing rates of BRAF reported in community practice at 0.1% in 14,445 patients—the lack of testing also poses a threat towards clinical trial enrollment and delivery of novel therapeutics to patients [106].

Table 2. Reported testing rates of clinically actionable and clinically relevant oncogenes in community practice.

Reported Study	EGFR	ALK	ROS1	MET	RET	NTRK	BRAF	KRAS	PD-L1 Expression
Inal et al. [66]	62%	23%	N/A	N/A	N/A	N/A	N/A	43%	N/A
Gutierrez et al. [67]	69%	65%	25%	15%	14%	N/A	18%	34%	N/A
Gierman et al. [68]	54%	51%	43%	N/A	N/A	N/A	29%	N/A	N/A
Presley et al. [69]	100%	95%	~15%	~15%	~15%	~15%	~15%	~15%	~15%
Illei et al. [94]	N/A	53.1%	N/A	N/A	N/A	N/A	N/A	N/A	N/A
Hussein et al. [95]	~60%	~50%	N/A	N/A	N/A	N/A	N/A	N/A	N/A
Mason et al. [29]	94%	92%	85%	N/A	N/A	N/A	N/A	N/A	56%
Audibert et al. [105]	68%	67%	32%	6%	8%	0%	12%	0%	N/A
Khozin et al. [142]	64%	61%	N/A	N/A	N/A	N/A	N/A	N/A	8.3%
Nadler et al. 2018 [143]	37%	35%	N/A	N/A	N/A	N/A	N/A	N/A	1.2%
Nadler et al. 2019 [106]	35.5%	32.9%	5.7%	N/A	N/A	N/A	0.1%	N/A	5.7%

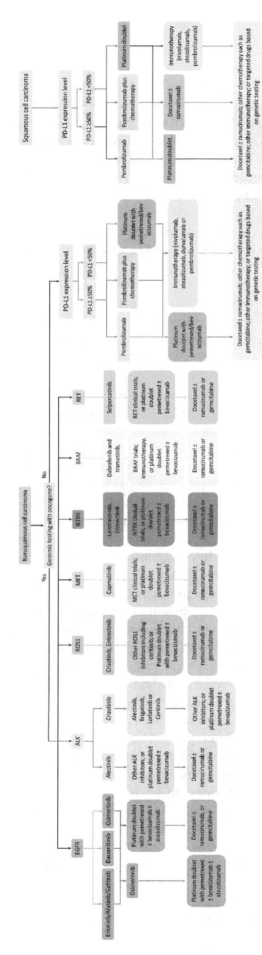

Figure 1. Genomic-informed and immunotherapy-focused management of NSCLC based on approved therapies. The role of immunotherapy is not clear in all of the actionable targets but is currently under investigation.

2.9. Immunotherapy

The availability and discovery of more and more targeted therapies makes it a priority that all advanced NSCLC patients are tested at presentation. However, when an actionable alteration is not available, treatment decisions may depend on PD-L1 expression, histology, or the onset of progressive disease. In these situations, immune checkpoint inhibitors have induced response through interaction with cytotoxic T cells, helper T cells, NK cells, macrophages, and other immune mechanisms. In 2015, the first results of monoclonal antibodies against programmed death ligand-1 (PD-1) in the refractory setting showed efficacy of nivolumab, PD-1 inhibitor, with OS (12.2 months) as compared to second-line chemotherapy (9.5 months) [18–20]. This led to the FDA approval of nivolumab in advanced NSCLC. Similar approval of pembrolizumab, a PD-1 inhibitor, was contingent upon results from KEYNOTE-001 that showed ORR of 19.4 in refractory NSCLC patients [21]. Soon after, two PD-L1 inhibitors, atezolizumab for stage IV metastatic disease and durvalumab for stage III disease, were also approved based on positive ORRs and OS [22,144]. However, the preliminary analysis reported that PD-L1 expression may be a potential biomarker of response and resistance with only 6.6% of patients whose tumors were negative to PD-L1 responding to durvalumab [22]. In the front-line setting, pembrolizumab was the first immune checkpoint inhibitor (ICI) to demonstrate median PFS of 10.3 months (vs. 6 months) and a response rate of 44.8% (vs. 27.8%) based on the results of KEYNOTE-024 as compared to chemotherapy [145], and it can be utilized as a monotherapy or in combination with chemotherapy depending on PD-L1 expression and the performance status of the patient at presentation [146]. The addition of chemotherapy to pembrolizumab resulted in an increased OS at 12 months of 69.2% (vs. 49.4%) and a median PFS of 8.8 months (vs. 4.9 months), with a comparable adverse event rate of 67.2% vs. 65.8% [147]. These results were surprisingly not recreated when nivolumab was evaluated as a monotherapy, showing a median PFS of 4.2 months with nivolumab vs. 5.9 months, and a similar OS benefit of 14.4 months vs. 13.2 months in the chemotherapy control group [23]. However, it did have success in combination with ipilimumab, showing an improvement in overall survival of 17.1 months vs. 13.9 months with chemotherapy, and a nominal duration of response of 23.3 months (vs. 6.2 months) for the front line setting [148].

Nivolumab plus ipilimumab remains a controversial choice due to grade 3 and 4 adverse events in 32.8% of patients [148]. Atezolizumab monotherapy achieved similar approval with incremental improvements in OS [24], but durvalumab in combination and alone failed to improve survival [149]. While the availability of therapies is beneficial to patients, pembrolizumab is slowly becoming the first-choice option for front-line immunotherapy, partially due to its favorable toxicity profile and versatility as a monotherapy and in combination therapy [150]. However, the availability of therapies has not translated into practice and a retrospective observational study of 55,969 NSCLC patients from the community showed that only 1,344 patients received nivolumab or pembrolizumab in the metastatic setting [142]. More surprisingly, only 8% of these patients were tested for PD-L1 expression [142]. More so, an outcomes study of 423 patients with high PD-L1 who received first-line pembrolizumab monotherapy in the community showed that community clinical outcomes were comparable to clinical trial results with a median PFS of 6.8 months vs. 6.1 months and a median OS of 19.1 months vs. 20 months [151]. A larger study of 10,689 patients in the community showed that utilization of immunotherapy in the first-line is not yet implemented, with <1% of patients treated with immunotherapy in the first-line, but rates were improved in the second and third-line setting [143]. PD-L1 expression was equally underperformed and was tested in <1% of patients [143]. Furthermore, in a quality improvement study of 100 patients who received immunotherapy in the community, only 61% fully completed immunotherapy as planned and 81% had immune-related adverse events [152]. While it is concerning that the reported use of immunotherapy in the community practice is limited, based on experience from melanoma and immunotherapy, the rates are anticipated to slowly increase over time with more education and acceptance of various immunotherapy options [153].

While PD-L1 remains an imperfect biomarker, several subgroup analyses in the trials mentioned above show an increased benefit in patients with PD-L1 ≥1% or ≥50%. Therefore, PD-L1 testing should be considered in everyday decision-making, and currently four PD-L1 testing types are available: 22C3, 28-8, SP263, and SP142 [154]. The 22C3 IHC assays were developed alongside pembrolizumab in the Phase I trial as a biomarker for patients who may benefit from treatment [155]. Meanwhile, IHC 28-8 test was developed to be used in conjunction with nivolumab, and SP142 was developed for trial use with atezolizumab [18,19,156,157]. SP263 is the most recent assay that was developed for use with durvalumab, especially in the Stage III setting in NSCLC [156]. All four assays are FDA approved in their individual setting and while testing is not required to initiate treatment, it may support clinical decision-making [156]. Meta-analysis reports show that there is high concordance between 22C3, 28-8, and SP263 assays, but SP142 detected significantly lower PD-L1 expression [154,156]. At the same time, evidence shows that non-commercial laboratory-developed tests (LDTs) used by academic centers detect similar overall percentages of PD-L1 ($\geq$1%) at 63% (vs. 22C3 61%), but PD-L1 $\geq$50% were much lower at 23% (vs. 22C3 33%) suggesting LDTs are less sensitive than commercial tests [158]. LDTs are becoming more and more utilized in practice and offer a potential solution to the complexity of commercial PD-L1 tests. However, the lack of PD-L1 testing and the difficulty of immune-related toxicities is a challenge that is more difficult to address, and we believe that the integration of community practice with the academic site model is one solution to this grave issue.

3. Integration of Personalized Therapy and Molecular Testing in the Community through an Academic Site to Community Practice Network

Advances in targeted therapy and immunotherapy have lowered the costs of molecular testing, making it a viable practice in the academic sites and the community [159]. While academic sites have benefited from a close knowledge of clinical trials and novel therapies, the drive of personalized medicine has not been uniform, with the majority of patients in the community lacking appropriate testing and assignment to therapy [66–69,94,95,106,142,143,152]. This is especially concerning as the majority of patients or approximately 85% with cancer are treated in the community setting and 50% of collaborative group trial accruals occur in the community [160]. Several models have been proposed to integrate community oncologists into the academic paradigm of personalized medicine, with the most promising being the establishment of interpersonal relationships between community oncologists and academic site physicians through molecular tumor board (MTB) teams [161–165]. The establishment of an MTB team would allow for the proper evaluation of imaging, histopathology, and genomic information that is required to make the appropriate therapeutic decision [166]. One reported study involving 1725 patients who were evaluated through a cloud-based virtual molecular tumor board (VMTB) showed that oncologists chose the VMTB-derived therapies over others, resulting in an increase of matched therapies [165]. Such a model also allows for the dissemination of information regarding available CLIA-certified vendors and platforms for both tissue and liquid biopsy testing that are imperative to improving testing rates and outcomes [167]. The MTB model can be scaled into the community through virtual or physical collaboration, and would further improve collaboration between community sites and academic sites through the interactions between pathologists, oncologists, primary care physicians, radiologists, and pulmonologists in the decision-making process (Figure 2). This team-based approach can be utilized in all cancers, especially during crises such as the recent pandemic of novel coronavirus [168]. The improvement in the relationships with various experts and free-flow of information from the academic site to the community will invariably yield improvements in patient outcomes.

Another available tool in building the community and academic network is the incorporation of guidelines and pathways into everyday practice. As the majority of oncologists in the community see a number of patients with varying histologies, it is often difficult to keep track of various therapies available, especially for lung cancer. While guidelines such as the National Comprehensive Cancer Network (NCCN) and the American Society of Clinical Oncology provide guidelines regarding the use of immunotherapy and targeted therapy, as well as genomic testing for FDA approved alterations [169], the results in our review show that the gaps in testing rates still remain prevalent and these guidelines are often difficult to interpret during a busy community practice. One proposed solution to this challenge is the implementation of vendor-based oncology clinical pathways (OCPs) that guide physicians in their decision-making based on query questions regarding the patient case [170]. A number of studies have shown that the use of OCPs not only maintains or improves outcomes, but they lower overhead costs for community practice [171–174]. While guidelines offer multiple recommendations that are difficult to interpret, clinical pathways create a local structure and framework from guidelines or evidence, with the goal of providing the single best therapeutic decision that provides value to the patient (Figure 3) [175]. The advantage of OCPs is not only the availability of decision-making support but the collection of analytics data that can be analyzed for research purposes and continuous quality improvement [176]. An OCP implemented in the community not only evaluates the performance of the community practice, but gives the tools to the community to drive improvements in testing rates and personalized therapy. The wide majority of community practice patients do not consider enrollment in clinical trials, as they are unaware of the option [177]. The pathways incorporate the clinical trials open within the entire enterprise, where trial decisions are placed ahead of other recommendations and always count as on-pathway, which encourages trial enrollment and integrates clinical trials into community practice. Our community practice utilizes the ClinicaPath (formerly ViaOncology) pathway systems in the decision-making process, but there are several vendors available [170].

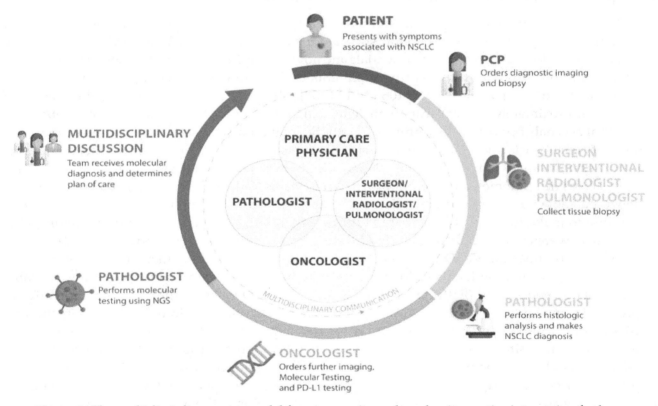

Figure 2. The multidisciplinary care model for community and academic practice integration for lung cancer decision-making.

One recent development in our enterprise is the implementation of a standardized electronic health record (EHR) system in the community that mirrors the academic site medical records in a single system and allows for optimization of testing results and physician referrals for clinical trials. The standardization of molecular testing results and reporting in a fast and reliable manner through the medical record is an important barrier for community oncology practice towards improving testing rates [178]. The cohesiveness of a singular EHR not only results in clinical decision support, but allows the community oncologists to participate in the clinical and translational research process through the evaluation of retrospective patient cohorts in a collaborative model that encompasses a multi-disciplinary team of pathologists, radiologists, and other specialties. The seamless amalgamation of high level genomic and treatment data from the community can be quickly extrapolated from the EHR and utilized in translational studies including evaluation of testing rates and therapy outcomes. This also helps in identifying patients that would be eligible for enrollment in clinical trials available at partnering academic sites, as evidenced by the top accrual rates of the adjuvant EVEREST study in renal cell carcinoma at City of Hope [179]. This is an especially significant strategy to implement in order to enroll and treat older cancer patients who are primarily seen at community sites [180]. Furthermore, the establishment of integrated clinical research has been shown to translate to wider awareness and acceptance of research results, and in 2013, the NCI formed the NCI Community Oncology Research Program (NCORP) [181]. First-cycle results showed that NCORP improved cancer care delivery and access in the community, but challenges remain in growing the program to more organizations across the nation [182]. The evolution of cancer care has to be met with advancements in cancer care and genomic testing access and delivery in community practice. However, the ultimate development of a successful community-based research program requires funding to empower local physicians, infrastructure to support implementation, collaboration between academic and community investigators, and flexibility in operations and organizations.

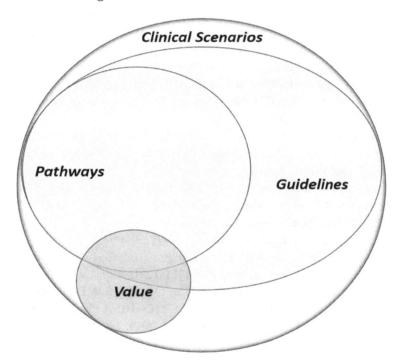

Figure 3. Advantage of guidelines and pathways in clinical scenarios. Patient outcomes are reliant on adherence to evidence-based medicine, which can be facilitated by guidelines and enhanced by pathways.

4. Conclusions

The advancements in lung cancer therapy and genomic testing have transformed the lung cancer decision-making process in the last decade. Next-generation sequencing has expanded from a few genes tested with routine testing to broad-based sequencing that has identified a plethora of oncogenes that are involved in driving the progression of NSCLC [183–185]. While targeted therapy was initially implemented in the first-line setting, the availability of a number of second- and third-generation TKIs has transitioned from a model of systemic therapy in the refractory setting to a framework of a number of TKIs administered in sequence based on resistance mechanisms and clinical progression of the individual patient [186]. The promise of personalized medicine continues to be realized through the development of ground-breaking immune checkpoint inhibitors and upcoming trials show promise for chimeric antigen receptor (CAR) T-cell therapy [187]. To further realize this mission of precision medicine and to deliver improved outcomes, rigorous clinical data science, and translational research of the care delivery model and access have to be expanded beyond academic sites and into community practice. As we have brought to attention in this review, the community practice, while currently lagging behind academic sites in delivery oncology care, can be systematically and procedurally integrated with academic centers in a unified model for lung cancer decision-making and clinical collaboration. Our identified tools and collaborative concepts, including pathways and MTBs, can be realized in any community setting to enhance communication and trial enrollment.

Author Contributions: Conceptualization, R.S., S.R., P.K, I.M.; Writing—original draft preparation, S.R., I.M., R.P., R.S., P.K.; Writing—review and editing, S.R., I.M., R.P., R.S., P.K., B.L. and T.T. All authors have read and agreed to the published version of the manuscript.

Acknowledgments: We would like to express our deepest gratitude for philanthropic funding by the Tenenblatt Family.

References

1. Siegel, R.L.; Miller, K.D.; Jemal, A. Cancer statistics, 2020. *CA A Cancer J. Clin.* **2020**, *70*, 7–30. [CrossRef]
2. Molina, J.R.; Yang, P.; Cassivi, S.D.; Schild, S.E.; Adjei, A.A. Non-small cell lung cancer: Epidemiology, risk factors, treatment, and survivorship. *Mayo Clin. Proc.* **2008**, *83*, 584–594. [CrossRef]
3. Cancer Stat Facts: Lung and Bronchus Cancer, Statistics at a Glance. Available online: https://seer.cancer.gov/statfacts/html/lungb.html (accessed on 20 May 2020).
4. Zhou, C.; Wu, Y.L.; Chen, G.; Feng, J.; Liu, X.Q.; Wang, C.; Zhang, S.; Wang, J.; Zhou, S.; Ren, S.; et al. Erlotinib versus chemotherapy as first-line treatment for patients with advanced EGFR mutation-positive non-small-cell lung cancer (OPTIMAL, CTONG-0802): A multicentre, open-label, randomised, phase 3 study. *Lancet Oncol.* **2011**, *12*, 735–742. [CrossRef]
5. Shaw, A.T.; Kim, D.W.; Nakagawa, K.; Seto, T.; Crino, L.; Ahn, M.J.; De Pas, T.; Besse, B.; Solomon, B.J.; Blackhall, F.; et al. Crizotinib versus chemotherapy in advanced ALK-positive lung cancer. *N. Engl. J. Med.* **2013**, *368*, 2385–2394. [CrossRef] [PubMed]
6. Mok, T.S.; Wu, Y.-L.; Ahn, M.-J.; Garassino, M.C.; Kim, H.R.; Ramalingam, S.S.; Shepherd, F.A.; He, Y.; Akamatsu, H.; Theelen, W.S.M.E.; et al. Osimertinib or Platinum–Pemetrexed in EGFR T790M–Positive Lung Cancer. *N. Engl. J. Med.* **2016**, *376*, 629–640. [CrossRef]
7. Shaw, A.T.; Riely, G.J.; Bang, Y.J.; Kim, D.W.; Camidge, D.R.; Solomon, B.J.; Varella-Garcia, M.; Iafrate, A.J.; Shapiro, G.I.; Usari, T.; et al. Crizotinib in ROS1-rearranged advanced non-small-cell lung cancer (NSCLC): Updated results, including overall survival, from PROFILE 1001. *Ann. Oncol.* **2019**, *30*, 1121–1126. [CrossRef]
8. Drilon, A.; Oxnard, G.; Wirth, L.; Besse, B.; Gautschi, O.; Tan, S.W.D.; Loong, H.; Bauer, T.; Kim, Y.J.; Horiike, A.; et al. PL02.08 Registrational Results of LIBRETTO-001: A Phase 1/2 Trial of LOXO-292 in Patients with RET Fusion-Positive Lung Cancers. *J. Thoracic Oncol.* **2019**, *14*, S6–S7. [CrossRef]
9. Drilon, A.; Siena, S.; Dziadziuszko, R.; Barlesi, F.; Krebs, M.G.; Shaw, A.T.; de Braud, F.; Rolfo, C.; Ahn, M.-J.; Wolf, J.; et al. Entrectinib in ROS1 fusion-positive non-small-cell lung cancer: Integrated analysis of three phase 1–2 trials. *Lancet Oncol.* **2020**, *21*, 261–270. [CrossRef]
10. Drilon, A.; Laetsch, T.W.; Kummar, S.; DuBois, S.G.; Lassen, U.N.; Demetri, G.D.; Nathenson, M.; Doebele, R.C.; Farago, A.F.; Pappo, A.S.; et al. Efficacy of Larotrectinib in TRK Fusion–Positive Cancers in Adults and Children. *N. Engl. J. Med.* **2018**, *378*, 731–739. [CrossRef]
11. Planchard, D.; Besse, B.; Groen, H.J.M.; Souquet, P.J.; Quoix, E.; Baik, C.S.; Barlesi, F.; Kim, T.M.; Mazieres, J.; Novello, S.; et al. Dabrafenib plus trametinib in patients with previously treated BRAF(V600E)-mutant metastatic non-small cell lung cancer: An open-label, multicentre phase 2 trial. *Lancet Oncol.* **2016**, *17*, 984–993. [CrossRef]
12. Wolf, J.; Seto, T.; Han, J.-Y.; Reguart, N.; Garon, E.B.; Groen, H.J.M.; Tan, D.S.-W.; Hida, T.; Jonge, M.J.D.; Orlov, S.V.; et al. Capmatinib (INC280) in METΔex14-mutated advanced non-small cell lung cancer (NSCLC): Efficacy data from the phase II GEOMETRY mono-1 study. *J. Clin. Oncol.* **2019**, *37*, 9004. [CrossRef]
13. Soria, J.-C.; Ohe, Y.; Vansteenkiste, J.; Reungwetwattana, T.; Chewaskulyong, B.; Lee, K.H.; Dechaphunkul, A.; Imamura, F.; Nogami, N.; Kurata, T.; et al. Osimertinib in Untreated EGFR-Mutated Advanced Non–Small-Cell Lung Cancer. *N. Engl. J. Med.* **2017**, *378*, 113–125. [CrossRef] [PubMed]

14. Camidge, D.R.; Kim, H.R.; Ahn, M.-J.; Yang, J.C.-H.; Han, J.-Y.; Lee, J.-S.; Hochmair, M.J.; Li, J.Y.-C.; Chang, G.-C.; Lee, K.H.; et al. Brigatinib versus Crizotinib in ALK-Positive Non–Small-Cell Lung Cancer. *N. Engl. J. Med.* **2018**, *379*, 2027–2039. [CrossRef]

15. Kuan, F.-C.; Kuo, L.-T.; Chen, M.-C.; Yang, C.-T.; Shi, C.-S.; Teng, D.; Lee, K.-D. Overall survival benefits of first-line EGFR tyrosine kinase inhibitors in EGFR-mutated non-small-cell lung cancers: A systematic review and meta-analysis. *Br. J. Cancer* **2015**, *113*, 1519–1528. [CrossRef] [PubMed]

16. Govindan, R.; Fakih, M.; Price, T.; Falchook, G.; Desai, J.; Kuo, J.; Strickler, J.; Krauss, J.; Li, B.; Denlinger, C.; et al. Phase 1 Study of AMG 510, a Novel Molecule Targeting KRAS G12C Mutant Solid Tumors. *ESMO 2019 Congress* **2019**, *30* (Suppl. 5), 159–193. [CrossRef]

17. Jänne, P. A phase 1 clinical trial evaluating the pharmacokinetics (PK), safety, and clinical activity of MRTX849, a mutant-selective small molecule KRAS G12C inhibitor, in advanced solid tumors. In Proceedings of the AACR-NCI-EORTC International Conference on Molecular Targets and Cancer Therapeutics, Boston, MA, USA, 26–30 October 2019.

18. Brahmer, J.; Reckamp, K.L.; Baas, P.; Crinò, L.; Eberhardt, W.E.E.; Poddubskaya, E.; Antonia, S.; Pluzanski, A.; Vokes, E.E.; Holgado, E.; et al. Nivolumab versus Docetaxel in Advanced Squamous-Cell Non–Small-Cell Lung Cancer. *N. Engl. J. Med.* **2015**, *373*, 123–135. [CrossRef]

19. Borghaei, H.; Paz-Ares, L.; Horn, L.; Spigel, D.R.; Steins, M.; Ready, N.E.; Chow, L.Q.; Vokes, E.E.; Felip, E.; Holgado, E.; et al. Nivolumab versus Docetaxel in Advanced Nonsquamous Non-Small-Cell Lung Cancer. *N. Engl. J. Med.* **2015**, *373*, 1627–1639. [CrossRef] [PubMed]

20. Horn, L.; Spigel, D.R.; Vokes, E.E.; Holgado, E.; Ready, N.; Steins, M.; Poddubskaya, E.; Borghaei, H.; Felip, E.; Paz-Ares, L.; et al. Nivolumab Versus Docetaxel in Previously Treated Patients With Advanced Non-Small-Cell Lung Cancer: Two-Year Outcomes From Two Randomized, Open-Label, Phase III Trials (CheckMate 017 and CheckMate 057). *J. Clin. Oncol.* **2017**, *35*, 3924–3933. [CrossRef] [PubMed]

21. Herbst, R.S.; Baas, P.; Kim, D.W.; Felip, E.; Pérez-Gracia, J.L.; Han, J.Y.; Molina, J.; Kim, J.H.; Arvis, C.D.; Ahn, M.J.; et al. Pembrolizumab versus docetaxel for previously treated, PD-L1-positive, advanced non-small-cell lung cancer (KEYNOTE-010): A randomised controlled trial. *Lancet* **2016**, *387*, 1540–1550. [CrossRef]

22. Garassino, M.C.; Cho, B.C.; Kim, J.H.; Mazières, J.; Vansteenkiste, J.; Lena, H.; Corral Jaime, J.; Gray, J.E.; Powderly, J.; Chouaid, C.; et al. Durvalumab as third-line or later treatment for advanced non-small-cell lung cancer (ATLANTIC): An open-label, single-arm, phase 2 study. *Lancet Oncol.* **2018**, *19*, 521–536. [CrossRef]

23. Carbone, D.P.; Reck, M.; Paz-Ares, L.; Creelan, B.; Horn, L.; Steins, M.; Felip, E.; van den Heuvel, M.M.; Ciuleanu, T.-E.; Badin, F.; et al. First-Line Nivolumab in Stage IV or Recurrent Non–Small-Cell Lung Cancer. *N. Engl. J. Med.* **2017**, *376*, 2415–2426. [CrossRef] [PubMed]

24. Spigel, D.; de Marinis, F.; Giaccone, G.; Reinmuth, N.; Vergnenegre, A.; Barrios, C.H.; Morise, M.; Felip, E.; Andric, Z.G.; Geater, S.; et al. LBA78-IMpower110: Interim overall survival (OS) analysis of a phase III study of atezolizumab (atezo) vs platinum-based chemotherapy (chemo) as first-line (1L) treatment (tx) in PD-L1–selected NSCLC. *Ann. Oncol.* **2019**, *30*, v915. [CrossRef]

25. Cottrell, T.R.; Taube, J.M. PD-L1 and Emerging Biomarkers in Immune Checkpoint Blockade Therapy. *Cancer J.* **2018**, *24*, 41–46. [CrossRef] [PubMed]

26. Davis, A.A.; Patel, V.G. The role of PD-L1 expression as a predictive biomarker: An analysis of all US Food and Drug Administration (FDA) approvals of immune checkpoint inhibitors. *J. Immunother. Cancer* **2019**, *7*, 278. [CrossRef] [PubMed]

27. Lantuejoul, S.; Sound-Tsao, M.; Cooper, W.A.; Girard, N.; Hirsch, F.R.; Roden, A.C.; Lopez-Rios, F.; Jain, D.; Chou, T.-Y.; Motoi, N.; et al. PD-L1 Testing for Lung Cancer in 2019: Perspective From the IASLC Pathology Committee. *J. Thorac. Oncol.* **2020**, *15*, 499–519. [CrossRef]

28. Garon, E.B.; Hellmann, M.D.; Rizvi, N.A.; Carcereny, E.; Leighl, N.B.; Ahn, M.J.; Eder, J.P.; Balmanoukian, A.S.; Aggarwal, C.; Horn, L.; et al. Five-Year Overall Survival for Patients With Advanced Non-Small-Cell Lung Cancer Treated With Pembrolizumab: Results From the Phase I KEYNOTE-001 Study. *J. Clin. Oncol.* **2019**, *37*, 2518–2527. [CrossRef] [PubMed]

29. Mason, C.; Ellis, P.G.; Lokay, K.; Barry, A.; Dickson, N.; Page, R.; Polite, B.; Salgia, R.; Savin, M.; Shamah, C.; et al. Patterns of Biomarker Testing Rates and Appropriate Use of Targeted Therapy in the First-Line, Metastatic Non-Small Cell Lung Cancer Treatment Setting. *J. Clin. Pathw.* **2018**, *4*, 49–54. [CrossRef]

30.   Dillman, R.O.; Seagren, S.L.; Propert, K.J.; Guerra, J.; Eaton, W.L.; Perry, M.C.; Carey, R.W.; Frei, E.F., 3rd;
      Green, M.R. A randomized trial of induction chemotherapy plus high-dose radiation versus radiation alone
      in stage III non-small-cell lung cancer. *N. Engl. J. Med.* **1990**, *323*, 940–945. [CrossRef] [PubMed]

31.   Curran, W.J., Jr.; Paulus, R.; Langer, C.J.; Komaki, R.; Lee, J.S.; Hauser, S.; Movsas, B.; Wasserman, T.;
      Rosenthal, S.A.; Gore, E.; et al. Sequential vs. concurrent chemoradiation for stage III non-small cell lung
      cancer: Randomized phase III trial RTOG 9410. *J. Natl. Cancer Inst.* **2011**, *103*, 1452–1460. [CrossRef]
      [PubMed]

32.   Schiller, J.H.; Harrington, D.; Belani, C.P.; Langer, C.; Sandler, A.; Krook, J.; Zhu, J.; Johnson, D.H. Comparison
      of four chemotherapy regimens for advanced non-small-cell lung cancer. *N. Engl. J. Med.* **2002**, *346*, 92–98.
      [CrossRef]

33.   Evans, J.P. The Human Genome Project at 10 years: A teachable moment. *Genet. Med.* **2010**, *12*, 477.
      [CrossRef] [PubMed]

34.   Salgia, R. Mutation testing for directing upfront targeted therapy and post-progression combination therapy
      strategies in lung adenocarcinoma. *Expert Rev. Mol. Diagn.* **2016**, *16*, 737–749. [CrossRef] [PubMed]

35.   Ashley, E.A. Towards precision medicine. *Nat. Rev. Genet.* **2016**, *17*, 507–522. [CrossRef] [PubMed]

36.   Kris, M.G.; Natale, R.B.; Herbst, R.S.; Lynch, T.J., Jr.; Prager, D.; Belani, C.P.; Schiller, J.H.; Kelly, K.;
      Spiridonidis, H.; Sandler, A.; et al. Efficacy of gefitinib, an inhibitor of the epidermal growth factor receptor
      tyrosine kinase, in symptomatic patients with non-small cell lung cancer: A randomized trial. *Jama* **2003**,
      290, 2149–2158. [CrossRef]

37.   Fukuoka, M.; Yano, S.; Giaccone, G.; Tamura, T.; Nakagawa, K.; Douillard, J.Y.; Nishiwaki, Y.; Vansteenkiste, J.;
      Kudoh, S.; Rischin, D.; et al. Multi-institutional randomized phase II trial of gefitinib for previously treated
      patients with advanced non-small-cell lung cancer (The IDEAL 1 Trial) [corrected]. *J. Clin. Oncol.* **2003**, *21*,
      2237–2246. [CrossRef] [PubMed]

38.   Lindeman, N.I.; Cagle, P.T.; Beasley, M.B.; Chitale, D.A.; Dacic, S.; Giaccone, G.; Jenkins, R.B.;
      Kwiatkowski, D.J.; Saldivar, J.S.; Squire, J.; et al. Molecular testing guideline for selection of lung cancer
      patients for EGFR and ALK tyrosine kinase inhibitors: Guideline from the College of American Pathologists,
      International Association for the Study of Lung Cancer, and Association for Molecular Pathology. *J. Thorac.
      Oncol.* **2013**, *8*, 823–859. [CrossRef]

39.   Blumenthal, G.M.; Karuri, S.W.; Zhang, H.; Zhang, L.; Khozin, S.; Kazandjian, D.; Tang, S.; Sridhara, R.;
      Keegan, P.; Pazdur, R. Overall response rate, progression-free survival, and overall survival with targeted
      and standard therapies in advanced non-small-cell lung cancer: US Food and Drug Administration trial-level
      and patient-level analyses. *J. Clin. Oncol.* **2015**, *33*, 1008–1014. [CrossRef]

40.   Simeone, J.C.; Nordstrom, B.L.; Patel, K.; Klein, A.B. Treatment patterns and overall survival in metastatic
      non-small-cell lung cancer in a real-world, US setting. *Future Oncol.* **2019**, *15*, 3491–3502. [CrossRef]

41.   Arbour, K.C.; Riely, G.J. Systemic Therapy for Locally Advanced and Metastatic Non-Small Cell Lung Cancer:
      A Review. *Jama* **2019**, *322*, 764–774. [CrossRef]

42.   Buyse, M.E.; Squifflet, P.; Laporte, S.; Fossella, F.V.; Georgoulias, V.; Pujol, J.; Kubota, K.; Monnier, A.;
      Kudoh, S.; Douillard, J. Prediction of survival benefits from progression-free survival in patients with
      advanced non small cell lung cancer: Evidence from a pooled analysis of 2,838 patients randomized in 7
      trials. *J. Clin. Oncol.* **2008**, *26*, 8019. [CrossRef]

43.   Ramalingam, S.S.; Vansteenkiste, J.; Planchard, D.; Cho, B.C.; Gray, J.E.; Ohe, Y.; Zhou, C.;
      Reungwetwattana, T.; Cheng, Y.; Chewaskulyong, B.; et al. Overall Survival with Osimertinib in Untreated,
      EGFR-Mutated Advanced NSCLC. *N. Engl. J. Med.* **2020**, *382*, 41–50. [CrossRef] [PubMed]

44.   Pacheco, J.M.; Gao, D.; Smith, D.; Purcell, T.; Hancock, M.; Bunn, P.; Robin, T.; Liu, A.; Karam, S.;
      Gaspar, L.; et al. Natural History and Factors Associated with Overall Survival in Stage IV ALK-Rearranged
      Non-Small Cell Lung Cancer. *J. Thorac Oncol.* **2019**, *14*, 691–700. [CrossRef] [PubMed]

45.   Gadgeel, S.; Rodríguez-Abreu, D.; Speranza, G.; Esteban, E.; Felip, E.; Dómine, M.; Hui, R.; Hochmair, M.J.;
      Clingan, P.; Powell, S.F.; et al. Updated Analysis From KEYNOTE-189: Pembrolizumab or Placebo Plus
      Pemetrexed and Platinum for Previously Untreated Metastatic Nonsquamous Non-Small-Cell Lung Cancer.
      J. Clin. Oncol. **2020**, *38*, 1505–1517. [CrossRef] [PubMed]

46.   Mambetsariev, I.; Wang, Y.; Chen, C.; Nadaf, S.; Pharaon, R.; Fricke, J.; Amanam, I.; Amini, A.; Bild, A.;
      Chu, P.; et al. Precision medicine and actionable alterations in lung cancer: A single institution experience.
      PLoS ONE **2020**, *15*, e0228188. [CrossRef] [PubMed]

47. Dietel, M.; Savelov, N.; Salanova, R.; Micke, P.; Bigras, G.; Hida, T.; Piperdi, B.; Burke, T.; Khambata-Ford, S.; Deitz, A. 130O Real-world prevalence of PD-L1 expression in locally advanced or metastatic non-small cell lung cancer (NSCLC): The global, multicentre EXPRESS study. *J. Thorac. Oncol.* **2018**, *13*, S74–S75. [CrossRef]

48. Gómez, X.E.; Soto, A.; Gómez, M.A. Survival and prognostic factors in non-small cell lung cancer patients with mutation of the EGFR gene treated with tyrosine kinase inhibitors in a peruvian hospital. *Am. J. Cancer Res.* **2019**, *9*, 1009–1016.

49. Ciardiello, F.; Tortora, G. EGFR Antagonists in Cancer Treatment. *N. Engl. J. Med.* **2008**, *358*, 1160–1174. [CrossRef]

50. Lynch, T.J.; Bell, D.W.; Sordella, R.; Gurubhagavatula, S.; Okimoto, R.A.; Brannigan, B.W.; Harris, P.L.; Haserlat, S.M.; Supko, J.G.; Haluska, F.G.; et al. Activating mutations in the epidermal growth factor receptor underlying responsiveness of non-small-cell lung cancer to gefitinib. *N. Engl. J. Med.* **2004**, *350*, 2129–2139. [CrossRef]

51. Paez, J.G.; Jänne, P.A.; Lee, J.C.; Tracy, S.; Greulich, H.; Gabriel, S.; Herman, P.; Kaye, F.J.; Lindeman, N.; Boggon, T.J.; et al. EGFR mutations in lung cancer: Correlation with clinical response to gefitinib therapy. *Science* **2004**, *304*, 1497–1500. [CrossRef]

52. Pao, W.; Miller, V.; Zakowski, M.; Doherty, J.; Politi, K.; Sarkaria, I.; Singh, B.; Heelan, R.; Rusch, V.; Fulton, L.; et al. EGF receptor gene mutations are common in lung cancers from "never smokers" and are associated with sensitivity of tumors to gefitinib and erlotinib. *Proc. Natl. Acad. Sci. USA* **2004**, *101*, 13306–13311. [CrossRef]

53. Rosell, R.; Carcereny, E.; Gervais, R.; Vergnenegre, A.; Massuti, B.; Felip, E.; Palmero, R.; Garcia-Gomez, R.; Pallares, C.; Sanchez, J.M.; et al. Erlotinib versus standard chemotherapy as first-line treatment for European patients with advanced EGFR mutation-positive non-small-cell lung cancer (EURTAC): A multicentre, open-label, randomised phase 3 trial. *Lancet Oncol.* **2012**, *13*, 239–246. [CrossRef]

54. Wu, Y.L.; Zhou, C.; Liam, C.K.; Wu, G.; Liu, X.; Zhong, Z.; Lu, S.; Cheng, Y.; Han, B.; Chen, L.; et al. First-line erlotinib versus gemcitabine/cisplatin in patients with advanced EGFR mutation-positive non-small-cell lung cancer: Analyses from the phase III, randomized, open-label, ENSURE study. *Ann. Oncol.* **2015**, *26*, 1883–1889. [CrossRef] [PubMed]

55. Wu, Y.L.; Zhou, C.; Hu, C.P.; Feng, J.; Lu, S.; Huang, Y.; Li, W.; Hou, M.; Shi, J.H.; Lee, K.Y.; et al. Afatinib versus cisplatin plus gemcitabine for first-line treatment of Asian patients with advanced non-small-cell lung cancer harbouring EGFR mutations (LUX-Lung 6): An open-label, randomised phase 3 trial. *Lancet Oncol.* **2014**, *15*, 213–222. [CrossRef]

56. Yang, J.C.; Wu, Y.L.; Schuler, M.; Sebastian, M.; Popat, S.; Yamamoto, N.; Zhou, C.; Hu, C.P.; O'Byrne, K.; Feng, J.; et al. Afatinib versus cisplatin-based chemotherapy for EGFR mutation-positive lung adenocarcinoma (LUX-Lung 3 and LUX-Lung 6): Analysis of overall survival data from two randomised, phase 3 trials. *Lancet Oncol.* **2015**, *16*, 141–151. [CrossRef]

57. Kazandjian, D.; Blumenthal, G.M.; Yuan, W.; He, K.; Keegan, P.; Pazdur, R. FDA Approval of Gefitinib for the Treatment of Patients with Metastatic EGFR Mutation-Positive Non-Small Cell Lung Cancer. *Clin. Cancer Res.* **2016**, *22*, 1307–1312. [CrossRef]

58. Han, J.Y.; Park, K.; Kim, S.W.; Lee, D.H.; Kim, H.Y.; Kim, H.T.; Ahn, M.J.; Yun, T.; Ahn, J.S.; Suh, C.; et al. First-SIGNAL: First-line single-agent iressa versus gemcitabine and cisplatin trial in never-smokers with adenocarcinoma of the lung. *J. Clin. Oncol.* **2012**, *30*, 1122–1128. [CrossRef]

59. Sequist, L.V.; Yang, J.C.; Yamamoto, N.; O'Byrne, K.; Hirsh, V.; Mok, T.; Geater, S.L.; Orlov, S.; Tsai, C.M.; Boyer, M.; et al. Phase III study of afatinib or cisplatin plus pemetrexed in patients with metastatic lung adenocarcinoma with EGFR mutations. *J. Clin. Oncol.* **2013**, *31*, 3327–3334. [CrossRef]

60. Mok, T.; Ahn, M.-J.; Han, J.-Y.; Kang, J.H.; Katakami, N.; Kim, H.; Hodge, R.; Ghiorghiu, D.C.; Cantarini, M.; Wu, Y.-L.; et al. CNS response to osimertinib in patients (pts) with T790M-positive advanced NSCLC: Data from a randomized phase III trial (AURA3). *J. Clin. Oncol.* **2017**, *35*, 9005. [CrossRef]

61. Sun, M.; Behrens, C.; Feng, L.; Ozburn, N.; Tang, X.; Yin, G.; Komaki, R.; Varella-Garcia, M.; Hong, W.K.; Aldape, K.D.; et al. HER family receptor abnormalities in lung cancer brain metastases and corresponding primary tumors. *Clin. Cancer Res.* **2009**, *15*, 4829–4837. [CrossRef]

62. Daniele, L.; Cassoni, P.; Bacillo, E.; Cappia, S.; Righi, L.; Volante, M.; Tondat, F.; Inghirami, G.; Sapino, A.; Scagliotti, G.V.; et al. Epidermal growth factor receptor gene in primary tumor and metastatic sites from non-small cell lung cancer. *J. Thorac Oncol.* **2009**, *4*, 684–688. [CrossRef]

63. Leonetti, A.; Sharma, S.; Minari, R.; Perego, P.; Giovannetti, E.; Tiseo, M. Resistance mechanisms to osimertinib in EGFR-mutated non-small cell lung cancer. *Br. J. Cancer* **2019**, *121*, 725–737. [CrossRef] [PubMed]

64. Yang, J.C.; Schuler, M.; Popat, S.; Miura, S.; Heeke, S.; Park, K.; Märten, A.; Kim, E.S. Afatinib for the Treatment of NSCLC Harboring Uncommon EGFR Mutations: A Database of 693 Cases. *J. Thorac Oncol.* **2020**, *15*, 803–815. [CrossRef] [PubMed]

65. Heymach, J.; Negrao, M.; Robichaux, J.; Carter, B.; Patel, A.; Altan, M.; Gibbons, D.; Fossella, F.; Simon, G.; Lam, V.; et al. OA02.06 A Phase II Trial of Poziotinib in EGFR and HER2 exon 20 Mutant Non-Small Cell Lung Cancer (NSCLC). *J. Thoracic Oncol.* **2018**, *13*, S323–S324. [CrossRef]

66. Inal, C.; Yilmaz, E.; Cheng, H.; Zhu, C.; Pullman, J.; Gucalp, R.A.; Keller, S.M.; Perez-Soler, R.; Piperdi, B. Effect of reflex testing by pathologists on molecular testing rates in lung cancer patients: Experience from a community-based academic center. *J. Clin. Oncol.* **2014**, *32*, 8098. [CrossRef]

67. Gutierrez, M.E.; Choi, K.; Lanman, R.B.; Licitra, E.J.; Skrzypczak, S.M.; Pe Benito, R.; Wu, T.; Arunajadai, S.; Kaur, S.; Harper, H.; et al. Genomic Profiling of Advanced Non-Small Cell Lung Cancer in Community Settings: Gaps and Opportunities. *Clin. Lung Cancer* **2017**, *18*, 651–659. [CrossRef]

68. Gierman, H.J.; Goldfarb, S.; Labrador, M.; Weipert, C.M.; Getty, B.; Skrzypczak, S.M.; Catasus, C.; Carbral, S.; Singaraju, M.; Singleton, N.; et al. Genomic testing and treatment landscape in patients with advanced non-small cell lung cancer (aNSCLC) using real-world data from community oncology practices. *J. Clin. Oncol.* **2019**, *37*, 1585. [CrossRef]

69. Presley, C.J.; Tang, D.; Soulos, P.R.; Chiang, A.C.; Longtine, J.A.; Adelson, K.B.; Herbst, R.S.; Zhu, W.; Nussbaum, N.C.; Sorg, R.A.; et al. Association of Broad-Based Genomic Sequencing With Survival Among Patients With Advanced Non-Small Cell Lung Cancer in the Community Oncology Setting. *Jama* **2018**, *320*, 469–477. [CrossRef]

70. Soda, M.; Choi, Y.L.; Enomoto, M.; Takada, S.; Yamashita, Y.; Ishikawa, S.; Fujiwara, S.; Watanabe, H.; Kurashina, K.; Hatanaka, H.; et al. Identification of the transforming EML4-ALK fusion gene in non-small-cell lung cancer. *Nature* **2007**, *448*, 561–566. [CrossRef]

71. Shaw, A.T.; Yeap, B.Y.; Mino-Kenudson, M.; Digumarthy, S.R.; Costa, D.B.; Heist, R.S.; Solomon, B.; Stubbs, H.; Admane, S.; McDermott, U.; et al. Clinical features and outcome of patients with non-small-cell lung cancer who harbor EML4-ALK. *J. Clin. Oncol.* **2009**, *27*, 4247–4253. [CrossRef]

72. Koivunen, J.P.; Mermel, C.; Zejnullahu, K.; Murphy, C.; Lifshits, E.; Holmes, A.J.; Choi, H.G.; Kim, J.; Chiang, D.; Thomas, R.; et al. EML4-ALK fusion gene and efficacy of an ALK kinase inhibitor in lung cancer. *Clin. Cancer Res.* **2008**, *14*, 4275–4283. [CrossRef]

73. Liao, B.C.; Lin, C.C.; Shih, J.Y.; Yang, J.C. Treating patients with ALK-positive non-small cell lung cancer: Latest evidence and management strategy. *Ther. Adv. Med. Oncol.* **2015**, *7*, 274–290. [CrossRef] [PubMed]

74. Choi, Y.L.; Soda, M.; Yamashita, Y.; Ueno, T.; Takashima, J.; Nakajima, T.; Yatabe, Y.; Takeuchi, K.; Hamada, T.; Haruta, H.; et al. EML4-ALK mutations in lung cancer that confer resistance to ALK inhibitors. *N. Engl. J. Med.* **2010**, *363*, 1734–1739. [CrossRef] [PubMed]

75. Sasaki, T.; Koivunen, J.; Ogino, A.; Yanagita, M.; Nikiforow, S.; Zheng, W.; Lathan, C.; Marcoux, J.P.; Du, J.; Okuda, K.; et al. A novel ALK secondary mutation and EGFR signaling cause resistance to ALK kinase inhibitors. *Cancer Res.* **2011**, *71*, 6051–6060. [CrossRef]

76. Lovly, C.M.; Pao, W. Escaping ALK inhibition: Mechanisms of and strategies to overcome resistance. *Sci. Transl. Med.* **2012**, *4*, 120ps122. [CrossRef] [PubMed]

77. Katayama, R.; Shaw, A.T.; Khan, T.M.; Mino-Kenudson, M.; Solomon, B.J.; Halmos, B.; Jessop, N.A.; Wain, J.C.; Yeo, A.T.; Benes, C.; et al. Mechanisms of acquired crizotinib resistance in ALK-rearranged lung Cancers. *Sci. Transl. Med.* **2012**, *4*, 120ra117. [CrossRef]

78. Katayama, R.; Khan, T.M.; Benes, C.; Lifshits, E.; Ebi, H.; Rivera, V.M.; Shakespeare, W.C.; Iafrate, A.J.; Engelman, J.A.; Shaw, A.T. Therapeutic strategies to overcome crizotinib resistance in non-small cell lung cancers harboring the fusion oncogene EML4-ALK. *Proc. Natl. Acad. Sci. USA* **2011**, *108*, 7535–7540. [CrossRef]

79. Doebele, R.C.; Pilling, A.B.; Aisner, D.L.; Kutateladze, T.G.; Le, A.T.; Weickhardt, A.J.; Kondo, K.L.; Linderman, D.J.; Heasley, L.E.; Franklin, W.A.; et al. Mechanisms of resistance to crizotinib in patients with ALK gene rearranged non-small cell lung cancer. *Clin. Cancer Res.* **2012**, *18*, 1472–1482. [CrossRef]

80. Shaw, A.T.; Kim, D.-W.; Mehra, R.; Tan, D.S.W.; Felip, E.; Chow, L.Q.M.; Camidge, D.R.; Vansteenkiste, J.; Sharma, S.; De Pas, T.; et al. Ceritinib in ALK-Rearranged Non–Small-Cell Lung Cancer. *N. Engl. J. Med.* **2014**, *370*, 1189–1197. [CrossRef]

81. Camidge, D.R.; Dziadziuszko, R.; Peters, S.; Mok, T.; Noe, J.; Nowicka, M.; Gadgeel, S.M.; Cheema, P.; Pavlakis, N.; de Marinis, F.; et al. Updated Efficacy and Safety Data and Impact of the EML4-ALK Fusion Variant on the Efficacy of Alectinib in Untreated ALK-Positive Advanced Non-Small Cell Lung Cancer in the Global Phase III ALEX Study. *J. Thorac Oncol.* **2019**, *14*, 1233–1243. [CrossRef]

82. Hida, T.; Nokihara, H.; Kondo, M.; Kim, Y.H.; Azuma, K.; Seto, T.; Takiguchi, Y.; Nishio, M.; Yoshioka, H.; Imamura, F.; et al. Alectinib versus crizotinib in patients with ALK-positive non-small-cell lung cancer (J-ALEX): An open-label, randomised phase 3 trial. *Lancet* **2017**, *390*, 29–39. [CrossRef]

83. Peters, S.; Camidge, D.R.; Shaw, A.T.; Gadgeel, S.; Ahn, J.S.; Kim, D.-W.; Ou, S.-H.I.; Pérol, M.; Dziadziuszko, R.; Rosell, R.; et al. Alectinib versus Crizotinib in Untreated ALK-Positive Non–Small-Cell Lung Cancer. *N. Engl. J. Med.* **2017**, *377*, 829–838. [CrossRef] [PubMed]

84. Zhang, S.; Anjum, R.; Squillace, R.; Nadworny, S.; Zhou, T.; Keats, J.; Ning, Y.; Wardwell, S.D.; Miller, D.; Song, Y.; et al. The Potent ALK Inhibitor Brigatinib (AP26113) Overcomes Mechanisms of Resistance to First- and Second-Generation ALK Inhibitors in Preclinical Models. *Clin. Cancer Res.* **2016**, *22*, 5527–5538. [CrossRef] [PubMed]

85. Amanam, I.; Gupta, R.; Mambetsariev, I.; Salgia, R. The brigatinib experience: A new generation of therapy for ALK-positive non-small-cell lung cancer. *Future Oncol.* **2018**, *14*, 1897–1908. [CrossRef]

86. Kim, D.W.; Tiseo, M.; Ahn, M.J.; Reckamp, K.L.; Hansen, K.H.; Kim, S.W.; Huber, R.M.; West, H.L.; Groen, H.J.M.; Hochmair, M.J.; et al. Brigatinib in Patients With Crizotinib-Refractory Anaplastic Lymphoma Kinase-Positive Non-Small-Cell Lung Cancer: A Randomized, Multicenter Phase II Trial. *J. Clin. Oncol.* **2017**, *35*, 2490–2498. [CrossRef] [PubMed]

87. Sakamoto, H.; Tsukaguchi, T.; Hiroshima, S.; Kodama, T.; Kobayashi, T.; Fukami, T.A.; Oikawa, N.; Tsukuda, T.; Ishii, N.; Aoki, Y. CH5424802, a selective ALK inhibitor capable of blocking the resistant gatekeeper mutant. *Cancer Cell.* **2011**, *19*, 679–690. [CrossRef]

88. Rivera, V.M.; Wang, F.; Anjum, R.; Zhang, S.; Squillace, R.; Keats, J.; Miller, D.; Ning, Y.; Wardwell, S.D.; Moran, L.; et al. Abstract 1794: AP26113 is a dual ALK/EGFR inhibitor: Characterization against EGFR T790M in cell and mouse models of NSCLC. *Cancer Res.* **2012**, *72*, 1794. [CrossRef]

89. Camidge, R.; Kim, H.R.; Ahn, M.J.; Yang, J.C.H.; Han, J.Y.; Hochmair, M.J.; Lee, K.H.; Delmonte, A.; Garcia Campelo, M.R.; Kim, D.W.; et al. Brigatinib vs crizotinib in patients with ALK inhibitor-naive advanced ALK+ NSCLC: Updated results from the phase III ALTA-1L trial. *Ann. Oncol.* **2019**, *30*, ix195–ix196. [CrossRef]

90. Horn, L.; Infante, J.R.; Reckamp, K.L.; Blumenschein, G.R.; Leal, T.A.; Waqar, S.N.; Gitlitz, B.J.; Sanborn, R.E.; Whisenant, J.G.; Du, L.; et al. Ensartinib (X-396) in ALK-Positive Non–Small Cell Lung Cancer: Results from a First-in-Human Phase I/II, Multicenter Study. *Clin. Cancer Res.* **2018**, *24*, 2771–2779. [CrossRef]

91. Shaw, A.T.; Solomon, B.J.; Besse, B.; Bauer, T.M.; Lin, C.C.; Soo, R.A.; Riely, G.J.; Ou, S.I.; Clancy, J.S.; Li, S.; et al. ALK Resistance Mutations and Efficacy of Lorlatinib in Advanced Anaplastic Lymphoma Kinase-Positive Non-Small-Cell Lung Cancer. *J. Clin. Oncol.* **2019**, *37*, 1370–1379. [CrossRef]

92. Barrows, S.M.; Wright, K.; Copley-Merriman, C.; Kaye, J.A.; Chioda, M.; Wiltshire, R.; Torgersen, K.M.; Masters, E.T. Systematic review of sequencing of ALK inhibitors in ALK-positive non-small-cell lung cancer. *Lung Cancer (Auckl)* **2019**, *10*, 11–20. [CrossRef]

93. Xu, H.; Ma, D.; Yang, G.; Li, J.; Hao, X.; Xing, P.; Yang, L.; Xu, F.; Wang, Y. Sequential therapy according to distinct disease progression patterns in advanced ALK-positive non-small-cell lung cancer after crizotinib treatment. *Chin. J. Cancer Res.* **2019**, *31*, 349–356. [CrossRef]

94. Illei, P.B.; Wong, W.; Wu, N.; Chu, L.; Gupta, R.; Schulze, K.; Gubens, M.A. ALK Testing Trends and Patterns Among Community Practices in the United States. *JCO Precis. Oncol.* **2018**, *2*, 1–11. [CrossRef]

95. Hussein, M.; Richards, D.A.; Ulrich, B.; Korytowsky, B.; Pandya, D.; Cogswell, J.; Batenchuk, C.; Burns, V. ORAL01.02: Biopsies in Initial Diagnosis of Non–Small Cell Lung Cancer in US Community Oncology Practices: Implications for First-Line Immunotherapy: Topic: Medical Oncology. *J. Thorac. Oncol.* **2016**, *11*, S249–S250. [CrossRef]

96. Leighl, N.B.; Page, R.D.; Raymond, V.M.; Daniel, D.B.; Divers, S.G.; Reckamp, K.L.; Villalona-Calero, M.A.; Dix, D.; Odegaard, J.I.; Lanman, R.B.; et al. Clinical Utility of Comprehensive Cell-Free DNA Analysis to Identify Genomic Biomarkers in Patients with Newly Diagnosed Metastatic Non-Small Cell Lung Cancer. *Clin. Cancer Res.* **2019**. [CrossRef] [PubMed]

97. Rikova, K.; Guo, A.; Zeng, Q.; Possemato, A.; Yu, J.; Haack, H.; Nardone, J.; Lee, K.; Reeves, C.; Li, Y.; et al. Global survey of phosphotyrosine signaling identifies oncogenic kinases in lung cancer. *Cell* **2007**, *131*, 1190–1203. [CrossRef] [PubMed]

98. Korpanty, G.J.; Graham, D.M.; Vincent, M.D.; Leighl, N.B. Biomarkers That Currently Affect Clinical Practice in Lung Cancer: EGFR, ALK, MET, ROS-1, and KRAS. *Front. Oncol.* **2014**, *4*, 204. [CrossRef] [PubMed]

99. Gainor, J.F.; Tseng, D.; Yoda, S.; Dagogo-Jack, I.; Friboulet, L.; Lin, J.J.; Hubbeling, H.G.; Dardaei, L.; Farago, A.F.; Schultz, K.R.; et al. Patterns of Metastatic Spread and Mechanisms of Resistance to Crizotinib in ROS1-Positive Non-Small-Cell Lung Cancer. *JCO Precis Oncol.* **2017**, *2017*. [CrossRef] [PubMed]

100. Dagogo-Jack, I.; Shaw, A.T. Expanding the Roster of ROS1 Inhibitors. *J. Clin. Oncol.* **2017**, *35*, 2595–2597. [CrossRef]

101. Shaw, A.T.; Ou, S.H.; Bang, Y.J.; Camidge, D.R.; Solomon, B.J.; Salgia, R.; Riely, G.J.; Varella-Garcia, M.; Shapiro, G.I.; Costa, D.B.; et al. Crizotinib in ROS1-rearranged non-small-cell lung cancer. *N. Engl. J. Med.* **2014**, *371*, 1963–1971. [CrossRef]

102. Lim, S.M.; Kim, H.R.; Lee, J.S.; Lee, K.H.; Lee, Y.G.; Min, Y.J.; Cho, E.K.; Lee, S.S.; Kim, B.S.; Choi, M.Y.; et al. Open-Label, Multicenter, Phase II Study of Ceritinib in Patients With Non-Small-Cell Lung Cancer Harboring ROS1 Rearrangement. *J. Clin. Oncol.* **2017**, *35*, 2613–2618. [CrossRef]

103. Doebele, R.; Ahn, M.; Siena, S.; Drilon, A.; Krebs, M.; Lin, C.; De Braud, F.; John, T.; Tan, D.; Seto, T.; et al. OA02.01 Efficacy and Safety of Entrectinib in Locally Advanced or Metastatic ROS1 Fusion-Positive Non-Small Cell Lung Cancer (NSCLC). *J. Thorac. Oncol.* **2018**, *13*, S321–S322. [CrossRef]

104. Ou, S.; Shaw, A.; Riely, G.; Chiari, R.; Bauman, J.; Clancy, J.; Thurm, H.; Peltz, G.; Abbattista, A.; Solomon, B. OA02.03 Clinical Activity of Lorlatinib in Patients with ROS1+ Advanced Non-Small Cell Lung Cancer: Phase 2 Study Cohort EXP-6. *J. Thorac. Oncol.* **2018**, *13*, S322–S323. [CrossRef]

105. Research, F.o.C. Trends in the Molecular Diagnosis of Lung Cancer, Results from an Online Market Research Survey. Available online: https://www.focr.org/sites/default/files/pdf/FINAL%202017%20Friends%20NSCLC%20White%20Paper.pdf (accessed on 20 May 2020).

106. Nadler, E.; Pavilack, M.; Clark, J.; Espirito, J.; Fernandes, A. Biomarker Testing Rates in Patients with Advanced Non-Small Cell Lung Cancer Treated in the Community. *J. Cancer Ther.* **2019**, *10*, 971–984. [CrossRef]

107. Rijavec, E.; Coco, S.; Genova, C.; Rossi, G.; Longo, L.; Grossi, F. Liquid Biopsy in Non-Small Cell Lung Cancer: Highlights and Challenges. *Cancers (Basel)* **2019**, *12*, 17. [CrossRef] [PubMed]

108. de Melo Gagliato, D.; Jardim, D.L.F.; Falchook, G.; Tang, C.; Zinner, R.; Wheler, J.J.; Janku, F.; Subbiah, V.; Piha-Paul, S.A.; Fu, S.; et al. Analysis of MET genetic aberrations in patients with breast cancer at MD Anderson Phase I unit. *Clin. Breast Cancer* **2014**, *14*, 468–474. [CrossRef] [PubMed]

109. Cappuzzo, F.; Marchetti, A.; Skokan, M.; Rossi, E.; Gajapathy, S.; Felicioni, L.; Del Grammastro, M.; Sciarrotta, M.G.; Buttitta, F.; Incarbone, M.; et al. Increased MET gene copy number negatively affects survival of surgically resected non-small-cell lung cancer patients. *J. Clin. Oncol. Off. J. Am. Soc. Clin. Oncol.* **2009**, *27*, 1667–1674. [CrossRef] [PubMed]

110. Carracedo, A.; Egervari, K.; Salido, M.; Rojo, F.; Corominas, J.M.; Arumi, M.; Corzo, C.; Tusquets, I.; Espinet, B.; Rovira, A.; et al. FISH and immunohistochemical status of the hepatocyte growth factor receptor (c-Met) in 184 invasive breast tumors. *Breast Cancer Res.* **2009**, *11*, 402. [CrossRef]

111. Drilon, A.; Cappuzzo, F.; Ou, S.-H.I.; Camidge, D.R. Targeting MET in Lung Cancer: Will Expectations Finally Be MET? *J. Thorac. Oncol.* **2017**, *12*, 15–26. [CrossRef]

112. Ghadjar, P.; Blank-Liss, W.; Simcock, M.; Hegyi, I.; Beer, K.T.; Moch, H.; Aebersold, D.M.; Zimmer, Y. MET Y1253D-activating point mutation and development of distant metastasis in advanced head and neck cancers. *Clin. Exp. Metastasis* **2009**, *26*, 809–815. [CrossRef]

113. Cipriani, N.A.; Abidoye, O.O.; Vokes, E.; Salgia, R. MET as a target for treatment of chest tumors. *Lung Cancer* **2009**, *63*, 169–179. [CrossRef]

114. Schmidt, L.; Duh, F.M.; Chen, F.; Kishida, T.; Glenn, G.; Choyke, P.; Scherer, S.W.; Zhuang, Z.; Lubensky, I.; Dean, M.; et al. Germline and somatic mutations in the tyrosine kinase domain of the MET proto-oncogene in papillary renal carcinomas. *Nat. Genet.* **1997**, *16*, 68–73. [CrossRef] [PubMed]

115. Ma, P.C.; Jagadeeswaran, R.; Jagadeesh, S.; Tretiakova, M.S.; Nallasura, V.; Fox, E.A.; Hansen, M.; Schaefer, E.; Naoki, K.; Lader, A.; et al. Functional expression and mutations of c-Met and its therapeutic inhibition with SU11274 and small interfering RNA in non-small cell lung cancer. *Cancer Res.* **2005**, *65*, 1479–1488. [CrossRef]

116. Ma, P.C.; Kijima, T.; Maulik, G.; Fox, E.A.; Sattler, M.; Griffin, J.D.; Johnson, B.E.; Salgia, R. c-MET mutational analysis in small cell lung cancer: Novel juxtamembrane domain mutations regulating cytoskeletal functions. *Cancer Res.* **2003**, *63*, 6272–6281. [PubMed]

117. Comprehensive molecular profiling of lung adenocarcinoma. *Nature* **2014**, *511*, 543–550. [CrossRef] [PubMed]

118. Comprehensive genomic characterization of squamous cell lung cancers. *Nature* **2012**, *489*, 519–525. [CrossRef]

119. Paik, P.K.; Drilon, A.; Fan, P.-D.; Yu, H.; Rekhtman, N.; Ginsberg, M.S.; Borsu, L.; Schultz, N.; Berger, M.F.; Rudin, C.M.; et al. Response to MET Inhibitors in Patients with Stage IV Lung Adenocarcinomas Harboring MET Mutations Causing Exon 14 Skipping. *Cancer Discov.* **2015**, *5*, 842–849. [CrossRef]

120. Drilon, A.; Clark, J.W.; Weiss, J.; Ou, S.I.; Camidge, D.R.; Solomon, B.J.; Otterson, G.A.; Villaruz, L.C.; Riely, G.J.; Heist, R.S.; et al. Antitumor activity of crizotinib in lung cancers harboring a MET exon 14 alteration. *Nat. Med.* **2020**, *26*, 47–51. [CrossRef]

121. Felip, E.; Horn, L.; Patel, J.D.; Sakai, H.; Scheele, J.; Bruns, R.; Paik, P.K. Tepotinib in patients with advanced non-small cell lung cancer (NSCLC) harboring MET exon 14-skipping mutations: Phase II trial. *J. Clin. Oncol.* **2018**, *36*, 9016. [CrossRef]

122. Nakamura, Y.; Niki, T.; Goto, A.; Morikawa, T.; Miyazawa, K.; Nakajima, J.; Fukayama, M. c-Met activation in lung adenocarcinoma tissues: An immunohistochemical analysis. *Cancer Sci* **2007**, *98*, 1006–1013. [CrossRef]

123. Cappuzzo, F.; Janne, P.A.; Skokan, M.; Finocchiaro, G.; Rossi, E.; Ligorio, C.; Zucali, P.A.; Terracciano, L.; Toschi, L.; Roncalli, M.; et al. MET increased gene copy number and primary resistance to gefitinib therapy in non-small-cell lung cancer patients. *Ann. Oncol.* **2009**, *20*, 298–304. [CrossRef]

124. Strickler, J.H.; Weekes, C.D.; Nemunaitis, J.; Ramanathan, R.K.; Heist, R.S.; Morgensztern, D.; Angevin, E.; Bauer, T.M.; Yue, H.; Motwani, M.; et al. First-in-Human Phase I, Dose-Escalation and -Expansion Study of Telisotuzumab Vedotin, an Antibody-Drug Conjugate Targeting c-Met, in Patients With Advanced Solid Tumors. *J. Clin. Oncol.* **2018**, *36*, 3298–3306. [CrossRef] [PubMed]

125. Wang, R.; Hu, H.; Pan, Y.; Li, Y.; Ye, T.; Li, C.; Luo, X.; Wang, L.; Li, H.; Zhang, Y.; et al. RET fusions define a unique molecular and clinicopathologic subtype of non-small-cell lung cancer. *J. Clin. Oncol.* **2012**, *30*, 4352–4359. [CrossRef] [PubMed]

126. Drilon, A.; Rekhtman, N.; Arcila, M.; Wang, L.; Ni, A.; Albano, M.; Van Voorthuysen, M.; Somwar, R.; Smith, R.S.; Montecalvo, J.; et al. Cabozantinib in patients with advanced RET-rearranged non-small-cell lung cancer: An open-label, single-centre, phase 2, single-arm trial. *Lancet Oncol.* **2016**, *17*, 1653–1660. [CrossRef]

127. Gainor, J.F.; Lee, D.H.; Curigliano, G.; Doebele, R.C.; Kim, D.-W.; Baik, C.S.; Tan, D.S.-W.; Lopes, G.; Gadgeel, S.M.; Cassier, P.A.; et al. Clinical activity and tolerability of BLU-667, a highly potent and selective RET inhibitor, in patients (pts) with advanced RET-fusion+ non-small cell lung cancer (NSCLC). *J. Clin. Oncol.* **2019**, *37*, 9008. [CrossRef]

128. Nakagawara, A. Trk receptor tyrosine kinases: A bridge between cancer and neural development. *Cancer Lett.* **2001**, *169*, 107–114. [CrossRef]

129. Vaishnavi, A.; Capelletti, M.; Le, A.T.; Kako, S.; Butaney, M.; Ercan, D.; Mahale, S.; Davies, K.D.; Aisner, D.L.; Pilling, A.B.; et al. Oncogenic and drug-sensitive NTRK1 rearrangements in lung cancer. *Nat. Med.* **2013**, *19*, 1469–1472. [CrossRef]

130. Doebele, R.C.; Drilon, A.; Paz-Ares, L.; Siena, S.; Shaw, A.T.; Farago, A.F.; Blakely, C.M.; Seto, T.; Cho, B.C.; Tosi, D.; et al. Entrectinib in patients with advanced or metastatic NTRK fusion-positive solid tumours: Integrated analysis of three phase 1-2 trials. *Lancet Oncol.* **2020**, *21*, 271–282. [CrossRef]

131. Drilon, A.; Li, G.; Dogan, S.; Gounder, M.; Shen, R.; Arcila, M.; Wang, L.; Hyman, D.M.; Hechtman, J.; Wei, G.; et al. What hides behind the MASC: Clinical response and acquired resistance to entrectinib after ETV6-NTRK3 identification in a mammary analogue secretory carcinoma (MASC). *Ann. Oncol.* **2016**, *27*, 920–926. [CrossRef]

132. Russo, M.; Misale, S.; Wei, G.; Siravegna, G.; Crisafulli, G.; Lazzari, L.; Corti, G.; Rospo, G.; Novara, L.; Mussolin, B.; et al. Acquired Resistance to the TRK Inhibitor Entrectinib in Colorectal Cancer. *Cancer Discov.* **2016**, *6*, 36–44. [CrossRef]

133. Drilon, A.; Nagasubramanian, R.; Blake, J.F.; Ku, N.; Tuch, B.B.; Ebata, K.; Smith, S.; Lauriault, V.; Kolakowski, G.R.; Brandhuber, B.J.; et al. A Next-Generation TRK Kinase Inhibitor Overcomes Acquired Resistance to Prior TRK Kinase Inhibition in Patients with TRK Fusion–Positive Solid Tumors. *Cancer Discov.* **2017**, *7*, 963–972. [CrossRef]

134. Hyman, D.; Kummar, S.; Farago, A.; Geoerger, B.; Mau-Sorensen, M.; Taylor, M.; Garralda, E.; Nagasubramanian, R.; Natheson, M.; Song, L.; et al. Abstract CT127: Phase I and expanded access experience of LOXO-195 (BAY 2731954), a selective next-generation TRK inhibitor (TRKi). *Cancer Res.* **2019**, *79*, CT127. [CrossRef]

135. Marchetti, A.; Felicioni, L.; Malatesta, S.; Sciarrotta, M.G.; Guetti, L.; Chella, A.; Viola, P.; Pullara, C.; Mucilli, F.; Buttitta, F. Clinical Features and Outcome of Patients With Non–Small-Cell Lung Cancer Harboring BRAF Mutations. *J. Clin. Oncol.* **2011**, *29*, 3574–3579. [CrossRef] [PubMed]

136. Planchard, D.; Smit, E.F.; Groen, H.J.M.; Mazieres, J.; Besse, B.; Helland, Å.; Giannone, V.; D'Amelio, A.M., Jr.; Zhang, P.; Mookerjee, B.; et al. Dabrafenib plus trametinib in patients with previously untreated BRAF(V600E)-mutant metastatic non-small-cell lung cancer: An open-label, phase 2 trial. *Lancet Oncol.* **2017**, *18*, 1307–1316. [CrossRef]

137. Mao, C.; Qiu, L.X.; Liao, R.Y.; Du, F.B.; Ding, H.; Yang, W.C.; Li, J.; Chen, Q. KRAS mutations and resistance to EGFR-TKIs treatment in patients with non-small cell lung cancer: A meta-analysis of 22 studies. *Lung Cancer* **2010**, *69*, 272–278. [CrossRef] [PubMed]

138. Johnson, M.L.; Sima, C.S.; Chaft, J.; Paik, P.K.; Pao, W.; Kris, M.G.; Ladanyi, M.; Riely, G.J. Association of KRAS and EGFR mutations with survival in patients with advanced lung adenocarcinomas. *Cancer* **2013**, *119*, 356–362. [CrossRef]

139. Shepherd, F.A.; Lacas, B.; Le Teuff, G.; Hainaut, P.; Janne, P.A.; Pignon, J.P.; Le Chevalier, T.; Seymour, L.; Douillard, J.Y.; Graziano, S.; et al. Pooled Analysis of the Prognostic and Predictive Effects of TP53 Comutation Status Combined With KRAS or EGFR Mutation in Early-Stage Resected Non-Small-Cell Lung Cancer in Four Trials of Adjuvant Chemotherapy. *J. Clin. Oncol.* **2017**, *35*, 2018–2027. [CrossRef]

140. AACR Project GENIE: Powering Precision Medicine through an International Consortium. *Cancer Discov.* **2017**, *7*, 818–831. [CrossRef]

141. Christensen, J.G.; Hallin, J.; Engstrom, L.D.; Hargis, L.; Calinisan, A.; Aranda, R.; Briere, D.M.; Sudhakar, N.; Bowcut, V.; Baer, B.R.; et al. The KRASG12C Inhibitor, MRTX849, Provides Insight Toward Therapeutic Susceptibility of KRAS Mutant Cancers in Mouse Models and Patients. *Cancer Discov.* **2019**, *10*, 54–71. [CrossRef]

142. Khozin, S.; Abernethy, A.P.; Nussbaum, N.C.; Zhi, J.; Curtis, M.D.; Tucker, M.; Lee, S.E.; Light, D.E.; Gossai, A.; Sorg, R.A.; et al. Characteristics of Real-World Metastatic Non-Small Cell Lung Cancer Patients Treated with Nivolumab and Pembrolizumab During the Year Following Approval. *Oncologist* **2018**, *23*, 328–336. [CrossRef]

143. Nadler, E.; Espirito, J.L.; Pavilack, M.; Boyd, M.; Vergara-Silva, A.; Fernandes, A. Treatment Patterns and Clinical Outcomes Among Metastatic Non-Small-Cell Lung Cancer Patients Treated in the Community Practice Setting. *Clin. Lung Cancer* **2018**, *19*, 360–370. [CrossRef] [PubMed]

144. Fehrenbacher, L.; Spira, A.; Ballinger, M.; Kowanetz, M.; Vansteenkiste, J.; Mazieres, J.; Park, K.; Smith, D.; Artal-Cortes, A.; Lewanski, C.; et al. Atezolizumab versus docetaxel for patients with previously treated non-small-cell lung cancer (POPLAR): A multicentre, open-label, phase 2 randomised controlled trial. *Lancet* **2016**, *387*, 1837–1846. [CrossRef]

145. Reck, M.; Rodríguez-Abreu, D.; Robinson, A.G.; Hui, R.; Csőszi, T.; Fülöp, A.; Gottfried, M.; Peled, N.; Tafreshi, A.; Cuffe, S.; et al. Updated Analysis of KEYNOTE-024: Pembrolizumab Versus Platinum-Based Chemotherapy for Advanced Non-Small-Cell Lung Cancer With PD-L1 Tumor Proportion Score of 50% or Greater. *J. Clin. Oncol.* **2019**, *37*, 537–546. [CrossRef] [PubMed]

146. Zhou, Y.; Lin, Z.; Zhang, X.; Chen, C.; Zhao, H.; Hong, S.; Zhang, L. First-line treatment for patients with advanced non-small cell lung carcinoma and high PD-L1 expression: Pembrolizumab or pembrolizumab plus chemotherapy. *J. Immunother. Cancer* **2019**, *7*, 120. [CrossRef] [PubMed]

147. Gandhi, L.; Rodríguez-Abreu, D.; Gadgeel, S.; Esteban, E.; Felip, E.; De Angelis, F.; Domine, M.; Clingan, P.; Hochmair, M.J.; Powell, S.F.; et al. Pembrolizumab plus Chemotherapy in Metastatic Non–Small-Cell Lung Cancer. *N. Engl. J. Med.* **2018**, *378*, 2078–2092. [CrossRef]

148. Hellmann, M.D.; Paz-Ares, L.; Bernabe Caro, R.; Zurawski, B.; Kim, S.-W.; Carcereny Costa, E.; Park, K.; Alexandru, A.; Lupinacci, L.; de la Mora Jimenez, E.; et al. Nivolumab plus Ipilimumab in Advanced Non–Small-Cell Lung Cancer. *N. Engl. J. Med.* **2019**, *381*, 2020–2031. [CrossRef]

149. Rizvi, N.A.; Cho, B.C.; Reinmuth, N.; Lee, K.H.; Luft, A.; Ahn, M.J.; van den Heuvel, M.M.; Cobo, M.; Vicente, D.; Smolin, A.; et al. Durvalumab With or Without Tremelimumab vs Standard Chemotherapy in First-line Treatment of Metastatic Non-Small Cell Lung Cancer: The MYSTIC Phase 3 Randomized Clinical Trial. *JAMA Oncol.* **2020**, *6*, 661–674. [CrossRef]

150. Theelen, W.S.M.E.; Baas, P. Pembrolizumab monotherapy for PD-L1 ≥50% non-small cell lung cancer, undisputed first choice? *Ann. Transl. Med.* **2019**, *7*, S140. [CrossRef]

151. Velcheti, V.; Chandwani, S.; Chen, X.; Pietanza, M.C.; Piperdi, B.; Burke, T. Outcomes of first-line pembrolizumab monotherapy for PD-L1-positive (TPS ≥50%) metastatic NSCLC at US oncology practices. *Immunotherapy* **2019**, *11*, 1541–1554. [CrossRef]

152. Shivakumar, L.; Weldon, C.B.; Lucas, L.; Perloff, T. Identifying obstacles to optimal integration of cancer immunotherapies in the community setting. *J. Clin. Oncol.* **2019**, *37*, 87. [CrossRef]

153. Krimphove, M.J.; Tully, K.H.; Friedlander, D.F.; Marchese, M.; Ravi, P.; Lipsitz, S.R.; Kilbridge, K.L.; Kibel, A.S.; Kluth, L.A.; Ott, P.A.; et al. Adoption of immunotherapy in the community for patients diagnosed with metastatic melanoma. *J. Immunother. Cancer* **2019**, *7*, 289. [CrossRef]

154. Ancevski Hunter, K.; Socinski, M.A.; Villaruz, L.C. PD-L1 Testing in Guiding Patient Selection for PD-1/PD-L1 Inhibitor Therapy in Lung Cancer. *Mol. Diagn. Ther.* **2018**, *22*, 1–10. [CrossRef] [PubMed]

155. Roach, C.; Zhang, N.; Corigliano, E.; Jansson, M.; Toland, G.; Ponto, G.; Dolled-Filhart, M.; Emancipator, K.; Stanforth, D.; Kulangara, K. Development of a Companion Diagnostic PD-L1 Immunohistochemistry Assay for Pembrolizumab Therapy in Non-Small-cell Lung Cancer. *Appl. Immunohistochem. Mol. Morphol. AIMM* **2016**, *24*, 392–397. [CrossRef] [PubMed]

156. Büttner, R.; Gosney, J.R.; Skov, B.G.; Adam, J.; Motoi, N.; Bloom, K.J.; Dietel, M.; Longshore, J.W.; López-Ríos, F.; Penault-Llorca, F.; et al. Programmed Death-Ligand 1 Immunohistochemistry Testing: A Review of Analytical Assays and Clinical Implementation in Non-Small-Cell Lung Cancer. *J. Clin. Oncol.* **2017**, *35*, 3867–3876. [CrossRef]

157. Rittmeyer, A.; Barlesi, F.; Waterkamp, D.; Park, K.; Ciardiello, F.; von Pawel, J.; Gadgeel, S.M.; Hida, T.; Kowalski, D.M.; Dols, M.C.; et al. Atezolizumab versus docetaxel in patients with previously treated non-small-cell lung cancer (OAK): A phase 3, open-label, multicentre randomised controlled trial. *Lancet* **2017**, *389*, 255–265. [CrossRef]

158. Velcheti, V.; Patwardhan, P.D.; Liu, F.X.; Chen, X.; Cao, X.; Burke, T. Real-world PD-L1 testing and distribution of PD-L1 tumor expression by immunohistochemistry assay type among patients with metastatic non-small cell lung cancer in the United States. *PLoS ONE* **2018**, *13*, e0206370. [CrossRef]

159. Gong, J.; Pan, K.; Fakih, M.; Pal, S.; Salgia, R. Value-based genomics. *Oncotarget Adv. Publ.* **2018**, *9*, 15792. [CrossRef] [PubMed]

160. Ellis, L.M.; Bernstein, D.S.; Voest, E.E.; Berlin, J.D.; Sargent, D.; Cortazar, P.; Garrett-Mayer, E.; Herbst, R.S.; Lilenbaum, R.C.; Sima, C.; et al. American Society of Clinical Oncology perspective: Raising the bar for clinical trials by defining clinically meaningful outcomes. *J. Clin. Oncol.* **2014**, *32*, 1277–1280. [CrossRef]

161. Chu, L.; Kelly, K.; Gandara, D.; Lara, P.; Borowsky, A.; Meyers, F.; McPherson, J.; Erlich, R.; Almog, N.; Schrock, A.; et al. P3.13-26 Outcomes of Patients with Metastatic Lung Cancer Presented in a Multidisciplinary Molecular Tumor Board. *J. Thoracic Oncol.* **2018**, *13*, S986. [CrossRef]

162. Koopman, B.; Wekken, A.J.v.d.; Elst, A.t.; Hiltermann, T.J.N.; Vilacha, J.F.; Groves, M.R.; Berg, A.v.d.; Hiddinga, B.I.; Hijmering-Kappelle, L.B.M.; Stigt, J.A.; et al. Relevance and Effectiveness of Molecular Tumor Board Recommendations for Patients With Non–Small-Cell Lung Cancer With Rare or Complex Mutational Profiles. *JCO Precis. Oncol.* **2020**, *4*, 393–410. [CrossRef]

163. Planchard, D.; Faivre, L.; Sullivan, I.; Kahn-charpy, V.; Lacroix, L.; Auger, N.; Adam, J.; De Montpreville, V.T.; Dorfmuller, P.; Pechoux, C.L.; et al. 3081 Molecular Tumor Board (MTB) in non-small cell lung cancers (NSCLC) to optimize targeted therapies: 4 years' experience at Gustave Roussy. *Eur. J. Cancer* **2015**, *51*, S624. [CrossRef]

164. Rolfo, C.; Manca, P.; Salgado, R.; Van Dam, P.; Dendooven, A.; Machado Coelho, A.; Ferri Gandia, J.; Rutten, A.; Lybaert, W.; Vermeij, J.; et al. Multidisciplinary molecular tumour board: A tool to improve clinical practice and selection accrual for clinical trials in patients with cancer. *ESMO Open* **2018**, *3*, e000398. [CrossRef]

165. Pishvaian, M.J.; Blais, E.M.; Bender, R.J.; Rao, S.; Boca, S.M.; Chung, V.; Hendifar, A.E.; Mikhail, S.; Sohal, D.P.S.; Pohlmann, P.R.; et al. A virtual molecular tumor board to improve efficiency and scalability of delivering precision oncology to physicians and their patients. *JAMIA Open* **2019**, *2*, 505–515. [CrossRef]

166. Lesslie, M.; Parikh, J.R. Implementing a Multidisciplinary Tumor Board in the Community Practice Setting. *Diagnostics (Basel)* **2017**, *7*, 55. [CrossRef] [PubMed]

167. El-Deiry, W.S.; Goldberg, R.M.; Lenz, H.-J.; Shields, A.F.; Gibney, G.T.; Tan, A.R.; Brown, J.; Eisenberg, B.; Heath, E.I.; Phuphanich, S.; et al. The current state of molecular testing in the treatment of patients with solid tumors, 2019. *CA A Cancer J. Clin.* **2019**, *69*, 305–343. [CrossRef] [PubMed]

168. Wang, T.; Liu, S.; Joseph, T.; Lyou, Y. Managing Bladder Cancer Care during the COVID-19 Pandemic Using a Team-Based Approach. *J. Clin. Med.* **2020**, *9*, 1574. [CrossRef] [PubMed]

169. Bironzo, P.; Di Maio, M. A review of guidelines for lung cancer. *J. Thorac Dis.* **2018**, *10*, S1556–S1563. [CrossRef]

170. Daly, B.; Zon, R.T.; Page, R.D.; Edge, S.B.; Lyman, G.H.; Green, S.R.; Wollins, D.S.; Bosserman, L.D. Oncology Clinical Pathways: Charting the Landscape of Pathway Providers. *J. Oncol. Pract.* **2018**, *14*, e194–e200. [CrossRef]

171. Neubauer, M.A.; Hoverman, J.R.; Kolodziej, M.; Reisman, L.; Gruschkus, S.K.; Hoang, S.; Alva, A.A.; McArthur, M.; Forsyth, M.; Rothermel, T.; et al. Cost effectiveness of evidence-based treatment guidelines for the treatment of non-small-cell lung cancer in the community setting. *J. Oncol. Pract.* **2010**, *6*, 12–18. [CrossRef]

172. Hoverman, J.R.; Cartwright, T.H.; Patt, D.A.; Espirito, J.L.; Clayton, M.P.; Garey, J.S.; Kopp, T.J.; Kolodziej, M.; Neubauer, M.A.; Fitch, K.; et al. Pathways, outcomes, and costs in colon cancer: Retrospective evaluations in two distinct databases. *J. Oncol. Pract.* **2011**, *7*, 52s–59s. [CrossRef]

173. Kreys, E.D.; Koeller, J.M. Documenting the benefits and cost savings of a large multistate cancer pathway program from a payer's perspective. *J. Oncol. Pract.* **2013**, *9*, e241–e247. [CrossRef] [PubMed]

174. Jackman, D.M.; Zhang, Y.; Dalby, C.; Nguyen, T.; Nagle, J.; Lydon, C.A.; Rabin, M.S.; McNiff, K.K.; Fraile, B.; Jacobson, J.O. Cost and Survival Analysis Before and After Implementation of Dana-Farber Clinical Pathways for Patients With Stage IV Non-Small-Cell Lung Cancer. *J. Oncol. Pract.* **2017**, *13*, e346–e352. [CrossRef]

175. Lawal, A.K.; Rotter, T.; Kinsman, L.; Machotta, A.; Ronellenfitsch, U.; Scott, S.D.; Goodridge, D.; Plishka, C.; Groot, G. What is a clinical pathway? Refinement of an operational definition to identify clinical pathway studies for a Cochrane systematic review. *BMC Med.* **2016**, *14*, 35. [CrossRef] [PubMed]

176. Zon, R.T.; Edge, S.B.; Page, R.D.; Frame, J.N.; Lyman, G.H.; Omel, J.L.; Wollins, D.S.; Green, S.R.; Bosserman, L.D. American Society of Clinical Oncology Criteria for High-Quality Clinical Pathways in Oncology. *J. Oncol. Pract.* **2017**, *13*, 207–210. [CrossRef] [PubMed]

177. Comis, R.L.; Miller, J.D.; Aldigé, C.R.; Krebs, L.; Stoval, E. Public attitudes toward participation in cancer clinical trials. *J. Clin. Oncol.* **2003**, *21*, 830–835. [CrossRef] [PubMed]

178. Ohno-Machado, L.; Kim, J.; Gabriel, R.A.; Kuo, G.M.; Hogarth, M.A. Genomics and electronic health record systems. *Hum. Mol. Genet.* **2018**, *27*, R48–R55. [CrossRef] [PubMed]

179. Salgia, N.; Philip, E.; Ziari, M.; Yap, K.; Pal, S. Advancing the Science and Management of Renal Cell Carcinoma: Bridging the Divide between Academic and Community Practices. *J. Clin. Med.* **2020**, *9*, 1508. [CrossRef]

180. Liu, J.; Gutierrez, E.; Tiwari, A.; Padam, S.; Li, D.; Dale, W.; Pal, S.; Stewart, D.; Subbiah, S.; Bosserman, L.; et al. Strategies to Improve Participation of Older Adults in Cancer Research. *J. Clin. Med.* **2020**, *9*, 1571. [CrossRef]

181. Zon, R.T.; Bruinooge, S.S.; Lyss, A.P. The Changing Face of Research in Community Practice. *J. Oncol. Pract.* **2014**, *10*, 155–160. [CrossRef] [PubMed]

182. Geiger, A.M.; O'Mara, A.M.; McCaskill-Stevens, W.J.; Adjei, B.; Tuovenin, P.; Castro, K.M. Evolution of Cancer Care Delivery Research in the NCI Community Oncology Research Program. *JNCI J. Natl. Cancer Inst.* **2019**. [CrossRef]

183. Herbst, R.S.; Morgensztern, D.; Boshoff, C. The biology and management of non-small cell lung cancer. *Nature* **2018**, *553*, 446–454. [CrossRef]

184. Aggarwal, C.; Thompson, J.C.; Black, T.A.; Katz, S.I.; Fan, R.; Yee, S.S.; Chien, A.L.; Evans, T.L.; Bauml, J.M.; Alley, E.W.; et al. Clinical Implications of Plasma-Based Genotyping With the Delivery of Personalized Therapy in Metastatic Non-Small Cell Lung Cancer. *JAMA Oncol.* **2019**, *5*, 173–180. [CrossRef] [PubMed]

185. Jonna, S.; Subramaniam, D.S. Molecular diagnostics and targeted therapies in non-small cell lung cancer (NSCLC): An update. *Discov. Med.* **2019**, *27*, 167–170. [PubMed]

186. Doroshow, D.B.; Herbst, R.S. Treatment of Advanced Non-Small Cell Lung Cancer in 2018. *JAMA Oncol.* **2018**, *4*, 569–570. [CrossRef] [PubMed]

5

Modular Strategies to Build Cell-Free and Cell-Laden Scaffolds towards Bioengineered Tissues and Organs

Aurelio Salerno [1,*], Giuseppe Cesarelli [1,2], Parisa Pedram [1,2] and Paolo Antonio Netti [1,2,3]

[1]   Center for Advanced Biomaterials for Healthcare, Istituto Italiano di Tecnologia (IIT@CRIB), 80125 Naples, Italy; Giuseppe.Cesarelli@unina.it (G.C.); Parisa.Pedram@iit.it (P.P.); nettipa@unina.it (P.A.N.)

[2]   Department of Chemical, Materials and Industrial Production Engineering, University of Naples Federico II, 80125 Naples, Italy

[3]   Interdisciplinary Research Center on Biomaterials (CRIB), University of Naples Federico II, 80125 Naples, Italy

*   Correspondence: asalerno@unina.it

Abstract: Engineering three-dimensional (3D) scaffolds for functional tissue and organ regeneration is a major challenge of the tissue engineering (TE) community. Great progress has been made in developing scaffolds to support cells in 3D, and to date, several implantable scaffolds are available for treating damaged and dysfunctional tissues, such as bone, osteochondral, cardiac and nerve. However, recapitulating the complex extracellular matrix (ECM) functions of native tissues is far from being achieved in synthetic scaffolds. Modular TE is an intriguing approach that aims to design and fabricate ECM-mimicking scaffolds by the bottom-up assembly of building blocks with specific composition, morphology and structural properties. This review provides an overview of the main strategies to build synthetic TE scaffolds through bioactive modules assembly and classifies them into two distinct schemes based on microparticles (µPs) or patterned layers. The µPs-based processes section starts describing novel techniques for creating polymeric µPs with desired composition, morphology, size and shape. Later, the discussion focuses on µPs-based scaffolds design principles and processes. In particular, starting from random µPs assembly, we will move to advanced µPs structuring processes, focusing our attention on technological and engineering aspects related to cell-free and cell-laden strategies. The second part of this review article illustrates layer-by-layer modular scaffolds fabrication based on discontinuous, where layers' fabrication and assembly are split, and continuous processes.

Keywords: additive manufacturing; bioprinting; drug delivery; microparticles; scaffold; soft lithography; vascularization

1. Introduction to Tissue Engineering Scaffolds and Bottom-Up Fabrication

Traumas, diseases and population ageing are major reasons for damage and failure of human body tissues and organs, which require medical treatments for their restoration or replacement. Despite the intrinsic body capability of repairing small injuries given sufficient time, to date, tissue growth in large (centimeter-size) defects requires complex, expensive and patient-painful autografts, allografts or xenografts [1,2]. In the case of bone, autograft and allograft implantation produces the best clinical results, but it requires secondary surgery and has a limited supply. The main advantage of a xenograft is its abundant supply and no need for secondary surgery, but poor implantation results and problems of infection from donors are critical issues [2]. Besides, the neo-tissue generated within the interstitial spaces of these grafts is often different from the native tissue and requires large remodeling time for the complete biological and biomechanical integration with surrounding tissues. For these reasons, the development of novel solutions for tissues and organs bioengineering is extremely demanding in the medical field.

Tissue engineering (TE), an important biomedical engineering field, aims to solve this important challenge by combining scaffolds and bioactive molecules for the artificial reconstruction of functional, three-dimensional (3D) tissues and organs [3]. Biomedical scaffolds are porous, implantable biomaterials, shaped to promptly restore the natural tissue anatomy and mechanical functions. The scaffolds must also be capable of controlling foreign body reaction and new-tissue formation by targeted presentation and delivery of key molecules, e.g., anti-inflammatory, growth factors, and proteins. Indeed, these molecules help scaffolds to reduce inflammation, recruit and direct differentiation of stem cells from surrounding tissues and ultimately, promote functional tissue integration in situ [4–6].

Scaffolds design and fabrication have evolved greatly in the past twenty years due to the large knowledge accumulated on materials design, processing and characterization of cell/scaffold interactions. In the natural tissues, cells and extracellular matrix (ECM) organize into 3D structures from sub-cellular to tissue level. Consequently, to engineer functional tissues and organs successfully, scaffolds must capture the essence of this cells/ECM organization and must provide a porous structure able to facilitate cells distribution and guide 3D tissue regeneration [7–9]. Scaffolds pore size and shape, pore wall morphology, porosity, surface area and pore interconnectivity, are probably the most important architectural parameters, as they have been shown to directly impact cells migration and colonization, new ECM biosynthesis and organization, oxygen and nutrients transport to cells, as well as metabolic wastes removal in the whole cell/scaffold construct [10–16]. The scaffold material must be selected and/or designed with a degradation and resorption rate such that scaffold strength is retained until the tissue-engineered transplant is fully remodeled by the host tissue and can assume its own structural role [17,18]. More importantly, controlling mechanical properties at cellular and sub-cellular levels is important to emulate as closely as possible the in vivo cell behavior and tissue growth [19,20]. Nevertheless, controlling the morphological and biomechanical properties of porous scaffolds is not enough for the success of scaffolds-based therapies, as there is also the need to load matricellular and soluble molecules inside scaffolds' matrix as biochemical regulators of cells behavior [21]. Indeed, it is reported that porous scaffolds releasing biochemical signals following a precise dose and time intervals to target sites stimulate cells' functions (e.g., adhesion, proliferation and migration) [22–25], promote the biosynthesis of new ECM [26] and, ultimately, guide tissue growth, morphogenesis [27] and vascularization [28–30].

Increasing scaffolds' design complexity is therefore extremely demanding and scientists face some important challenges, such as: (1) engineering of scaffold microarchitecture to mimic the ECM structure, (2) imprinting topological and biochemical patterns inside scaffolds pores to guide cells' growth and tissue morphogenesis, and (3) developing automated processes for the precise and reliable control of scaffolds' features and geometry.

Porous bioactive scaffolds can be fabricated by combining biomaterials and growth factors through different processing techniques. This review focuses the attention on modular approaches where samples are built by the "bottom-up" assembly of smaller units or "modules", each one specifically designed for distinct tasks [31–33]. Bottom up approaches have the potential to build scaffolds mimicking the complex molecular and structural microenvironment of the native ECM of every kind of tissues by the proper assembly of micro- and nano-structured modules with well-defined morphological and biochemical properties [34].

Several processing techniques are available for modules fabrication, including fluidic emulsion [35], electrofluidodynamic processes [36], and advanced computer aided manufacturing [37,38]. All of these approaches offer, nowadays, a wide library of materials, each one characterized by different composition, shape, nano- and micro-topography, and porous architecture. The assembly of individual modules, such as microparticles (µPs) or patterned layers, by packing, stacking, and printing, allows for achieving multifunctional scaffolds for tissue and organ bioengineering. As will be discussed in the next sections, cell-free or cell-laden µPs can be packed together in a mold giving rise to a sintered matrix by contact points union [39]. Sintering can be obtained by heat or proper plasticizers, in the case of cell-free samples, and by promoting cells/cells and cells/ECM interlocking to obtain hybrid structures [34]. μPs can also be used as cell and/or drug carriers to be loaded inside hydrogel pastes for printing more ordered and complex structures [40]. Layer-by-layer scaffolds' fabrication uses medical imaging combined with computer-aided design (CAD) and automated scaffolds' manufacturing processes to produce customized cell-free or cell-laden scaffolds characterized by a highly controlled structure and reliable properties. This broad category of fabrication techniques includes discontinuous processes, based on the assembly (stacking/sintering) of layered structures obtained by mold replication methods [37]. Alternatively, continuous processes, named additive manufacturing (AM), are used to construct scaffolds by joining/printing biomaterials and cells [38].

The focus of this review is to describe and discuss the advancement of current bottom-up techniques for creating adaptive scaffolds built from μPs or prepared using layer-by-layer assembly techniques, focusing on cell-free and cell-laden strategies. The advantages of each approach to controlling scaffolds' microstructural properties and drug release capability will be discussed, outlining some of the most promising results achieved for regenerating different tissues and organs, such as bone and cartilage, blood vessels, and derma.

2. Microparticles (μPs) as Building Blocks for Modular Tissue Engineering Scaffolds

Nowadays, μPs are essential elements of clinical and regenerative medicine applications such as cell culture μ-scaffolds for in vivo cell delivery and in vitro tissue biofabrication, and drug delivery carriers for biosensing and diagnostic purposes [41–43]. Both synthetic and natural polymeric biomaterials have been investigated for μPs design and engineering. Indeed, chemical and physical polymers properties can be easily manipulated to design and fabricate μPs with tailored morphological properties, size-shape distribution, and degradation rate. Furthermore, scaffolds prepared from synthetic polymeric μPs offer better chemical stability and mechanical properties than those prepared by using natural polymers, especially for load bearing applications. Common examples of the main synthetic polymers for μPs' fabrication which can be mentioned are PCL, poly-lactic acid (PLA), polylactic-co-glycolic acid (PLGA), poly-ethylene glycol (PEG), and their composites with ceramic fillers like calcium phosphate, alumina, and hydroxyapatite [4,44–48]. Natural polymers, conversely, have a chemical composition and structure resembling that of native biological tissues. This aspect is extremely fascinating for μPs' fabrication as it makes it possible to achieve materials faithfully replicating the ECM microenvironment functions. Natural polymeric μPs can be classified into two main groups: protein-based, such as silk, collagen, and fibrin, and polysaccharide-based, like agarose, chitosan, and hyaluronic acid. These kinds of μPs have advantages like excellent biocompatibility, immunogenicity, and degradation rate that can be tuned by varying μPs' materials composition, molecular weight, and crosslinking degree. In the next section, an overview will be provided about μPs' fabrication, highlighting the most advanced techniques to control μPs' composition, structure, and size-shape distribution. Furthermore, the use of μPs as building blocks for cell-free and cell-laden scaffolds fabrication and their use as μ-scaffolds for in vitro cell culture and tissue production will be described in detail.

2.1. μPs Fabrication by Advanced Processes

Several conventional methods are used to prepare μPs, such as phase separation, spray drying, and batch emulsion techniques. The resulting polymeric material is often characterized by heterogeneous size distribution and limited control over their shape [49,50]. To overcome these limitations and achieve even highly complex μPs morphology and composition, new advanced techniques were implemented for μPs' fabrication in the past decades, as highlighted in Figure 1. Microfluidics is a revolutionary technique that manipulates fluids into microscale channels for fluid mixing, merging, splitting, and reaction [51]. Microfluidic emulsion is one of the most investigated techniques for the high-throughput production of monodisperse modular microstructures variable in size, shape, and composition. Microfluidic devices are generally made of transparent and chemically strong devices obtained by assembling glass capillaries or patterning channels in a silicone elastomer, e.g., polydimethylsiloxane (PDMS), through soft lithography methods (Figure 1a,b) [52]. Oil-in-water single emulsions generated with the assistance of the co-flow devices schematized in Figure 1a,b enabled the production of uniform and size-controlled droplets by simple modulation of flow rate of continuous and disperse phases. These droplets can be conveniently converted into uniform beads (Figure 1c) or beads with core-shell, patchy, and Janus architectures (Figure 1d) by the adequate choice of solutions' compositions and controlling the solvent evaporation and phase separation mechanism [45,53]. For instance, using PLGA/PCL as model materials, the authors showed that the core-shell, patchy, and Janus types of particles can be produced with a high yield and a narrow size distribution by precisely controlling interfacial tensions and spreading coefficients between immiscible phases of the generated droplets. As a direct consequence, μPs' hydrophilicity, degradation rate, and drug delivery properties can be tuned depending on the specific application [45].

The formation of multiple emulsions within these microfluidic devices may enable the fabrication of μPs with multiples cores and drug delivery capability (Figure 1e). More importantly, these methods are able to improve loading efficiency of hydrophobic polymeric μPs by changing their polarity [54]. Microfluidic flow-focusing devices were fabricated to generate droplets of different sizes and shapes and narrow size distribution in either PDMS or glass capillary devices [55]. Indicating the diameter of an undeformed (regular) spherical droplet as dS = (6V/π)1/3, non-spherical droplets are obtained when dS is larger than at least one of the dimensions of the outlet channel, as the confinement hinder shape relaxation of droplets into spheres after breakup. As a direct consequence, in wide channels, when w > dS (w = width) while the height h < dS, the drops assume a discoid shape with rounded borders (Figure 1f). For channels with both h and w smaller than dS, the droplet makes contact with all channel walls and assumes a rod-like morphology (Figure 1g). As shown in Figure 1h, microfluidic approaches were also used for preparing porous μPs with a large surface area, good mechanical strength, and high interconnectivity to be suitable as μ-scaffolds for cells' culture [53]. This was achieved by injecting an unstable water-in-oil emulsion, made of gelatin and poly (vinyl alcohol) (PVA) as discontinuous phase in a PLGA solution in dichloromethane that served as continuous phase. The resultant water-oil-in-water droplets were subsequently solidified by solvent extraction and evaporation in a collection phase (water), generating porous μPs.

Lithography-based processes, such as those reported in Figure 1, are the subsequent example to manufacture precisely shaped polymeric μPs. Flow-lithography processes (e.g., continuous or stop-flow-lithography) enable for continuously synthesizing a variety of different shapes and sizes using several oligomers and produce multifunctional Janus particles. These approaches use ultraviolet (UV) light combined with light-transparent PDMS devices for the selective photopolymerization of a fluidic bead with the aid of proper masks (Figure 1i). Particles' shape in the x–y plane is determined by the transparency masks pattern (Figure 1j–l); whereas the z-plane projection is dependent on the height of the channel used and the thickness of the oxygen inhibition layer [47]. For instance, polyethylene glycol diacrylate (PEGDA) microgels were synthesized with tunable shapes such as triangles, squares, and hexagons, showing good fidelity to the original mask features (Figure 1j–l) [47]. The fundamental limitations of the flow-lithography technique are mainly dependent on the optical resolution and the depth-of-field of the microscope objective used as well, as it requires a short polymerization time or slow flow rate to avoid smearing of the patterned feature in the hydrogels. The main limitation of this technique is the use of prepolymer solutions with high concentrations of monomer and/or photoinitiator, necessary for reducing μPs' setting time that may induce a possible cytotoxic effect. A stop-flow-lithography (SFL) process was recently proposed to overcome this limitation. This process involves stopping the liquid flow, polymerizing the patterned solution, and the flowing of the particles out of the device. This workflow proved suitable for fabricating cell-laden PEGDA particles with controlled shapes and size for TE (Figure 1m,n) [56]. Nevertheless, flow-lithography processes are mainly limited to materials that can polymerize under UV light (hydrogels) and therefore, cannot be used for synthetic materials such as thermoplastic polymers.

Recent advances in micro/nanotechnology have allowed fabrication of µPs made of thermoplastic polymers with uniform sizes and well-defined shapes and composition, which are otherwise impossible to fabricate using conventional µPs' manufacturing methods, providing new building blocks libraries for modular TE. In particular, soft-lithography techniques involve the use of elastomeric PDMS stamps with topological microfeatures to fabricate µPs with precise control over size and geometry in a simple, versatile, and cost-effective modality (Figure 1o) [57–59]. After solvent evaporation, the dried polymer is deposited on selective portions of the mold in the form of particles, and it is removed from the PDMS mold by stamping it onto a PVA sacrificial layer at temperatures and pressures in the range of 80–120 °C and 30–90 KPa, respectively [58]. The µPs are released from the mold by dissolving the PVA layer in water. The versatility of these fabrication methods has been demonstrated using materials of biomedical interest including thermoplastic polymers such as PCL and PLGA (Figure 1p–r) [59], polyethylene glycol dimethacrylate (PEGDMA) hydrogels, and chitosan. An advancement in this fabrication technique was reported recently by McHugh and co-workers that developed a microfabrication method, termed StampEd Assembly of polymer Layers (SEAL), for fabricating modular micrometric structures, such as injectable pulsatile drug-delivery PLGA µPs with complex geometry at a high resolution (Figure 1s,t) [60]. In another study, de Alteriis and co-workers used microspheres to obtain shaped µPs by a soft-lithography approach [46]. This was achieved by positioning PLGA microspheres into PDMS mold cavities with different shapes and deforming them under gentle process conditions, i.e., at room temperature using a solvent/non-solvent vapor mixture. By this approach, it was also possible to preserve the microstructure and bioactivity of molecules loaded inside the µPs (Figure 1u). In conclusion, all of the discussed advanced µPs' fabrication methods may open new avenues for the fabrication of multifunctional building blocks for modular TE applications.

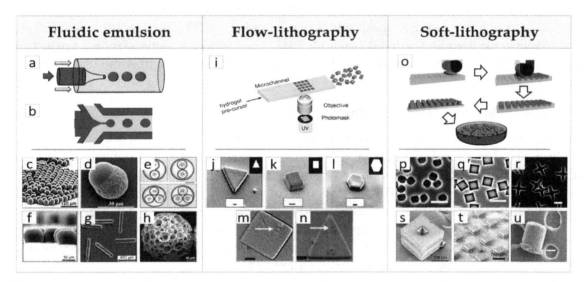

Figure 1. Microfluidic emulsion: Fabrication of microparticles (µPs) with advanced processes. (**a**) Co-flow and (**b**) flow-focusing pictures of fluidic emulsion devices. Effect of processing conditions on µPs morphology, composition and structure: (**c**) spherical monodisperse µPs, (**d**) Janus µPs, (**e**) core-shell µPs with dual and triple cores, (**f**) disks and (**g**) rods µPs obtained by controlling the dimension of the outlet channel, (**h**) highly porous polylactic-co-glycolic acid (PLGA) spherical µPs prepared by double emulsion. Flow-lithography: (**i**) Picture of the flow-lithography continuous process for making shape-controlled µPs by exposure of precursor solution to patterned ultraviolet (UV) light. Morphology of (**j**) triangles, (**k**) squares and (**l**) hexagons µPs prepared by the continuous flow-lithography process. Single-cell encapsulated within (**m**) square and (**n**) triangular µPs prepared by the stop-flow-lithography (SFL) process. Soft-lithography: (**o**) Schematic drawing of the soft-lithography and lift-out molding fabrication protocol of µPs: (**p,q,r**) effect of mold type on µPs shape. Morphology of µPs obtained by the StampEd Assembly of polymer Layers (SEAL) process before (**s**) and (**t**) after sealing. (**u**) Morphology of vascular endothelial growth factor (VEGF)-loaded PLGA microsphere after solvent vapor shaping

process. **c, f, g** Reproduced with permission from Reference [55] (Xu, Angewandte Chemie International Edition; Published by John Wiley and Sons, 2005); **d** Reproduced with permission from Reference [45] (Cao, RCS. Advances; published by Royal Society of Chemistry, 2015); **e, i** Reproduced with permission from Reference [54] (Baah, Microfluid Nanofluid; published by Springer Nature, 2014); **h** Reproduced with permission from Reference [53] (Choi, Small; published by John Wiley and Sons, 2010); **j, l** Reproduced with permission from Reference [47] (Dendukuri, Nature Materials; published by Springer Nature, 2006); **m, n** Reproduced with permission from Reference [56] (Panda, Lab Chip; published by Royal Society of Chemistry, 2008); **o** Reproduced with permission from Reference [57] (Canelas, Nanomed Nanobiotechnol; published by John Wiley and Sons, 2009); **p, q, r** Reproduced with permission from Reference [59] (Guan, Biomaterials; published by Elsevier Ltd, 2006); **s, t** Reproduced with permission from Reference [60] (Kevin J. McHugh, Science; published by American Association for the Advancement of Science, 2017); **u** Reproduced with permission from Reference [46] (Renato de Alteriis, Scientific Reports; published by Springer Nature, 2015).

2.2. μPs as Building Blocks for In Vitro and In Vivo Modular Tissue Engineering (TE) Scaffolds

The use of μPs for engineering biological tissues may follow two main approaches. In the first approach, named cell-free, μPs are used as building blocks and assembled together to form a sintered porous scaffold. Therefore, the scaffold can be used for in vitro cell culture studies before in vivo implantation. Alternatively, the scaffold is directly implanted in vivo to deliver bioactive molecules and to promptly restore tissue anatomy and functions. In the second approach, named cell-laden, μPs are used as μ-scaffolds for in vitro cell expansion and proliferation. The as-obtained cell-laden μ-scaffolds are subsequently assembled in vitro inside bioreactors to stimulate cell biosynthesis and material degradation, finally leaving a biological tissue replicating native tissues' composition and structure. Both approaches require building blocks assembly into 3D large (centimeter scale) structures by two main ways: random and ordered assembly [61]. The following sections will describe techniques of μPs' assembly for cell-free and cell-laden TE strategies, bringing to light some of the most relevant results achieved to date.

2.2.1. Porous Scaffolds Prepared by the Random/Ordered Assembly of μPs

The literature review has evidenced a plethora of works reporting the design and fabrication of scaffolds by using biodegradable and biocompatible μPs, demonstrating the possibility to achieve tailored porous structure, full interconnected porosity, high mechanical stiffness and, ultimately, drug loading and controlled release features. In a typical process, researchers prepared bioactive and biodegradable μPs using traditional or advanced methods, such as those described in the previous section. The μPs were then poured into appropriate molds and sintered together to form a continuous matrix. As shown in Figure 2a, the resultant scaffolds have a particles-aggregated structure while their size and shape replicated the mold (cylinder) geometry [4].

A scaffold's morphology as well as its pore structures were correlated to the size and shape of the μPs and the sintering process. Sintering depended on the motion of polymeric chains from the μPs surface to contact points that leads to chain inter-diffusion and the subsequent formation of connecting necks between μPs. This mechanism depends on polymer plasticization and can be promoted by heat, organic solvents, or high-pressure fluids [62–67]. For instance, PCL scaffolds were fabricated using thermal sintering of spherical μPs with two different size ranges, smaller (300–500 μm) and larger (500–630 μm) at 60 °C for 1 h. A double emulsion process was also implemented for bovine serum albumin (BSA) encapsulation inside the depots of smaller (50–180 μm) PCL particles for drug delivery purposes. The authors reported the decrease of scaffolds' porosity and pore size as well as the increase of compression moduli with the decrease of μPs' size. This effect is ascribable to an enhanced μPs' compaction and a concomitant higher number of fusion points between smaller μPs [4]. However, low porosity and pore size may result in decreased cell adhesion and colonization. The use of porous μPs enable to overcome this limitation and achieve higher scaffolds' porosity. This aspect was studied by

Qutachi and co-workers, who fabricated highly porous PLGA µPs by the double emulsion technique, where phosphate buffered saline (PBS) was used as the internal aqueous phase. Hydrolysis treatment on µPs using 30% 0.25 M NaOH:70% absolute ethanol enabled the formation of a double-scale sintered matrix at body temperature that can therefore be used as a minimally invasive injectable scaffold (Figure 2b) [62].

The optimization of the sintering step is a critical aspect for scaffolds prepared by µPs' assembly. Indeed, sintering not only affects the integrity of the scaffold structure, but also influences some key properties, such as porosity and mechanical stiffness. Borden et al. addressed this aspect for melt-sintered scaffolds [68], while Brown et al. [69] and Hyeong Jeon et al. [63] addressed it for solvent-sintered scaffolds and for a high-pressure CO_2 sintering, respectively. As shown in Figure 2c, the mechanical properties of PLGA scaffolds increased with the increase of fusion time from 2 to 4 h, while higher treatment times produced the complete collapse of the pore structure due to the extensive polymer melting. Overall, these scaffolds, with a range in modulus from 137.44 to 296.87 MPa, appeared to be capable of sustaining loads in the mid-range of cancellous bone [68]. The solvent/non-solvent chemical sintering, is an alternative strategy for sintering a wide range of polymeric µPs at a low temperature for developing TE scaffolds and drug delivery vehicles [69]. Polymers such as polyphosphazenes, exhibiting glass transition temperatures from −8 to 41 °C, and PLGA were tested to optimize solvent/non-solvent mixtures and the treatment time based on the affinity between polymer and solvent mixtures. The authors reported that the solvent/non-solvent sintering technique produced scaffolds with median pore size and porosity similar to the heat-sintered microspheres [69]. Nevertheless, the use of potentially toxic organic solvents is a critical issue for this approach. A low-temperature organic solvent-free approach was proposed for µPs' sintered scaffolds fabrication [62,63]. This approach used high-pressurized CO_2 to produce scaffolds from a large variety of polymeric materials, such as PCL, PLGA, and PLA [63]. For instance, it was reported that the optimal CO_2 pressure for PLGA scaffolds was in the 15–25 MPa range, and that sintering increased with pressure due to the enhanced polymer plasticization, representing a useful way to tune scaffolds' porosity and mechanical properties [63].

As pointed out in the Introduction section, engineering tissues and organs requires combinations of biomaterials, cells, and bioactive signaling cues. The design of bioactive molecules releasing scaffolds has to consider that the spatial patterning of bioactive signals is vital to some of the most fundamental aspects of life, from embryogenesis to wound healing, all involving concentration gradients of signaling molecules that have to be replicated by scaffolds. µPs have been long studied as drug delivery systems for a variety of molecules as they enable an easy control of the release kinetics of loaded therapeutics. Alendronate (AL)- and dexamethasone (Dex)-loaded PLGA-based scaffolds were proposed by Shi and co-workers for bone regeneration [70]. These molecules were chosen as AL is a bisphosphonate able to promote the activity and maturation of osteoblasts and mesenchymal stem cells (MSCs) differentiation, while Dex is a glucocorticoid with osteogenic properties. Scaffolds' capability to release AL and Dex up to two months in a sustained fashion resulted in a marked osteogenic differentiation of MSCs in vitro and in vivo, as evidenced by significantly higher expression of bone-related proteins and genes, such as alkaline phosphatase activity (ALP), type-I collagen, osteocalcin, and bone morphogenic protein (BMP)-2, if compared to unloaded scaffold. Additionally, drug-loaded scaffolds showed significantly higher new bone formation at eight weeks implantation into rabbit femurs bone defects [70]. Jaklenec et al. used PLGA µPs loaded with dyes to demonstrate the feasibility of creating spatially controlled particles' distribution inside porous scaffolds (Figure 2d) [71]. In another study, Singh and co-workers developed a two-syringe pumping device for the controlled deposition of functional microspheres to create gradients of releasing molecules for interfacial tissues' regeneration [72]. By controlling suspensions composition and flow rates during pumping, it was possible to engineer multiple gradient configurations, such as the bi-layered and multi-layered concentration profiles. The authors further used this technique to prepare a PLGA microspheres scaffold containing opposing gradients of BMP-2 and transforming growth factor (TGFb1) for osteochondral interface TE (Figure 2e) [73]. After six weeks of in vitro culture, MSCs-seeded scaffolds evidence regionalized gene expression of major osteogenic and chondrogenic markers.

Overall, scaffolds based on the assembly of µPs are versatile for a wide range of TE applications, from soft to hard tissues. For instance, the use of synthetic polymers resulted in high mechanical stiffness and a slow degradation rate for in vivo load-bearing implantation, such as bone [74] and osteochondral tissue [75]. Conversely, soft biopolymeric chitosan µPs scaffolds were proposed as a 3D, functional neuronal networks' regeneration platform [76]. Even if all of these studies clearly evidenced the potential of µPs-based scaffolds in TE applications, some key issues are still to be addressed for their successful clinical translation. As previously discussed, biological tissues are characterized by hierarchical-ordered architectures at both nano- and micro-metric size scales, that can be replicated only in part by µPs' random assembly. Furthermore, µPs-based scaffolds require multiple steps of fabrication, from µPs' fabrication up to assembly and sintering. Therefore, the possibility to reduce scaffolds' fabrication time by automated processes will be a great step towards clinical implementation.

One of the most investigated methods to obtain ordered scaffolds from sintered µPs is selective laser sintering (SLS). As shown in Figure 2f–h, this powder-based AM technique enabled patient-specific implantable scaffolds with interconnected multi-scaled porosity [77]. SLS employs a CO_2 laser beam to selectively sinter a powder bead, based on a computer-aided design (CAD) scaffold model. Du and co-workers fabricated PCL and PCL-hydroxyapatite scaffolds for bone TE [78]. Both in vitro and in vivo evaluations demonstrated that these scaffolds not only promoted cell adhesion, supported cell proliferation, and induced cell differentiation in vitro, but also evidenced in vivo bone formation and vascularization. This effect was higher for composite scaffold as the hydroxyapatite increased surface roughness and positively charged the PCL surface. The same authors also explored the fabrication of bioinspired multilayer scaffolds mimicking the complex hierarchical architecture of the osteochondral tissue that was used to repair osteochondral defects of a rabbit model [78]. It is, however, important to point out that SLS techniques create ordered structures (Figure 2g) inside randomly assembled µPs (Figure 2h), while they cannot manipulate µPs and allow their precise positioning inside the scaffold structure. One of the first attempts to solve this aspect and to fabricate porous µPs'-sintered scaffolds with highly ordered pore structure at the µPs-scale was recently proposed by Rossi and co-workers [79]. The authors prepared PCL µPs with size in the 425–500 µm range and used alignment PDMS molds for precise particle positioning and sintering. Final scaffolds were achieved by the stacking of three µPs layers followed by a solvent bonding step (Figure 2i). If compared to randomly assembled scaffolds, the ordered scaffolds showed a better vascularization in the inner core, as evidenced by the deeper blood vessel penetration and the larger diameter of the infiltrating vessels [79]. This approach was tested with large µPs (500 µm), as smaller µPs require the implementation of new advanced automated manufacturing. Nevertheless, these recent results pave the way on the importance on µPs' scaffold design features and provide the basis for the future development in this extremely promising scaffold design research field.

2.2.2. Porous µPs as µ-Scaffolds for In Vitro Tissue Building

In the past decade, researchers in TE have focused the attention on the possibility of recreating large implantable living and functional tissues in vitro by assembling cell-laden µ-scaffolds. The advantage of this approach relies on the fact that porous micro-sized scaffolds can be designed and modularly assembled to guide the correct spatial composition and organization of the de-novo synthesized cell/ECM construct. Furthermore, by this approach, it is possible to overcome limitations related to cells culturing in 3D thick scaffolds, such as cells' seeding efficiency and oxygen and nutrients' transport inside the scaffold core. The capability of recreating in vitro fully biologic centimeter-sized tissues was validated for a large variety of applications. For instance, Urciuolo and co-workers [80] have studied the fabrication of a dermis-equivalent tissue by culturing human dermal fibroblasts (HDFs) onto gelatin µ-scaffolds. The developed process involved two main steps: (Step 1) dynamic cell-seeding of fibroblasts on porous µ-scaffolds using a spinner flask bioreactor for up to nine days to obtain micro-tissue precursors (μTPs). (Step 2) assembly of μTPs and maturation in a specifically designed chamber for up to 28 days [80]. Following this strategy, a 3D functional dermal tissue has been created and used as a base platform to study natural and pathologic tissue morphogenesis mechanisms, such as follicle-like structure formation [81] and tissue vascularization [82], as well as to study dermis remodeling and epidermis senescence after UV radiation exposure [83]. The feasibility of using cell-laden μ-scaffolds to fabricate highly complex biomimetic tissues was also explored in the case of bone [84], cardiac tissue [85], and liver tissues [86]. For example, Chen et al. cultured human amniotic MSCs onto gelatin μ-scaffolds for up to eight days, after which, cells were induced to undergo osteogenic differentiation in the same culture flask and cultured for up to 28 days. These bone-like μ-tissues were finally used as building blocks to fabricate a macroscopic cylindrical bone construct (2 cm in diameter, 1 cm height) evidencing good cell viability and homogenous distribution of cellular content (Figure 2j) [87]. The modularity of this approach was explored by Scott et al., who combined human liver cancer cell line, HepG2, and different types of PEG μPs to study the effect of porosity and drug delivery on cells' behavior (Figure 2k) [88]. In particular, the authors considered three types of PEG microspheres: the first type provided μ-scaffolds mechanical support, the second type provided controlled delivery of the sphingosine 1-phosphate (S1P), an angiogenesis-promoting molecule, and the third type served as a slowly dissolving non-cytotoxic porogen. After components' centrifugation into a mold and incubation at 37 °C overnight, μPs fused together and, within two days of culture, macropores formed thanks to the dissolution of the porogenic particles. The S1P delivery combined with the structural properties allowed HepG2 cells' migration through the scaffolds' macropores (Figure 2j).

AM processes are successfully used to obtain cell-laden μ-scaffolds with ordered structures for biomedical applications. Among these techniques, bioprinting is the most popular as it allows the fabrication of living constructs with custom-made architectures by the controlled deposition of cell-laden μ-scaffolds bioinks [40,89]. In a recent study, Levato and co-workers seeded MSCs onto PLA μ-scaffolds via static culture or spinner flask expansion and loaded these samples in gelatin methacrylamide-gellan gum bioinks [40]. The optimization of the composite material formulation and printing conditions enabled the fabrication of highly ordered constructs with enhanced mechanical properties and high cell-seeded densities (Figure 2l). Process flexibility was also validated by designing and fabricating bi-layered osteochondral scaffolds (Figure 2l). Tan et al. presented a similar approach for the recreation of vascular tubular tissues, based on the micropipette extrusion bioprinting method (Figure 2m) [89]. The selected bioink was made of cell-laden PLGA porous microspheres encapsulated within agarose-collagen hydrogels. Furthermore, the authors demonstrated the possibility to use concomitantly C2C12 and Rat2 cell-laden μ-scaffolds.

Manipulation of cell-laden μ-scaffolds at the micro-scale was also investigated to obtain precisely designed 3D structures for TE. The μ-scaffolds were soaked in an inert medium (mineral oil) while their assembly was obtained by geometrical constraints, specifically by the use of guiding structures or by more complex mechanisms, such as magnetic actuation. The picture in Figure 2n highlights 3D structures obtained by assembling cell-laden μ-scaffolds fabricated by soft-lithography (Figure 1) and starting from a UV-photo-cross-linkable metacrylated gelatin solution [90]. The assembly process was controlled by geometrical constraint or by using a syringe needle swiped uniaxially against the linear array of ring-shaped μ-scaffolds [90]. Liu and co-workers combined μ-scaffolds shape and magnetic field for the construction of artificial bioarchitectures [91]. Magnetite-alginate-chitosan composite microcapsule robots characterized by magnetization along the central axis were magnetically actuated to grab the building components during the transportation and assembly processes. Position and orientation remote control of the cell-laden μ-scaffolds offered a non-invasive and dynamical manipulation system for the creation of complex 3D structures for TE.

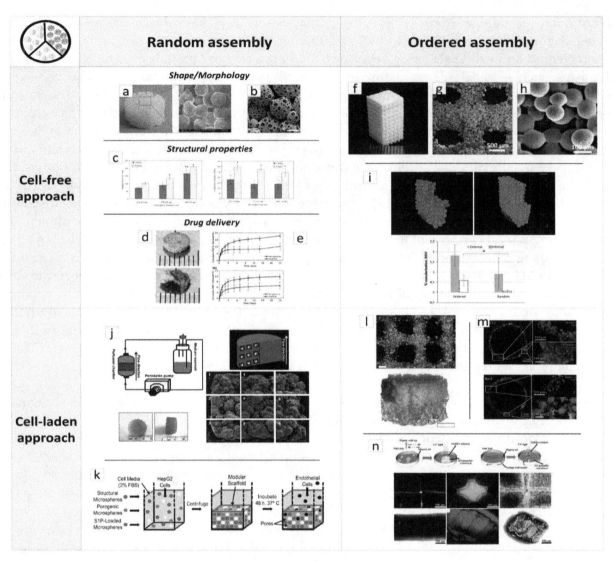

Figure 2. Overview of µPs applications in tissue engineering (TE) scaffold-based strategies classified by random (left column) and ordered (right column) assemblies, cell-free (first row) and cell-laden (second row) approaches. (**a**) morphology of µPs' sintered polycaprolactone (PCL) scaffold obtained by thermal sintering. (**b**) Morphology of porous µPs' sintered PLGA scaffold obtained by chemical sintering. (**c**) Effect of µPs' diameter and thermal sintering time on mean pore size and compressive modulus of PLGA-sintered scaffolds. (**d**) Optical images of sintered scaffolds with homogeneous and heterogeneous spatial distribution of loaded µPs. (**e**) Release profiles of bone morphogenic protein (BMP)-2 and transforming growth factor (TGF) b1 from µPs'-sintered scaffolds for osteochondral interface TE. (**f**) Optical image of ordered scaffold obtained by selective laser sintering (SLS) and made of PCL µPs. (**g,h**) morphology of SLS scaffold evidencing the order and random structures, respectively. (**i**) Comparison of random and ordered PCL scaffolds on degree of vascularization in vivo. Results proved that the internal vascularization of the ordered scaffolds has significantly better vascularization in the inner core if compared to the random scaffold. (**j**) Culture device used to generate three-dimensional (3D) bone in vitro by cell-laden µPs' assembly and morphological and optical visualization of corresponding tissue. (**k**) Assembly of cells and multifunctional poly-ethylene glycol (PEG) µPs to study cells migration in vitro as a function of scaffolds porosity and sphingosine 1-phosphate (S1P) release. (**l,m**) Porous scaffolds obtained by µPs' printing for osteochondral and vascular tissues repair, respectively. (**n**) Schematic of assembly processes of cell-laden µ-scaffolds obtained by soft-lithography process and resulting cell-laden constructs. **a** Reproduced with permission from Reference [4] (Luciani, Biomaterials; published by Elsevier Ltd., 2008); **b** Reproduced with permission from Reference [62] (Qutachi, Acta

Biomaterialia; published by Elsevier Ltd., 2014); c Reproduced with permission from Reference [68] (Borden, Biomaterials; published by Elsevier Science Ltd., 2002); d Reproduced with permission from Reference [71] (Jaklenec, Biomaterials; published by Elsevier Ltd., 2008); e Reproduced with permission from Reference [73] (Dormer, Annals of Biomedical Engineering; published by Springer Nature, 2010); f–h Reproduced with permission from Reference [77] (Du, Colloids and Surfaces B: Biointerfaces; published by Elsevier B.V, 2015); i Reproduced with permission from Reference [79] (Rossi, Journal of Materials Science Materials in Medicine; published by Springer Nature, 2016); j Reproduced with permission from Reference [87] (Chen, Biomaterials; published by Elsevier Ltd., 2011); k Reproduced with permission from Reference [88] (Scott, Acta Biomaterialia; published by Elsevier Ltd., 2009); l Reproduced with permission from Reference [40] (Levato, Biofabrication; published by Institute of Physics Publishing, 2014); m Reproduced with permission from Reference [89] (Tan, Scientific Reports; published by Springer Nature, 2016); n Reproduced with permission from Reference [90] (Xiao, Materials Letters; published by Elsevier Ltd., 2018).

3. Layer-by-Layer Approaches for Scaffolds' Fabrication

A valid alternative to modular µPs-based scaffolds is micro/nanostructured modular scaffolds obtained by layer-by-layer assembly processes, as layers' assembly into 3D modular scaffolds enables the fabrication of geometrically and topographically complex architectures. The layer-by-layer scaffolds' fabrication approaches that are the subject of this review are divided into two groups: discontinuous and continuous processes. Discontinuous processes involve layers' fabrication and assembly in two distinct processing steps. Conversely, the continuous processes steps are almost totally automatized and take place simultaneously. This part of the review will outline and discuss some of the most useful and efficient techniques for layer-by-layer scaffolds' fabrication, highlighting the most promising results in tissue and organ regeneration.

3.1. Discontinuous Processes

Discontinuous processes involve the separate fabrication of scaffolds' layers followed by their assembly into 3D structures. These two steps often increase processing times but take advantage of the possibility to use micro/nanofabrication technologies for scaffolds' features creation. This was mainly achieved by replication methods, such as those highlighted in Figure 3, where layers are obtained by replicating the features of master molds. As shown, replication methods can be divided into two main groups based on mold type, namely elastomeric (PDMS) and rigid molds, and two sub-groups, depending on polymers processing (solution/temperature plasticization). We also report suitable assembly techniques for the fabricated layers considering the absence (cell-free)/presence of biological matter (cell-laden). However, we would like to point out herein that layers' fabrication and assembly are not confined to only one set of methods and could be combined properly depending on the application.

Common methods to fabricate two-dimensional (2D) layers involved the deposition of pre-polymer or polymer solutions onto PDMS mold by casting or spin-coating, followed by a consolidation step. For instance, Gallego et al. have presented a multilayer micromolding technique to fabricate and assemble PCL scaffolds [92]. Layers were fabricated via spin-coating of a PCL solution in tetrahydrofuran and dimethylsulfoxide (1:3:6 w/w/w ratio) at 4000 rpm for 1 min. Later, solvent was extracted overnight and 10 µm thick PCL layers, with 45×45 µm^2 pores were achieved. One of the previously obtained layers was then transferred onto a glass slide and manually stacked to another layer for 3D scaffold building. By following this approach, the authors obtained up to 100 µm thick PCL scaffolds characterized by 81% porosity, which were suitable for studying the effect of pores size and architecture on cell behavior in vitro. A similar approach was used by Sodha et al. for preparing PCL scaffolds with 200 µm circular or star-shaped pores for retinal transplantation [93].

2D layers			3D scaffolds	
Fabrication process	**Main features**	**Composition**	**Layers assembling/bonding**	**Main outcomes**
Elastomeric mould — *Consolidation from solution* — Spin coating/solvent evaporation [92]	✓ Layer thickness: 10 μm ✓ Dual-scale pores: large (45 x 45 μm², square); small (≈1μm, round)	✓ PCL ✓ Cell-free	Manual stacking followed by thermal bonding at 70°C for 2 min under 52 psi pressure	✓ Scaffolds thickness up to 100 μm ✓ 81% porosity ✓ Scaffolds with different layers orientations ✓ Platform for studying in vitro cell/scaffold interactions
Solution casting/solvent evaporation [94]	✓ Layer thickness: 25 μm ✓ Dual scale pores: large (100 x 500 μm², rectangular); small (< 100 nm, round)	✓ Poly(NIPAAm-co-HEMAHex)/alginate/gelatin ✓ Cell-free	Manual stacking followed by thermal bonding at 60°C for 10 min under compression	✓ Anisotropic mechanical properties and high stiffness ✓ Myoblasts elongation and orientation along scaffolds patterning
Solution casting/freeze drying [37, 95]	✓ Layer thickness: 500 μm ✓ Dual scale pores: large (≥100 μm, channels); small (10-50μm, round) [37]	✓ Chitosan–gelatin ✓ Cell-free	HUVEC or SMC cell seeding, manual stacking, Cell/ECM mediated bonding	✓ Controlled endothelialisation by interactive HUVEC/SMC layers stacking
	✓ Layer thickness: 2 mm ✓ Dual scale pores: large (500 μm, liver lobule-like); small (100-200 μm, round) ✓ Porosity (70-90%) [95]	✓ Silk fibroin–gelatin ✓ Cell-free	Stacking mould with alignment wires followed by polymeric solution bonding at RT	✓ Scaffolds thickness up to 1 cm ✓ Complex 3D microfluidic channels design
Solution casting/gelation [97, 98]	✓ Layer thickness: 140 μm ✓ Hepatic lobule-like mesh with 300-μm-diameter central pore and smaller cylindrical pores (150 μm distanced) [97]	✓ HepG2 or NIH3T3 cell-laden alginate	Stacking container, Alginate solution bonding with calcium chloride for 30 s	✓ 420 μm thick scaffolds ✓ 3D model for studying cells interaction in co-culture
	✓ Layer thickness: 200 μm ✓ Hexagonal pores (100-250-500 μm) [98]	✓ HUVEC/HepG2 cell-laden collagen	Stacking container, Cell/ECM mediated bonding after 4 days culture	✓ Construct thickness up to 2 mm and customized modular tissue assembly ✓ HUVEC migration and scaffold vascularization model
Pre-polymer solution casting + UV crosslinking [99]	✓ Layer thickness: 150-300 μm ✓ Dual scale-pores: channels luminal section and microstructured pores (10 - 20 μm) induced by porogen leaching	✓ POMaC ✓ Cell-free	Stage+microscope alignement and stacking followed by polymeric and UV crosslinking for 4 min	✓ Up to 2 cm-thick scaffold ✓ 3D platforms for in vitro and in vivo models of cardiac and hepatic tissues studies
Thermal processing — Microembossing [101, 102]	✓ Layer thickness: 60 μm ✓ 120 μm wide pores	✓ PLGA ✓ Cell-free	hMSCs or mouse ES cells seeding, manual stacking followed by layers pressing and bonding with CO₂ or N₂ at 0.69-1.73 MPa, 37°C for 15 min	✓ Up to 2 cm-thick scaffold ✓ 3D platforms for studying the effect of pore geometry and pore size as well as biomolecules release on tissue growth
Rigid mould — *Consolidation from solution* — Polymeric solution casting/phase separation [104]	✓ Layer thickness: 20-100 μm ✓ 75% porosity, 2-10 μm rounded pores and 45 μm ridge height.	✓ PLLA ✓ Cell-free	C2C12 pre-myoblast cell seeding, manual stacking w/o rolling, external fixation without bonding	✓ 4 layers planar or tubular scaffolds ✓ In vitro study of cell behaviour in 3D conditions
Polymeric solution electrodeposition [105]	✓ Layer thickness: 300 μm ✓ Hepatic lobule structure with 1.5 and 2 mm outer diameter	✓ Ca-Alginate ✓ RLC-18 cell-laden	Stacking mould without bonding	✓ 600 μm scaffolds thickness (2 layers) ✓ In vitro model of liver tissue
Pre-polymer solution casting followed by thermal curing [106]	✓ Layer thickness: 100 μm ✓ Rectangular pores (500x350 μm²)	✓ APS ✓ Cell-free	Dip coating in pre-polymeric solution and manual stacking followed by curing at 165°C for 2h.	✓ 200 μm scaffolds thickness (2 layers) ✓ Struts offset configuration ✓ Design of vascularized myocardial grafts by modular assembly of scaffold and microfluidic base separated by a rapidly degradable interface.
Pre-polymer solution casting followed by UV crosslinking [107]	✓ 87/125 μm thick layers ✓ Micropores (362 x 564 μm², rectangular)	✓ PLT32o and PGS ✓ Cell-free	Manual stacking with struts offset followed by solvent treatment and bonding	✓ Up to 2 mm thick scaffolds ✓ Elastomeric mechanical properties ✓ In vitro and in vivo Cardiac TE
Thermal processing — Microembossing [108, 109]	✓ Layer thickness: 20 μm ✓ Layer 1: channels (20 x 30 μm, rectangular) ✓ Layer 2: micropores (20 μm diameter) [108]	✓ PCGA ✓ Cell-free	Layers plasticization by vaporised solvent followed by stacking chamber and pressing for bonding	✓ Up to 60 μm scaffolds thickness ✓ In vitro model to study single cell population
	✓ 500 μm thick layers ✓ Micropores (300 μm diameter) [109]	✓ PCL and SPCL ✓ Cell-free	Layer dipping into polymeric solution followed by manual staking and bonding for 20 min	✓ 1.5 mm scaffolds thickness ✓ 88% porosity ✓ In vitro platform for bone TE

Figure 3. Discontinuous processes overview scheme. Left side: two-dimensional (2D) layers' fabrication processes. Right side: three-dimensional (3D) scaffolds' assembly processes. APS: Poly (ester-amide),1:2 poly (1,3-diamino-2-hydroxypropane-co -polyol sebacate); ECM: Extracellular matrix; ES cells: Embryonic stem cells; hMSC: Human mesenchymal stem cell; HUVEC: Human umbilical vein endothelial cell; NIH3T3: Mouse embryo fibroblast cell line; PCGA: Poly (ε-caprolactone–co-glycolic acid); PCL Polycaprolactone; PGS: Poly (glycerol sebacate); PLGA: Polylactic-co-glycolic acid; PLLA: Poly(L-lactic acid); PLT32o: Poly (limonene thioether); Poly(NIPAAm-co-HEMAHex): Poly (N-isopropylacrylamide–co-2-hydroxyethylmethacrylate-6-hydroxyhexanoate); POMaC: Poly (octamethylene maleate (anhydride) citrate; RLC: Rat liver cells; SMC: Smooth muscle cell; SPCL: Starch-polycaprolactone; TE: Tissue engineering.

A valid alternative to spin-coating consists in solution infiltration through a vacuum. Rosellini et al. [94] in fact fabricated a biomimetic myocardial scaffold, based on a simplified model of an original ECM microarchitecture. Several 25 μm thick layers with 100×500 μm² rectangular pores were successfully fabricated and thermally assembled to promote layers' merging and achieve a mechanically consistent scaffold.

Freeze-drying has been proven as another effective solution-based consolidation method to increase layers' thickness and obtain additional porosity. For example, He and co-workers [95] have fabricated 2 mm thick cylindrical layers by pipetting a silk fibroin/gelatin solution onto a pre-frozen micropatterned PDMS mold. The frozen system is then freeze-dried for at least one day to extract the residual solvent, preserving the fabricated microstructure. Results showed the possibility to modulate layers porosity, in the 70–90% range, and pores size, from 125 to 225 μm by changing the concentration of the polymer in solution, to control cell behavior. A solution-mediated bonding was used to prepare microstructured scaffolds mimicking the liver lobule architecture for liver TE purposes. The use of freeze-drying for polymeric layers' setting was also explored by Wang et al. [37], who fabricated porous scaffolds for vascular TE purposes. The authors used a microfluidic molding method to obtain 500 μm thick chitosan/gelatin layers (100 μm microstructures thickness) pipetting a 1:1 solution between a PDMS mold covered by a glass slide. The final layer was achieved by cooling and freeze-drying. An interesting aspect of their approach was that, before scaffolds' assembly, the layers were seeded with human umbilical vein endothelial cells (HUVECs) or smooth muscle cells (SMCs) with bonding promoted in this case by the cell/cell and cell/ECM interactions. Morphological and histological analysis demonstrated the possibility to create a complete branching vascular network and direct SMCs growth into fiber-like bundles inside the microstructured channels. A similar approach was implemented by He et al., who fabricated agarose/collagen layers by solvent casting and thermal gelation [96]. These layers were seeded with HUVECs/collagen suspension, disposed inside an alignment mold, and bonded with the aid of a thin layer of agarose to obtain a fully perfusable 3D construct.

To explore the advantages of combining layers and cells, Son et al. [97] have presented an evolution of the aforementioned methods using cell-laden solutions and a solution cross-linking assembly method to fabricate a 3D construct which mimics the hepatic liver lobule with sinusoids. To accomplish this purpose, a cell-laden alginate suspension was casted on a plasma-cleaned PDMS mold. Then, the system was incubated into a humidifier with a cross-linking reagent to induce gelation and achieve 8×8.7 mm layers with thicknesses up to 200 μm. The authors fabricated a PDMS chamber for layer stacking and used a small amount of alginate solution and cross-linker at layers' edges for bonding. The results show that layers maintained their structure during cell proliferation, while the manipulation techniques did not result in cell loss. Furthermore, cells show high viability because scaffolds' lateral and central pores ensure oxygen and nutrients' transport in the entire 3D structure. HepG2 cell-loaded constructs exhibited increased hepatic secretion and, when used in combination with mouse embryo fibroblast cell line (NIH3T3), allowed for studying cells interactions in 3D co-culture experiments. This approach was also used to test different porous structures, namely hexagonal pores with size in the 100–500 μm range, and by using collagen as layers' material [98]. A patterned cellulose filter substrate was used for collagen layer manipulation and the scaffold was assembled by alternating cell-free and HUVECs-laden collagen sheets to study cells' migration and scaffold vascularization [98].

Solution-based layers' fabrication was also implemented by using pre-polymer mixtures, which can be consolidated by UV radiation, as reported by Zhang and co-workers, for the microfabrication of the AngioChip scaffold [99]. Layers were fabricated from a mixture of poly (ethylene glycol) dimethyl ether (PEGDM) and poly (octamethylene maleate (anhydride) citrate) (POMaC), that was injected in a patterned PDMS prior to UV cross-linking and solution consolidation. Later, the as-obtained layers (5×3.1 mm² surface and 150–300 μm thickness) were demolded, stacked, and bonded by an additional UV treatment. The key feature of this micro-construct is the presence of a built-in endothelialized branched network, suitable to assess cardiac and hepatic tissues' responses to drugs delivered through the internal vasculature. For example, the generation of an angiogenic stimulus (thymosin β4) in vitro allowed endothelial cells' migration through the scaffold micro-holes as a first step of blood vessel formation in vitro. AngioChip also enabled fast anastomosis in vivo and tissue remodeling during the first week.

Processing biomaterials and bioactive molecules from organic solvent solutions require the removal of solvent residues from the final scaffolds, as these residues could be toxic for cells and tissues. In this context, previous researchers have also documented that PDMS could be used as a mold to produce micro-patterned layers from thermally plasticized polymers [100]. Yang et al. [101] have in fact presented several protocols to fabricate PLGA layers (120 μm wide pores and 60 μm thick) by PDMS micro-embossing at a temperature close to the PLGA glass transition temperature. The final porous scaffolds were obtained by stacking layers with the help of an alignment mold followed by compressed CO2 bonding for 1 h. This solvent-free approach was successfully applied to cell-seeded PLGA layers, demonstrating that CO2 bonding ensured proper human MSCs viability and functions [101]. Later, Xie and co-workers also demonstrated the possibility of bonding PLGA layers using N_2, which resulted in enhanced embryonic stem (ES) cells' viability with respect to CO_2 [102].

Although we have explained the motivations that have directed several researchers to choose elastomeric PDMS mold for layers' fabrication, features distortion during the process may be a critical issue. This problem arises because PDMS may swell and deform in contact with a broad range of organic solvents [103] or during compression [101]. As shown in Figure 3, rigid molds are the suitable alternative to overcome this limitation and fabricate layers for TE applications through replication techniques from solution and thermal processing.

Regarding solution-based processes, the first examples we introduce are those presented by Papenburg et al., who fabricated layers of different biocompatible polymers through solution casting/phase separation on a silicon mold [104]. Morphological analysis evidenced 80% porosity and high pore interconnection, low closed isolated pores, and a minor dense outer layer. However, this process leads to films with micropattern dimensions differing to the mold pattern because of film shrinking during the solvent extraction process [104]. Manual stacking and residual solvent bonding enabled the achievement of 3D scaffolds. In a further work, settled layers were seeded with C2C12 pre-myoblasts cells and rolled up to form a hollow cylinder without bonding to evaluate the effect of static and dynamic culture conditions on nutrient transport and cell behavior in vitro [104].

Recently, Liu et al. proposed an electrodeposition process for the preparation of rat liver cell (RLC-18)-laden alginate layers for an in vitro liver application [105]. The process involves the casting of a solution onto a rigid mold, fabricated through photolithographic techniques, with an architecture mimicking the hepatic lobule morphology. Then, the solution was electrodeposited for 15 s to obtain 300 μm thick cell-laden hydrogel layers, whose cells remain viable during all the microfabrication steps and proliferate over time. Two layers were subsequently stacked in an appropriate mold, similar to the process described in Reference [97], to obtain a 3D scaffold.

As for the "Angiochip" device [99], cell-free scaffolds for vascular TE purposes represent interesting examples of modules fabricated by solution consolidation [106,107]. In the work by Ye and co-workers, a modular strategy was proposed to build a slowly degradable poly(ester-amide),1:2 poly (1,3-diamino-2-hydroxypropane-co -polyol sebacate) (APS) bilayer scaffold connected to a microfluidic base through a rapidly degradable porous poly (glycerol sebacate) (PGS) module fabricated by an acrylic template [106]. As-obtained four-layer scaffolds increased the 3D permeability to oxygen and nutrients in vitro and degraded in vivo with a rate suitable to enhance scaffold vascularization. The fabrication of layer-by-layer heart scaffolds by photo-cross-linkable poly (limonene thioether) (PLT32o) prepolymer was reported by Fisher et al., with the aim to provide long in vivo half-life [107]. Layers with rectangular micropores (362 × 564 μm^2) were obtained by replica molding (REM) of polycarbonate molds and were assembled to form 3D scaffolds with elastomeric mechanical behavior and were able to retain structural integrity until one month in vivo.

Micro-embossing in rigid molds is the last discontinuous process described in this section. This process was widely used by Ryu and co-workers, who fabricated silicon molds to realize patterned layers with interconnecting structures made of thermoplastic materials such as PLGA, poly (p-dioxanone), and Monocryl® [108]. Morphological analyses showing the possibility of embossing structures of different aspect ratios were presented and discussed. Technological points of interest for the process, mainly mold-microstructures detachment and modulation of polymers bulk properties were also addressed. Porous scaffolds were fabricated by layers' stacking and bonding using a novel solvent vapor-mediated assembly process. Briefly, two layers were placed in an assembly chamber at a pre-defined temperature followed by a solvent vapor injection. Layers bonding was then achieved bringing the layers in contact under pressure. By this approach, it was possible to preserve layers' features and eventually incorporate bioactive molecules. As a result, 60 μm thick scaffolds with rectangular pores (20 × 30 μm) were achieved and tested as a 3D platform for single-cells' culture and characterization. In another work, Lima et al. [109] produced PCL and starch-polycaprolactone (SPCL) thicker layers (500 μm) with 300 μm circular pores and 300 thick pillars using a stainless-steel mold. Layers were manually stacked and bonded by using a PCL solution in chloroform, finally achieving 1.5 mm thick scaffolds with 88% porosity for in vitro bone TE.

3.2. Continuous Processes

Scaffolds' fabrication has evolved significantly by continuous processes due to the impressive evolution in the fields of materials science, cells engineering, and AM materials/cells processing platforms. AM are bottom-up processes where the basic components are assembled layer-by-layer to make objects from 3D model data. For example, the common workflow starts with the 3D virtual reconstruction of the defect to regenerate and can end with a patient-specific scaffold implantation to the site of injury [110]. To date, several AM systems available in market are capable of performing multiple operations simultaneously in the same work, e.g., extruding a synthetic polymer strand from a nozzle and embedding a cell-laden hydrogel in a predefined position. In addition, other important features of AM are scaffolds' reproducibility and consistency, as well as the possibility to create complex shaped 3D structures that are necessary for patient-specific treatments.

Regarding the application fields, AM techniques have still proven versatile and of great impact in regenerating several tissues. Indeed, the level of control offered by these techniques is a key technological aspect to increase our knowledge regarding biophysical and biochemical cues governing tissues' formation and functions. Through this section, we will show relevant results published in recent literature about AM scaffolds, pointing out advantages of the implemented manufacture technique and promising results.

Bone is a dynamic tissue characterized by heterogeneous and anisotropic structures and compositions that are required to support biomechanical and biological bone functions. The hierarchical structure of bone is composed of nanostructures made of organic (e.g., collagen) fibers and inorganic (HA) crystals that form the macroscopic cortical and cancellous bone structures passing through a series of intermediate microstructures, like lamellae, osteons, and harvesian channels. Scaffolds for bone regeneration must mimic bone morphology and structure. Concomitantly, these scaffolds must promote bone deposition (ostoconductive) and must be capable of delivering growth factors, such as BMPs and TGFs, to promote recruited cells' osteogenic differentiation (osteoinductive).

Advances in bone scaffolds' fabrication by AM processes have tried to replicate bone biological and biomechanical complexities. An example of this biomimetic approach is proposed by Kang and co-workers, who developed an innovative AM platform named "integrated tissue–organ printer" (ITOP) [110]. The ITOP is equipped with multi-cartridges capable of printing concomitantly synthetic polymers and cell-laden hydrogels with a resolution down to 2 μm for biomaterials and down to 50 μm for cells (Figure 4a). These features were used to fabricate a calvarial bone construct (8 mm diameter × 1.2 mm thickness) made of a PCL and tricalcium phosphate (TCP) nanoparticles blend and stem cells-loaded hydrogels, embedded in predefined positions (Figure 4b). After 10 days of in vitro osteogenic culture, the bioprinted bone is implanted in a calvarial bone defect region to study maturation up to five months. Histological (Figure 4c) and immunohistological images clearly show new bone formation even in the defect central portion; moreover, the presence of blood vessels demonstrates the absence of tissue necrosis confirming regeneration effectiveness. These promising results suggested the potential utility of printed living tissue constructs in translational applications.

Other recent examples have demonstrated, in vivo, successful calvarial bone regeneration using printed scaffolds made of hydroxyapatite (HA) or PCL/PLGA/HA composite, respectively [111,112]. Furthermore, the advantage of printing techniques to process multiple bioinks in a single scaffold was used to bioactivate the scaffold with BMP-2 peptide or μ-RiboNucleic Acid (μ-RNA) conjugates to enhance stem cells' osteoinduction to stimulate in vivo bone formation.

The regeneration of interface tissues, as osteocartilagenous anatomical regions, requires scaffolds displaying compositional and structural complexity that are only achievable with AM processes. In this context, an interesting fabrication approach is presented by Mekhileri and co-workers [113]. The authors have combined a commercial printer (BioScaffolder) with a custom-made device capable of handling pre-loaded μ-tissues (Figure 4d). The fabricated polymer strands are about 225 μm with a maximum resolution of 25 μm. μ-tissues could be positioned in scaffolds' pores once the fabrication process is finished or could be integrated during the fabrication process (inset of Figure 4d), demonstrating the possibility to fabricate large hybrid constructs with a predetermined architecture and mechanical stability. μ-tissues were produced with dimension of 700 μm to 1.4 mm, without undifferentiated or necrotic cells in the central regions at 28 days of in vitro culture and the chosen dimension was 1 mm for the integration into scaffolds due to design and handling considerations. Using this approach, the authors presented a proof of concept scaffold for joint resurfacing purposes (Figure 4e,f), in which two different natural hydrogels' microspheres were used to simulate the biphasic bone and cartilage portions. The process enabled the manipulation and positioning of the μ-tissues inside the scaffold (Figure 4g), while adjacent μ-tissues fusion is observed at 35 days of in vitro culture in chondrogenic differentiation media (Figure 4h).

A wide range of materials was used for AM purposes in this field, with encouraging results. For example, Gao and co-workers [114] have synthesized a strong copolymer hydrogel with large stretchability (up to 860%) and high compressive strength (up to 8.4 MPa). The material had a rapid thermoreversible sol-gel transition behavior that makes it suitable for graded scaffold printing. Furthermore, this gradient hydrogel scaffold printed with TGF β1 and β-tricalciumphosphate for chondral and bone layers respectively, promotes simultaneous regeneration of cartilage and subchondral bone in a rat model [114]. In another work, Deng and co-workers [115] used 3D printing process to prepare lithium (Li)- and silicon (Si)-containing scaffolds to study the effect of ions' release on osteochondral tissue repair in rabbits. The release of Li and Si ions synergistically exerted a positive effect on cartilage through the activation of hypoxia-inducible factor (HIF-1α) pathway and preservation of chondrocytes from an osteoarthritic environment. Concomitantly, Li and Si ions released from the scaffold improve subchondral bone reconstruction through activating Wnt signal pathways.

The versatility of AM techniques in terms of materials choice and structure design enabled the use of additive manufactured scaffolds in other important fields, such as cardiac and nerve tissues' regeneration. One of the most interesting works concerns a scaffold for cardiac remodeling after myocardial infarction, which is proposed by Yang and co-workers [116]. This device was fabricated by employing the fused deposition modeling (FDM) technology, whose typical resolution is of hundreds of microns [117], to obtain a stacked construction of PGS/PCL blend with regular crisscrossed strands and interconnected micropores (Figure 4i). The PGS/PCL scaffolds exhibited improved elasticity and toughness, if compared to raw PCL and PGS scaffolds respectively, and mechanical properties similar to heart tissue. Moreover, the PGS/PCL mixture was filled with NaCl particles with the goal to leach them out to generate an additional interconnected microporosity for oxygen and nutrients' transport and neovascularization. The study was conducted to first assess the in vitro and in vivo scaffolds' behavior, demonstrating an interesting therapeutic effect in rodents with respect to scaffold-free and PCL or PGS scaffolds implanted after myocardial infarction (Figure 4j), and later to study an annular-shaped scaffold whose results indicate a promising application for preventing ventricular dilation (Figure 4k). Moreover, those 3D-printed PGS/PCL scaffolds possess interesting shape-memory properties after rolling, folding, and compression. This feature holds promise for minimal invasiveness delivery via, for example, a catheter or mini-thoracotomy, in case of future surgical translation.

Another interesting example in this field is that of Boffito and co-workers [118], who have used a custom-made AM equipment to fabricate polyurethane (PU) scaffolds seeded with human cardiac progenitor cells (CPCs). PU scaffolds grafted with laminin-1 supported CPCs differentiation in cardiomyocytes while preliminary in vivo subcutaneous implantation experiments evidenced a minimal inflammatory response and adequate angiogenesis, suggesting their future use as implantable patches for myocardial TE.

Regarding the neural TE field, here we reported the results of the study of Koffler and co-workers [119], who have developed a "microscale continuous projection printing method" (μCPP) (Figure 4l) to fabricate, in a very short time (less than 2 s), a 2 mm-thick biomimetic scaffold for spinal cord injury repair (Figure 4m,n). Materials used for fabrication were mixtures of PEG and gelatin methacrylate. This material, in fact retained its structure over four weeks in vivo and exhibited an acceptable inflammatory response. The chosen material was then processed to obtain scaffolds mimicking the spinal cord structure (Figure 4m,n) and which were seeded with neural progenitor cells (NPCs) before implantation. After six weeks in vivo, injured host axons regenerate into 3D biomimetic scaffolds and synapse onto NPCs implanted into the device (Figure 4o). Furthermore, implanted NPCs extend axons out of the scaffold and into the host spinal cord below the injury to restore synaptic transmission and significantly improve spinal cord functionality.

The advantage of NPCs-laden 3D-printed biocompatible scaffold on nerve tissue repair is also highlighted in Reference [120], where clusters of induced pluripotent stem cell (iPSC)-derived spinal NPCs and oligodendrocyte progenitor cells (OPCs) are placed in precise positions within 3D-printed hydrogel scaffolds during assembly. A combination of transplanted neuronal and glial cells enhance functional axonal connections' formation across areas of the damaged central nervous system. Finally, the combination of cells and growth factor therapies, such as scaffolds releasing neurotrophin-3 growth factor [121], may represent a possible further step towards complete nerve tissue repair.

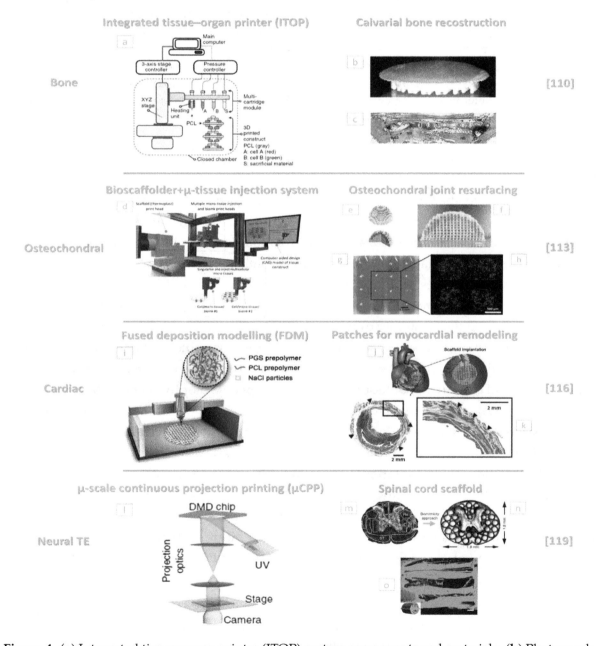

Figure 4. (**a**) Integrated tissue–organ printer (ITOP) system components and materials. (**b**) Photograph of the printed calvarial bone construct. (**c**) Histological image of the printed calvarial construct after in vivo implantation. (**d**) Image of the bioscaffolder + micro-tissue injection system (inset: working

concept overview of the micro-tissue injection system) used for the preparation of the osteochondral joint resurfacing device. (**e**) Computer-aided design (CAD) images and (**f**) optical image of an assembled hemispherical construct. (**g**) Image of μ-tissues in 3D printed PCL fibers and (**h**) resulting 4′,6-diamidino-2-phenylindole (DAPI) (blue) and Aggrecan (purple) antibodies staining of the construct showing cells distribution and μ-tissues fusion at 35 days of in vitro chondrogenic culture. (**i**) Fused deposition modeling (FDM) machine overview and materials for the elastic cardiac patch fabrication. (**j**) Illustration of the scaffold implantation site after induced myocardial infarction in rats. (**k**) Representative Masson's trichrome stained heart section four weeks after implantation. Black boxes denote higher magnification area of the left panel. Black arrows indicate the annular-shaped PGS-PCL scaffolds. Scale bars: 2.0 mm. (**l**) Microscale continuous projection printing (μCPP) system used to fabricate PEG–gelatin methacrylate scaffolds loaded with neural progenitor cells (NPCs) for nerve regeneration. (**m**) Spinal cord structure evidencing fascicles regions (motor systems are shown in green and sensory systems are shown in blue) and (**n**) corresponding scaffold. (**o**) Image of the NPCs-loaded scaffold after four weeks in vivo showing channels filled with green fluorescent protein (GFP)-expressing NPCs. (**a**–**c**) Reproduced with permission from Reference [110] (Kang, Nature Biotechnology; published by Springer Nature, 2016). (**d**–**h**) Reproduced with permission from Reference [113] (Mekhileri, Biofabrication; published by IOP Publishing, 2018). (**i**–**k**) Reproduced with permission from Reference [116] (Yang, Advanced Healthcare Materials; published by John Wiley and Sons, 2019). (**l**–**o**) Reproduced with permission from Reference [119] (Koffler, Nature Medicine; published by Springer Nature, 2019).

4. Conclusions

Over the last decade, there has been an impressive advancement on scaffolds-based formulations and strategies for bioengineer functional tissues and organs in vitro and in vivo. In this context, bottom-up approaches based on the rational assembly of modular units, in the form of cell-free/cell-laden μPs and/or layers, are, nowadays, the most promising and used approaches. Polymeric μPs offer the advantage in scaffolds' design of morphology and shape control, full pores interconnectivity, high mechanical properties, and biomolecules encapsulation and release. Furthermore, cell-laden μ-scaffolds demonstrated the capability to self-assemble in vitro to form μTPs made up of endogenous ECM and tunable in size and shape. These μTPs can be further assembled in large 3D patches. After μPs degradation, the resulting tissue can be used for in vitro study of complex tissue morphogenesis or for screening normal and dysfunctional tissues' response to specific biophysical and biochemical factors.

Soft-lithography and AM techniques enabled the CAD of cell-free scaffolds and cell-laden constructs down to nano-scale resolution, thereby overcoming limitations related to in vitro cell seeding and micro-architectural features' control. Although it was possible the fabrication of patient-specific devices suitable for clinical implantation, the regeneration of even complex biological tissues aided by these scaffolds is still far from being achieved and requires extensive research efforts on materials design and processing, automated systems integration, and processing times acceleration.

In conclusion, all the results highlighted in this work indicate that the next decades challenge will be to obtain a technology platform that enables users to fabricate ECM-mimicking architectures capable of controlling cell activities and directing their fate for clinical translation and successful engineering of tissues and organs.

Author Contributions: Conceptualization, A.S. and P.A.N.; writing—original draft preparation, A.S., G.C. and P.P.; writing—review and editing, A.S., G.C., P.P. and P.A.N.; visualization, A.S., G.C. and P.P.

Abbreviations

AL	Alendronate
ALP	Alkaline phosphatase activity
AM	Additive manufacturing
APS	Poly (ester-amide),1:2 poly (1,3-diamino-2-hydroxypropane-co -polyol sebacate)
3D	Three-dimensional
BMP	Bone morphogenic protein
BSA	Bovine serum albumin
CAD	Computer-aided design
CPC	Cardiac progenitor cell
Dex	Dexamethasone
ECM	Extracellular matrix
ES cells	Embryonic stem cells
FDM	Fused deposition modeling
HA	Hydroxyapatite
HDF	Human dermal fibroblast
HIF	Hypoxia-inducible factor
hMSC	Human mesenchymal stem cell
HUVEC	Human umbilical vein endothelial cell
ITOP	Integrated tissue–organ printer
μCPP	Microscale continuous projection printing method
μP	Microparticle
μTP	Micro-tissue precursor
MSC	Mesenchymal stem cell
NIH3T3	Mouse embryo fibroblast cell line
NPC	Neural progenitor cell
OPC	Oligodendrocyte progenitor cell
Pa	Pascal
PBS	Phosphate-buffered saline
PCGA	Poly (ε-caprolcatone–co-glycolic acid)
PCL	Polycaprolactone
PDMS	Polydimethylsiloxane
PEG	Poly-ethylene glycol
PEGDM	Poly (ethylene glycol) dimethyl ether
PEGDA	Polyethylene glycol diacrylate
PEGDMA	Polyethylen glycol dimethacrylate
PGS	Poly (glycerol sebacate)
PLA	Poly-lactic acid
PLGA	Polylactic-co-glycolic acid
PLLA	Poly(L-lactic acid)
PLT32o	Poly (limonene thioether)
Poly(NIPAAm-co-HEMAHex)	Poly (N-isopropylacrylamide–co-2-hydroxyethylmethacrylate-6-hydroxyhexanoate)
POMaC	Poly (octamethylene maleate (anhydride) citrate
PSC	Pluripotent stem cell
PU	Polyurethane
PVA	Poly (vinyl alcohol)
REM	Replica molding
RLC	Rat liver cells
RNA	RiboNucleic Acid
S1P	Sphingosine 1-phosphate
SEAL	StampEd Assembly of polymer Layers
SLS	Selective laser sintering
SMC	Smooth muscle cell
SPCL	Starch-polycaprolactone

TCP   Tricalcium phosphate
TE   Tissue engineering
TGF   Transforming growth factor
UV   Ultraviolet
VEGF   Vascular endothelial growth factor

References

1.   O'Brien, F.J. Biomaterials & scaffolds for tissue engineering. *Mater. Today* **2011**, *14*, 88–95.
2.   Trappmann, B.; Gautrot, J.E.; Connelly, J.T.; Strange, D.G.T.; Li, Y.; Oyen, M.L.; Stuart, M.A.C.; Boehm, H.; Li, B.; Vogel, V.; et al. Extracellular-matrix tethering regulates stem-cell fate. *Nat. Mater.* **2012**, *11*, 642–649. [CrossRef] [PubMed]
3.   Stratton, S.; Shelke, N.B.; Hoshino, K.; Rudraiah, S.; Kumbar, S.G. Bioactive polymeric scaffolds for tissue engineering. *Bioact. Mater.* **2016**, *1*, 93–108. [CrossRef] [PubMed]
4.   Luciani, A.; Coccoli, V.; Orsi, S.; Ambrosio, L.; Netti, P.A. PCL microspheres based functional scaffolds by bottom-up approach with predefined microstructural properties and release profiles. *Biomaterials* **2008**, *29*, 4800–4807. [CrossRef] [PubMed]
5.   Netti, P.A. *Biomedical Foams for Tissue Engineering Applications*; Woodhead Publishing series in biomaterials; Woodhead Publishing: Cambridge, UK, 2014; ISBN 978-0-85709-703-3.
6.   Moioli, E.K.; Clark, P.A.; Xin, X.; Lal, S.; Mao, J.J. Matrices and scaffolds for drug delivery in dental, oral and craniofacial tissue engineering. *Adv. Drug Deliv. Rev.* **2007**, *59*, 308–324. [CrossRef]
7.   Schantz, J.-T.; Chim, H.; Whiteman, M. Cell Guidance in Tissue Engineering: SDF-1 Mediates Site-Directed Homing of Mesenchymal Stem Cells within Three-Dimensional Polycaprolactone Scaffolds. *Tissue Eng.* **2007**, *13*, 2615–2624. [CrossRef]
8.   Iannone, M.; Ventre, M.; Pagano, G.; Giannoni, P.; Quarto, R.; Netti, P.A. Defining an optimal stromal derived factor-1 presentation for effective recruitment of mesenchymal stem cells in 3D: Optimal SDF-1 Presentation for MSCs Recruitment. *Biotechnol. Bioeng.* **2014**, *111*, 2303–2316. [CrossRef]
9.   Sundararaghavan, H.G.; Saunders, R.L.; Hammer, D.A.; Burdick, J.A. Fiber alignment directs cell motility over chemotactic gradients. *Biotechnol. Bioeng.* **2013**, *110*, 1249–1254. [CrossRef]
10. Ma, J.; Both, S.K.; Yang, F.; Cui, F.-Z.; Pan, J.; Meijer, G.J.; Jansen, J.A.; van den Beucken, J.J.J.P. Concise Review: Cell-Based Strategies in Bone Tissue Engineering and Regenerative Medicine. *STEM CELLS Transl. Med.* **2014**, *3*, 98–107. [CrossRef]
11. Badylak, S.F.; Taylor, D.; Uygun, K. Whole-Organ Tissue Engineering: Decellularization and Recellularization of Three-Dimensional Matrix Scaffolds. *Annu. Rev. Biomed. Eng.* **2011**, *13*, 27–53. [CrossRef]
12. Loh, Q.L.; Choong, C. Three-Dimensional Scaffolds for Tissue Engineering Applications: Role of Porosity and Pore Size. *Tissue Eng. Part B Rev.* **2013**, *19*, 485–502. [CrossRef] [PubMed]
13. Reinwald, Y.; Johal, R.; Ghaemmaghami, A.; Rose, F.; Howdle, S.; Shakesheff, K.; Howdle, S.; Shakesheff, K. Interconnectivity and permeability of supercritical fluid-foamed scaffolds and the effect of their structural properties on cell distribution. *Polymers* **2014**, *55*, 435–444. [CrossRef]
14. Harley, B.A.C.; Kim, H.-D.; Zaman, M.H.; Yannas, I.V.; Lauffenburger, D.A.; Gibson, L.J. Microarchitecture of Three-Dimensional Scaffolds Influences Cell Migration Behavior via Junction Interactions. *Biophys. J.* **2008**, *95*, 4013–4024. [CrossRef] [PubMed]
15. Bai, F.; Wang, Z.; Lu, J.; Liu, J.; Chen, G.; Lv, R.; Wang, J.; Lin, K.; Zhang, J.; Huang, X. The Correlation between the Internal Structure and Vascularization of Controllable Porous Bioceramic Materials In Vivo: A Quantitative Study. *Tissue Eng. Part A* **2010**, *16*, 3791–3803. [CrossRef]
16. Perez, R.A.; Mestres, G. Role of pore size and morphology in musculo-skeletal tissue regeneration. *Mater. Sci. Eng. C* **2016**, *61*, 922–939. [CrossRef]
17. Hutmacher, D.W. Scaffolds in tissue engineering bone and cartilage. *Biomaterials* **2000**, *21*, 2529–2543. [CrossRef]
18. Zhang, H.; Zhou, L.; Zhang, W. Control of Scaffold Degradation in Tissue Engineering: A Review. *Tissue Eng. Part B Rev.* **2014**, *20*, 492–502. [CrossRef]
19. Huang, J.; Gräter, S.V.; Corbellini, F.; Rinck, S.; Bock, E.; Kemkemer, R.; Kessler, H.; Ding, J.; Spatz, J.P.; Rinck-Jahnke, S. Impact of Order and Disorder in RGD Nanopatterns on Cell Adhesion. *Nano Lett.* **2009**, *9*, 1111–1116. [CrossRef]

20. Sun, A.X.; Lin, H.; Fritch, M.R.; Shen, H.; Alexander, P.G.; Dehart, M.; Tuan, R.S. Chondrogenesis of human bone marrow mesenchymal stem cells in 3-dimensional, photocrosslinked hydrogel constructs: Effect of cell seeding density and material stiffness. *Acta Biomater.* **2017**, *58*, 302–311. [CrossRef]

21. Swinehart, I.T.; Badylak, S.F. Extracellular matrix bioscaffolds in tissue remodeling and morphogenesis: ECM Bioscaffolds in Development and Healing. *Dev. Dyn.* **2016**, *245*, 351–360. [CrossRef]

22. Chaudhuri, O.; Gu, L.; Klumpers, D.; Darnell, M.; Bencherif, S.A.; Weaver, J.C.; Huebsch, N.; Lee, H.; Lippens, E.; Duda, G.N.; et al. Hydrogels with tunable stress relaxation regulate stem cell fate and activity. *Nat. Mater.* **2016**, *15*, 326–334. [CrossRef] [PubMed]

23. Baker, B.M.; Trappmann, B.; Wang, W.Y.; Sakar, M.S.; Kim, I.L.; Shenoy, V.B.; Burdick, J.A.; Chen, C.S. Cell-mediated fibre recruitment drives extracellular matrix mechanosensing in engineered fibrillar microenvironments. *Nat. Mater.* **2015**, *14*, 1262–1268. [CrossRef] [PubMed]

24. Subbiah, R.; Guldberg, R.E. Materials Science and Design Principles of Growth Factor Delivery Systems in Tissue Engineering and Regenerative Medicine. *Adv. Healthc. Mater.* **2019**, *8*, 1801000. [CrossRef] [PubMed]

25. Lee, K.; Silva, E.A.; Mooney, D.J. Growth factor delivery-based tissue engineering: General approaches and a review of recent developments. *J. R. Soc. Interface* **2011**, *8*, 153–170. [CrossRef] [PubMed]

26. Fusco, S.; Panzetta, V.; Embrione, V.; Netti, P.A. Crosstalk between focal adhesions and material mechanical properties governs cell mechanics and functions. *Acta Biomater.* **2015**, *23*, 63–71. [CrossRef] [PubMed]

27. Hoffman-Kim, D.; Mitchel, J.A.; Bellamkonda, R.V. Topography, cell response, and nerve regeneration. *Annu. Rev. Biomed. Eng.* **2010**, *12*, 203–231. [CrossRef]

28. Carmeliet, P.; Conway, E.M. Growing better blood vessels. *Nat. Biotechnol.* **2001**, *19*, 1019–1020. [CrossRef]

29. Richardson, T.P.; Peters, M.C.; Ennett, A.B.; Mooney, D.J. Polymeric system for dual growth factor delivery. *Nat. Biotechnol.* **2001**, *19*, 1029–1034. [CrossRef]

30. Patel, Z.S.; Young, S.; Tabata, Y.; Jansen, J.A.; Wong, M.E.; Mikos, A.G. Dual delivery of an angiogenic and an osteogenic growth factor for bone regeneration in a critical size defect model. *Bone* **2008**, *43*, 931–940. [CrossRef]

31. Nichol, J.W.; Khademhosseini, A. Modular Tissue Engineering: Engineering Biological Tissues from the Bottom Up. *Soft Matter* **2009**, *5*, 1312–1319. [CrossRef]

32. Elbert, D.L. Bottom-up tissue engineering. *Curr. Opin. Biotechnol.* **2011**, *22*, 674–680. [CrossRef] [PubMed]

33. Kesireddy, V.; Kasper, F.K. Approaches for building bioactive elements into synthetic scaffolds for bone tissue engineering. *J. Mater. Chem. B* **2016**, *4*, 6773–6786. [CrossRef] [PubMed]

34. Leferink, A.; Schipper, D.; Arts, E.; Vrij, E.; Rivron, N.; Karperien, M.; Mittmann, K.; Van Blitterswijk, C.; Moroni, L.; Truckenmuller, R. Engineered Micro-Objects as Scaffolding Elements in Cellular Building Blocks for Bottom-Up Tissue Engineering Approaches. *Adv. Mater.* **2014**, *26*, 2592–2599. [CrossRef] [PubMed]

35. Huang, C.-C.; Wei, H.-J.; Yeh, Y.-C.; Wang, J.-J.; Lin, W.-W.; Lee, T.-Y.; Hwang, S.-M.; Choi, S.-W.; Xia, Y.; Chang, Y.; et al. Injectable PLGA porous beads cellularized by hAFSCs for cellular cardiomyoplasty. *Biomaterials* **2012**, *33*, 4069–4077. [CrossRef] [PubMed]

36. Maya, I.C.; Guarino, V. Introduction to electrofluidodynamic techniques. Part I. In *Electrofluidodynamic Technologies (EFDTs) for Biomaterials and Medical Devices*; Elsevier BV: Amsterdam, The Netherlands, 2018; pp. 1–17.

37. Wang, L.; Chen, Y.; Qian, J.; Tan, Y.; Huangfu, S.; Ding, Y.; Ding, S.; Jiang, B. A bottom-up method to build 3d scaffolds with predefined vascular network. *J. Mech. Med. Boil.* **2013**, *13*, 1340008. [CrossRef]

38. Giannitelli, S.; Accoto, D.; Trombetta, M.; Rainer, A. Current trends in the design of scaffolds for computer-aided tissue engineering. *Acta Biomater.* **2014**, *10*, 580–594. [CrossRef]

39. Cheng, D.; Hou, J.; Hao, L.; Cao, X.; Gao, H.; Fu, X.; Wang, Y. Bottom-up topography assembly into 3D porous scaffold to mediate cell activities. *J. Biomed. Mater. Res. B Appl. Biomater.* **2016**, *104*, 1056–1063. [CrossRef]

40. Levato, R.; Visser, J.; Planell, J.A.; Engel, E.; Malda, J.; Mateos-Timoneda, M.A. Biofabrication of tissue constructs by 3D bioprinting of cell-laden microcarriers. *Biofabrication* **2014**, *6*, 035020. [CrossRef]

41. Xu, Y.; Kim, C.-S.; Saylor, D.M.; Koo, D. Polymer degradation and drug delivery in PLGA-based drug-polymer applications: A review of experiments and theories. *J. Biomed. Mater. Res. B Appl. Biomater.* **2017**, *105*, 1692–1716. [CrossRef]

42. Cho, D.-I.D.; Yoo, H.J. Microfabrication Methods for Biodegradable Polymeric Carriers for Drug Delivery System Applications: A Review. *J. Microelectromech. Syst.* **2015**, *24*, 10–18. [CrossRef]

43.   Edmondson, R.; Broglie, J.J.; Adcock, A.F.; Yang, L. Three-Dimensional Cell Culture Systems and Their Applications in Drug Discovery and Cell-Based Biosensors. *ASSAY Drug Dev. Technol.* **2014**, *12*, 207–218. [CrossRef] [PubMed]

44.   Salerno, A.; Levato, R.; Mateos-Timoneda, M.A.; Engel, E.; Netti, P.A.; Planell, J.A. Modular polylactic acid microparticle-based scaffolds prepared via microfluidic emulsion/solvent displacement process: Fabrication, characterization, and in vitro mesenchymal stem cells interaction study. *J. Biomed. Mater. Res. A* **2013**, *101A*, 720–732. [CrossRef] [PubMed]

45.   Cao, X.; Li, W.; Ma, T.; Dong, H. One-step fabrication of polymeric hybrid particles with core–shell, patchy, patchy Janus and Janus architectures via a microfluidic-assisted phase separation process. *RSC Adv.* **2015**, *5*, 79969–79975. [CrossRef]

46.   De Alteriis, R.; Vecchione, R.; Attanasio, C.; De Gregorio, M.; Porzio, M.; Battista, E.; Netti, P.A. A method to tune the shape of protein-encapsulated polymeric microspheres. *Sci. Rep.* **2015**, *5*, 12634. [CrossRef]

47.   Dendukuri, D.; Pregibon, D.C.; Collins, J.; Hatton, T.A.; Doyle, P.S. Continuous-flow lithography for high-throughput microparticle synthesis. *Nat. Mater.* **2006**, *5*, 365–369. [CrossRef] [PubMed]

48.   Vallet-Regí, M.; Salinas, A.J. Ceramics as bone repair materials. In *Bone Repair Biomaterials*; Elsevier: Amsterdam, The Netherlands, 2019; pp. 141–178, ISBN 978-0-08-102451-5.

49.   Xia, Y.; Pack, D.W. Uniform biodegradable microparticle systems for controlled release. *Chem. Eng. Sci.* **2015**, *125*, 129–143. [CrossRef]

50.   Campos, E.; Branquinho, J.; Carreira, A.S.; Carvalho, A.; Coimbra, P.; Ferreira, P.; Gil, M.H. Designing polymeric microparticles for biomedical and industrial applications. *Eur. Polym. J.* **2013**, *49*, 2005–2021. [CrossRef]

51.   Ma, S.; Mukherjee, N. Microfluidics Fabrication of Soft Microtissues and Bottom-Up Assembly. *Adv. Biosyst.* **2018**, *2*, 1800119. [CrossRef]

52.   Li, W.; Zhang, L.; Ge, X.; Xu, B.; Zhang, W.; Qu, L.; Choi, C.-H.; Xu, J.; Zhang, A.; Lee, H.; et al. Microfluidic fabrication of microparticles for biomedical applications. *Chem. Soc. Rev.* **2018**, *47*, 5646–5683. [CrossRef]

53.   Choi, S.-W.; Yeh, Y.-C.; Zhang, Y.S.; Sung, H.-W.; Xia, Y. Uniform beads with controllable pore sizes for biomedical applications. *Small* **2010**, *6*, 1492–1498. [CrossRef]

54.   Baah, D.; Floyd-Smith, T. Microfluidics for particle synthesis from photocrosslinkable materials. *Microfluid. Nanofluid.* **2014**, *17*, 431–455. [CrossRef]

55.   Xu, S.; Nie, Z.; Seo, M.; Lewis, P.; Kumacheva, E.; Stone, H.A.; Garstecki, P.; Weibel, D.B.; Gitlin, I.; Whitesides, G.M. Generation of Monodisperse Particles by Using Microfluidics: Control over Size, Shape, and Composition. *Angew. Chem.* **2005**, *117*, 3865. [CrossRef]

56.   Panda, P.; Ali, S.; Lo, E.; Chung, B.G.; Hatton, T.A.; Khademhosseini, A.; Doyle, P.S. Stop-flow lithography to generate cell-laden microgel particles. *Lab Chip* **2008**, *8*, 1056–1061. [CrossRef] [PubMed]

57.   Canelas, D.A.; Herlihy, K.P.; DeSimone, J.M. Top-down particle fabrication: Control of size and shape for diagnostic imaging and drug delivery: Top-down particle fabrication. *Wiley Interdiscip. Rev. Nanomed. Nanobiotechnol.* **2009**, *1*, 391–404. [CrossRef] [PubMed]

58.   Higuita, N.; Dai, Z.; Kaletunç, G.; Hansford, D.J. Fabrication of pH-sensitive microparticles for drug delivery applications using soft lithography techniques. In Proceedings of the Mater. *Res. Soc. Symp. Proc.* **2008**, *1095*, 7–12.

59.   Guan, J.; Ferrell, N.; Lee, L.J.; Hansford, D.J. Fabrication of polymeric microparticles for drug delivery by soft lithography. *Biomaterials* **2006**, *27*, 4034–4041. [CrossRef] [PubMed]

60.   McHugh, K.J.; Nguyen, T.D.; Linehan, A.R.; Yang, D.; Behrens, A.M.; Rose, S.; Tochka, Z.L.; Tzeng, S.Y.; Norman, J.J.; Anselmo, A.C.; et al. Fabrication of fillable microparticles and other complex 3D microstructures. *Science* **2017**, *359*, 1138–1142. [CrossRef]

61.   Wang, H.; Leeuwenburgh, S.C.G.; Li, Y.; Jansen, J.A. The Use of Micro- and Nanospheres as Functional Components for Bone Tissue Regeneration. *Tissue Eng. Part B Rev.* **2012**, *18*, 24–39. [CrossRef]

62.   Qutachi, O.; Vetsch, J.R.; Gill, D.; Cox, H.; Scurr, D.J.; Hofmann, S.; Müller, R.; Quirk, R.A.; Shakesheff, K.M.; Rahman, C.V. Injectable and porous PLGA microspheres that form highly porous scaffolds at body temperature. *Acta Biomater.* **2014**, *10*, 5090–5098. [CrossRef]

63.   Jeon, J.H.; Bhamidipati, M.; Sridharan, B.; Scurto, A.M.; Berkland, C.J.; Detamore, M.S. Tailoring of processing parameters for sintering microsphere-based scaffolds with dense-phase carbon dioxide. *J. Biomed. Mater. Res. B Appl. Biomater.* **2013**, *101B*, 330–337. [CrossRef]

64. Bhamidipati, M.; Sridharan, B.; Scurto, A.M.; Detamore, M.S. Subcritical CO2 sintering of microspheres of different polymeric materials to fabricate scaffolds for tissue engineering. *Mater. Sci. Eng. C* **2013**, *33*, 4892–4899. [CrossRef] [PubMed]

65. Ghanbar, H.; Luo, C.; Bakhshi, P.; Day, R.; Edirisinghe, M. Preparation of porous microsphere-scaffolds by electrohydrodynamic forming and thermally induced phase separation. *Mater. Sci. Eng. C* **2013**, *33*, 2488–2498. [CrossRef] [PubMed]

66. Mikael, P.E.; Amini, A.R.; Basu, J.; Arellano-Jimenez, M.J.; Laurencin, C.T.; Sanders, M.M.; Carter, C.B.; Nukavarapu, S.P. Functionalized carbon nanotube reinforced scaffolds for bone regenerative engineering: Fabrication, in vitro and in vivo evaluation. *Biomed. Mater.* **2014**, *9*, 35001. [CrossRef] [PubMed]

67. Lv, Q.; Nair, L.; Laurencin, C.T. Fabrication, characterization, and in vitro evaluation of poly(lactic acid glycolic acid)/nano-hydroxyapatite composite microsphere-based scaffolds for bone tissue engineering in rotating bioreactors. *J. Biomed. Mater. Res. A* **2009**, *91A*, 679–691. [CrossRef]

68. Borden, M. Structural and human cellular assessment of a novel microsphere-based tissue engineered scaffold for bone repair. *Biomaterials* **2003**, *24*, 597–609. [CrossRef]

69. Brown, J.L.; Nair, L.S.; Laurencin, C.T. Solvent/non-solvent sintering: A novel route to create porous microsphere scaffolds for tissue regeneration. *J. Biomed. Mater. Res. Part B Appl. Biomater.* **2008**, *86*, 396–406. [CrossRef]

70. Shi, X.; Ren, L.; Tian, M.; Yu, J.; Huang, W.; Du, C.; Wang, D.-A.; Wang, Y. In vivo and in vitro osteogenesis of stem cells induced by controlled release of drugs from microspherical scaffolds. *J. Mater. Chem.* **2010**, *20*, 9140. [CrossRef]

71. Jaklenec, A.; Wan, E.; Murray, M.E.; Mathiowitz, E. Novel scaffolds fabricated from protein-loaded microspheres for tissue engineering. *Biomaterials* **2008**, *29*, 185–192. [CrossRef]

72. Singh, M.; Morris, C.P.; Ellis, R.J.; Detamore, M.S.; Berkland, C. Microsphere-Based Seamless Scaffolds Containing Macroscopic Gradients of Encapsulated Factors for Tissue Engineering. *Tissue Eng. Part C Methods* **2008**, *14*, 299–309. [CrossRef]

73. Dormer, N.H.; Singh, M.; Wang, L.; Berkland, C.J.; Detamore, M.S. Osteochondral interface tissue engineering using macroscopic gradients of bioactive signals. *Ann. Biomed. Eng.* **2010**, *38*, 2167–2182. [CrossRef]

74. Jiang, T.; Nukavarapu, S.P.; Deng, M.; Jabbarzadeh, E.; Kofron, M.D.; Doty, S.B.; Abdel-Fattah, W.I.; Laurencin, C.T. Chitosan–poly (lactide-co-glycolide) microsphere-based scaffolds for bone tissue engineering: In vitro degradation and in vivo bone regeneration studies. *Acta Biomater.* **2010**, *6*, 3457–3470. [CrossRef] [PubMed]

75. Gupta, V.; Lyne, D.V.; Laflin, A.D.; Zabel, T.A.; Barragan, M.; Bunch, J.T.; Pacicca, D.M.; Detamore, M.S. Microsphere-Based Osteochondral Scaffolds Carrying Opposing Gradients of Decellularized Cartilage And Demineralized Bone Matrix. *ACS Biomater. Sci. Eng.* **2017**, *3*, 1955–1963. [CrossRef]

76. Tedesco, M.T.; Di Lisa, D.; Massobrio, P.; Colistra, N.; Pesce, M.; Catelani, T.; Dellacasa, E.; Raiteri, R.; Martinoia, S.; Pastorino, L. Soft chitosan microbeads scaffold for 3D functional neuronal networks. *Biomaterials* **2018**, *156*, 159–171. [CrossRef] [PubMed]

77. Du, Y.; Liu, H.; Shuang, J.; Wang, J.; Ma, J.; Zhang, S. Microsphere-based selective laser sintering for building macroporous bone scaffolds with controlled microstructure and excellent biocompatibility. *Colloids Surf. B Biointerfaces* **2015**, *135*, 81–89. [CrossRef] [PubMed]

78. Du, Y.; Liu, H.; Yang, Q.; Wang, S.; Wang, J.; Ma, J.; Noh, I.; Mikos, A.G.; Zhang, S. Selective laser sintering scaffold with hierarchical architecture and gradient composition for osteochondral repair in rabbits. *Biomaterials* **2017**, *137*, 37–48. [CrossRef]

79. Rossi, L.; Attanasio, C.; Vilardi, E.; De Gregorio, M.; Netti, P.A. Vasculogenic potential evaluation of bottom-up, PCL scaffolds guiding early angiogenesis in tissue regeneration. *J. Mater. Sci. Mater. Electron.* **2016**, *27*, 107. [CrossRef]

80. Urciuolo, F.; Imparato, G.; Totaro, A.; Netti, P.A. Building a Tissue in Vitro from the Bottom Up: Implications in Regenerative Medicine. *Methodist DeBakey Cardiovasc. J.* **2013**, *9*, 213–217. [CrossRef]

81. Casale, C.; Imparato, G.; Urciuolo, F.; Netti, P.A. Endogenous human skin equivalent promotes in vitro morphogenesis of follicle-like structures. *Biomaterials* **2016**, *101*, 86–95. [CrossRef]

82. Mazio, C.; Casale, C.; Imparato, G.; Urciuolo, F.; Attanasio, C.; De Gregorio, M.; Rescigno, F.; Netti, P.A. Pre-vascularized dermis model for fast and functional anastomosis with host vasculature. *Biomaterials* **2019**, *192*, 159–170. [CrossRef]

83. Casale, C.; Imparato, G.; Urciuolo, F.; Rescigno, F.; Scamardella, S.; Escolino, M.; Netti, P.A. Engineering a human skin equivalent to study dermis remodelling and epidermis senescence in vitro after UVA exposure. *J. Tissue Eng. Regen. Med.* **2018**, *12*, 1658–1669. [CrossRef]

84. Totaro, A.; Salerno, A.; Imparato, G.; Domingo, C.; Urciuolo, F.; Netti, P.A. PCL-HA microscaffolds for in vitro modular bone tissue engineering: PCL-HA microscaffolds for bone tissue engineering. *J. Tissue Eng. Regen. Med.* **2017**, *11*, 1865–1875. [CrossRef] [PubMed]

85. Totaro, A.; Urciuolo, F.; Imparato, G.; Netti, P.A. Engineered cardiac micromodules for the in vitro fabrication of 3D endogenous macro-tissues. *Biofabrication* **2016**, *8*, 025014. [CrossRef] [PubMed]

86. Yajima, Y.; Yamada, M.; Utoh, R.; Seki, M. Collagen Microparticle-Mediated 3D Cell Organization: A Facile Route to Bottom-up Engineering of Thick and Porous Tissues. *ACS Biomater. Sci. Eng.* **2017**, *3*, 2144–2154. [CrossRef]

87. Chen, M.; Wang, X.; Ye, Z.; Zhang, Y.; Zhou, Y.; Tan, W.-S. A modular approach to the engineering of a centimeter-sized bone tissue construct with human amniotic mesenchymal stem cells-laden microcarriers. *Biomaterials* **2011**, *32*, 7532–7542. [CrossRef]

88. Scott, E.A.; Nichols, M.D.; Kuntz-Willits, R.; Elbert, D.L. Modular scaffolds assembled around living cells using poly(ethylene glycol) microspheres with macroporation via a non-cytotoxic porogen. *Acta Biomater.* **2010**, *6*, 29–38. [CrossRef] [PubMed]

89. Tan, Y.J.; Tan, X.; Yeong, W.Y.; Tor, S.B. Hybrid microscaffold-based 3D bioprinting of multi-cellular constructs with high compressive strength: A new biofabrication strategy. *Sci. Rep.* **2016**, *6*, 39140. [CrossRef] [PubMed]

90. Xiao, W.; Xi, H.; Li, J.; Wei, D.; Li, B.; Liao, X.; Fan, H. Fabrication and assembly of porous micropatterned scaffolds for modular tissue engineering. *Mater. Lett.* **2018**, *228*, 360–364. [CrossRef]

91. Liu, Y.; Li, G.; Lu, H.; Yang, Y.; Liu, Z.; Shang, W.; Shen, Y. Magnetically Actuated Heterogeneous Microcapsule-Robot for the Construction of 3D Bioartificial Architectures. *ACS Appl. Mater. Interfaces* **2019**, *11*, 25664–25673. [CrossRef]

92. Gallego, D.; Ferrell, N.; Sun, Y.; Hansford, D.J. Multilayer micromolding of degradable polymer tissue engineering scaffolds. *Mater. Sci. Eng. C* **2008**, *28*, 353–358. [CrossRef]

93. Sodha, S.; Wall, K.; Redenti, S.; Klassen, H.; Young, M.J.; Tao, S.L. Microfabrication of a Three-Dimensional Polycaprolactone Thin-Film Scaffold for Retinal Progenitor Cell Encapsulation. *J. Biomater. Sci. Polym. Ed.* **2011**, *22*, 443–456. [CrossRef]

94. Rosellini, E.; Vozzi, G.; Barbani, N.; Giusti, P.; Cristallini, C. Three-dimensional microfabricated scaffolds with cardiac extracellular matrix-like architecture. *Int. J. Artif. Organs* **2010**, *33*, 885–894. [CrossRef] [PubMed]

95. He, J.; Liu, Y.; Hao, X.; Mao, M.; Zhu, L.; Li, D. Bottom-up generation of 3D silk fibroin–gelatin microfluidic scaffolds with improved structural and biological properties. *Mater. Lett.* **2012**, *78*, 102–105. [CrossRef]

96. He, J.; Zhu, L.; Liu, Y.; Li, D.; Jin, Z. Sequential assembly of 3D perfusable microfluidic hydrogels. *J. Mater. Sci. Mater. Electron.* **2014**, *25*, 2491–2500. [CrossRef] [PubMed]

97. Son, J.; Bae, C.Y.; Park, J.-K. Freestanding stacked mesh-like hydrogel sheets enable the creation of complex macroscale cellular scaffolds. *Biotechnol. J.* **2016**, *11*, 585–591. [CrossRef]

98. Son, J.; Bang, M.S.; Park, J.-K. Hand-Maneuverable Collagen Sheet with Micropatterns for 3D Modular Tissue Engineering. *ACS Biomater. Sci. Eng.* **2019**, *5*, 339–345. [CrossRef]

99. Zhang, B.; Lai, B.F.L.; Xie, R.; Huyer, L.D.; Montgomery, M.; Radisic, M. Microfabrication of AngioChip, a biodegradable polymer scaffold with microfluidic vasculature. *Nat. Protoc.* **2018**, *13*, 1793–1813. [CrossRef]

100. Lee, B.-K.; Lee, B.-Y. Investigation of thermoplastic hot embossing process using soft polydimethylsiloxane (PDMS) micromold. *J. Mech. Sci. Technol.* **2015**, *29*, 5063–5067. [CrossRef]

101. Yang, Y.; Xie, Y.; Kang, X.; Lee, L.J.; Kniss, D.A. Assembly of Three-Dimensional Polymeric Constructs Containing Cells/Biomolecules Using Carbon Dioxide. *J. Am. Chem. Soc.* **2006**, *128*, 14040–14041. [CrossRef]

102. Xie, Y.; Yang, Y.; Kang, X.; Li, R.; Volakis, L.I.; Zhang, X.; Lee, L.J.; Kniss, D.A. Bioassembly of three-dimensional embryonic stem cell-scaffold complexes using compressed gases. *Biotechnol. Prog.* **2009**, *25*, 535–542. [CrossRef]

103. Wang, Y.; Balowski, J.; Phillips, C.; Phillips, R.; Sims, C.E.; Allbritton, N.L. Benchtop micromolding of polystyrene by soft lithography. *Lab Chip* **2011**, *11*, 3089–3097. [CrossRef]

104. Papenburg, B.J.; Liu, J.; Higuera, G.A.; Barradas, A.M.; De Boer, J.; Van Blitterswijk, C.A.; Wessling, M.; Stamatialis, D. Development and analysis of multi-layer scaffolds for tissue engineering. *Biomaterials* **2009**, *30*, 6228–6239. [CrossRef] [PubMed]

105. Liu, Z.; Lu, M.; Takeuchi, M.; Yue, T.; Hasegawa, Y.; Huang, Q.; Fukuda, T. In vitro mimicking the morphology of hepatic lobule tissue based on Ca-alginate cell sheets. *Biomed. Mater.* **2018**, *13*, 035004. [CrossRef] [PubMed]

106. Ye, X.; Lu, L.; Kolewe, M.E.; Hearon, K.; Fischer, K.M.; Coppeta, J.; Freed, L.E. Scalable units for building cardiac tissue. *Adv. Mater.* **2014**, *26*, 7202–7208. [CrossRef] [PubMed]

107. Fischer, K.M.; Morgan, K.Y.; Hearon, K.; Sklaviadis, D.; Tochka, Z.L.; Fenton, O.S.; Anderson, D.G.; Langer, R.; Freed, L.E. Poly (Limonene Thioether) Scaffold for Tissue Engineering. *Adv. Healthc. Mater.* **2016**, *5*, 813–821. [CrossRef] [PubMed]

108. Ryu, W.; Hammerick, K.E.; Kim, Y.B.; Kim, J.B.; Fasching, R.; Prinz, F.B. Three-dimensional biodegradable microscaffolding: Scaffold characterization and cell population at single cell resolution. *Acta Biomater.* **2011**, *7*, 3325–3335. [CrossRef] [PubMed]

109. Lima, M.J.; Pirraco, R.P.; Sousa, R.A.; Neves, N.M.; Marques, A.P.; Bhattacharya, M.; Correlo, V.M.; Reis, R.L. Bottom-up approach to construct microfabricated multi-layer scaffolds for bone tissue engineering. *Biomed. Microdevices* **2014**, *16*, 69–78. [CrossRef]

110. Kang, H.-W.; Lee, S.J.; Ko, I.K.; Kengla, C.; Yoo, J.J.; Atala, A. A 3D bioprinting system to produce human-scale tissue constructs with structural integrity. *Nat. Biotechnol.* **2016**, *34*, 312–319. [CrossRef]

111. Chen, G.; Sun, Y.; Lu, F.; Jiang, A.; Subedi, D.; Kong, P.; Wang, X.; Yu, T.; Chi, H.; Song, C.; et al. A three-dimensional (3D) printed biomimetic hierarchical scaffold with a covalent modular release system for osteogenesis. *Mater. Sci. Eng. C* **2019**, *104*, 109842. [CrossRef]

112. Moncal, K.K.; Aydin, R.S.T.; Abu-Laban, M.; Heo, D.N.; Rizk, E.; Tucker, S.M.; Lewis, G.S.; Hayes, D.; Ozbolat, I.T. Collagen-infilled 3D printed scaffolds loaded with miR-148b-transfected bone marrow stem cells improve calvarial bone regeneration in rats. *Mater. Sci. Eng. C* **2019**, *105*, 110128. [CrossRef]

113. Mekhileri, N.V.; Lim, K.S.; Brown, G.C.J.; Mutreja, I.; Schon, B.S.; Hooper, G.J.; Woodfield, T.B.F.; Lim, K. Automated 3D bioassembly of micro-tissues for biofabrication of hybrid tissue engineered constructs. *Biofabrication* **2018**, *10*, 024103. [CrossRef]

114. Gao, F.; Xu, Z.; Liang, Q.; Liu, B.; Li, H.; Wu, Y.; Zhang, Y.; Lin, Z.; Wu, M.; Ruan, C.; et al. Direct 3D Printing of High Strength Biohybrid Gradient Hydrogel Scaffolds for Efficient Repair of Osteochondral Defect. *Adv. Funct. Mater.* **2018**, *28*, 1706644. [CrossRef]

115. Deng, C.; Yang, Q.; Sun, X.; Chen, L.; Feng, C.; Chang, J.; Wu, C. Bioactive scaffolds with Li and Si ions-synergistic effects for osteochondral defects regeneration. *Appl. Mater. Today* **2018**, *10*, 203–216. [CrossRef]

116. Yang, Y.; Lei, D.; Huang, S.; Yang, Q.; Song, B.; Guo, Y.; Shen, A.; Yuan, Z.; Li, S.; Qing, F.; et al. Elastic 3D-Printed Hybrid Polymeric Scaffold Improves Cardiac Remodeling after Myocardial Infarction. *Adv. Healthc. Mater.* **2019**, *8*, e1900065. [CrossRef] [PubMed]

117. Zhang, B.; Seong, B.; Nguyen, V.; Byun, D. 3D printing of high-resolution PLA-based structures by hybrid electrohydrodynamic and fused deposition modeling techniques. *J. Micromech. Microeng.* **2016**, *26*, 25015. [CrossRef]

118. Boffito, M.; Di Meglio, F.; Mozetic, P.; Giannitelli, S.M.; Carmagnola, I.; Castaldo, C.; Nurzynska, D.; Sacco, A.M.; Miraglia, R.; Montagnani, S.; et al. Surface functionalization of polyurethane scaffolds mimicking the myocardial microenvironment to support cardiac primitive cells. *PLoS ONE* **2018**, *13*, e0199896. [CrossRef]

119. Koffler, J.; Zhu, W.; Qu, X.; Platoshyn, O.; Dulin, J.N.; Brock, J.; Graham, L.; Lu, P.; Sakamoto, J.; Marsala, M.; et al. Biomimetic 3D-printed scaffolds for spinal cord injury repair. *Nat. Med.* **2019**, *25*, 263–269. [CrossRef]

120. Joung, D.; Truong, V.; Neitzke, C.C.; Guo, S.-Z.; Walsh, P.J.; Monat, J.R.; Meng, F.; Park, S.H.; Dutton, J.R.; Parr, A.M.; et al. 3D Printed Stem-Cell Derived Neural Progenitors Generate Spinal Cord Scaffolds. *Adv. Funct. Mater.* **2018**, *28*, 1801850. [CrossRef]

121. Chen, X.; Zhao, Y.; Li, X.; Xiao, Z.; Yao, Y.; Chu, Y.; Farkas, B.; Romano, I.; Brandi, F.; Dai, J. Functional Multichannel Poly (Propylene Fumarate)-Collagen Scaffold with Collagen-Binding Neurotrophic Factor 3 Promotes Neural Regeneration After Transected Spinal Cord Injury. *Adv. Healthc. Mater.* **2018**, *7*, 1800315. [CrossRef]

6

The *Reeler* Mouse: A Translational Model of Human Neurological Conditions, or Simply a Good Tool for Better Understanding Neurodevelopment?

Laura Lossi [1], Claudia Castagna [1], Alberto Granato [2],* and Adalberto Merighi [1],*

[1]   Department of Veterinary Sciences, University of Turin, I-10095 Grugliasco (TO), Italy; laura.lossi@unito.it (L.L.); claudia.castagna@unito.it (C.C.)

[2]   Department of Psychology, Catholic University of the Sacred Heart, I-20123 Milano (MI), Italy

*   Correspondence: alberto.granato@unicatt.it (A.G.); adalberto.merighi@unito.it (A.M.)

Abstract: The first description of the *Reeler* mutation in mouse dates to more than fifty years ago, and later, its causative gene (*reln*) was discovered in mouse, and its human orthologue (*RELN*) was demonstrated to be causative of lissencephaly 2 (LIS2) and about 20% of the cases of autosomal-dominant lateral temporal epilepsy (ADLTE). In both human and mice, the gene encodes for a glycoprotein referred to as reelin (Reln) that plays a primary function in neuronal migration during development and synaptic stabilization in adulthood. Besides LIS2 and ADLTE, *RELN* and/or other genes coding for the proteins of the Reln intracellular cascade have been associated substantially to other conditions such as spinocerebellar ataxia type 7 and 37, *VLDLR*-associated cerebellar hypoplasia, *PAFAH1B1*-associated lissencephaly, autism, and schizophrenia. According to their modalities of inheritances and with significant differences among each other, these neuropsychiatric disorders can be modeled in the homozygous (*reln*$^{-/-}$) or heterozygous (*reln*$^{+/-}$) *Reeler* mouse. The worth of these mice as translational models is discussed, with focus on their construct and face validity. Description of face validity, i.e., the resemblance of phenotypes between the two species, centers onto the histological, neurochemical, and functional observations in the cerebral cortex, hippocampus, and cerebellum of *Reeler* mice and their human counterparts.

Keywords: reelin; LIS2; ADLTE; autism; schizophrenia; translational models; GABAergic interneurons; dendritic spines; forebrain; cerebellum

1. Introduction

Neuronal migration and precise setting during neurogenesis depend, among others, on reelin (Reln), a 388 kDa glycoprotein secreted by certain neurons within the extracellular matrix [1,2]. The name was given to the protein after the detection of its coding gene, and the acknowledgement that its lack was causative of the mouse *Reeler* mutation [3], which was described, about half a century before, consisting in a form of ataxia [4]. The mutation is autosomic and shows recessive transmission. Consequently, only homozygous recessive *Reeler* mice (*reln*$^{-/-}$) are totally devoid of Reln and have a definite phenotype. Behaviorally, the latter consists of dystonia, ataxia, and tremor; structurally it primarily affects the design of the cerebral cortex, hippocampus, and cerebellum [5,6]. Contrarily to the mutants, the phenotype of heterozygous *Reeler* mice (*reln*$^{+/-}$) is normal, but, interestingly, these animals may be translational models of certain human neuropsychiatric disorders [7].

Shortly after the original discovery, it became clear that the mouse gene (*reln*) had a very high homology to that in humans (*RELN*) [8]. Then, a few years later, it was shown that autosomic recessive mutations of the *RELN* gene were linked to a form of lissencephaly with cerebellar hypoplasia (LCH) [9], with associated findings suggested that *RELN* was linked to some neuropsychiatric conditions [10], and *RELN* was demonstrated to be reduced in the cerebellum of autistic patients after Western blotting and immunodetection [11].

Determining a good translational mouse model for a neuropsychiatric condition needs construct, predictive, and face validity [12]. Rigorously, construct validity only relates to transgenic mice, but, in a broader definition, it also comprehends the syndromic models and the spontaneous DNA mutations linked to the phenotype under study. In other words, this factor defines the similarity of the disease between the mouse and the human disorder in terms of the causal gene(s) as e.g., deducted from gene association and linkage analysis. As mentioned above, LCH is a human monogenic condition caused by a mutation in *RELN*. Therefore, the *Reeler* mouse fully meets the criterion of construct validity for the condition. There is also evidence for genetics to be associated with the etiology of several neuropsychiatric conditions, such as autism and schizophrenia, but, as the result of their multidimensional clinical symptoms, causal gene(s), if any, persist to be undiscovered [13]. Nonetheless, there are numerous genes associated with the human autistic pathology after analysis of Mendelian disorders (syndromes), rare mutations, or association studies; see e.g., [14].

Predictive validity, i.e., the similarity of the response to cures in humans and mice is difficult to establish, in the nonexistence of a recognized therapy in humans [14]. Thus, in the context of this discussion, face validity, i.e., the resemblance of the model phenotype to that of the human disorder, is the most important parameter to consider.

Assessment of face validity in neuroscience translational studies requires a careful consideration of their behavioral and structural phenotypes. Broadly speaking, there are contradictory opinions as regarding the repetition in mouse of the human behavioral neuropsychiatric changes. This was, to some extent, predictable, as only a few trials, such as e.g., pre-pulse inhibition (PPI), which records sensory-motor responses, are highly comparable with only minimal modifications in the two species [15]. Notably, the issue has been the subject of several reviews on rodent models of autism, e.g., [16]. The conclusion of these surveys was that, although most of the models that have been used in drug discovery display behaviors with face validity for the human symptoms (i.e., deficits in social communication and restricted interests/repetitive behaviors), many drugs that were found to be useful in ameliorating these autism-related behaviors in mice were ineffective in humans.

Therefore, it becomes imperative to compare the structural alterations of the brains in the two species to substantiate or invalidate the models. We here summarize the state-of-art knowledge on the translational validity of homozygous ($reln^{-/-}$) and heterozygous ($reln^{+/-}$) *Reeler* mice with reference to the most common neuropsychiatric conditions directly or indirectly related to *RELN*. Because of its importance, we will primarily focus onto the brain structural modifications at magnetic resonance imaging (MRI) and histopathology in the two species.

2. The Reelin Gene and Protein

In humans, *RELN*, which has 94.2% homology with the mouse orthologue [8], is in chromosome 7q22 [17] and encodes for REELIN (RELN), a large glycoprotein of the extracellular matrix. The murine gene (*reln*) that also encodes for Reelin (Reln) was originally identified as the mutated gene in the *Reeler* mouse, which displays, among others, irregular lamination of the cerebral and cerebellar cortices, with an inversion of the regular 'inside-out' design observed in mammals [3,18]. The mouse and the human proteins have a similar size of 388 kDa. The structure of the protein recalls that of certain cell adhesion molecules, which specific cell types produce during brain and spinal cord development.

In the neocortex, the Cajal–Retzius cells synthesize the glycoprotein and secrete it into the extracellular space [19]. Then, in post mitotic migrating neurons, Reln activates a specific signaling pathway that is required for proper positioning of these neurons. Northern blot hybridization showed that other areas of the fetal and postnatal brain also express the protein, with levels particularly high in cerebellum.

Reln is part of a signal transduction pathway that includes the apolipoprotein E2 (ApoER2), the very low-density lipoprotein receptors (VLDLR) and the cytoplasmic protein Dab1 [20]. Notably, the brain phenotype of mice with disruptions of *mDab1* or of both *apoER2* and *vldlr* closely resemble the brain of the *Reeler* mouse [21]. Another gene that interacts with the components of the Reln signaling pathways is platelet-activating factor acetyl hydrolase IB subunit α *(PAFAH1B1)*, also referred to as *LIS1* [22].

3. *RELN*-Related Human Neurological Conditions and Their Mouse Counterparts

Several human neurological conditions have a direct or indirect link with *RELN* and its encoded protein, as well as with the components of the RELN signaling pathway (Figure 1 and Table 1). We will briefly describe these conditions below, aiming to put in the better perspective those features that may be useful for well understanding the translational relevance of the *Reeler* mouse.

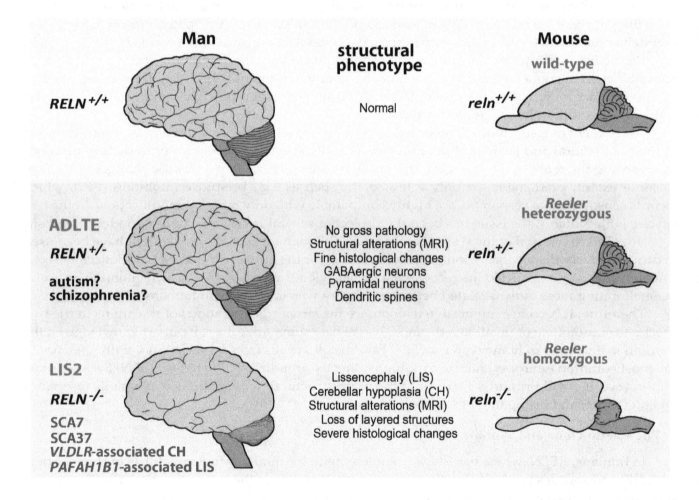

Figure 1. Summary of the most relevant human pathologies modeled in the *Reeler* mouse. The monogenic conditions provoked by the *RELN* gene, i.e., ADLTE and LIS2, are in red, those related to genes encoding for the proteins of the Reln intracellular cascade or only tentatively linked to RELN are indicated in blue. Autism and schizophrenia, which have a complex multifactorial etiology, are in black with an interrogative mark to underline the still tentative association of the two disorders with *RELN*. Abbreviations: ADLTE autosomal-dominant lateral temporal epilepsy, LIS2 lissencephaly 2, PAFAH1B1 platelet-activating factor acetyl hydrolase IB subunit α, *RELN* reelin gene (human), *reln* reelin gene (mouse), SCA37 spinocerebellar ataxia type 37, SCA7 spinocerebellar ataxia type 7, VLDLR very low-density lipoprotein receptor.

Table 1. Summary list of the human neurological conditions related to the *RELN* gene.

Disease	Transmission	Causative Gene(s)	*Reeler* Mutants of Translational Interest	Other Mouse Models
LIS 2	Autosomal recessive	*RELN*	Homozygous	see text
ADLTE	Autosomal dominant	*RELN* (in 17.5% of cases)	Heterozygous	*LG11*-mutated
VLDLR-associated cerebellar hypoplasia	Autosomal recessive	*VLDLR*	Homozygous	*VLDLR* knock-out
SCA37	Autosomal dominant	*DAB1*	Homozygous	*DAB1* knock-out *apoER2* knock-out
PAFAH1B1-associated lissencephaly	Autosomal dominant	*PAFAH1B1*	Homozygous	*Lis1*$^{+/-}$
SCA7	Autosomal dominant	*ATXN7*	Homozygous	SCA7 knock-in
Autism	Isolated cases Multifactorial	see https://omim.org # 209850	Heterozygous	see text
Schizophrenia	Autosomal dominant	see https://omim.org # 181500	Heterozygous	see text

Note that only LIS2 and autosomal-dominant lateral temporal epilepsy (ADLTE) have a demonstrated link with *RELN*. *RELN* may be relevant for *LIS1*.

3.1. Neurological Conditions Caused by RELN Mutations

Several diseases are based on mutations of *RELN* or of genes encoding for proteins associated with the RELN signaling pathways. Among these, lissencephaly 2 (LIS2) and autosomal-dominant lateral temporal epilepsy (ADLTE) are of relevance to the present discussion as they have a clear genetic link with *RELN*.

3.1.1. Human Lissencephalies and the Homozygous *Reeler* Mouse

Human lissencephalies are a group of cortical malformations that are consequent to neuronal migration disorders. Broadly speaking, the structural phenotype in lissencephalies ranges from a thickened cortex and complete absence of sulci (agyria) to a thickened cortex with a few, shallow sulci (pachygyria) [23]. The main feature of classic lissencephaly, formerly referred to as type I lissencephaly but today named lissencephaly 1 (LIS1), is a marked thickening of the cerebral cortex with a posterior to anterior grade of severity. An anomalous neuronal migration in the interval between the ninth to the thirteenth week of pregnancy causes LIS1, resulting in an assortment of agyria, mixed agyria/pachygyria, and pachygyria. An abnormally thick and ill ordered cortex with four highly disorganized layers, diffuse neuronal heterotopia, enlarged cerebral ventricles of anomalous shape, and, often, hypoplasia of the corpus callosum are typical of LIS1 [24]. The basal ganglia are normal, except that the anterior limb of the internal capsule is usually not noticeable, and, most often, the cerebellum is normal as well.

Lissencephalies are now classified based on brain imaging results and molecular investigation [25], as they have been associated with mutations in several genes such as *LIS1* (*PAFAH1B1*; MIM#601545), *DCX* (Doublecortin; MIM#300121), *ARX* (Aristaless-related homeobox gene; MIM#300382), *RELN* (Reelin; MIM#600514), *VLDLR* (MIM#224050) and *TUBA1A* (αtubulin 1a) [26]. Some rare forms of lissencephaly (LCH) are associated with a disproportionately small cerebellum.

Lissencephaly 2

a) Humans

Lissencephaly 2 (LIS2) also referred to lissencephaly syndrome, Norman–Roberts type or Norman–Roberts syndrome (OMIM #257320) is associated with *LIS1* but displays several specific clinical features. In 2000, Hong and colleagues were the first to describe an autosomal recessive form of lissencephaly that, at MRI, also exhibited severe alterations of the cerebellum, hippocampus, and brainstem. More specifically, these alterations consisted of a thickening of the cerebral cortex with a simplified convolutional pattern that was particularly evident in the frontal and temporal lobes, whereas the parietal and occipital lobes were almost normal. The hippocampus was unfolded and flattened, lacking definable upper and lower blades. The corpus callosum was thin and the lateral ventricles enlarged. The cerebellum was clearly smaller than in the normal brain, hypoplastic, and devoid of folia. Authors also showed that the responsible gene mapped to chromosome 7q22 and that the condition was associated with two independent mutations in *RELN*, resulting in low or undetectable amounts of RELN after Western blots analysis of the patients' serum [9]. Two other unrelated groups of patients, later, presented the same type of LIS2 [27]. They were children that, at MRI, displayed a 5–10 mm thick cerebral cortex, a malformed hippocampus and a very hypoplastic cerebellum, almost completely devoid of folia. As LIS2 is a rare disease, there are very limited histopathological data on the condition. To our knowledge, the only post-mortem description of a male fetus with Norman–Roberts syndrome reported the occurrence of a four-layered cerebral cortex (Figure 2A,B), a well-developed cerebellum with organized folia, and heterotopia of the dentate nucleus [28].

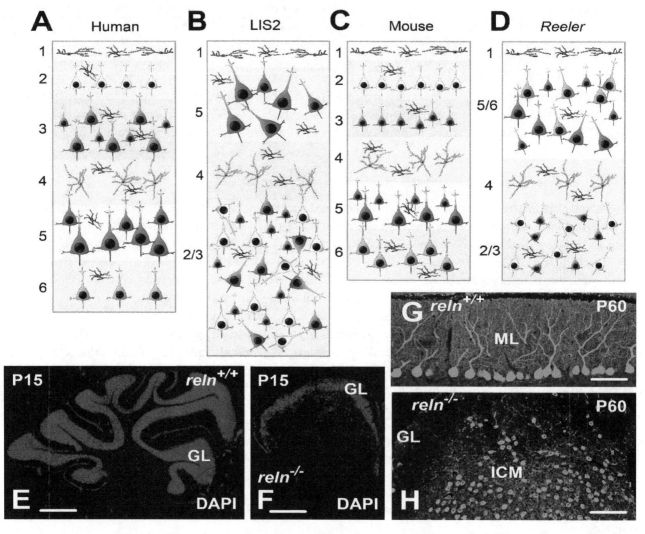

Figure 2. Structural alterations in human, LIS2, and homozygous *Reeler* mouse (**A–D**); modifications of the neocortex architecture in human LIS2 (**B**); and *Reeler* mutation (**D**); compared to healthy controls (**A,C**). After MRI imaging, the human LIS2 cortex is thicker than normal, whereas there are apparently no thickness changes in mouse. Note that in both species the pathological neocortex only consists of four layers, with an upside-down layer disposition mainly affecting the pyramidal neurons that are also irregularly oriented compared to their usual positioning in normal individuals/mice. Pyramidal neurons are in different color and sizes according to their position in cortical layers. Stellate spiny cells of layer 4 are orange. Inhibitory interneurons are black with a red nucleus. Cajal-Retzius cells of layer 1 are red.

(**E–H**): Structural alterations in the *Reeler* mouse cerebellum; (**E**) sagittal sections of the P15 cerebellum in a normal *reln*$^{+/+}$ mouse; and (**F**) a *Reeler reln*$^{-/-}$ mouse: the *Reeler* cerebellum is much smaller and devoid of folia, with a smooth surface. (**G**) Misalignment of the Purkinje neurons in the P60 cerebellum of the *Reeler* mouse. After calbindin 28 kDa immunostaining, the Purkinje neurons are well aligned in a monolayer below the molecular layer in *reln*$^{+/+}$ mice. They, instead, form a large internal cellular mass within the white matter in *reln*$^{-/-}$ mutants (**H**). Abbreviations: DAPI = 4′,6-Diamidine-2′-phenylindole; GL = granular layer of the cerebellar cortex; ICM = internal cellular mass; ML = molecular layer of the cerebellar cortex; P = postnatal day.

b) *Reeler* Homozygous Mice

Alterations in *Reeler* homozygous recessive mice fully recapitulate those in human LIS2 (Figure 1). Due to obvious technical and practical reasons, the amount of MRI data in mouse is by far less abundant than in patients, whereas mice have provided extensive histopathological information. The first MRI description of the neuroanatomical phenotypes in homozygous (and heterozygous) mice using morphometry and texture analysis, led to conclude that the structural features of the *Reeler* brain most closely copied the MRI phenotype of LIS2 patients [29]. Indeed, the *reln*$^{-/-}$ mice had a smaller brain, but larger lateral ventricles compared to wild-type littermates. Sharp differences existed in the olfactory bulbs, dorsomedial frontal and parietal cortex, certain districts of the temporal and occipital lobes, and the ventral hippocampus where gadolinium-based active staining demonstrated a general disorganization with differences in the thickness of individual hippocampal layers. The cerebellum also resulted profoundly affected by the mutation and appeared strongly hypoplastic. A subsequent study, based on the use of manganese-enhanced MRI (MEMRI) to better detect the cortical laminar architecture, compared the MEMRI signal intensity in the cerebral cortex of normal and mutant mice. The authors of this survey observed that signal was low in cortical layer 1, increased in layer 2, decreased in layer 3 until mid-layer 4, and increased again, peaking in layer 5, before decreasing through layer 6. In *Reeler* there were, instead, no appreciable changes in signal intensity, an observation consistent with the absence of cortical lamination after histological examination [30]. A more recent and very elegant study has employed diffusion tractography imaging (DTI) to perform an in vivo origin-to-ending reconstruction of the mouse somatosensory thalamo-cortical connections and demonstrated an extensive remodeling in *Reeler* mutants because of the highly disorganized cortical lamination [31].

In keeping with the results of imaging studies, at gross anatomical examination the *reln*$^{-/-}$ mouse brain was atrophic, as total volume in mutants decreased of about 19% when compared to normal mice [29]. Such a reduction was particularly evident in the cerebellum (Figure 2E,F) that also displayed a very limited degree of foliation. Therefore, also the gross anatomy of the *Reeler* brain closely resembled that of the LIS2 human brain.

In general, it seems that the histological anomalies in mutants depended on an abnormal migration of neurons, rather than an alteration in cell fate determination or axonal guidance. Among these anomalies, the most distinguishing ones are that the cerebral and cerebellar cortices lose their layered structure, in accordance with the MEMRI observations [30]; numerous neuronal nuclei disappeared or, at least, became hardly recognizable in several brain regions; and neurons often displayed an ectopic position. Table 2 summarizes the most important structural anomalies of the *reln*$^{-/-}$ CNS without taking into consideration the histological alterations in the cerebral cortex, hippocampus and cerebellum, as we will analytically discuss the phenotype of these brain areas in the following sections. Detailed descriptions of the morphological phenotype of the *Reeler* mouse CNS can be found e.g., in [29,32].

Table 2. Main histopathological changes in the homozygous *Reeler* mouse.

Division of CNS	Region/Division	Subdivision/Nucleus	Type(s) of Alteration	Ref
Forebrain	Olfactory bulb		• Slight disruption of the glomerular layer. • Numerical reduction and clustering of granule cells	[33,34]
	Striatum		• Decreased PV-immunoreactivity	[35]
	Diencephalon		• Misrouting of GnRH neurons to the cerebral cortex	[36]
		Mammilary bodies	• Alteration of projections to hippocampus	[37]
Midbrain	Rostral colliculus		• Loss of individual limits in the three more superficial layers • Spread of corticotectal projections • Anomalies of retinotectal projections	[38]
	Mesencephalic nucleus of V		• Spread of neurons along their route of migration	[39]
	Substantia nigra		• Anomalous clustering lateral to the ventral tegmental area	[40]
	Medulla oblongata and pons	Dorsal cochlear nucleus	• Partial loss of layered organization	[41]
		Inferior olivary nucleus	• Loss of folding - Swelling	[42]
		Somatic motorneurons (Nucleus ambiguous, facial and trigeminal)	• Slight displacement and loss of somatotopic organization (muscolotopy)	[6,43]
		Pontine nuclei	• Ventral shift	[44]
Spinal cord	Dorsal horn (laminae I-II)	Nociceptive	• Abnormal neuronal positioning	[45]
	Lateral horn	Preganglionic sympathetic and parasympathetic neurons	• Abnormal neuronal positioning	[46,47]

The Table does not list the histopathological observations on cerebral cortex, hippocampus, and cerebellum.

Very early observations demonstrated the occurrence of dendritic anomalies in cortical and hippocampal neurons of *Reeler* mice [48,49]. The discovery of *Reln* confirmed the dendritic pathology, as not only Reln but also the molecules of its signaling pathway resulted to be necessary for the correct maturation and differentiation of the dendritic branches and spines in hippocampal and neocortical pyramidal neurons [50,51].

Due to the complexity of the phenomena involved in dendritic maturation, one can argue that dendritic anomalies represented a consequence of the deep cytoarchitectonic derangement occurring in *Reeler* mice rather than a primary effect of the lack of Reln, but observations on heterozygous mice were not supportive of this interpretation [52,53]. Interestingly, the block of the Reln signaling by means of specific antibodies resulted in an increased complexity of branching in the apical dendrites of layer 2/3 cortical pyramidal neurons, whereas their basal arborizations remained unaffected [54].

There are many important issues related to the structure and role of the dendritic tree of neocortical and hippocampal pyramidal neurons that make the *Reeler* mouse an important tool for the study of (forebrain) neurodevelopment. Inputs to layer 5 neurons are processed by separate compartments, with the basal dendrites receiving bottom-up information and the apical dendrite being the recipient of a feedback input from higher cortical areas, see e.g., [55]. This framework is, however, even more complex because apical dendrites span most cortical layers before reaching layer 1, where the apical tuft is located [56]. Today we know well that the type and distribution of ion channels at the neurolemma ultimately determine the electrophysiological properties of a neuron.

Essential to the function of the long apical dendrite of the pyramidal neurons is the progressively increasing density of hyperpolarization-activated cyclic nucleotide–gated (HCN) channels, proceeding from proximal to distal segments [57]. Such a gradient critically contributes to the functional distinction between dendritic compartments. Although Reln signaling specifies this gradient [58], 17β-estradiol, which stimulates Reln expression, promoted the enrichment of HCN1 in the distal dendritic compartment of CA1 neurons without the intervention of Reln [59]. The evidence that Reln was involved in the trafficking and targeting of ion channels in cortical and hippocampal neurons suggested that their intrinsic electrophysiological properties could indeed be different in the *Reeler* mouse. However, an early study by Bliss and Chung [60] demonstrated that, despite the layering derangement, the basic synaptic organization of the hippocampus was largely unchanged in mutants.

More recently, Silva et al. [61] carried out an accurate survey dealing with the intrinsic electrophysiological properties of cortical neurons in *Reeler* mice. These authors showed that the firing pattern and synaptic responses of the pyramidal neurons were normal, but with an inverted radial distribution. Notably, these authors concluded that, although mispositioned, neurons maintained the membrane properties appropriate to their function.

The apparent discrepancy between the data demonstrating the role of Reln in the modulation of ion channels and the relative lack of anomalies in the intrinsic properties of cortical neurons in mutant mice might have several explanations. Other factors, such as neuronal activity [62] could be more effective than Reln for the modulation of membrane channel targeting. Furthermore, the complex machinery of the long apical dendrite is required when layer 5 neurons settle appropriately but might be useless for the same neurons displaced to more superficial cortical layers. Finally, future investigations based on refined electrophysiological techniques, such as direct dendritic recordings, will help to establish if indeed the cortical neurons in *Reeler* mice display subtler changes of their firing/intrinsic properties that those so far ascertained.

Reln signaling is also able to modulate key molecules of the cascade leading to synaptic plasticity, such as the NMDA receptors [63,64]. Therefore, several studies concentrated on the changes of synaptic plasticity in *Reeler* mutants. Ishida et al. [65] reported that the induction of long-term potentiation (LTP) was impaired in the CA1 region of the hippocampus, claiming that the malpositioning of some neuronal populations could account for such an alteration. On the other hand, both the overexpression of Reln in transgenic mice [66] and Reln supplementation strongly increased LTP [67]. Later, a defective LTP was observed in the hippocampus of *vldr*-deficient mice, but slice perfusion with Reln was able to enhance LTP in CA1 [68].

Most cortical neurons are spiny, glutamatergic pyramidal cells, whose migratory path during prenatal development follows an inside-out radial pattern from the ventricular zone to the final position [69]. Reln signaling is essential for the localization of pyramidal neurons to appropriate cortical layers, as reviewed in [70]. Consequently, the lack of Reln caused a disruption of the layered cortical organization, including abnormal positioning [71,72], as well as an increased percentage of inverted pyramidal cells [73,74] (Figure 2C,D).

Inhibitory GABAergic interneurons represent a minority population within the neocortex. Yet, their morphological, neurochemical and functional diversity likely plays a key role for the cortical function, see e.g., [75]. Unlike pyramidal neurons, interneurons originate in the ganglionic eminence of the ventral telencephalon and follow a tangential migratory path to the cortex [69]. While the malpositioning of the pyramidal neurons in *Reeler* mice is evident, it is not clear if the Reln signaling cascade also affects the migration of the interneurons. An answer to this latter issue came from observations on *Reeler* mutants crossed with mice expressing the green fluorescent protein (GFP) in inhibitory neurons. Thus, the results of these observations confirmed that also the cortical interneurons displayed an abnormal laminar position and morphology [76]. However, we still do not know whether interneurons' ectopy directly depends from Reln signaling or is rather the consequence of the malpositioning of principal pyramidal projection neurons. The debate on this issue is still open, as contradictory views exist in the literature. Namely, while some observations [77,78] argue against a direct role of Reln,

Hammond et al. [79] showed that only early-generated cortical interneurons were misplaced as a consequence of the ectopy of the pyramidal neurons, whereas the correct layering of late-generated interneurons seemed to be directly modulated by Reln signaling.

Other basic neurodevelopmental features, such as cortical [80] and cerebellar neurogenesis, seem to be as well regulated by the glycoprotein. Consequently, the minicolumnar organization of the cerebral neocortex appeared to be deeply affected by Reln deficiency [81] and some physiological counterparts of cortical connectivity, such as trans-synaptic signal propagation, were also impaired [82]. However, the outcome of Reln deficiency on the microcircuitry sustaining the cortical machinery is controversial and, surprisingly, the deep architectonic disorganization that follows the lack of the protein occurs in the absence of dramatic functional anomalies. Both early and more recent studies point out that the absence of Reln did not prevent the development of functionally appropriate cortical connections and maps [31,83–86]. In addition, when studied at the fine-scale electron microscopic level, the basic synaptic organization of misplaced cortical neurons was unchanged [87]. Therefore, although the laminar organization is thought to be critical for cortical computation [88,89], evidences obtained in *Reeler* mice led Guy and Staiger [90] to challenge the importance of cortical lamination, affirming that "future studies directed toward understanding cortical functions should rather focus on circuits specified by functional cell type composition than mere laminar location".

Macroscopically, the cerebellum of the *Reeler* mouse is smaller than that of age-matched littermates (Figure 2E,F); it is club-shaped with the main axis transverse to the mid plan of the body, and has an almost completely smooth surface, with just a few superficial grooves [91]. The architecture of the *Reeler* cerebellum is profoundly different from the normal pattern, firstly because of the impairment in the complicated series of migrations made by neurons to reach their destination in the mature organ. Trajectories of migrating neurons follow two opposite directions from the surface to the depth of the cerebellum and the other way around, depending from the species, the type(s) of neurons and the developmental stages (for details see e.g., [92]). Eventually, disturbances in the migration of the cerebellar neurons make that *Reeler* mice display a cerebellum that retains several features of immaturity.

The area of the cerebellar cortex in mutants was analyzed quantitatively during postnatal (P0–P25) development and resulted to be reduced compared to age-matched controls [93]. Reduction in the extension of the cortex was particularly evident in the molecular layer and the (internal) granular layer. Physiologically, as the cerebellum matured, the molecular layer became more and more populated by the parallel fibers, but, at P25, its increase in size was about one third in the mutants compared to $reln^{+/+}$ mice [93]. Post-migratory granule cells, which are born in the temporary subpial external granular layer, progressively populate the (internal) granular layer during normal cerebellar development. This process was disturbed in *Reeler*, to the extent that, from P0 to P10, the granular layer of $reln^{+/+}$ mice increased about five-folds in size, but only 2.6-fold in $reln^{-/-}$, where it was significantly reduced in size to 0.62-fold that of normal mice after P10 [93]. In a different way from the cortex, the medullary body was larger in the mutants than in wild-type mice. Its progressively increasing area mainly reflected the ongoing myelination of the axons of the Purkinje neurons that abandon the cortex moving across the white matter to reach the cerebellar nuclei, as well as the expansion of the incoming afferent and departing efferent fiber systems. The mass of the medullary body augmented in relation to postnatal age irrespectively of the lack of Reln ($reln^{-/-}$ 2.59, $reln^{+/+}$ 1.93-fold), but, at P25, *Reeler* mice had a larger medullary body than normal mice (1.88-fold) [93]. In brief, *Reeler* mice had a reduced cerebellar cortex but a bigger medullary body than their $reln^{+/+}$ littermates. The cerebellar hypoplasia was thus a consequence of a reduction in cortical magnitude and cellularity and the latter, in turn, resulted to be associated to measurable differences in the degree of cell proliferation and apoptosis, as well as imbalances in the timing of postnatal cortical maturation [93]. The same study led to conclude that density of proliferating cells was the most significant predictive factor to determine the cortical cellularity in *Reeler* [93]. Therefore, beside the well-defined consequences onto neuronal migration, the lack of Reln also caused a calculable deficit in neuronal expansion. Ultrastructurally, the cerebellar neurons underwent several different forms of programmed cell death during postnatal development and the deficit of Reln affected the kind and grade of neuronal death [94].

Perhaps the most striking histological feature in mutants is the lack of alignment of the Purkinje neurons to form a discrete intermediate layer in the cerebellar cortex (Figure 2G,H). Thus, in *Reeler*, only about 5% of the Purkinje neurons were in a normal position, 10% were still inside the cortex but in the granular layer, and the remaining 85% formed an internal cellular mass intermixed with the white matter [95–97]. Ultrastructurally, in *Reeler* there was a reduction in the density of the contacts between the Purkinje neurons and the parallel and climbing fibers, from P5 onward [98]. Functionally, both the normally placed Purkinje neurons and those ectopically dislocated in the granular layer displayed a 0–1 response to stimulation, indicating that, as in normal mice, they received a synaptic contact by a single climbing fiber. The Purkinje neurons in the internal cellular mass, instead, showed intensity-graded responses to electrical stimulation, as several climbing fibers provided them with a convergent input [95], likely as a failure of physiological pruning to occur [99]. Neurochemically, there were no obvious variations between normal mice and the mutants in the temporal expression of some widely diffused neuronal and glial markers (NeuN, vimentin, calbindin, GFAP, Smi32, GAD67) during postnatal development [93], but the Bergmann glia was misplaced in *Reeler* [100].

To conclude, the histological and electrophysiological observations in *Reeler* mutants suggest that similar structural and functional alterations may also occur in LIS2 patients, particularly in relation to the postnatal growth retardation, severe intellectual disability, and spasticity observed in affected subjects (see also https://www.orpha.net/).

Lissencephaly 3

TUBA1A mutations [101,102] cause lissencephaly 3 (LIS3), another human condition that has a mouse counterpart. TUBA1A chiefly occurs in cortical, hippocampal, cerebellar and brainstem post-mitotic neurons, with expression falling soon after birth but persisting through adulthood [103]. The mouse phenotype consists, among others, in a failure of the cerebellar Purkinje neurons to migrate, so that, similarly to *Reeler*, they remain entrapped into the medullary body, where they form a series of streaks intermingled with the neurons of the cerebellar nuclei [104]. Several other mutations of *TUBA1A* exist in humans. They give rise to a predominant phenotype of LCH, which also shows irregularities of the corpus callosum and the basal ganglia/internal capsule [105].

3.1.2. Autosomal-Dominant Lateral Temporal Epilepsy and the Heterozygous *Reeler* Mouse

ADLTE, also referred to as autosomal dominant epilepsy with auditory features, partial epilepsy with auditory aura or partial epilepsy with auditory features, is a genetic epileptic syndrome, clinically showing typical focal seizures in response to specific sounds. ADLTE is genetically heterogeneous, and mutations in the leucine-rich, glioma inactivated 1 gene (*LGI1*) account for fewer than 50% of affected families. Very recent observations demonstrated that heterozygous *RELN* mutations give rise to a classic ADLTE syndrome, clinically identical to that associated with mutations of *LGI1*. Seven different heterozygous missense mutations in *RELN* were, in fact, described in some unrelated families of Italian ancestry with familial temporal lobe epilepsy-7 (ETL7–OMIM #616436) [106]. Incidence was 17.5% over the total number of families studied that were specifically suffering by lateral temporal lobe epilepsy [106]. By three-dimensional modeling, the same authors anticipated that the outcomes of these mutations would be protein structural defects and misfolding. Some of the affected individuals displayed a reduction up to 50% of their serum levels of the 310 kDa RELN isoform in comparison to healthy subjects and thus, very likely, the mutations also resulted in a loss of function. In a subsequent study on the same patients, 1.5 T MRI scans were not useful in detecting structural anomalies of the brain [107]. Similarly, in a very recent study on an 18-year old ADLTE patient, 3T MRI brain scans could not provide relevant information on indistinct grey-white matter connections, voxel-based morphometry, and cortical thickness [108]. However, analysis of functional connectivity with high-density electroencephalography (HdEEG) revealed greater local synchrony in the left temporal (middle temporal gyrus), left frontal (supplementary motor area, superior frontal gyrus), and left parietal (gyrus angularis, gyrus supramarginalis) regions of the cerebral cortex and the cingulate cortex (middle cingulate gyrus) as compared to normal subjects [108].

As the discovery of RELN mutations in ADLTE is a quite recent finding, there are, at present, no observations on heterozygous *Reeler* mice focused to ascertain possible similarities with the human phenotype. Like ADLTE patients, $reln^{+/-}$ mice display a 50% reduction of Reln in their serum. Therefore, it would be interesting to investigate whether sound-triggered epileptic manifestations also occur in these animals. A very recent study has demonstrated that optogenetic stimulation of the parvalbumin (PV) immunoreactive GABAergic neurons of the mouse basal forebrain can modulate the cortical topography of auditory steady-state responses [109]. As the regional distribution of these neurons displayed relevant differences in $reln^{+/-}$ mice compared to wild-type animals [110,111], any phenotypic alteration may be of interest to shed additional light onto human ADLTE. Finally, a very latest report has provided proof of concept that HdEEG can be used to record electrical activity from the mouse brain in a model of juvenile myoclonic epilepsy [112]. Therefore, one can envisage applying such an approach to analyze the brain electrical pattern in $reln^{+/-}$ mice aiming to collect data for translational comparison with ADLTE.

3.2. Human Conditions Caused by Mutations of Genes of the Reln Intracellular Pathway and Their Mouse Correlates

In general, the brain phenotype of the human monogenetic conditions that are consequent to mutations of the genes coding for the proteins of the RELN intracellular signaling pathway is similar to that of the $reln^{-/-}$ mouse brain, except that, in certain cases, differently from *Reeler*, the human cerebellum is normal at MRI and gross anatomical observation (Figure 1). We will briefly describe these conditions below.

3.2.1. *VLDLR*-Associated Cerebellar Hypoplasia

VLDLR-associated cerebellar hypoplasia is an autosomal recessive genetic form of non-progressive congenital ataxia [113]. The main clinical symptom of the condition is a predominantly truncal ataxia with retarded ambulation, so that children either learn to walk after six years of age or never walk without aid. Dysarthria, strabismus, moderate-to-profound intellectual disability, and seizures are other features of the disorder. MRI findings comprise hypoplasia of the inferior portion of the cerebellum, affecting both the vermis and the hemispheres; pachygyria of the cerebral hemispheres with a negligibly but uniformly thickened cortex in the absence of a neat anteroposterior gradient, reduction is size of the brainstem, particularly the pons. The condition is monogenic, and due to mutations in *VLDLR*.

Vldlr only knock-out mice did not show the drastic brain phenotype that can be seen in double knock-out mice devoid of *vldlr* and *apoER2*, which, instead, recapitulate in full the phenotypic alterations of *Reeler* mutants or *dab1* knock-out mice [21,114]. As Reln interacts with both Vldlr and ApoER2, clear functional differences in how these two receptors transduce the glycoprotein signal have been postulated [114]. That the interaction of Reln with Vldrl occurs with much lower affinity than with ApoER2 [115] could explain the less severe phenotype of the *vldlr* knockout mice compared to *Reeler*. Remarkably, alterations that in mouse followed the knocking-out of *vldlr* were particularly noticeable in cerebellum and consisted in failure of the Purkinje neurons to form a well-defined monolayer and reduction of their dendritic arbor [114]. They thus recall in full the human MRI phenotype of *VLDLR*-associated cerebellar hypoplasia.

3.2.2. Spinocerebellar Ataxia Type 37

Spinocerebellar ataxia type 37 (SCA37) is a late onset syndrome that affects adults, with dysarthria, slowly progressive gait and limb ataxia, severe dysmetria in the lower extremities, mild dysmetria in the upper extremities, dysphagia, and abnormal ocular movements. In most cases, the first clinical signs encompass tumbles, dysarthria, or stiffness followed by a typical cerebellar syndrome. The early presence of altered vertical eye movements is a characteristic clinical feature of SCA37 that foregoes the symptoms of ataxia. The progression is slow and affected individuals usually become wheelchair bound between ten and thirty-three years after the onset of the disease [116]. At MRI, there is an initial atrophy of the vermis. Later, atrophy rapidly affects the entire cerebellum, without alterations of the brainstem [117]. Molecular analysis has shown that an unstable repeat insertion in *DAB1* is the cause of the cerebellar degeneration and, on the basis of the genetic and phenotypic evidence, the mutation has been proposed as the molecular basis for SCA37 [118].

Notably, the *dab1* deficient mice that derived from a spontaneous mutation called *Scrambler* or from gene knockout were phenotypically indistinguishable from the homozygous *Reeler* mice [119].

3.2.3. PAFAH1B1-Associated Lissencephaly/Subcortical Band Heterotopia

PAFAH1B1-associated lissencephaly/subcortical band heterotopia, also referred to as *LIS1*-associated lissencephaly/subcortical band heterotopia, encompasses Miller–Dieker syndrome (MDS), isolated lissencephaly sequence (ILS) and, infrequently, subcortical band heterotopia (SBH) [120]. MRI findings for lissencephaly are the absence or the abnormal broadening of cerebral gyri, and the aberrant thickness of the cerebral cortex. Less frequently, it may be possible to observe an enlargement of the lateral ventricles, mild hypoplasia of the corpus callosum and of the cerebellar vermis. In *PAFAH1B1*-associated SBH, just beneath the cortex of the parietal and occipital lobes there are subcortical bands of heterotopic gray matter separated from the superficial cerebral cortex by a thin layer of white matter. Histologically, the cerebral cortex in LIS1-associated lissencephaly consists of four layers: a poorly defined marginal zone, which, however, has a very high cell density; a superficial neuronal layer with diffusely scattered neurons; a deeper neuronal layer with relatively sparse neurons; and a deepest neuronal layer with neurons arranged in columns.

The architectural alterations of the human cerebral cortex and hippocampus can be somewhat recapitulated in genetically engineered mice. For example, the overexpression of *pafah1b1* disturbed neuronal migration and layer formation in the developing cerebral cortex [121], whereas *lis1* deficiency in homozygous mice resulted in early embryonic death and in heterozygous mice led to a derangement of the normal hippocampal organization with ectopy of the granule cells [122]. Of note, Lis1, the protein encoded by *Pafah1b*, is part of the Pafah1b complex and binds, downstream of the Vldlr receptor, to Dab1 that becomes phosphorylated in response to Reln [123].

3.3. Human Conditions Possibly Related to RELN Mutations and Their Mouse Correlates

3.3.1. Spinocerebellar Ataxia Type 7

Spinocerebellar ataxia type 7 (SCA7) is an autosomal-dominant neurodegenerative syndrome that outcomes from polyglutamine expansion of ataxin 7 (ATXN7). Remarkably, although ATXN7 has a widespread expression in SCA7 patients, the pathology primarily hits the cerebellum and the retina [124]. A recently published paper suggested that RELN might be a formerly unidentified factor accountable for the tissue specificity of SCA7 [125].

3.3.2. Autism and the Heterozygous Reeler Mouse

The disorders of the autistic spectrum (ASD), which are characterized by social, behavioral, and language insufficiencies, comprise Asperger syndrome, autism, and pervasive developmental disorder-not otherwise specified (PDD-NOS). Less than 20% of these disorders, acknowledged as "syndromic autism", derives from monogenetic diseases, most commonly fragile X syndrome and tuberous sclerosis. The remaining 80% of ASD cases are classified as "non-syndromic autism" and are widely investigated to find candidate genes that may contribute to pathology [126].

Genetics

At present autism cannot be considered, strictly speaking, a genetic disease, as one or more causative gene(s) has (have) not been found yet. The first gene association study implicating *RELN* in autism dates to 2001 [127]. However, subsequent gene population surveys yielded contrasting results [128–131]. Nonetheless, a more recent meta-analysis showed that at least one single nucleotide polymorphism (SNP) in *RELN* could be significantly associated with the risk of autism [132]. Therefore, results of SNP analysis appear to be compatible with the idea that heterozygous mutations in *RELN* may contribute to the onset of the disorder. Genetic studies on autism led to two main outcomes: 1. the more predominant existence of rare or de novo inherited mutations of a number of genes in autistic patients; 2. the discovery of certain common gene variants that contribute to the risk of autism but are also present, albeit at lower frequency, in the normal population [133]. When more than two de novo mutations occur in a gene, the latter becomes a very likely causative candidate of a disorder. There are four unique documented de novo mutations of *RELN* associated with autism [134–136], thus implicating *RELN* as a possible cause of ASD. However, although nonsense mutations are more frequent in autistic patients than in controls after whole-exome sequencing, there is not a striking gross increase of de novo mutations in the former [135]. To study autism heritability, one can also employ a different approach that distinguishes total narrow-sense heritability from that due to common gene variants. By this method, it was concluded that narrow-sense heritability of autism is ~52.4%, and that the main contribution heritability was due to common gene variants, whereas rare de novo mutations contribute only for about 2.6% of cases, but substantially influence individual liability to the condition [137]. Thus, *RELN* may primarily have a role in the individual *predisposition* to manifest autism rather than being one of the contributory causes of the disorder.

Further support for a RELN involvement in autism derived from the detection of reduced expression of the *RELN* transcript and protein in autistic individuals. Decreased RELN levels were apparent in the superior frontal cortex [10] and cerebellum of autistics as compared to controls [10,11,138]. In these areas, the levels of *RELN* mRNA were lower, as was the *DAB1* transcript, whereas *VLDLR* mRNA levels augmented.

Imaging

Imaging findings in autism have been recently reviewed [139]. Numerous observations join to prove that there is an atypical development of the brain in autistic children. Early cross-sectional studies demonstrated that the brain of these children had a higher volume than that of regularly developing subjects. However, growth curves in the two groups eventually met at later childhood. More specifically, in the 6–35-year interval, there was an initial period of brain overgrowth, and then growth slowed down or even stopped during early and late infancy to which a phase of fast reduction of the brain volume eventually followed [140]. Neuroimaging data also indicated that differences in the brain of autistic people started to be detectable within the first two years after birth, *before* clinical symptoms became obvious. There are conflicting views about the probability that an accelerated growth rate of the brain in this postnatal window goes together with the occurrence of early neurodevelopmental perturbations [139]. In relation to this, it is relevant that we still do not know when the initial neuropathological signs of autism occur, also from the paucity of studies on autistic children during the first year of life.

The mechanisms at the basis of the abnormal growth of the autistic brain are also unclear. Although most imaging studies have focused onto the gray matter of the cerebral cortex, there are data indicating that an increased amount of cerebrospinal fluid in the subarachnoid space [141] and/or a greater volume of the white matter [142] occurred in parallel to the enlargement of the autistic brain. As regarding the cerebral cortex, its surface, but not thickness, increased in the autistic brain [143].

To summarize, that an initial brain overgrowth may be a reliable biomarker for autism remains highly questionable. Thus, it seems more profitable to focus onto regional brain structural differences in a more effective search for new neuroanatomical findings of clinical relevance [139].

Before entering the description of regional MRI investigations in autism, it is important to stress that, at present, there are no specific and/or causative objective findings for the condition, but, instead, the very same regions altered in autism may be interested in other psychiatric conditions.

The individual constituents of the neural circuitries causal of ASD are well defined. They include regions of the fronto-temporal, fronto-parietal, and dorsolateral prefrontal cortex (PFC); parts of the limbic system; the fronto-striatal circuitry, and the cerebellum. Neuroimaging studies on these regions have employed different approaches such as the definition of a region-of-interest (ROI), voxel- or vertex-vise methods. Traditional ROI studies have reported atypical findings in brain areas that participate to social cognition such as the medial PFC, the anterior cingulate cortex (ACC), the inferior frontal cortex, the superior temporal sulcus, the amygdala, and the anterior insula.

The cerebellum was larger than in controls in several MRI studies on autistic patients older than three years [144], but not in younger children [143]. Differently from the cerebellum, the size of the vermis was smaller [145–147] or larger [146] or did not display any relevant difference [147], and such discrepancies possibly depend from the different clinical presentations of the condition [147,148]. It is also unclear whether there are differences in size of individual vermal lobules, as claimed by some authors [145], but not others [147]. Similarly, there were no differences between cerebellar hemispheres in one study [147], whereas another group has found the hemispheric size as the only significant structural dissimilarity between verbal and nonverbal subjects [149].

The still fuzzy picture emerging from the imaging studies onto the autistic brain makes it very difficult to compare the human and mouse data in the search for common biomarkers. To our knowledge, there are only two MRI studies on the brain of the heterozygous *Reeler* mouse. In the first, Badea and co-worker [29] reported that the total volume of the brain, the ventricular volume and the hippocampal volume correspondingly raised of about 6%, 82%, and 7% compared to normal control mice. However, after statistical analysis, they showed that these volumes were like those of *reln*$^{+/+}$ normal mice. They also measured the areas of different parts of the brain in comparison with wild-type mice and found no differences in hippocampus and cerebellum, but an enlargement of the lateral ventricles. A more recent paper confirmed the ventricular enlargement, but found a reduction of the cerebellar volume, whereas the volume of the motor cortex as well as its thickness was unchanged [150]. Therefore, given the paucity of data in mouse and the still unclear MRI pattern in human autistic subjects, one can only conclude that, at present, the cerebellum could be a part of the brain deserving further imaging investigations for translational purposes.

Histopathology

A series of histological alterations of the whole brain occur in the autistic brain. In the first histological surveys, the only cortical area showing qualitative structural abnormalities was the ACC that, in autistic patients, lacked architectural refinement and had only a coarse lamination [151]. However, in the following decades substantial amounts of data have been collected and the list of cerebral structures displaying histopathological changes in ASD has grown substantially to include a series of cortical regions, the amygdala, the cerebellum and the brainstem, see e.g., [152,153]. Below we will briefly summarize the most significant histopathological findings in human patients and compare them to those in the heterozygous *Reeler* mouse. However, the interpretation of both human and mouse finding needs often much caution, because not all studies used sound quantitative approaches and/or proper stereological procedures.

a) Changes Affecting the Whole Brain

The diffuse alterations observed in the brains of autistic subjects at postmortem included cortical dysplasia and neuronal heterotopia, with the formation of aggregates of neuronal cell bodies in anomalous positions [154]. Other alterations, i.e., differences in size of the neuronal nucleus and perikaryon, occurred at the cytological level. These differences started being evident in young children and became more apparent in adults, but then tended to re-equilibrate with time [155].

Remarkably, there might be some compensations between different areas, as in some parts of the brain neurons were bigger, but smaller in others.

In the autistic brain there was also an increase of the neuropil extension in certain but not all cortical areas that have been investigated so far [156]. It is unclear which neuropil component(s) is (are) responsible of these volumetric variations. Fewer dendrites were, in fact, immunostained for microtubule-associated protein 2 (MAP2) in the PFC [157] and a reduction of dendritic spines was reported in hippocampus [158], but other studies reached completely opposite conclusions after examination of the pyramidal neurons from layers 2 and 5 in the frontal, temporal, and parietal cortex [159]. The issue of dendrite and dendritic spines density is quite important in the general framework of this discussion, because these parameters have been widely investigated, primarily aiming to validate the heterozygous *Reeler* mouse as a translational model.

Alterations in neuronal differentiation and migration may also occur in the autistic nervous system and, thus, the consequences of a dysregulation of these processes may be at the basis of whole brain changes in autism [154]. In spite of this, there are only a few investigations on the expression of RELN in the brain of autistic patients and, after quantitative analysis, there was no alteration in the density of layer 1 RELN+ neurons in the superior temporal lobe of the autistic brain, although these neurons represent about 70% of the total layer 1 population [160].

b) Brain Regional Changes

Forebrain

Most of the histopathological observations on the brain of autistic patients focused on the cerebral cortex and hippocampus and, broadly speaking, alterations were almost exclusively restricted to neurons. The parameters considered have been size, number, and density of the different neuronal populations, often in relation to the cortical layers or the hippocampal subfields. A point of attention in considering these studies is that, in several cases, comparative brain volume evaluations between autistic patients and controls are missing, while they are, instead, essential to settle whether modifications in cell density reflect true differences in total cell counts.

Cerebral Cortex

The autistic pathology affects several regions of the cerebral cortex.

The PFC, which plays a major role in cognitive control, displayed a general overgrowth with an increase in the number of neurons, whereas glial cells were apparently unaffected. Among the GABAergic interneurons, there was a numerical increase of the PV-immunoreactive chandelier neurons, whereas the calbindin- and calretinin-expressing neurons were unaltered [153,161–163]. However, after qRT-PCR, the levels of the RELN and GAD67 mRNAs diminished in the post-mortem PFC from autistic patients in comparison to healthy controls [164].

In the inferior frontal cortex, changes affected the small-sized pyramidal neurons that did not display numerical alterations but were of smaller size [163].

The fusiform gyrus, which intervenes in facial recognition and social interactions, had a reduced neuronal density in layer 3, whereas neurons in layers 2, 5, and 6 were less numerous, being also smaller in layers 5 and 6 [165], but these alterations were not confirmed in [166].

In the frontoinsular cortex and ACC, both intervening in emotional regulation and self and others awareness, lamination was rudimental. In the former, von Economo neurons (VENs) of layer 5 increased in number [167–169], whereas in ACC neuronal density augmented in layers 1–2 of area 24a of the left hemisphere but diminished in layers 5–6 of area 24c; size, instead, diminished in all layers of area 24b [151,170].

The anterior midcingulate cortex also displayed a numerical increase of VENs, as well as of the pyramidal neurons of layer 5 that, however, were of smaller size [171].

Lastly, the entorhinal cortex, which has a role in memory, navigation and perception of time, displayed characteristic terminal swellings, referred to as spheroids [172] that were also observed in all hippocampal subfields (see below).

Another issue of interest is the possibility that there are alterations in the minicolumnar organization of the cerebral cortex in early age onset autism [156], as it might be the case in *Reeler* mice. Specifically, it appeared that minicolumns were smaller, more numerous and with lower neuronal density in several cortical areas of autistic (and Asperger's syndrome) patients, although these observations still need to be confirmed in full [156]. Under this perspective, it may be useful to here recall some of the results on the localization of the neural cell adhesion molecule 2 (NCAM2) in the *Reeler* mouse because the molecule has also been proposed as a predisposition gene for the development of autism [173]. In mutants, NCAM2 immunopositive and negative patches formed a mosaic filled with dendritic aggregates originating from two different populations of neurons in a fashion suggestive of a minicolumnar organization [174,175]. However, one must consider these findings with much caution, as that minicolumns are indeed the fundamental modular units of neocortical organization is currently still a matter of debate, see e.g., [176] for review.

Whereas the human cerebral cortex has been widely investigated in autism, investigations on the cerebral cortex of the heterozygous *Reeler* mouse have been relatively few but reported a reduction in the levels of GAD67 [53,177] like that observed in humans. Since the studies on hippocampus led to highly comparable results in the two species, it would be of importance to undertake rigorous investigations on the number and density of the cortical neurons in $reln^{+/-}$ mice, with attention to the different neurochemical populations of inhibitory interneurons. The results of these studies will be relevant, from one side, to validate the mouse model and, from the other, to confirm some numerical observations in humans that, as mentioned at beginning of this section, need validation using approaches more reliable than those often employed at histopathology.

Hippocampus and Amygdala

In humans, beside the widespread occurrence of spheroids, other general changes in hippocampus [151,158,172,178,179] consisted in a reduction of neuronal size and dendritic arbors, and these smaller neurons appeared to be more densely packed. There were also a series of specific modifications affecting the excitatory pyramidal neurons that were more numerous in CA1, but less abundant in all other adjacent hippocampal regions. The GABAergic inhibitory interneurons, instead, displayed a higher density, specifically the calbindin-immunoreactive neurons in the dentate gyrus, the parvalbumin-immunoreactive neurons in CA1 and CA3, and the calretinin-immunoreactive neurons in CA1 [151,158,172,178,179].

In the heterozygous *Reeler* mouse the hippocampus displayed reduced levels of GAD67, [53,177] that could be somewhat restored after stereotaxic injections of Reln [67,180]. These experiments indicated the existence of a causal link between the decrease in GAD67 expression and Reln haplodeficiency. In keeping with such a possibility, Reln supplementation could, at least partly, reverse such a decrease. Other experiments, in line with this interpretation, have confirmed that the decrease in the levels of GAD67 in heterozygous mice can be overturned, e.g., after administration of nicotine, which reduces the GAD67 promoter methylation and increases its transcription [177].

In heterozygous mice, pyramidal neurons displayed a reduction in the average length and width of their apical and basal dendritic spines [52], consistent with the decrease in the spread of the dendritic arbor of the same population of neurons in humans. Additionally, Reln supplementation was effective in promoting a full (apical) or partial (basal shaft) spine recovery [180]. These morphological observations are in line with a previous report showing that, in the forebrain, spines were hypertrophic in mice conditionally overexpressing Reln [66]. At electrophysiological recordings CA1 pyramidal neurons displayed reduced spontaneous inhibitory postsynaptic currents [181], an observation that was fully coherent with the reduction of the inhibitory input from the GABAergic interneurons observed histologically.

Synaptic plasticity is fundamental for hippocampal function. In CA1 of heterozygous mice, LTP was impaired [182] as well as long-term depression (LTD) [181], which returned to normal levels after the administration of Reln [180]. Additionally, in $reln^{+/-}$ and $reln^{-/-}$ mice, post tetanic potentiation (PTP), a form of short-term plasticity that depends on neurotransmitter release, was reduced in CA1 [180,183] and could be reversed by Reln [180].

Collectively these data indicate that the experimental administration of the glycoprotein was able to reverse the morphological, neurochemical, and physiological hippocampal deficits consequent to a reduction of brain Reln. Translationally, they are very important because they offer some cues for further investigations onto the autistic brain. It would be of interest to map the post-mortem distribution of hippocampal RELN in patients compared to healthy controls, to ascertain whether the pattern of immunoreactivity will be consistent between humans and mice.

In the autistic patients, several studies reported that the amygdala, which is involved in emotional learning, increased in size and displayed an augmented density of neurons within the medial, central, and cortical nuclei [151,184–187]. Neurons were, however, less numerous, although numerical variations could be age dependent. To our knowledge, Boyle et al have investigated in detail the amygdala of the homozygous *Reeler* mouse with a marker-based phenotypic approach [188], but there are no data on heterozygous mice.

Cerebellum

Analysis of cerebellar alterations in autism has attracted many efforts of the basic researchers and clinicians. The most consistent anatomic findings in autistic patients were a reduction in size of certain lobules of the cerebellar vermis (but see 3.3.2b Imaging) and a decrease in the number [186,189–192] and size [193,194] of the Purkinje neurons. The inhibitory GABAergic basket and stellate interneurons that connect with these neurons did not show quantitative differences compared to normal cerebella [195]. This observation is indicative of a late developmental death of the Purkinje neurons, as they differentiate well before the interneurons. In addition to structural observations, Western blots demonstrated a reduction of about 40% in the level of expression of RELN in autistic patients related to age and sex corresponding controls [11]. Quantitative RT-PCR also showed a drop of RELN and GAD67 mRNAs in the post-mortem autistic brain [164].

Notably many of the histological alterations in the human autistic cerebellum are like those described in $reln^{+/-}$ mice. These animals displayed a progressive loss of Purkinje neurons already during the first weeks of life [35], and inferior numbers of these cells were observed in adult subjects as well [196]. Human MRI studies did not allow, at present, to ascertain whether the cerebellar vermis is hit by the pathology in its entirety or, rather, only at specific lobuli. Therefore, our group has, at first, focused its attention on five different lobules, which receive diverse types of afferent functional inputs, to analyze the number and topological organization of the Purkinje neurons in $reln^{+/+}$ and $reln^{+/-}$ adult mice of both sexes [197]. We have thus shown that the Purkinje neurons: 1. Displayed a lower density in $reln^{+/-}$ males (14.37%) and $reln^{+/-}$ females (17.73%) compared to $reln^{+/+}$ males; 2. Were larger in $reln^{+/-}$ males than in the other phenotypes under study, and smaller in females (regardless of the *reln* genetic background) than in $reln^{+/+}$ males; 3. Were more messily arranged along the YZ axis of the vermis in $reln^{+/-}$ males than in $reln^{+/+}$ males and, except in central lobule, $reln^{+/-}$ females.

Very recently, as many observations have associated a number of synapse-related genes in the genesis of autism and other neuropsychiatric conditions [198,199], we have examined the expression of synaptophysin 1 (SYP1) and contactin 6 (CNTN6) in the vermis of $reln^{+/-}$ and $reln^{+/+}$ adult mice of both genders [200].

SYP1 is a pre-synaptic marker and CNTN6 is a marker of the synapses made by the parallel fibers onto the Purkinje neurons' dendrites. Notably, there is evidence, although still to be validated in full, that SYP1 is involved in the structural alterations of the autistic synapses [189,201], and very recent observations have shown that copy number variations [202] or a truncating variant [203] of

CNTN6 are found in autistic patients. In addition, *CNTN6* mutations may be a risk factor for several neurodevelopmental and neuropsychiatric disorders [150,199,204].

In line with these human studies, we have demonstrated that $reln^{+/-}$ mouse males displayed a statistically significant drop of 11.89% in SYP1 compared to sex-matched normal animals, whereas no modifications were detected comparing $reln^{+/+}$ and $reln^{+/-}$ females [200]. In $reln^{+/-}$ male and female mice, reductions in SYP1 levels were particularly evident in the molecular layer, whereas in heterozygous mice of both sexes a reduction in CNTN6 occurred in all the three cortical layers of the vermis. In addition, alterations in the levels of expression of SYP1 in the molecular layer of male $reln^{+/-}$ mice ensued across all lobules except lobule VII, but they were limited to lobule II for the granular layer and lobule VII for the Purkinje cell layer.

Thus, the widespread reduction of SYP1 and of CNTN6 in the molecular layer of $reln^{+/-}$ male mice well matched with the autistic phenotype in humans [150].

In the vermis (and the whole cerebellum), there is proof for a topographic segregation of the areas controlling motion versus those connected to cognitive and affective functions, and the diverse lobules are coupled with precise zones of the brain and spinal cord [205]. The CNS areas that handle sensorimotor inputs are directly or indirectly connected with the anterior lobe (lobules I–V of the vermis), lobule VIII, and, to a lesser grade, with lobule VI; on the contrary, cortical association areas that collect non-motor responses are linked to lobules VI and VII. Existing clinical data indicate that the vermis is the chief target of the limbic system, and physiological and behavioral observations implicate the vermis in the regulation of emotions [206]. Therefore, the neurochemical modifications of the cerebellar cortex in heterozygous mice are fully in line with the possibility that the social and communication aberrations typical of autism rest on anomalies of the limbic system and its connections [207,208].

At post-mortem, a numerical reduction of the Purkinje neurons in the posterior cerebellum was long ago described in autistic subjects [184,209], but it did not appear to disturb the vermis [189]. Hypoplasia in lobules VI and VII was initially detected in vivo using MRI [145], but subsequent observations proved the existence of two distinct autistic subtypes related to vermian hypoplasia or hyperplasia [146]. A systematic review and meta-analysis of the accounts of structural MRI has then established that the reduction in size of lobules VI–X (i.e., the lobules included in the posterior cerebellum) showed a remarkable heterogeneity that associated to differences in time of life and intelligence quotient (IQ) merely in lobules VI–VII [210]. Other observations showed that the posterior/inferior vermis, i.e., lobules VII, VIIIb (left), and IX, was more prone to pathological deviations [211], with a decrease of the gray matter after quantitative MRI [190,212,213]. Therefore, it appears that the cerebellar phenotype of the heterozygous *Reeler* mouse is fully compatible with that in humans and that a deeper structural and neurochemical characterization may be useful to direct the discovery of new biomarkers of translational interest.

3.3.3. Schizophrenia and the Heterozygous *Reeler* Mouse

Schizophrenia is a ruinous psychiatric condition that affects about 1% of the population. Its main clinical symptoms are hallucinations, delusions, and cognitive disturbances. These symptoms derive from brain dysfunctions that derive from genetic and environmental factors [214]. However, schizophrenia is not strictly a genetic disease, although gene deletions, duplications, and variations may be risk factors for the disorder. At present, the gene(s) that could be involved in the pathology remain elusive for the most (see OMIM #181500), but a microdeletion in a region of chromosome 22, called 22q11, was recently established to be involved in a small percentage of cases [215].

Genetic studies have shown a link between *RELN* and schizophrenia [216] and, over the past ten years, many SNPs in the *RELN* gene loci occurred in parallel with the beginning and/or severity of the clinical signs [217], but results still are under debate and need further verification [218]. One should perhaps emphasize that observations on gene expression have converged to show that the genes implicated in schizophrenia are more highly expressed during fetal than postnatal life [219], thus making more difficult to ascertain their true role in the etiology of the condition.

Imaging

Structural MRI findings in schizophrenia have been recently reviewed [220]. There is enough information to propose that the condition is associated with a continuing development of gray matter aberrations, chiefly throughout the first stages of the disease. Reduction of the depth of the cerebral cortex in the superior temporal and inferior frontal regions was reported in individuals that later became psychotic. In patients with first episode psychosis, there was, instead, a reduction in the thickness of the superior and inferior frontal cortex, and in the volume of the thalamus. In chronic schizophrenia, the gray matter decreased further in the frontal and temporal areas, cingulate cortices, and thalamus, particularly in patients with unfortunate outcomes. Structural modifications of the white matter occurred only in a small number of longitudinal studies.

As the human phenotype is still very far from clear, it is not surprising that the few MRI observations in *Reeler* mice are still insufficient to draw any definitive consideration of translational relevance (for MRI data on Reeler see 3.3.2 Imaging).

Histopathology

Although gross structural alterations of the brain were lacking, subtle pathological changes in specific populations of neurons and in cell-to-cell communication occurred in schizophrenic patients, see [221] for a recent review. Histopathology mainly consisted in modifications of the number and density of neurons at the level of the whole brain and/or specific neuronal subpopulations, and in morphological and neurochemical alterations of these neurons.

a) Cerebral Cortex

As discussed above for autism, the most widely investigated area of the brain has been the PFC that, in general terms, displayed an increased neuronal density and an altered neuroplasticity with age-related differences between normal and schizophrenic subjects. More specifically, a statistical meta-analysis of thirty papers published between 1993 and 2012, concluded that the density of cortical neurons increased with age irrespective of the condition, but the rate of accretion was much slower in the schizophrenics [222]. However, other cortical areas, such as e.g., the dorsal ACC, displayed no changes in neuronal and glial densities after stereological analysis [223].

The above-mentioned meta-analysis [222] has also taken into consideration the density of inhibitory neurons after immunolabeling with GAD67, PV, or calbindin, and found that it was greater in schizophrenic patients compared to controls before the age of 40, but lower thereafter.

Notably, both Reln and GAD67 mRNAs were downregulated in the PFC of schizophrenic subjects with no relation to neuronal damage [224]. In keeping with these observations, it appeared that in the PFC there was a vulnerability of the inhibitory circuits, with markers of the inhibitory interneurons showing some of the more consistent alterations [225]. More precisely, these alterations consisted in a reduction in the levels of the GAD67 mRNA and protein in subsets of GABAergic basket cells containing PV [222,226,227] or cholecystokinin (CCK) [226]. Notably, these two populations of basket cells are responsible of the inhibition of the pyramidal neurons giving rise, respectively, to the cortical θ and γ oscillations altered in schizophrenia. In addition, the pyramidal neurons targeted by the PV+ basket cells expressed lower levels of the $GABA_A$ receptor $\alpha 1$ [226].

It is also interesting that the levels of RELN and GAD67 mRNAs in microdissected GABAergic neurons of PFC layer 1 were lower in schizophrenics, but unchanged in layer 5 of the same patients [228]. In addition, in the dorsolateral division of the PFC, the GABAergic chandelier neurons targeting the axon initial segment of the pyramidal neurons displayed remarkable neurochemical alterations. These changes were particularly evident in layers 2/3, where immunoreactivity for the GABA membrane transporter GAT1 diminished, in parallel with an increase of the $GABA_A$ receptor $\alpha 2$ subunit in the axons of their target pyramidal neurons [229].

Occurrence of dendritic spine pathology was another prominent feature of the schizophrenic human brain [230,231]. Spine loss mainly affected the smaller spines of the pyramidal neurons in layer 3 of the neocortex and arose during development, possibly because of altered mechanisms of generation, pruning, and/or upkeep [230].

As already mentioned in the section dedicated to autism, investigations on the cerebral cortex of the heterozygous *Reeler* reported a reduction in the levels of GAD67 [53,177], in full accordance with the human studies. A study carried out on mice whose mothers were stressed during pregnancy showed that the downregulation of Reln and GAD67 was associated with a hypermethylation of their promoters [232], this being one the mechanisms in support for the contribution of an altered epigenetic control in the down-regulation of RELN expression in schizophrenia, see [233] for review.

b) Hippocampus

The human hippocampal pathology in schizophrenia is by far less clear than in the cortex. Some initial studies have, in fact, reported a decrease in area or overall volume of the hippocampus, or in the number, size, and density of neurons, as well as a disarray of the pyramidal cells, with greatest differences affecting the pyramidal cell density in left CA4; however, several other subsequent surveys were negative, see [234] for review. In any case, hippocampal alterations in schizophrenics are not specific, as they display several common traits with those in autism.

We have previously discussed the histological changes in the hippocampus of the heterozygous *Reeler* mice in relation to autism. These modifications recall, in toto or in part, those in schizophrenia. Additional information detailed, in individual hippocampal layers, the decrease of neuronal GAD67 in CA1, CA2 and dentate gyrus, and the reduction of PV immunoreactive interneurons in CA1 and CA2, in the perspective to validate these mice as a model of schizophrenia [111]. In translational terms, the aforementioned impairment of LTP in heterozygous mice [182] is of interest, as it also occurs in schizophrenic patients [235].

c) Cerebellum

In the cerebellum of schizophrenic patients, there was a loss of distal and terminal dendritic branches and a decrease in density of the dendritic spines of the Purkinje neurons [236]. Again, these histological alterations are not specific for the condition, being evident also in autism. In addition to such changes, in the schizophrenic cerebellum there were altered levels of expression of the general presynaptic marker SYP1, of complexin II, a marker of the excitatory synapses, but not of complexin I that, instead, labels the inhibitory synapses [237]. Thus, some of the structural changes described in the heterozygous *Reeler* mouse in relation to autism also in cerebellum recollected the human schizophrenic phenotype.

4. Does the Behavior of Heterozygous *Reeler* Mice Recall the Human Conditions Related to RELN?

The recapitulation of the behavioral modifications typical of human autism, schizophrenia, or epilepsy in heterozygous *Reeler* mice still is a subject of debate. The dissimilar outcome of behavioral experiments performed in different laboratories is not surprising, because neuropsychiatric behaviors in humans primarily regard social interaction, communication, and restricted interest, and these behaviors are, obviously, very difficult to measure objectively in mice [238].

It is perhaps worth mentioning here that most of our knowledge on the effects of Reln in the cognitive or behavioral field derives from work on mouse hippocampus. This is not surprising as this part of the brain, as discussed previously, has been the primary focus of numerous investigations also in human patients affected by neuropsychiatric disturbs. Several behaviors comparable to those observed in these human disturbs also occur in $reln^{+/-}$ mice [239–241], as well as the deficits in reversal learning after visual discrimination tasks that were hypothesized to follow a diminished visual attention [240]. In addition, testing $reln^{+/-}$ mice for anxiety-related behavior, motor impulsivity and morphine-induced analgesia yielded a different behavioral profile from that of wild-type littermates in that they displayed, starting form adolescence, a decreased inhibition and emotionality. To these modifications, a small increase of impulsive behavior and different pain thresholds also occurred in adult mice [242]. Heterozygous mice were also tested in a complex series of PPI protocols (unimodal and cross-modal) to conclude that they exhibited a multifaceted configuration of changes in startle reactivity and sensorimotor gating, with both resemblances to and dissimilarities from schizophrenia [243]. At least partly in line with these latter observations, other studies failed, incompletely or in full, to validate the behavioral analogies between neuropsychiatric patients and $reln^{+/-}$ mice [181,244–248]. For example, Salinger and co-workers were unsuccessful to find differences between $reln^{+/-}$ and $reln^{+/+}$ mice after testing gait, emotionality, social aggression, spatial working memory, novel-object detection, fear conditioning, and sensorimotor reflex modulation [244]. In another survey [246], heterozygous *Reeler* mice were evaluated for cognitive plasticity in an instrumental reversal learning task, impulsivity in an inhibitory control task, attentional function in a three-choice serial reaction time task, and working memory in a delayed matching-to-position task to conclude that there were no differences in comparison to $reln^{+/+}$ littermates in prefrontal-related cognitive trials. However, $reln^{+/-}$ mice were deficient in two operant tasks. From these observations, the authors concluded that heterozygous *Reeler* mice were *not* a good model for the essential prefrontal-dependent cognitive shortfalls detected in schizophrenia, although they could be useful to model learning deficits in a more general sense.

In another paper it was reported that heterozygous and wild-type mice displayed comparable levels of general activity, coordination, thermal nociception, startle responses, anxiety-like behavior, shock threshold; identical cued freezing behavior, and comparable spatial learning in Morris water maze tasks, albeit a significant decrease in contextual fear conditioned learning was observed in $reln^{+/-}$ mice only [181]. These authors have then hypothesized that the pharmacological administration of Reln in heterozygous mice could restore the response to PPI. They were unable to find differences in the acoustic startle reflex among treated and untreated animals, but Reln-treated $reln^{+/-}$ mice showed a substantial increase in the percent inhibition to 78-, 86- and 90-dB pre-pulse [180].

One study has specifically focused onto the $reln^{+/-}$ mouse behavioral phenotype in young (P50–70) and fully adult (older than P75) animals to conclude that they were not useful to model schizophrenia [245]. An ample series of behavioral test was used (Irwin test; rotarod; spontaneous locomotor activity; social behavior; light-dark transition; startle response and pre-pulse inhibition; hot plate). Heterozygous mice were like their wild-type littermates at either age, though completely adult male $reln^{+/-}$ mice were involved in social exploration for a longer time. In addition, performance on the rotarod deteriorated with age.

Indeed, age appeared to be a further issue of complexity. In fact, adult $reln^{+/-}$ mice did not display discernible changes in activity, motor coordination, anxiety, or environmental perception compared to wild-type littermate controls. However, juvenile animals displayed not as much of anxiety- and risk assessment-related behaviors in the elevated plus-maze [182,241]. In addition, in one of these two studies it was demonstrated that young $reln^{+/-}$ mice had a hippocampal-dependent shortfall in associative learning and impulsivity–anxiety-related behavior [182]. Additionally, one study, starting from the clinical observations that reported the occurrence of vocal and motor anomalies in autistic patients, has described that $reln^{+/-}$ mice had a general delay in the development of their repertoire of neonatal vocal and motor behaviors [249].

Finally, one must consider that gender apparently influenced some behaviors, although very few studies have focused on this issue. Among these studies, young heterozygous female mice were described to be more active in the light/dark transition test than the heterozygous males that were, instead, more aggressive than females during social interaction [241].

5. Usefulness of the *Reeler* Mouse in Translational Studies: Concluding Remarks

The analysis of the literature discussed above requires one trying to draw some conclusions about the true usefulness of the *Reeler* mouse in translational studies.

At first, it may perhaps be useful to remember that, as discussed, *RELN* is causative of LIS2 and a small percentage of ADLTE, whereas only tentative associations up to now hold for the other conditions here considered (see Figure 1 and Table 1).

Remarkably, both LIS2 and ADLTE are rare diseases. Very few cases of LIS2 (around ten) so far come about in the literature (see OMIM #257320). Similarly, patients with lateral temporal epilepsy (LTE) are only about 10% of all temporal epilepsies, and the real prevalence of ADLTE, which has been up to now reported in Europe, USA, and Japan, is unknown, but it may account for about 19% of familial idiopathic focal epilepsies [250,251]. When one considers the human conditions related to the Reln signaling pathway, one still encounters a group of rare diseases. The actual frequency of *VLDLR*-associated cerebellar hypoplasia is unknown, but initial reports regarded not more than twenty-five affected individuals in Canada and USA [113,252], although the condition occurs worldwide, *PAFAH1B1*-associated lissencephaly is very rare as the prevalence of classic lissencephaly ranges from 11.7 to 40 per million births [120]. To date, sixty-six affected individuals and seven asymptomatic individuals with the ATTTC repeat insertion within *DAB1* have been reported in ten relatives from the south of the Iberian Peninsula, and no individuals with SCA37 from other geographic areas have been described [116]. SCA7 has a prevalence of less than 1:100,000 and accounts for about 2% of all SCAs [253].

Therefore, one must deal with the paradox of the relatively little interest for translational studies on the very conditions for which the *Reeler* mouse and/or mice with mutations of the genes of the Reln pathway fully meet the criteria for construct and face validity. Thus, the homozygous Reeler mice appear to be more interesting to the neurobiologist than to the clinician and their study will surely be still rewarding in terms of our comprehension of neurodevelopment, as the model already helped to establish that many functional and circuit features of cortical neurons are relatively independent from positional cues and cortical lamination, e.g., [179].

Very differently, the prevalence of autism in the worldwide population is around 1% [254] and that of schizophrenia is just below [221]. As the two conditions are very diffuse in the human population, there is an obvious translational interest for the heterozygous *Reeler* mouse as a model for the two disorders. However, such an interest is again paradoxical, as the validity of these mice to extract information about the human pathologies remains dubious. The first explanation for this uncertainty lies, beyond any doubt, in the substantial lack of construct validity, which is the direct consequence of the complex genetic background of autism and schizophrenia. As regarding face validity, the present survey of the literature clearly points out that there are several similarities but also dissimilarities between the human and the mouse phenotypes. Among dissimilarities, one must consider the heterogeneity of results of the behavioral experiments in mouse. Further complexity derives by the vast array of clinical symptoms in humans. Structurally, most of the imaging and post-mortem findings in humans are not specific for each of the two conditions. However, one must consider that both the human and mouse phenotype converges to indicate the cerebral cortex, hippocampus, and cerebellum as the primary foci of the pathologies and the inhibitory interneurons as major players in the context of the circuitry involved.

A serious drawback to a full validation of the heterozygous *Reeler* mouse as a model of autism and/or schizophrenia lies in the observation that the alterations so far described in mouse are very subtle in both structural, functional and neurochemical terms. The relatively low resolution of current neuroimaging procedures, and the difficulty to obtain post-mortem samples amenable for neurochemical, electrophysiological, and fine (ultra) structural analyses make it very difficult to establish whether the alterations in heterozygous *Reeler* mice have a true biological significance that goes beyond mere statistics [255,256]. In the affirmative, one could take advantage of these alterations to discover novel biomarkers that will be helpful for an earlier and more precise diagnosis in the human practice.

Author Contributions: All authors contributed to write the manuscript.

Author Contributions: All authors contributed to write the manuscript.

Abbreviations

ACC	anterior cingulate cortex
ADLTE	autosomal-dominant lateral temporal epilepsy
ApoER2	apolipoprotein E2
ARX	aristaless-related homeobox gene
ASD	autism spectrum disorders
ATXN7	ataxin 7
CCK	cholecystokinin
CNS	central nervous system
CNTN6	contactin 6
DCX	doublecortin
DTI	diffusion tractography imaging
ETL7	temporal lobe epilepsy-7
GFP	green fluorescent protein
HCN	hyperpolarization-activated cyclic nucleotide–gated
HdEEG	high-density electroencephalography
ILS	isolated lissencephaly sequence
IQ	intelligence quotient
LCH	lissencephaly with cerebellar hypoplasia
LGI1	leucine-rich, glioma inactivated 1 gene
LIS1	lissencephaly 1
LIS2	lissencephaly 2
LIS3	lissencephaly 3
LTD	long-term depression
LTE	lateral temporal epilepsy
LTP	long-term potentiation
MAP2	microtubule-associated protein 2
MDS	Miller-Dieker syndrome
MEMRI	manganese-enhanced MRI
NCAM2	neural cell adhesion molecule 2
PAFAH1B1	platelet-activating factor acetylhydrolase IB subunit α
PDD-NOS	pervasive developmental disorder-not otherwise specified
PFC	prefrontal cortex
PPI	pre-pulse inhibition
PTP	post tetanic potentiation
PV	parvalbumin
RELN	Reelin gene (human)
Reln	Reelin gene (mouse)
RELN	Reelin glycoprotein (human)
Reln	Reelin glycoprotein (mouse)
ROI	region-of-interest
SBH	subcortical band heterotopia
SCA37	spinocerebellar ataxia type 37
SCA7	spinocerebellar ataxia type 7
SNP	single nucleotide polymorphism
SYP1	synaptophysin 1
TUBA1A	α tubulin 1A
VENs	von Economo neurons
VLDLR	very low-density lipoprotein receptor

References

1. Andersen, T.E.; Finsen, B.; Goffinet, A.M.; Issinger, O.G.; Boldyreff, B. A reeler mutant mouse with a new, spontaneous mutation in the reelin gene. *Brain Res. Mol. Brain Res.* **2002**, *105*, 153–156. [CrossRef]

2. Tissir, F.; Goffinet, A.M. Reelin and brain development. *Nat. Rev. Neurosci.* **2003**, *4*, 496–505. [CrossRef] [PubMed]

3. D'Arcangelo, G.; Miao, G.G.; Chen, S.C.; Soares, H.D.; Morgan, J.I.; Curran, T. A protein related to extracellular matrix proteins deleted in the mouse mutant reeler. *Nature* **1995**, *374*, 719–723. [CrossRef] [PubMed]

4. Falconer, D.S. Two new mutants, 'trembler' and 'reeler', with neurological actions in the house mouse (*Mus musculus* L.). *J. Genet.* **1951**, *50*, 192–201. [CrossRef]

5. Caviness, V.S.; Rakic, P. Mechanisms of Cortical Development: A View from Mutations in Mice. *Annu. Rev. Neurosci.* **1978**, *1*, 297–326. [CrossRef]

6. Goffinet, A.M. Events governing organization of postmigratory neurons: Studies on brain development in normal and reeler mice. *Brain Res. Rev.* **1984**, *7*, 261–296. [CrossRef]

7. Folsom, T.D.; Fatemi, S.H. The involvement of Reelin in neurodevelopmental disorders. *Neuropharmacology* **2013**, *68*, 122–135. [CrossRef]

8. DeSilva, U.; D'Arcangelo, G.; Braden, V.V.; Chen, J.; Miao, G.G.; Curran, T.; Green, E.D. The human reelin gene: Isolation, sequencing, and mapping on chromosome 7. *Genome Res.* **1997**, *7*, 157–164. [CrossRef]

9. Hong, S.E.; Shugart, Y.Y.; Huang, D.T.; Shahwan, S.A.; Grant, P.E.; Hourihane, J.O.; Martin, N.D.; Walsh, C.A. Autosomal recessive lissencephaly with cerebellar hypoplasia is associated with human RELN mutations. *Nat. Genet.* **2000**, *26*, 93–96. [CrossRef]

10. Fatemi, S.H. Reelin glycoprotein in autism and schizophrenia. *Int. Rev. Neurobiol.* **2005**, *71*, 179–187.

11. Fatemi, S.H.; Stary, J.M.; Halt, A.R.; Realmuto, G.R. Dysregulation of Reelin and Bcl-2 proteins in autistic cerebellum. *J. Autism Dev. Disord.* **2001**, *31*, 529–535. [CrossRef] [PubMed]

12. Robertson, H.R.; Feng, G. Annual Research Review: Transgenic mouse models of childhood-onset psychiatric disorders. *J. Child Psychol. Psychiatry* **2011**, *52*, 442–475. [CrossRef] [PubMed]

13. Miles, J.H. Autism spectrum disorders—A genetics review. *Genet. Med.* **2011**, *13*, 278–294. [CrossRef] [PubMed]

14. Vorstman, J.A.S.; Parr, J.R.; Moreno-De-Luca, D.; Anney, R.J.L.; Nurnberger, J.I., Jr.; Hallmayer, J.F. Autism genetics: Opportunities and challenges for clinical translation. *Nat. Rev. Genet.* **2017**, *18*, 362–376. [CrossRef]

15. Geyer, M.A. Developing translational animal models for symptoms of schizophrenia or bipolar mania. *Neurotox. Res.* **2008**, *14*, 71–78. [CrossRef]

16. Chadman, K.K. Animal models for autism in 2017 and the consequential implications to drug discovery. *Exp. Opin. Drug Discov.* **2017**, *12*, 1187–1194. [CrossRef]

17. Zaki, M.; Shehab, M.; El-Aleem, A.A.; Abdel-Salam, G.; Koeller, H.B.; Ilkin, Y.; Ross, M.E.; Dobyns, W.B.; Gleeson, J.G. Identification of a novel recessive RELN mutation using a homozygous balanced reciprocal translocation. *Am. J. Med. Genet. A* **2007**, *143*, 939–944. [CrossRef]

18. Hirotsune, S.; Takahara, T.; Sasaki, N.; Hirose, K.; Yoshiki, A.; Ohashi, T.; Kusakabe, M.; Murakami, Y.; Muramatsu, M.; Watanabe, S. The reeler gene encodes a protein with an EGF-like motif expressed by pioneer neurons. *Nat. Genet.* **1995**, *10*, 77–83. [CrossRef]

19. Ogawa, M.; Miyata, T.; Nakajima, K.; Yagyu, K.; Seike, M.; Ikenaka, K.; Yamamoto, H.; Mikoshiba, K. The reeler gene-associated antigen on Cajal-Retzius neurons is a crucial molecule for laminar organization of cortical neurons. *Neuron* **1995**, *14*, 899–912. [CrossRef]

20. D'Arcangelo, G. Reelin in the years: Controlling neuronal migration and maturation in the mammalian brain. *Adv. Neurosci.* **2014**, *2014*, 597395. [CrossRef]

21. Hiesberger, T.; Trommsdorff, M.; Howell, B.W.; Goffinet, A.; Mumby, M.C.; Cooper, J.A.; Herz, J. Direct binding of Reelin to VLDL receptor and ApoE receptor 2 induces tyrosine phosphorylation of disabled-1 and modulates tau phosphorylation. *Neuron* **1999**, *24*, 481–489. [CrossRef]

22. Assadi, A.H.; Zhang, G.; Beffert, U.; McNeil, R.S.; Renfro, A.L.; Niu, S.; Quattrocchi, C.C.; Antalffy, B.A.; Sheldon, M.; Armstrong, D.D.; et al. Interaction of reelin signaling and Lis1 in brain development. *Nat. Genet.* **2003**, *35*, 270–276. [CrossRef] [PubMed]

23. Bahi-Buisson, N.; Cavallin, M. Tubulinopathies overview. In *GeneReviews®*; Adam, M.P., Ardinger, H.H., Pagon, R.A., Wallace, S.E., Eds.; University of Washington: Seattle, WA, USA, 2016.

24. Lo, N.C.; Chong, C.S.; Smith, A.C.; Dobyns, W.B.; Carrozzo, R.; Ledbetter, D.H. Point mutations and an intragenic deletion in LIS1, the lissencephaly causative gene in isolated lissencephaly sequence and Miller-Dieker syndrome. *Hum. Mol. Genet.* **1997**, *6*, 157–164.

25. Kato, M.; Dobyns, W.B. Lissencephaly and the molecular basis of neuronal migration. *Hum. Mol. Genet.* **2003**, *12*, R89–R96. [CrossRef]

26. Lecourtois, M.; Poirier, K.; Friocourt, G.; Jaglin, X.; Goldenberg, A.; Saugier-Veber, P.; Chelly, J.; Laquerriere, A. Human lissencephaly with cerebellar hypoplasia due to mutations in TUBA1A: Expansion of the foetal neuropathological phenotype. *Acta Neuropathol.* **2010**, *119*, 779–789. [CrossRef]

27. Ross, M.E.; Swanson, K.; Dobyns, W.B. Lissencephaly with cerebellar hypoplasia (LCH): A heterogeneous group of cortical malformations. *Neuropediatrics* **2001**, *32*, 256–263. [CrossRef]

28. Sergi, C.; Zoubaa, S.; Schiesser, M. Norman-Roberts syndrome: Prenatal diagnosis and autopsy findings. *Prenat. Diagn.* **2000**, *20*, 505–509. [CrossRef]

29. Badea, A.; Nicholls, P.J.; Johnson, G.A.; Wetsel, W.C. Neuroanatomical phenotypes in the reeler mouse. *Neuroimage* **2007**, *34*, 1363–1374. [CrossRef]

30. Silva, A.C.; Lee, J.H.; Wu, C.W.H.; Tucciarone, J.; Pelled, G.; Aoki, I.; Koretsky, A.P. Detection of cortical laminar architecture using manganese-enhanced MRI. *J. Neurosci. Meth.* **2008**, *167*, 246–257. [CrossRef]

31. Harsan, L.A.; David, C.; Reisert, M.; Schnell, S.; Hennig, J.; von Elverfeld, D.; Staiger, J.F. Mapping remodeling of thalamocortical projections in the living reeler mouse brain by diffusion tractography. *Proc. Natl. Acad. Sci. USA* **2013**, *110*, E1797–E1806. [CrossRef]

32. Pappas, G.D.; Kriho, V.; Liu, W.S.; Tremolizzo, L.; Lugli, G.; Larson, J. Immunocytochemical localization of reelin in the olfactory bulb of the heterozygous reeler mouse: an animal model for schizophrenia. *Neurol. Res.* **2003**, *25*, 819–830. [CrossRef] [PubMed]

33. Katsuyama, Y.; Terashima, T. Developmental anatomy of reeler mutant mouse. *Dev. Growth Differ.* **2009**, *51*, 271–286. [CrossRef] [PubMed]

34. Wyss, J.M.; Stanfield, B.B.; Cowan, W.M. Structural abnormalities in the olfactory bulb of the Reeler mouse. *Brain Res.* **1980**, *188*, 566–571. [CrossRef]

35. Marrone, M.C.; Marinelli, S.; Biamonte, F.; Keller, F.; Sgobio, C.A.; Ammassari-Teule, M.; Bernardi, G.; Mercuri, N.B. Altered cortico-striatal synaptic plasticity and related behavioural impairments in reeler mice. *Eur. J. Neurosci.* **2006**, *24*, 2061–2070. [CrossRef]

36. Cariboni, A.; Rakic, S.; Liapi, A.; Maggi, R.; Goffinet, A.; Parnavelas, J.G. Reelin provides an inhibitory signal in the migration of gonadotropin-releasing hormone neurons. *Development* **2005**, *132*, 4709–4718. [CrossRef]

37. Stanfield, B.B.; Wyss, J.M.; Cowan, W.M. The projection of the supramammillary region upon the dentate gyrus in normal and reeler mice. *Brain Res.* **1980**, *198*, 196–203. [CrossRef]

38. Baba, K.; Sakakibara, S.; Setsu, T.; Terashima, T. The superficial layers of the superior colliculus are cytoarchitectually and myeloarchitectually disorganized in the reelin-deficient mouse, reeler. *Brain Res.* **2007**, *1140*, 205–215. [CrossRef]

39. Terashima, T. Distribution of mesencephalic trigeminal nucleus neurons in the reeler mutant mouse. *Anat. Rec.* **1996**, *244*, 563–571. [CrossRef]

40. Nishikawa, S.; Goto, S.; Yamada, K.; Hamasaki, T.; Ushio, Y. Lack of Reelin causes malpositioning of nigral dopaminergic neurons: Evidence from comparison of normal and Reln (rl) mutant mice. *J. Comp. Neurol.* **2003**, *461*, 166–173. [CrossRef]

41. Takaoka, Y.; Setsu, T.; Misaki, K.; Yamauchi, T.; Terashima, T. Expression of reelin in the dorsal cochlear nucleus of the mouse. *Brain Res. Dev. Brain Res.* **2005**, *159*, 127–134. [CrossRef]

42. Goffinet, A.M. The embryonic development of the inferior olivary complex in normal and reeler (rlORL) mutant mice. *J. Comp. Neurol.* **1983**, *219*, 10–24. [CrossRef] [PubMed]

43. Terashima, T.; Inoue, K.; Inoue, Y.; Mikoshiba, K.; Tsukada, Y. Observations on the brainstem-spinal descending systems of normal and reeler mutant mice by the retrograde HRP method. *J. Comp. Neurol.* **1984**, *225*, 95–104. [CrossRef] [PubMed]

44. Tanaka, Y.; Okado, H.; Terashima, T. Retrograde infection of precerebellar nuclei neurons by injection of a recombinant adenovirus into the cerebellar cortex of normal and reeler mice. *Arch. Histol. Cytol.* **2007**, *70*, 51–62. [CrossRef] [PubMed]

45. Villeda, S.A.; Akopians, A.L.; Babayan, A.H.; Basbaum, A.I.; Phelps, P.E. Absence of Reelin results in altered nociception and aberrant neuronal positioning in the dorsal spinal cord. *Neuroscience* **2006**, *139*, 1385–1396. [CrossRef] [PubMed]

46. Yip, J.W.; Yip, Y.P.; Nakajima, K.; Capriotti, C. Reelin controls position of autonomic neurons in the spinal cord. *Proc. Natl. Acad. Sci. USA* **2000**, *97*, 8612–8616. [CrossRef]

47. Phelps, P.E.; Rich, R.; Dupuy-Davies, S.; Rios, Y.; Wong, T. Evidence for a cell-specific action of Reelin in the spinal cord. *Dev. Biol.* **2002**, *244*, 180–198. [CrossRef]

48. Stanfield, B.B.; Cowan, W.M. The morphology of the hippocampus and dentate gyrus in normal and reeler mice. *J. Comp. Neurol.* **1979**, *185*, 393–422. [CrossRef]

49. Pinto Lord, M.C.; Caviness, V.S., Jr. Determinants of cell shape and orientation: A comparative Golgi analysis of cell-axon interrelationships in the developing neocortex of normal and reeler mice. *J. Comp. Neurol.* **1979**, *187*, 49–69. [CrossRef]

50. Niu, S.; Yabut, O.; D'Arcangelo, G. The Reelin signaling pathway promotes dendritic spine development in hippocampal neurons. *J. Neurosci.* **2008**, *28*, 10339–10348. [CrossRef]

51. Olson, E.C.; Kim, S.; Walsh, C.A. Impaired neuronal positioning and dendritogenesis in the neocortex after cell-autonomous Dab1 suppression. *J. Neurosci.* **2006**, *26*, 1767–1775. [CrossRef]

52. Niu, S.; Renfro, A.; Quattrocchi, C.C.; Sheldon, M.; D'Arcangelo, G. Reelin promotes hippocampal dendrite development through the VLDLR/ApoER2-Dab1 pathway. *Neuron* **2004**, *41*, 71–84. [CrossRef]

53. Liu, W.S.; Pesold, C.; Rodriguez, M.A.; Carboni, G.; Auta, J.; Lacor, P.; Larson, J.; Condie, B.G.; Guidotti, A.; Costa, E. Down-regulation of dendritic spine and glutamic acid decarboxylase 67 expressions in the reelin haploinsufficient heterozygous reeler mouse. *Proc. Natl. Acad. Sci. USA* **2001**, *98*, 3477–3482. [CrossRef] [PubMed]

54. Chameau, P.; Inta, D.; Vitalis, T.; Monyer, H.; Wadman, W.J.; van Hooft, J.A. The N-terminal region of reelin regulates postnatal dendritic maturation of cortical pyramidal neurons. *Proc. Natl. Acad. Sci. USA* **2009**, *106*, 7227–7232. [CrossRef] [PubMed]

55. Manita, S.; Suzuki, T.; Homma, C.; Matsumoto, T.; Odagawa, M.; Yamada, K.; Ota, K.; Matsubara, C.; Inutsuka, A.; Sato, M.; et al. Top-Down Cortical Circuit for Accurate Sensory Perception. *Neuron* **2015**, *86*, 1304–1316. [CrossRef] [PubMed]

56. Larkum, M.E.; Petro, L.S.; Sachdev RN, S.; Muckli, L. A Perspective on cortical layering and layer-spanning neuronal elements. *Front. Neuroanat.* **2018**, *12*, 56. [CrossRef]

57. Lörincz, A.; Notomi, T.; Tamás, G.; Shigemoto, R.; Nusser, Z. Polarized and compartment-dependent distribution of HCN1 in pyramidal cell dendrites. *Nat. Neurosci.* **2002**, *5*, 1185–1193. [CrossRef]

58. Kupferman, J.V.; Basu, J.; Russo, M.J.; Guevarra, J.; Cheung, S.K.; Siegelbaum, S.A. Reelin signaling specifies the molecular identity of the pyramidal neuron distal dendritic compartment. *Cell* **2014**, *158*, 1335–1347. [CrossRef]

59. Meseke, M.; Neumuller, F.; Brunne, B.; Li, X.; Anstotz, M.; Pohlkamp, T.; Rogalla, M.M.; Herz, J.; Rune, G.M.; Bender, R.A. distal dendritic enrichment of HCN1 channels in hippocampal CA1 is promoted by estrogen, but does not require Reelin. *eNeuro* **2018**, *5*. [CrossRef]

60. Bliss, T.V.; Chung, S.H. An electrophysiological study of the hippocampus of the 'reeler' mutant mouse. *Nature* **1974**, *252*, 153–155. [CrossRef]

61. Silva, L.R.; Gutnick, M.J.; Connors, B.W. Laminar distribution of neuronal membrane properties in neocortex of normal and reeler mouse. *J. Neurophysiol.* **1991**, *66*, 2034–2040. [CrossRef]

62. Shah, M.M.; Hammond, R.S.; Hoffman, D.A. Dendritic ion channel trafficking and plasticity. *Trends Neurosci.* **2010**, *33*, 307–316. [CrossRef] [PubMed]

63. Chen, Y.; Beffert, U.; Ertunc, M.; Tang, T.S.; Kavalali, E.T.; Bezprozvanny, I.; Herz, J. Reelin modulates NMDA receptor activity in cortical neurons. *J. Neurosci.* **2005**, *25*, 8209–8216. [CrossRef] [PubMed]

64. Beffert, U.; Weeber, E.J.; Durudas, A.; Qiu, S.; Masiulis, I.; Sweatt, J.D.; Li, W.P.; Adelmann, G.; Frotscher, M.; Hammer, R.E.; et al. Modulation of synaptic plasticity and memory by Reelin involves differential splicing of the lipoprotein receptor Apoer2. *Neuron* **2005**, *47*, 567–579. [CrossRef] [PubMed]

65. Ishida, A.; Shimazaki, K.; Terashima, T.; Kawai, N. An electrophysiological and immunohistochemical study of the hippocampus of the reeler mutant mouse. *Brain Res.* **1994**, *662*, 60–68. [CrossRef]

66. Pujadas, L.; Gruart, A.; Bosch, C.; Delgado, L.; Teixeira, C.M.; Rossi, D.; De Lecea, L.; Martinez, A.; Delgado-Garcia, J.M.; Soriano, E. Reelin regulates postnatal neurogenesis and enhances spine hypertrophy and long-term potentiation. *J. Neurosci.* **2010**, *30*, 4636–4649. [CrossRef]

67. Rogers, J.T.; Rusiana, I.; Trotter, J.; Zhao, L.; Donaldson, E.; Pak, D.T.; Babus, L.W.; Peters, M.; Banko, J.L.; Chavis, P.; et al. Reelin supplementation enhances cognitive ability, synaptic plasticity, and dendritic spine density. *Learn. Mem.* **2011**, *18*, 558–564. [CrossRef]

68. Weeber, E.J.; Beffert, U.; Jones, C.; Christian, J.M.; Forster, E.; Sweatt, J.D.; Herz, J. Reelin and ApoE receptors cooperate to enhance hippocampal synaptic plasticity and learning. *J. Biol. Chem.* **2002**, *277*, 39944–39952. [CrossRef]

69. Parnavelas, J.G. The origin and migration of cortical neurones: New vistas. *Trends Neurosci.* **2000**, *23*, 126–131. [CrossRef]

70. D'Arcangelo, G. Reelin mouse mutants as models of cortical development disorders. *Epilepsy Behav.* **2006**, *8*, 81–90. [CrossRef]

71. Caviness, V.S., Jr. Patterns of cell and fiber distribution in the neocortex of the reeler mutant mouse. *J. Comp. Neurol* **1976**, *170*, 435–447. [CrossRef]

72. Terashima, T.; Takayama, C.; Ichikawa, R.; Inoue, Y. Dendritic arbolization of large pyramidal neurons in the motor cortex of normal and reeler mutant mouse. *Okajimas Folia Anat. Jpn.* **1992**, *68*, 351–363. [CrossRef] [PubMed]

73. Landrieu, P.; Goffinet, A. Inverted pyramidal neurons and their axons in the neocortex of reeler mutant mice. *Cell Tissue Res.* **1981**, *218*, 293–301. [CrossRef] [PubMed]

74. Terashima, T.; Inoue, K.; Inoue, Y.; Mikoshiba, K.; Tsukada, Y. Distribution and morphology of corticospinal tract neurons in reeler mouse cortex by the retrograde HRP method. *J. Comp. Neurol.* **1983**, *218*, 314–326. [CrossRef] [PubMed]

75. Markram, H.; Toledo-Rodriguez, M.; Wang, Y.; Gupta, A.; Silberberg, G.; Wu, C. Interneurons of the neocortical inhibitory system. *Nat. Rev. Neurosci.* **2004**, *5*, 793–807. [CrossRef] [PubMed]

76. Yabut, O.; Renfro, A.; Niu, S.; Swann, J.W.; Marin, O.; D'Arcangelo, G. Abnormal laminar position and dendrite development of interneurons in the reeler forebrain. *Brain Res.* **2007**, *1140*, 75–83. [CrossRef]

77. Hevner, R.F.; Daza, R.A.; Englund, C.; Kohtz, J.; Fink, A. Postnatal shifts of interneuron position in the neocortex of normal and reeler mice: Evidence for inward radial migration. *Neuroscience* **2004**, *124*, 605–618. [CrossRef]

78. Pla, R.; Borrell, V.; Flames, N.; Marin, O. Layer acquisition by cortical GABAergic interneurons is independent of Reelin signaling. *J. Neurosci.* **2006**, *26*, 6924–6934. [CrossRef]

79. Hammond, V.; So, E.; Gunnersen, J.; Valcanis, H.; Kalloniatis, M.; Tan, S.S. Layer positioning of late-born cortical interneurons is dependent on Reelin but not p35 signaling. *J. Neurosci.* **2006**, *26*, 1646–1655. [CrossRef]

80. Lakoma, J.; Garcia-Alonso, L.; Luque, J.M. Reelin sets the pace of neocortical neurogenesis. *Development* **2011**, *138*, 5223–5234. [CrossRef]

81. Nishikawa, S.; Goto, S.; Hamasaki, T.; Yamada, K.; Ushio, Y. Involvement of reelin and Cajal-Retzius cells in the developmental formation of vertical columnar structures in the cerebral cortex: Evidence from the study of mouse presubicular cortex. *Cereb. Cortex* **2002**, *12*, 1024–1030. [CrossRef]

82. Nishibe, M.; Katsuyama, Y.; Yamashita, T. Developmental abnormality contributes to cortex-dependent motor impairments and higher intracortical current requirement in the reeler homozygous mutants. *Brain Struct. Funct.* **2018**, *223*, 2575–2587. [CrossRef] [PubMed]

83. Simmons, P.A.; Lemmon, V.; Pearlman, A.L. Afferent and efferent connections of the striate and extrastriate visual cortex of the normal and reeler mouse. *J. Comp. Neurol.* **1982**, *211*, 295–308. [CrossRef] [PubMed]

84. Wagener, R.J.; David, C.; Zhao, S.; Haas, C.A.; Staiger, J.F. The somatosensory cortex of reeler mutant mice shows absent layering but intact formation and behavioral activation of columnar somatotopic maps. *J. Neurosci.* **2010**, *30*, 15700–15709. [CrossRef] [PubMed]

85. Pielecka-Fortuna, J.; Wagener, R.J.; Martens, A.K.; Goetze, B.; Schmidt, K.F.; Staiger, J.F.; Lowel, S. The disorganized visual cortex in reelin-deficient mice is functional and allows for enhanced plasticity. *Brain Struct. Funct.* **2015**, *220*, 3449–3467. [CrossRef]

86. Guy, J.; Wagener, R.J.; Mock, M.; Staiger, J.F. persistence of functional sensory maps in the absence of cortical layers in the somsatosensory cortex of Reeler mice. *Cereb. Cortex* **2015**, *25*, 2517–2528. [CrossRef]

87. Prume, M.; Rollenhagen, A.; Lubke, J.H.R. Structural and synaptic organization of the adult reeler mouse somatosensory neocortex: A comparative fine-scale electron microscopic study of Reeler with wild type mice. *Front. Neuroanat.* **2018**, *12*, 80. [CrossRef]
88. Grossberg, S. Towards a unified theory of neocortex: Laminar cortical circuits for vision and cognition. *Prog. Brain Res.* **2007**, *165*, 79–104.
89. D'Souza, R.D.; Burkhalter, A.A. Laminar Organization for Selective Cortico-Cortical Communication. *Front. Neuroanat.* **2017**, *11*, 71. [CrossRef]
90. Guy, J.; Staiger, J.F. The Functioning of a Cortex without Layers. *Front. Neuroanat.* **2017**, *11*, 54. [CrossRef]
91. Mikoshiba, K.; Nagaike, K.; Kohsaka, S.; Takamatsu, K.; Aoki, E.; Tsukada, Y. Developmental studies on the cerebellum from reeler mutant mouse in vivo and in vitro. *Dev. Biol.* **1980**, *79*, 64–80. [CrossRef]
92. Altman, J.; Bayer, S.A. *Development of the Cerebellar System in Relation to Its Evolution, Structure and Functions*; CRC Press: Boca Raton, FL, USA, 1997.
93. Cocito, C.; Merighi, A.; Giacobini, M.; Lossi, L. alterations of cell proliferation and apoptosis in the hypoplastic Reeler cerebellum. *Front. Cell. Neurosci.* **2016**, *10*, 141. [CrossRef] [PubMed]
94. Castagna, C.; Merighi, A.; Lossi, L. Cell death and neurodegeneration in the postnatal development of cerebellar vermis in normal and Reeler mice. *Ann. Anat.* **2016**, *207*, 76–90. [CrossRef] [PubMed]
95. Mariani, J.; Crepel, F.; Mikoshiba, K.; Changeux, J.P.; Sotelo, C. Anatomical, physiological and biochemical studies of the cerebellum from Reeler mutant mouse. *Philos. Trans. R. Soc. B* **1977**, *281*, 1–28. [CrossRef] [PubMed]
96. Heckroth, J.A.; Goldowitz, D.; Eisenman, L.M. Purkinje cell reduction in the reeler mutant mouse: A quantitative immunohistochemical study. *J. Comp. Neurol.* **1989**, *279*, 546–555. [CrossRef]
97. Yuasa, S.; Kitoh, J.; Oda, S.; Kawamura, K. Obstructed migration of Purkinje cells in the developing cerebellum of the reeler mutant mouse. *Anat. Embryol.* **1993**, *188*, 317–329. [CrossRef]
98. Castagna, C.; Aimar, P.; Alasia, S.; Lossi, L. Post-natal development of the Reeler mouse cerebellum: An ultrastructural study. *Ann. Anat.* **2014**, *196*, 224–235. [CrossRef]
99. Mariani, J. Extent of multiple innervation of Purkinje cells by climbing fibers in the olivocerebellar system of weaver, reeler, and staggerer mutant mice. *J. Neurobiol.* **1982**, *13*, 119–126. [CrossRef]
100. Terashima, T.; Inoue, K.; Inoue, Y.; Mikoshiba, K.; Tsukada, Y. Observations on Golgi epithelial cells and granule cells in the cerebellum of the reeler mutant mouse. *Brain Res.* **1985**, *350*, 103–112. [CrossRef]
101. Keays, D.A.; Tian, G.; Poirier, K.; Huang, G.J.; Siebold, C.; Cleak, J.; Oliver, P.L.; Fray, M.; Harvey, R.J.; Molnár, Z.; et al. Mutations in αtubulin cause abnormal neuronal migration in mice and lissencephaly in humans. *Cell* **2007**, *128*, 45–57. [CrossRef]
102. Bahi-Buisson, N.; Poirier, K.; Fourniol, F.; Saillour, Y.; Valence, S.; Lebrun, N.; Hully, M.; Bianco, C.F.; Boddaert, N.; Elie, C.; et al. The wide spectrum of tubulinopathies: What are the key features for the diagnosis? *Brain* **2014**, *137*, 1676–1700. [CrossRef]
103. Aiken, J.; Buscaglia, G.; Bates, E.A.; Moore, J.K. The α-tubulin gene TUBA1A in brain development: A key ingredient in the neuronal isotype blend. *J. Dev. Biol.* **2017**, *5*, 8. [CrossRef] [PubMed]
104. Goncalves, F.G.; Freddi, T.A.L.; Taranath, A.; Lakshmanan, R.; Goetti, R.; Feltrin, F.S.; Mankad, K.; Teixeira, S.R.; Hanagandi, P.B.; Arrigoni, F. Tubulinopathies. *Top. Magn. Reson. Imaging* **2018**, *27*, 395–408. [CrossRef] [PubMed]
105. Romaniello, R.; Arrigoni, F.; Fry, A.E.; Bassi, M.T.; Rees, M.I.; Borgatti, R.; Pilz, D.T.; Cushion, T.D. Tubulin genes and malformations of cortical development. *Eur. J. Med. Genet.* **2018**, *61*, 744–754. [CrossRef] [PubMed]
106. Dazzo, E.; Fanciulli, M.; Serioli, E.; Minervini, G.; Pulitano, P.; Binelli, S.; Di, B.C.; Luisi, C.; Pasini, E.; Striano, S.; et al. Heterozygous reelin mutations cause autosomal-dominant lateral temporal epilepsy. *Am. J. Hum. Genet.* **2015**, *96*, 992–1000. [CrossRef]
107. Michelucci, R.; Pulitano, P.; Di Bonaventura, C.; Binelli, S.; Luisi, C.; Pasini, E.; Striano, S.; Striano, P.; Coppola, G.; La Neve, A.; et al. The clinical phenotype of autosomal dominant lateral temporal lobe epilepsy related to reelin mutations. *Epilepsy Behav.* **2017**, *68*, 103–107. [CrossRef]
108. Ceská, K.; Aulická, Š.; Horák, O.; Danhofer, P.; Ríha, P.; Marecek, R.; Šenkyrík, J.; Rektor, I.; Brázdil, M.; Oslejsková, H. Autosomal dominant temporal lobe epilepsy associated with heterozygous reelin mutation: 3 T brain MRI study with advanced neuroimaging methods. *Epilepsy Behav. Case Rep.* **2019**, *11*, 39–42. [CrossRef]

109. Hwang, E.; Brown, R.E.; Kocsis, B.; Kim, T.; McKenna, J.T.; McNally, J.M.; Han, H.B.; Choi, J.H. Optogenetic stimulation of basal forebrain parvalbumin neurons modulates the cortical topography of auditory steady-state responses. *Brain Struct. Funct.* **2019**, *224*, 1505–1518. [CrossRef]

110. Ammassari-Teule, M.; Sgobio, C.; Biamonte, F.; Marrone, C.; Mercuri, N.B.; Keller, F. Reelin haploinsufficiency reduces the density of PV+neurons in circumscribed regions of the striatum and selectively alters striatal-based behaviors. *Psychopharmacology* **2009**, *204*, 511–521. [CrossRef]

111. Nullmeier, S.; Panther, P.; Dobrowolny, H.; Frotscher, M.; Zhao, S.; Schwegler, H.; Wolf, R. Region-specific alteration of GABAergic markers in the brain of heterozygous reeler mice. *Eur. J. Neurosci.* **2011**, *33*, 689–698. [CrossRef]

112. Ding, L.; Satish, S.; Zhou, C.; Gallagher, M.J. Cortical activation in generalized seizures. *Epilepsia* **2019**, *60*, 1932–1941. [CrossRef]

113. Boycott, K.M.; Bonnemann, C.; Herz, J.; Neuert, S.; Beaulieu, C.; Scott, J.N.; Venkatasubramanian, A.; Parboosingh, J.S. Mutations in VLDLR as a cause for autosomal recessive cerebellar ataxia with mental retardation (dysequilibrium syndrome). *J. Child Neurol.* **2009**, *24*, 1310–1315. [CrossRef] [PubMed]

114. Trommsdorff, M.; Gotthardt, M.; Hiesberger, T.; Shelton, J.; Stockinger, W.; Nimpf, J.; Hammer, R.E.; Richardson, J.A.; Herz, J. Reeler/Disabled-like disruption of neuronal migration in knockout mice lacking the VLDL receptor and ApoE receptor 2. *Cell* **1999**, *97*, 689–701. [CrossRef]

115. Korwek, K.M.; Trotter, J.H.; LaDu, M.J.; Sullivan, P.M.; Weeber, E.J. ApoE isoform-dependent changes in hippocampal synaptic function. *Mol. Neurodegener.* **2009**, *4*, 21. [CrossRef] [PubMed]

116. Matilla-Dueñas, A.; Volpini, V. Spinocerebellar ataxia type 37. In *GeneReviews®*; Adam, M.P., Ardinger, H.H., Pagon, R.A., Wallace, S.E., Eds.; University of Washington: Seattle, WA, USA, 2019.

117. Serrano-Munuera, C.; Corral-Juan, M.; Stevanin, G.; San Nicolás, H.; Roig, C.; Corral, J.; Campos, B.; De Jorge, L.; Morcillo-Suárez, C.; Navarro, A.; et al. New subtype of spinocerebellar ataxia with altered vertical eye movements mapping to chromosome 1p32 subtype of SCA with altered vertical eye movements. *JAMA Neurol.* **2013**, *70*, 764–771. [CrossRef] [PubMed]

118. Seixas, A.I.; Loureiro, J.R.; Costa, C.; Ordóñez-Ugalde, A.S.; Marcelino, H.; Oliveira, C.L.; Loureiro, J.L.; Dhingra, A.; Brandão, E.; Cruz, V.T.; et al. A Pentanucleotide ATTTC Repeat Insertion in the Non-coding Region of DAB1, Mapping to SCA37, Causes Spinocerebellar Ataxia. *Am. J. Hum. Genet.* **2017**, *101*, 87–103. [CrossRef] [PubMed]

119. Ware, M.L.; Fox, J.W.; González, J.L.; Davis, N.M.; De Rouvroit, C.L.; Russo, C.J.; Chua, S.C.; Goffinet, A.M.; Walsh, C.A. Aberrant splicing of a mouse disabled homolog, mdab1, in the scrambler Mouse. *Neuron* **1997**, *19*, 239–249. [CrossRef]

120. Dobyns, W.B.; Das, S. PAFAH1B1-Associated Lissencephaly/Subcortical Band Heterotopia. In *GeneReviews®*; Adam, M.P., Ardinger, H.H., Pagon, R.A., Wallace, S.E., Eds.; University of Washington: Seattle, WA, USA, 2014.

121. Katayama, K.I.; Hayashi, K.; Inoue, S.; Sakaguchi, K.; Nakajima, K. Enhanced expression of Pafah1b1 causes over-migration of cerebral cortical neurons into the marginal zone. *Brain Struct. Funct.* **2017**, *222*, 4283–4291. [CrossRef]

122. Hunt, R.F.; Dinday, M.T.; Hindle-Katel, W.; Baraban, S.C. LIS1 Deficiency Promotes Dysfunctional synaptic integration of granule cells generated in the developing and adult dentate gyrus. *J. Neurosci.* **2012**, *32*, 12862–12875. [CrossRef]

123. Zhang, G.; Assadi, A.H.; McNeil, R.S.; Beffert, U.; Wynshaw-Boris, A.; Herz, J.; Clark, G.D.; D'Arcangelo, G. The Pafah1b complex interacts with the Reelin receptor VLDLR. *PLoS ONE* **2007**, *2*, e252. [CrossRef]

124. Enevoldson, T.P.; Sanders, M.D.; Harding, A.E. Autosomal dominant cerebellar ataxia with pigmentary macular dystrophy. A clinical and genetic study of eight families. *Brain* **1994**, *117*, 445–460. [CrossRef]

125. McCullough, S.D.; Xu, X.; Dent, S.Y.; Bekiranov, S.; Roeder, R.G.; Grant, P.A. Reelin is a target of polyglutamine expanded ataxin-7 in human spinocerebellar ataxia type 7 (SCA7) astrocytes. *Proc. Natl. Acad. Sci. USA* **2012**, *109*, 21319–21324. [CrossRef] [PubMed]

126. Lammert, D.B.; Howell, B.W. RELN Mutations in Autism Spectrum Disorder. *Front. Cell Neurosci.* **2016**, *10*, 84. [CrossRef] [PubMed]

127. Persico, A.M.; D'Agruma, L.; Maiorano, N.; Totaro, A.; Militerni, R.; Bravaccio, C.; Wassink, T.H.; Schneider, C.; Melmed, R.; Trillo, S.; et al. Reelin gene alleles and haplotypes as a factor predisposing to autistic disorder. *Mol. Psychiatry* **2001**, *6*, 150–159. [CrossRef] [PubMed]

128. Zhang, H.; Liu, X.; Zhang, C.; Mundo, E.; Macciardi, F.; Grayson, D.R.; Guidotti, A.R.; Holden, J.J.A. Reelin gene alleles and susceptibility to autism spectrum disorders. *Mol. Psychiatry* **2002**, *7*, 1012–1017. [CrossRef] [PubMed]

129. Holt, R.; Barnby, G.; Maestrini, E.; Bacchelli, E.; Brocklebank, D.; Sousa, I.S.; Mulder, E.J.; Kantojärvi, K.; Järvelä, I.; Klauck, S.M.; et al. Linkage and candidate gene studies of autism spectrum disorders in European populations. *Eur. J. Hum. Genet.* **2010**, *18*, 1013–1019. [CrossRef] [PubMed]

130. Devlin, B.; Bennett, P.; Dawson, G.; Figlewicz, D.A.; Grigorenko, E.L.; McMahon, W.; Minshew, N.; Pauls, D.; Smith, M.; Spence, M.A.; et al. Alleles of a reelin CGG repeat do not convey liability to autism in a sample from the CPEA network. *Am. J. Med. Genet.* **2004**, *126*, 46–50. [CrossRef]

131. Bonora, E.; Beyer, K.S.; Lamb, J.A.; Parr, J.R.; Klauck, S.M.; Benner, A.; Paolucci, M.; Abbott, A.; Ragoussis, I.; Poustka, A.; et al. Analysis of reelin as a candidate gene for autism. *Mol. Psychiatry* **2003**, *8*, 885–892. [CrossRef]

132. Wang, Z.; Hong, Y.; Zou, L.; Zhong, R.; Zhu, B.; Shen, N.; Chen, W.; Lou, J.; Ke, J.; Zhang, T.; et al. Reelin gene variants and risk of autism spectrum disorders: An integrated meta-analysis. *Am. J. Med. Genet.* **2014**, *165*, 192–200. [CrossRef]

133. Parihar, R.; Ganesh, S. Autism genes: The continuum that connects us all. *J. Genet.* **2016**, *95*, 481–483. [CrossRef]

134. De Rubeis, S.; He, X.; Goldberg, A.P.; Poultney, C.S.; Samocha, K.; Ercument Cicek, A.; Kou, Y.; Liu, L.; Fromer, M.; Walker, S.; et al. Synaptic, transcriptional and chromatin genes disrupted in autism. *Nature* **2014**, *515*, 209–215. [CrossRef]

135. Neale, B.M.; Kou, Y.; Liu, L.; Ma'ayan, A.; Samocha, K.E.; Sabo, A.; Lin, C.F.; Stevens, C.; Wang, L.S.; Makarov, V.; et al. Patterns and rates of exonic de novo mutations in autism spectrum disorders. *Nature* **2012**, *485*, 242–245. [CrossRef] [PubMed]

136. Iossifov, I.; O'Roak, B.J.; Sanders, S.J.; Ronemus, M.; Krumm, N.; Levy, D.; Stessman, H.A.; Witherspoon, K.T.; Vives, L.; Patterson, K.E.; et al. The contribution of de novo coding mutations to autism spectrum disorder. *Nature* **2014**, *515*, 216–221. [CrossRef] [PubMed]

137. Gaugler, T.; Klei, L.; Sanders, S.J.; Bodea, C.A.; Goldberg, A.P.; Lee, A.B.; Mahajan, M.; Manaa, D.; Pawitan, Y.; Reichert, J.; et al. Most genetic risk for autism resides with common variation. *Nat. Genet.* **2014**, *46*, 881–885. [CrossRef] [PubMed]

138. Fatemi, S.H. Reelin mutations in mouse and man: From reeler mouse to schizophrenia, mood disorders, autism and lissencephaly. *Mol. Psychiatry* **2001**, *6*, 129–133. [CrossRef]

139. Ecker, C. The neuroanatomy of autism spectrum disorder: An overview of structural neuroimaging findings and their translatability to the clinical setting. *Autism* **2017**, *21*, 18–28. [CrossRef]

140. Lange, N.; Travers, B.G.; Bigler, E.D.; Prigge, M.B.; Froehlich, A.L.; Nielsen, J.A.; Cariello, A.N.; Zielinski, B.A.; Anderson, J.S.; Fletcher, P.T.; et al. Longitudinal volumetric brain changes in autism spectrum disorder ages 6–35 years. *Autism Res.* **2015**, *8*, 82–93. [CrossRef]

141. Shen, M.D.; Nordahl, C.W.; Young, G.S.; Wootton-Gorges, S.L.; Lee, A.; Liston, S.E.; Harrington, K.R.; Ozonoff, S.; Amaral, D.G. Early brain enlargement and elevated extra-axial fluid in infants who develop autism spectrum disorder. *Brain* **2013**, *136*, 2825–2835. [CrossRef]

142. Schumann, C.M.; Bloss, C.S.; Barnes, C.C.; Wideman, G.M.; Carper, R.A.; Akshoomoff, N.; Pierce, K.; Hagler, D.; Schork, N.; Lord, C.; et al. Longitudinal magnetic resonance imaging study of cortical development through early childhood in autism. *J. Neurosci.* **2010**, *30*, 4419–4427. [CrossRef]

143. Hazlett, H.C.; Poe, M.D.; Gerig, G.; Styner, M.; Chappell, C.; Smith, R.G.; Vachet, C.; Piven, J. Early brain overgrowth in autism associated with an increase in cortical surface area before age 2 years. *Arch. Gen. Psychiatry* **2011**, *68*, 467–476. [CrossRef]

144. Minshew, N.J.; Sweeney, J.A.; Bauman, M.L.; Webb, S.J. Neurologic aspects of autism. In *Handbook of Autism and Pervasive Developmental Disorders*; Volkmar, F.R., Paul, R., Klin, A., Cohen, D., Eds.; John Wiley & Sons, Inc.: Hoboken, NJ, USA, 2005; pp. 473–514. [CrossRef]

145. Courchesne, E.; Yeung-Courchesne, R.; Hesselink, J.R.; Jernigan, T.L. Hypoplasia of cerebellar vermal lobules VI and VII in autism. *N. Engl. J. Med.* **1988**, *318*, 1349–1354. [CrossRef]

146. Courchesne, E.; Saitoh, O.; Townsend, J.; Yeung-Courchesne, R.; Press, G.; Lincoln, A.; Haas, R.; Schreibman, L. Cerebellar hypoplasia and hyperplasia in infantile autism. *Lancet* **1994**, *343*, 63–64. [CrossRef]

147. Scott, J.A.; Schumann, C.M.; Goodlin-Jones, B.L.; Amaral, D.G. A comprehensive volumetric analysis of the cerebellum in children and adolescents with autism spectrum disorder. *Autism Res.* **2009**, *2*, 246–257. [CrossRef] [PubMed]

148. Piven, J.; Saliba, K.; Bailey, J.; Arndt, S. An MRI study of autism: The cerebellum revisited. *Neurology* **1997**, *49*, 546–551. [CrossRef] [PubMed]

149. Lucibello, S.; Verdolotti, T.; Giordano, F.M.; Lapenta, L.; Infante, A.; Piludu, F.; Tartaglione, T.; Chieffo, D.; Colosimo, C.; Mercuri, E.; et al. Brain morphometry of preschool age children affected by autism spectrum disorder: Correlation with clinical findings. *Clin. Anat.* **2019**, *32*, 143–150. [CrossRef] [PubMed]

150. Oguro-Ando, A.; Zuko, A.; Kleijer, K.T.E.; Burbach, J.P.H. A current view on contactin-4,-5, and-6: Implications in neurodevelopmental disorders. *Mol. Cell. Neurosci.* **2017**, *81*, 72–83. [CrossRef] [PubMed]

151. Kemper, T.L.; Bauman, M.L. The contribution of neuropathologic studies to the understanding of autism. *Neurol. Clin.* **1993**, *11*, 175–187. [CrossRef]

152. Amaral, D.G.; Schumann, C.M.; Nordahl, C.W. Neuroanatomy of autism. *Trends Neurosci.* **2008**, *31*, 137–145. [CrossRef]

153. Varghese, M.; Keshav, N.; Jacot-Descombes, S.; Warda, T.; Wicinski, B.; Dickstein, D.L.; Harony-Nicolas, H.; De Rubeis, S.; Drapeau, E.; Buxbaum, J.D.; et al. Autism spectrum disorder: Neuropathology and animal models. *Acta Neuropathol.* **2017**, *134*, 537–566. [CrossRef]

154. Wegiel, J.; Kuchna, I.; Nowicki, K.; Imaki, H.; Wegiel, J.; Marchi, E.; Ma, S.Y.; Chauhan, A.; Chauhan, V.; Bobrowicz, T.W.; et al. The neuropathology of autism: Defects of neurogenesis and neuronal migration, and dysplastic changes. *Acta Neuropathol.* **2010**, *119*, 755–770. [CrossRef]

155. Wegiel, J.; Flory, M.; Kuchna, I.; Nowicki, K.; Ma, S.Y.; Imaki, H.; Wegiel, J.; Frackowiak, J.; Kolecka, B.M.; Wierzba-Bobrowicz, T.; et al. Neuronal nucleus and cytoplasm volume deficit in children with autism and volume increase in adolescents and adults. *Acta Neuropathol. Commun.* **2015**, *3*, 2. [CrossRef]

156. Casanova, M.F. Neuropathological and genetic findings in autism: The significance of a putative minicolumnopathy. *Neuroscientist* **2006**, *12*, 435–441. [CrossRef] [PubMed]

157. Mukaetova-Ladinska, E.B.; Arnold, H.; Jaros, E.; Perry, R.; Perry, E. Depletion of MAP2 expression and laminar cytoarchitectonic changes in dorsolateral prefrontal cortex in adult autistic individuals. *Neuropathol. Appl. Neurobiol.* **2004**, *30*, 615–623. [CrossRef] [PubMed]

158. Raymond, G.V.; Bauman, M.L.; Kemper, T.L. Hippocampus in autism: A Golgi analysis. *Acta Neuropathol.* **1996**, *91*, 117–119. [CrossRef] [PubMed]

159. Hutsler, J.J.; Zhang, H. Increased dendritic spine densities on cortical projection neurons in autism spectrum disorders. *Brain Res.* **2010**, *1309*, 83–94. [CrossRef] [PubMed]

160. Camacho, J.; Ejaz, E.; Ariza, J.; Noctor, S.C.; Martínez-Cerdeño, V.N. RELN-expressing neuron density in layer I of the superior temporal lobe is similar in human brains with autism and in age-matched controls. *Neurosci. Lett.* **2014**, *579*, 163–167. [CrossRef]

161. Courchesne, E.; Mouton, P.R.; Calhoun, M.E.; Semendeferi, K.; Ahrens-Barbeau, C.; Hallet, M.J.; Barnes, C.C.; Pierce, K. Neuron number and size in prefrontal cortex of children with autism. *JAMA* **2011**, *306*, 2001–2010. [CrossRef]

162. Hashemi, E.; Ariza, J.; Rogers, H.; Noctor, S.C.; Martínez-Cerdeño, V.N. The number of parvalbumin-expressing interneurons is decreased in the prefrontal cortex in autism. *Cereb. Cortex* **2017**, *27*, 1931–1943.

163. Jacot-Descombes, S.; Uppal, N.; Wicinski, B.; Santos, M.; Schmeidler, J.; Giannakopoulos, P.; Heinsein, H.; Schmitz, C.; Hof, P.R. Decreased pyramidal neuron size in Brodmann areas 44 and 45 in patients with autism. *Acta Neuropathol.* **2012**, *124*, 67–79. [CrossRef]

164. Zhubi, A.; Chen, Y.; Guidotti, A.; Grayson, D.R. Epigenetic regulation of RELN and GAD1 in the frontal cortex (FC) of autism spectrum disorder (ASD) subjects. *Int. J. Dev. Neurosci.* **2017**, *62*, 63–72. [CrossRef]

165. Van Kooten, I.A.J.; Palmen, S.J.M.C.; Von Cappeln, P.; Steinbusch, H.W.M.; Korr, H.; Heinsen, H.; Hof, P.R.; Van Engeland, H.; Schmitz, C. Neurons in the fusiform gyrus are fewer and smaller in autism. *Brain* **2008**, *131*, 987–999. [CrossRef]

166. Oblak, A.L.; Rosene, D.L.; Kemper, T.L.; Bauman, M.L.; Blatt, G.J. Altered posterior cingulate cortical cyctoarchitecture, but normal density of neurons and interneurons in the posterior cingulate cortex and fusiform gyrus in autism. *Autism Res.* **2011**, *4*, 200–211. [CrossRef] [PubMed]

167. Kennedy, D.P.; Semendeferi, K.; Courchesne, E. No reduction of spindle neuron number in frontoinsular cortex in autism. *Brain Cogn.* **2007**, *64*, 124–129. [CrossRef] [PubMed]

168. Allman, J.M.; Watson, K.K.; Tetreault, N.A.; Hakeem, A.Y. Intuition and autism: A possible role for Von Economo neurons. *Trends Cogn. Sci.* **2005**, *9*, 367–373. [CrossRef] [PubMed]

169. Santos, M.; Uppal, N.; Butti, C.; Wicinski, B.; Schmeidler, J.; Giannakopoulos, P.; Heinsen, H.; Schmitz, C.; Hof, P.R. Von Economo neurons in autism: A stereologic study of the frontoinsular cortex in children. *Brain Res.* **2011**, *1380*, 206–217. [CrossRef] [PubMed]

170. Simms, M.L.; Kemper, T.L.; Timbie, C.M.; Bauman, M.L.; Blatt, G.J. The anterior cingulate cortex in autism: Heterogeneity of qualitative and quantitative cytoarchitectonic features suggests possible subgroups. *Acta Neuropathol.* **2009**, *118*, 673–684. [CrossRef] [PubMed]

171. Uppal, N.; Wicinski, B.; Buxbaum, J.D.; Heinsen, H.; Schmitz, C.; Hof, P.R. Neuropathology of the Anterior Midcingulate Cortex in Young Children with Autism. *J. Neuropathol. Exp. Neurol.* **2014**, *73*, 891–902. [CrossRef] [PubMed]

172. Weidenheim, K.M.; Goodman, L.; Dickson, D.W.; Gillberg, C.; Råstam, M.; Rapin, I. Etiology and Pathophysiology of Autistic Behavior: Clues from Two Cases with an Unusual Variant of Neuroaxonal Dystrophy. *J. Child Neurol.* **2001**, *16*, 809–819. [CrossRef]

173. Hussman, J.P.; Chung, R.H.; Griswold, A.J.; Jaworski, J.M.; Salyakina, D.; Ma, D.; Konidari, I.; Whitehead, P.L.; Vance, J.M.; Martin, E.R.; et al. A noise-reduction GWAS analysis implicates altered regulation of neurite outgrowth and guidance in autism. *Mol. Autism* **2011**, *2*, 1. [CrossRef]

174. Ichinohe, N.; Knight, A.; Ogawa, M.; Ohshima, T.; Mikoshiba, K.; Yoshihara, Y.; Terashima, T.; Rockland, K.S. Unusual Patch–Matrix Organization in the Retrosplenial Cortex of the Reeler Mouse and *Shaking Rat Kawasaki*. *Cereb. Cortex* **2007**, *18*, 1125–1138. [CrossRef]

175. Ichinohe, N. Small-Scale Module of the Rat Granular retrosplenial cortex: An example of the minicolumn-like structure of the cerebral cortex. *Front. Neuroanat.* **2012**, *5*, 69. [CrossRef]

176. Lui, J.; Hansen, D.; Kriegstein, A. Development and Evolution of the Human Neocortex. *Cell* **2011**, *146*, 18–36. [CrossRef] [PubMed]

177. Romano, E.; Fuso, A.; Laviola, G. Nicotine restores Wt-like levels of reelin and GAD67 gene expression in brain of heterozygous reeler mice. *Neurotox. Res.* **2013**, *24*, 205–215. [CrossRef] [PubMed]

178. Bailey, A.; Luthert, P.; Dean, A.; Harding, B.; Janota, I.; Montgomery, M.; Rutter, M.; Lantos, P. A clinicopathological study of autism. *Brain* **1998**, *121*, 889–905. [CrossRef] [PubMed]

179. Lawrence, Y.A.; Kemper, T.L.; Bauman, M.L.; Blatt, G.J. Parvalbumin-, calbindin-, and calretinin-immunoreactive hippocampal interneuron density in autism. *Acta Neurol. Scand.* **2010**, *121*, 99–108. [CrossRef] [PubMed]

180. Rogers, J.T.; Zhao, L.; Trotter, J.H.; Rusiana, I.; Peters, M.M.; Li, Q.; Donaldson, E.; Banko, J.L.; Keenoy, K.E.; Rebeck, G.W.; et al. Reelin supplementation recovers sensorimotor gating, synaptic plasticity and associative learning deficits in the heterozygous reeler mouse. *J. Psychopharmacol.* **2013**, *27*, 386–395. [CrossRef]

181. Qiu, S.; Zhao, L.F.; Korwek, K.M.; Weeber, E.J. Differential Reelin-Induced Enhancement of NMDA and AMPA Receptor Activity in the Adult Hippocampus. *J. Neurosci.* **2006**, *26*, 12943. [CrossRef]

182. Qiu, S.; Korwek, K.M.; Pratt-Davis, A.R.; Peters, M.; Bergman, M.Y.; Weeber, E.J. Cognitive disruption and altered hippocampus synaptic function in Reelin haploinsufficient mice. *Neurobiol. Learn. Mem.* **2006**, *85*, 228–242. [CrossRef]

183. Hellwig, S.; Hack, I.; Kowalski, J.; Brunne, B.; Jarowyj, J.; Unger, A.; Bock, H.H.; Junghans, D.; Frotscher, M. Role for Reelin in neurotransmitter release. *J. Neurosci.* **2011**, *31*, 2352–2360. [CrossRef]

184. Bauman, M.; Kemper, T.L. Histoanatomic observations of the brain in early infantile autism. *Neurology* **1985**, *35*, 866–874. [CrossRef]

185. Schumann, C.M.; Amaral, D.G. Stereological Analysis of Amygdala Neuron Number in Autism. *J. Neurosci.* **2006**, *26*, 7674–7679. [CrossRef]

186. Wegiel, J.; Flory, M.; Kuchna, I.; Nowicki, K.; Ma, S.Y.; Imaki, H.; Wegiel, J.; Cohen, I.L.; London, E.; Wisniewski, T.; et al. Stereological study of the neuronal number and volume of 38 brain subdivisions of subjects diagnosed with autism reveals significant alterations restricted to the striatum, amygdala and cerebellum. *Acta Neuropathol. Commun.* **2014**, *2*, 141. [CrossRef] [PubMed]

187. Morgan, J.T.; Barger, N.; Amaral, D.G.; Schumann, C.M. Stereological study of amygdala glial populations in adolescents and adults with autism spectrum disorder. *PLoS ONE* **2014**, *9*, e110356. [CrossRef] [PubMed]

188. Boyle, M.P.; Bernard, A.; Thompson, C.L.; Ng, L.; Boe, A.; Mortrud, M.; Hawrylycz, M.J.; Jones, A.R.; Hevner, R.F.; Lein, E.S. Cell-type-specific consequences of reelin deficiency in the mouse neocortex, hippocampus, and amygdala. *J. Comp. Neurol.* **2011**, *519*, 2061–2089. [CrossRef] [PubMed]

189. Fatemi, S.H.; Aldinger, K.A.; Ashwood, P.; Bauman, M.L.; Blaha, C.D.; Blatt, G.J.; Chauhan, A.; Chauhan, V.; Dager, S.R.; Dickson, P.E.; et al. Consensus paper: Pathological role of the cerebellum in autism. *Cerebellum* **2012**, *11*, 777–807. [CrossRef] [PubMed]

190. D'Mello, A.M.; Crocetti, D.; Mostofsky, S.H.; Stoodley, C.J. Cerebellar gray matter and lobular volumes correlate with core autism symptoms. *Neuroimage Clin.* **2015**, *7*, 631–639. [CrossRef]

191. Hampson, D.R.; Blatt, G.J. Autism spectrum disorders and neuropathology of the cerebellum. *Front. Neurosci.* **2015**, *9*, 420. [CrossRef] [PubMed]

192. Skefos, J.; Cummings, C.; Enzer, K.; Holiday, J.; Weed, K.; Levy, E.; Yuce, T.; Kemper, T.; Bauman, M. Regional alterations in purkinje cell density in patients with autism. *PLoS ONE* **2014**, *9*, e81255. [CrossRef]

193. Fatemi, S.H.; Halt, A.R.; Realmuto, G.; Earle, J.; Kist, D.A.; Thuras, P.; Merz, A. Purkinje cell size is reduced in cerebellum of patients with autism. *Cell. Mol. Neurobiol.* **2002**, *22*, 171–175. [CrossRef]

194. Wegiel, J.; Kuchna, I.; Nowicki, K.; Imaki, H.; Wegiel, J.; Ma, S.Y.; Azmitia, E.C.; Banerjee, P.; Flory, M.; Cohen, I.L.; et al. Contribution of olivofloccular circuitry developmental defects to atypical gaze in autism. *Brain Res.* **2013**, *1512*, 106–122. [CrossRef]

195. Whitney, E.R.; Kemper, T.L.; Rosene, D.L.; Bauman, M.L.; Blatt, G.J. Density of cerebellar basket and stellate cells in autism: Evidence for a late developmental loss of Purkinje cells. *J. Neurosci. Res.* **2009**, *87*, 2245–2254. [CrossRef]

196. Maloku, E.; Covelo, I.R.; Hanbauer, I.; Guidotti, A.; Kadriu, B.; Hu, Q.; Davis, J.M.; Costa, E. Lower number of cerebellar Purkinje neurons in psychosis is associated with reduced reelin expression. *Proc. Natl. Acad. Sci. USA* **2010**, *107*, 4407–4411. [CrossRef] [PubMed]

197. Magliaro, C.; Cocito, C.; Bagatella, S.; Merighi, A.; Ahluwalia, A.; Lossi, L. The number of Purkinje neurons and their topology in the cerebellar vermis of normal and reln haplodeficient mouse. *Ann. Anat.* **2016**, *207*, 68–75. [CrossRef] [PubMed]

198. Keller, R.; Basta, R.; Salerno, L.; Elia, M. Autism, epilepsy, and synaptopathies: A not rare association. *Neurol. Sci.* **2017**, *38*, 1353–1361. [CrossRef] [PubMed]

199. Mercati, O.; Huguet, G.; Danckaert, A.; André-Leroux, G.; Maruani, A.; Bellinzoni, M.; Rolland, T.; Gouder, L.; Mathieu, A.; Buratti, J.; et al. CNTN6 mutations are risk factors for abnormal auditory sensory perception in autism spectrum disorders. *Mol. Psychiatry* **2016**, *22*, 625–633. [CrossRef] [PubMed]

200. Castagna, C.; Merighi, A.; Lossi, L. Decreased expression of synaptophysin 1 (SYP1 major synaptic vesicle protein p38) and contactin 6 (CNTN6/NB3) in the cerebellar vermis of reln haplodeficient mice. *Cell. Mol. Neurobiol.* **2019**, *39*, 833–856. [CrossRef] [PubMed]

201. Sundberg, M.; Tochitsky, I.; Buchholz, D.E.; Winden, K.; Kujala, V.; Kapur, K.; Cataltepe, D.; Turner, D.; Han, M.J.; Woolf, C.J.; et al. Purkinje cells derived from TSC patients display hypoexcitability and synaptic deficits associated with reduced FMRP levels and reversed by rapamycin. *Mol. Psychiatry* **2018**, *23*, 2167–2183. [CrossRef]

202. Tassano, E.; Uccella, S.; Giacomini, T.; Severino, M.; Fiorio, P.; Gimelli, G.; Ronchetto, P. Clinical and molecular characterization of two patients with CNTN6 copy number variations. *Cytogenet. Genome Res.* **2018**, *156*, 144–149. [CrossRef]

203. Garcia-Ortiz, J.E.; Zarazúa-Niño, A.I.; Hernández-Orozco, A.A.; Reyes-Oliva, E.A.; Pérez-Ávila, C.E.; Becerra-Solano, L.E.; Galán-Huerta, K.A.; Rivas-Estilla, A.M.; Córdova-Fletes, C. Case Report: Whole exome sequencing unveils an inherited truncating variant in CNTN6 (p. Ser189Ter) in a mexican child with autism spectrum disorder. *J. Autism Dev. Disord.* **2019**. [CrossRef]

204. Hu, J.; Liao, J.; Sathanoori, M.; Kochmar, S.; Sebastian, J.; Yatsenko, S.A.; Surti, U. CNTN6 copy number variations in 14 patients: A possible candidate gene for neurodevelopmental and neuropsychiatric disorders. *J. Neurodev. Disord.* **2015**, *7*, 26. [CrossRef]

205. Stoodley, C.J.; Schmahmann, J.D. Evidence for topographic organization in the cerebellum of motor control versus cognitive and affective processing. *Cortex* **2010**, *46*, 831–844. [CrossRef]

206. Schmahmann, J.D.; Weilburg, J.B.; Sherman, J.C. The neuropsychiatry of the cerebellum—insights from the clinic. *Cerebellum* **2007**, *6*, 254–267. [CrossRef] [PubMed]

207. Catani, M.; Jones, D.K.; Daly, E.; Embiricos, N.; Deeley, Q.; Pugliese, L.; Curran, S.; Robertson, D.; Murphy, D.G. Altered cerebellar feedback projections in Asperger syndrome. *Neuroimage* **2008**, *41*, 1184–1191. [CrossRef] [PubMed]

208. Catani, M.; Dell'Acqua, F.; de Schotten, M.T. A revised limbic system model for memory, emotion and behaviour. *Neurosci. Biobehav. Rev.* **2013**, *37*, 1724–1737. [CrossRef] [PubMed]

209. Bauman, M.L. Microscopic neuroanatomic abnormalities in autism. *Pediatrics* **1991**, *87*, 791–796.

210. Stanfield, A.C.; McIntosh, A.M.; Spencer, M.D.; Philip, R.; Gaur, S.; Lawrie, S.M. Towards a neuroanatomy of autism: A systematic review and meta-analysis of structural magnetic resonance imaging studies. *Eur. Psychiatry* **2008**, *23*, 289–299. [CrossRef]

211. Limperopoulos, C.; Bassan, H.; Gauvreau, K.; Robertson, R.L., Jr.; Sullivan, N.R.; Benson, C.B.; Avery, L.; Stewart, J.; Soul, J.S.; Ringer, S.A.; et al. Does cerebellar injury in premature infants contribute to the high prevalence of long-term cognitive, learning, and behavioral disability in survivors? *Pediatrics* **2007**, *120*, 584–593. [CrossRef]

212. D'Mello, A.M.; Stoodley, C.J. Cerebro-cerebellar circuits in autism spectrum disorder. *Front. Neurosci.* **2015**, *9*, 408. [CrossRef]

213. Stoodley, C.J. Distinct regions of the cerebellum show gray matter decreases in autism, ADHD, and developmental dyslexia. *Front. Syst. Neurosci.* **2014**, *8*, 92. [CrossRef]

214. Insel, T.R. Rethinking schizophrenia. *Nature* **2010**, *468*, 187–193. [CrossRef]

215. Van, L.; Boot, E.; Bassett, A.S. Update on the 22q11.2 deletion syndrome and its relevance to schizophrenia. *Curr. Opin. Psychiatry* **2017**, *30*, 191–196. [CrossRef]

216. Ishii, K.; Kubo, K.I.; Nakajima, K. Reelin and Neuropsychiatric Disorders. *Front. Cell. Neurosci.* **2016**, *10*, 229. [CrossRef] [PubMed]

217. Luo, X.; Chen, S.; Xue, L.; Chen, J.H.; Shi, Y.W.; Zhao, H. SNP variation of RELN gene and schizophrenia in a chinese population: A hospital-based case-control study. *Front. Genet.* **2019**, *10*, 175. [CrossRef] [PubMed]

218. Tost, H.; Weinberger, D.R. RELN rs7341475 and schizophrenia risk: Confusing, yet somehow intriguing. *Biol. Psychiatry* **2011**, *69*, e19. [CrossRef] [PubMed]

219. Weinberger, D.R. Future of Days Past: Neurodevelopment and Schizophrenia. *Schizophr. Bull.* **2017**, *43*, 1164–1168. [CrossRef]

220. Dietsche, B.; Kircher, T.; Falkenberg, I. Structural brain changes in schizophrenia at different stages of the illness: A selective review of longitudinal magnetic resonance imaging studies. *Aust. N. Z. J. Psychiatry* **2017**, *51*, 500–508. [CrossRef]

221. Kahn, R.S.; Sommer, I.E.; Murray, R.M.; Meyer-Lindenberg, A.; Weinberger, D.R.; Cannon, T.D.; O'Donovan, M.; Correll, C.U.; Kane, J.M.; Van Os, J.; et al. Schizophrenia. *Nat. Rev. Dis. Primers* **2015**, *1*, 15067. [CrossRef]

222. Bakhshi, K.; Chance, S.A. The neuropathology of schizophrenia: A selective review of past studies and emerging themes in brain structure and cytoarchitecture. *Neuroscience* **2015**, *303*, 82–102. [CrossRef]

223. Hoistad, M.; Heinsen, H.; Wicinski, B.; Schmitz, C.; Hof, P.R. Stereological assessment of the dorsal anterior cingulate cortex in schizophrenia: Absence of changes in neuronal and glial densities. *Neuropathol. Appl. Neurobiol.* **2013**, *39*, 348–361. [CrossRef]

224. Guidotti, A.; Auta, J.; Davis, J.M.; Di-Giorgi-Gerevini, V.; Dwivedi, Y.; Grayson, D.R.; Impagnatiello, F.; Pandey, G.; Pesold, C.; Sharma, R.; et al. Decrease in reelin and glutamic acid decarboxylase67 (GAD67) expression in schizophrenia and bipolar disorder: A postmortem brain study. *Arch. Gen. Psychiatry* **2000**, *57*, 1061–1069. [CrossRef]

225. Dienel, S.J.; Lewis, D.A. Alterations in cortical interneurons and cognitive function in schizophrenia. *Neurobiol. Dis.* **2019**, *131*, 104208. [CrossRef]

226. Curley, A.A.; Lewis, D.A. Cortical basket cell dysfunction in schizophrenia. *J. Physiol.* **2012**, *590*, 715–724. [CrossRef] [PubMed]

227. Lewis, D.A.; Curley, A.A.; Glausier, J.R.; Volk, D.W. Cortical parvalbumin interneurons and cognitive dysfunction in schizophrenia. *Trends Neurosci.* **2012**, *35*, 57–67. [CrossRef] [PubMed]

228. Ruzicka, W.B.; Zhubi, A.; Veldic, M.; Grayson, D.R.; Costa, E.; Guidotti, A. Selective epigenetic alteration of layer I GABAergic neurons isolated from prefrontal cortex of schizophrenia patients using laser-assisted microdissection. *Mol. Psychiatry* **2007**, *12*, 385–397. [CrossRef] [PubMed]

229. Lewis, D.A. The chandelier neuron in schizophrenia. *Dev. Neurobiol.* **2011**, *71*, 118–127. [CrossRef] [PubMed]

230. Glausier, J.R.; Lewis, D.A. Dendritic spine pathology in schizophrenia. *Neuroscience* **2013**, *251*, 90–107. [CrossRef]

231. MacDonald, M.L.; Alhassan, J.; Newman, J.T.; Richard, M.; Gu, H.; Kelly, R.M.; Sampson, A.R.; Fish, K.N.; Penzes, P.; Wills, Z.P.; et al. Selective loss of smaller spines in schizophrenia. *AJP* **2017**, *174*, 586–594. [CrossRef]

232. Matrisciano, F.; Tueting, P.; Dalal, I.; Kadriu, B.; Grayson, D.R.; Davis, J.M.; Nicoletti, F.; Guidotti, A. Epigenetic modifications of GABAergic interneurons are associated with the schizophrenia-like phenotype induced by prenatal stress in mice. *Neuropharmacology* **2013**, *68*, 184–194. [CrossRef]

233. Guidotti, A.; Grayson, D.R.; Caruncho, H.J. Epigenetic RELN dysfunction in schizophrenia and related neuropsychiatric disorders. *Front. Cell. Neurosci.* **2016**, *10*, 89. [CrossRef]

234. Gothelf, D.; Soreni, N.; Nachman, R.P.; Tyano, S.; Hiss, Y.; Reiner, O.; Weizman, A. Evidence for the involvement of the hippocampus in the pathophysiology of schizophrenia. *Eur. Neuropsychopharmacol.* **2000**, *10*, 389–395. [CrossRef]

235. Konradi, C.; Yang, C.K.; Zimmerman, E.I.; Lohmann, K.M.; Gresch, P.; Pantazopoulos, H.; Berretta, S.; Heckers, S. Hippocampal interneurons are abnormal in schizophrenia. *Schizophr. Res.* **2011**, *131*, 165–173. [CrossRef]

236. Mavroudis, I.A.; Petrides, F.; Manani, M.; Chatzinikolaou, F.; Ciobica, A.S.; Padurariu, M.; Kazis, D.; Njau, S.N.; Costa, V.G.; Baloyannis, S.J. Purkinje cells pathology in schizophrenia. A morphometric approach. *Rom. J. Morphol. Embryol.* **2017**, *58*, 419–424. [PubMed]

237. Eastwood, S.L.; Cotter, D.; Harrison, P.J. Cerebellar synaptic protein expression in schizophrenia. *Neuroscience* **2001**, *105*, 219–229. [CrossRef]

238. Bey, A.L.; Jiang, Y.H. Overview of mouse models of autism spectrum disorders. *Curr. Protoc. Pharmacol.* **2014**, *66*, 5–26. [PubMed]

239. Tueting, P.; Costa, E.; Dwivedi, Y.; Guidotti, A.; Impagnatiello, F.; Manev, R.; Pesold, C. The phenotypic characteristics of heterozygous reeler mouse. *Neuroreport* **1999**, *10*, 1329–1334. [CrossRef]

240. Brigman, J.L.; Padukiewicz, K.E.; Sutherland, M.L.; Rothblat, L.A. Executive functions in the heterozygous reeler mouse model of schizophrenia. *Behav. Neurosci.* **2006**, *120*, 984–988. [CrossRef]

241. Ognibene, E.; Adriani, W.; Macri, S.; Laviola, G. Neurobehavioural disorders in the infant reeler mouse model: Interaction of genetic vulnerability and consequences of maternal separation. *Behav. Brain Res.* **2007**, *177*, 142–149. [CrossRef]

242. Ognibene, E.; Adriani, W.; Granstrem, O.; Pieretti, S.; Laviola, G. Impulsivity–anxiety-related behavior and profiles of morphine-induced analgesia in heterozygous reeler mice. *Brain Res.* **2007**, *1131*, 173–180. [CrossRef]

243. Barr, A.M.; Fish, K.N.; Markou, A.; Honer, W.G. Heterozygous reeler mice exhibit alterations in sensorimotor gating but not presynaptic proteins. *Eur. J. Neurosci.* **2008**, *27*, 2568–2574. [CrossRef]

244. Salinger, W.L.; Ladrow, P.; Wheeler, C. Behavioral phenotype of the reeler mutant mouse: Effects of RELN gene dosage and social isolation. *Behav. Neurosci.* **2003**, *117*, 1257–1275. [CrossRef]

245. Podhorna, J.; Didriksen, M. The heterozygous reeler mouse: Behavioural phenotype. *Behav. Brain Res.* **2004**, *153*, 43–54. [CrossRef]

246. Krueger, D.D.; Howell, J.L.; Hebert, B.F.; Olausson, P.; Taylor, J.R.; Nairn, A.C. Assessment of cognitive function in the heterozygous reeler mouse. *Psychopharmacology* **2006**, *189*, 95–104. [CrossRef] [PubMed]

247. Michetti, C.; Romano, E.; Altabella, L.; Caruso, A.; Castelluccio, P.; Bedse, G.; Gaetani, S.; Canese, R.; Laviola, G.; Scattoni, M.L. Mapping pathological phenotypes in reelin mutant mice. *Front. Pediatr.* **2014**, *2*, 95. [CrossRef] [PubMed]

248. Teixeira, C.M.; Martín, E.D.; Sahún, I.; Masachs, N.; Pujadas, L.; Corvelo, A.; Bosch, C.; Rossi, D.; Martinez, A.; Maldonado, R.; et al. Overexpression of Reelin Prevents the Manifestation of Behavioral Phenotypes Related to Schizophrenia and Bipolar Disorder. *Neuropsychopharmacology* **2011**, *36*, 2395–2405. [CrossRef] [PubMed]

249. Romano, E.; Michetti, C.; Caruso, A.; Laviola, G.; Scattoni, M.L. Characterization of neonatal vocal and motor repertoire of reelin mutant mice. *PLoS ONE* **2013**, *8*, e64407. [CrossRef] [PubMed]

250. Ottman, R.; Risch, N.; Hauser, W.A.; Pedley, T.A.; Lee, J.H.; Barker-Cummings, C.; Lustenberger, A.; Nagle, K.J.; Lee, K.S.; Scheuer, M.L.; et al. Localization of a gene for partial epilepsy to chromosome 10q. *Nat. Genet.* **1995**, *10*, 56–60. [CrossRef] [PubMed]

251. Michelucci, R.; Pasini, E.; Nobile, C. Lateral temporal lobe epilepsies: Clinical and genetic features. *Epilepsia* **2009**, *50*, 52–54. [CrossRef] [PubMed]

252. Boycott, K.M.; Flavelle, S.; Bureau, A.; Glass, H.C.; Fujiwara, T.M.; Wirrell, E.; Davey, K.; Chudley, A.E.; Scott, J.N.; McLeod, D.R.; et al. Homozygous deletion of the very low density lipoprotein receptor gene causes autosomal recessive cerebellar hypoplasia with cerebral gyral simplification. *Am. J. Hum. Genet.* **2005**, *77*, 477–483. [CrossRef]

253. Garden, G. Spinocerebellar Ataxia Type 7. In *GeneReviews®*; Adam, M.P., Ardinger, H.H., Pagon, R.A., Wallace, S.E., Eds.; University of Washington: Seattle, WA, USA, 1993.

254. Lai, M.C.; Lombardo, M.V.; Baron-Cohen, S. Autism. *Lancet* **2014**, *383*, 896–910. [CrossRef]

255. Marino, M.J. The use and misuse of statistical methodologies in pharmacology research. *Biochem. Pharmacol.* **2014**, *87*, 78–92. [CrossRef]

256. Motulsky, H.J. Common misconceptions about data analysis and statistics. *Br. J. Pharmacol.* **2015**, *172*, 2126–2132. [CrossRef]

7

Small Cell Lung Cancer from Traditional to Innovative Therapeutics: Building a Comprehensive Network to Optimize Clinical and Translational Research

Shanmuga Subbiah, Arin Nam, Natasha Garg, Amita Behal, Prakash Kulkarni and Ravi Salgia *

Department of Medical Oncology and Therapeutics Research, City of Hope National Medical Center, Duarte, CA 91010, USA; ssubbiah@coh.org (S.S.); anam@coh.org (A.N.); ngarg@coh.org (N.G.); abehal@coh.org (A.B.); pkulkarni@coh.org (P.K.)
* Correspondence: rsalgia@coh.org

Abstract: Small cell lung cancer (SCLC) is an aggressive, complex disease with a distinct biology that contributes to its poor prognosis. Management of SCLC is still widely limited to chemotherapy and radiation therapy, and research recruitment still poses a considerable challenge. Here, we review the current standard of care for SCLC and advances made in utilizing immunotherapy. We also highlight research in the development of targeted therapies and emphasize the importance of a team-based approach to make clinical advances. Building an integrative network between an academic site and community practice sites optimizes biomarker and drug target discovery for managing and treating a difficult disease like SCLC.

Keywords: small cell lung cancer; translational research; immunotherapy; clinical trials; team medicine; community practice

1. Introduction

Lung cancer is the leading cause of cancer deaths in both men and women in the United States [1]. Small cell lung cancer (SCLC) is a subtype of lung cancer that has an incidence of 13% and is strongly associated with smoking [2,3]. A distinct biology, aggressive clinical course with distant metastasis, and poor survival outcomes characterize SCLC. The disease is classified into extensive stage and limited stage. While limited stage SCLC (LS-SCLC) is disease confined to one hemithorax that can be enclosed within a radiation field, extensive stage SCLC (ES-SCLC) is more prevalent (66%) and includes malignant pleural or pericardial effusions along with distant metastasis [4]. Despite the bleak prognosis, standard chemotherapies for patients with SCLC have not changed significantly in the last 30 years. However, recently, immunotherapy with checkpoint inhibitors have shown promising efficacy in advanced disease [5,6]. The lack of advances in SCLC therapies are partly due to disease complexity, research recruitment, and resource utilization. Thus, collaborative efforts between academic and community practices that combine knowledge, skills, experiences, and expertise of academicians, clinicians, and researchers, can accelerate advances in treatment and patient care. Academic centers are critical in the advancement of cancer treatment, but community hospital care plays an equally important and complementary role. Indeed, academic–community collaboration, or 'team medicine', has become an emerging culture to advance and shape clinical care.

In this article, we first highlight the current standard treatments in SCLC as well as recent advances in immunotherapies. We also review potential targeted therapies and underscore the importance of a team-based approach toward SCLC based on our experience at the City of Hope (COH).

2. Current Standard Therapies

2.1. Radiation Therapy

For LS-SCLC the standard of care is chemotherapy with concurrent radiation therapy [7]. Two meta-analyses established that concurrent cisplatin and etoposide treatment combined with radiation therapy improves survival compared to chemotherapy alone [8,9], although the dosage (once daily vs. twice daily) of radiation with chemotherapy remains equivocal. One study showed a significant survival advantage of patients who received 1.5 Gy in 30 fractions twice daily compared to 1.8 Gy in 25 fractions after a median follow-up of 8 years [10]. However, a more recent trial that randomized patients to receiving 1.5 Gy twice daily fractions (45 Gy dose) or 2 Gy once daily fractions (66 Gy dose) concurrently with platinum based chemotherapy showed that survival outcomes did not differ between the regimens, although the trial was not powered for equivalence [11]. The ongoing trial of CALGB 30,610 comparing 45 Gy twice daily to 70 Gy once daily (NCT00632853) is likely to shed more light on this issue.

2.2. Chemotherapy

Regardless of the stage, platinum with etoposide (EP) is the standard of care for patients with SCLC in the United States. Outside the United States, some patients are given platinum with irinotecan as an alternative treatment [12–14]. The overall response rates (ORR) range from 40–70% with up to 10% of the patients achieving complete radiographic response, and the median overall survival (OS) spans 7–12 months, with a two-year survival rate of less than 5% [15]. Eventually, however, most SCLC tumors become resistant to chemotherapy resulting in disease progression. For patients with disease relapse, topotecan as a single agent is the only approved second-line drug that has demonstrated increased survival compared to supportive care [16,17]. Nonetheless, the ORR of patients treated with topotecan is only about 5% [18] and even worse, in SCLC patients who develop disease recurrence within 3 months of the first-line platinum doublet chemotherapy, in which case topotecan is ineffective. Other chemotherapeutic agents such as gemcitabine, docetaxel, paclitaxel, temozolomide, irinotecan, and vinorelbine, may be used in certain cases based on limited clinical evidence [19–24]. Amrubicin is an anthracycline agent that has been developed more recently and approved only in Japan for second-line therapy [25]. Unfortunately, beyond second-line therapy, currently there are no standard guidelines of care although, newer immunotherapies appear promising in some patients.

2.3. Surgery

Compared to non-small cell lung cancer (NSCLC), SCLC is rarely treated surgically. However, over the years the fraction of SCLC patients treated surgically has increased considerably from 14.9% in 2004 to 28.5% in 2013. This is at least in part due to availability of better diagnostic tools in the form of positron emission tomography (PET) scans and increasing usage of low-dose computed tomography (CT) screening. Randomized trials reported in the late 1960s and early 1970s showed no survival advantage for surgery alone or in combination with radiation therapy compared with radiation therapy alone [26,27]. Subsequently, it was reported that chemotherapy given sequentially with radiation and then randomized to surgery vs. non-surgical group did not show any benefit to surgery [28]. However, recently there have been increasing numbers of retrospective studies showing survival benefit of surgery compared to non-surgical therapy [29–32]. For example, a meta-analysis published by Liu et al. [33], which included two randomized control trials described above and thirteen retrospective studies for a total of 41,483 patients, concluded that surgical resection significantly improved overall survival when compared to non-surgical treatment (hazard ratio (HR) = 0.56, $p < 0.001$) for retrospective studies, and in the two randomized trials there was no survival advantage to the surgical arm. This meta-analysis also showed that lobectomy was associated with superior OS compared with sub lobar resection (HR = 0.64, $p < 0.001$). Based on these data, the National Comprehensive Cancer Network (NCCN) also recommends surgery for T1-2N0M0 SCLC provided preoperative evaluation of mediastinal lymph nodes are done. Unfortunately, there are no ongoing randomized trials evaluating surgery in SCLC, since less than 5% of patients present with stage I SCLC. However, a collaborative engagement with community clinic sites where majority of cancer patients are seen and academic institutes similar to COH should help accrue enough patients to conduct a prospective trial.

3. Novel Therapies

Immunotherapy for SCLC was considered viable due to frequent somatic mutations as a result of smoking and the presence of paraneoplastic disorders [34–36]. Furthermore, in light of the remarkable success seen in NSCLC, parallel studies undertaken in SCLC have also shown considerable promise for immunotherapies that include antibodies against programmed cell death protein 1 (PD-1), programmed death-ligand 1 (PD-L1), and cytotoxic T-lymphocyte antigen 4 (CTLA4; Figure 1) [37,38] discussed below.

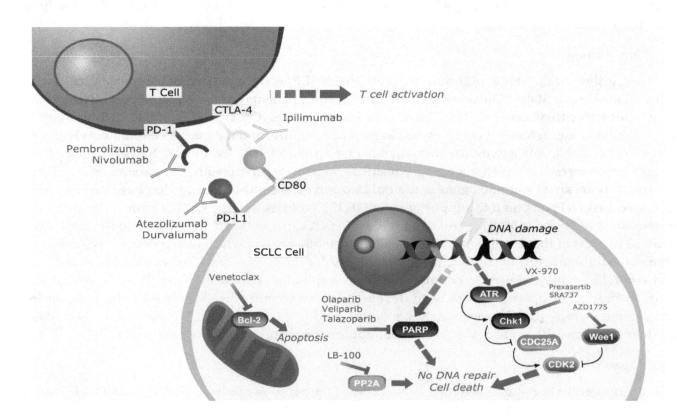

Figure 1. Current investigational immunotherapies and targeted therapies for small cell lung cancer SCLC.

3.1. Atezolizumab

In treatment-naïve ES-SCLC patients, a recently published a phase III trial involving 403 patients, IMpower-133, combining atezolizumab with carboplatin and etoposide (EP) demonstrated an improved progression-free survival (PFS) as well as overall survival (OS) [39]. More specifically, the patients who did not progress after 4 cycles of induction therapy, received atezolizumab or placebo as maintenance every 3 weeks until disease progression or intolerable toxicity. Median OS for those treated with atezolizumab was 12.3 months compared to 10.3 months for the placebo group, with a hazard ratio for death of 0.70. Median PFS was also improved in the atezolizumab group, which was 5.2 months vs. 4.3 months, with a hazard ratio for disease progression at 0.77, resulting in the approval of atezolizumab with EP for ES-SCLC in the first-line setting. However, blood-based tumor mutational burden (TMB) was not associated with clinical benefit in this study.

3.2. Durvalumab

Another phase III trial, the CASPIAN trial, which used durvalumab as the immunotherapy in combination with platinum with etoposide to treat treatment-naïve ES-SCLC patients, also showed improvement in OS compared to platinum-etoposide alone (13 months vs. 10.3 months, with a hazard ratio of 0.73) [40]. Based on these results, the Food and Drug Administration (FDA) also approved durvalumab for ES-SCLC.

3.3. Ipilimumab and Nivolumab

In contrast to atezolizumab or durvalumab, ipilimumab (an anti-cytotoxic T-lymphocyte-associated protein 4 (CTLA4) antibody) in combination with chemotherapy prolongs PFS, but does not improve OS in treatment-naïve ES-SCLC [41]. However, maintenance therapy in such patients with nivolumab/ipilimumab combination or nivolumab alone did not show improvement in OS, according to results from the phase III CheckMate 451 study presented at the recent European Lung Cancer Congress 2019 [42]. Another trial CheckMate 032 assessed nivolumab as a single agent or in combination with ipilimumab in previously treated SCLC and found that ORR with single agent nivolumab was 11% compared to 22% in the cohort with combination of nivolumab with ipilimumab. The median OS for nivolumab alone was 4.1 months, and for nivolumab with ipilimumab, it was 6 months to 7.8 months based on the doses received [43]. Because the long-term survival benefits with nivolumab alone demonstrated better outcomes compared to previous agents used in the third-line setting, nivolumab received FDA approval for third-line treatment of SCLC.

3.4. Pembrolizumab

Pembrolizumab was studied in relapsed SCLC patients in the KEYNOTE-028 and KEYNOTE-158 trials. In KEYNOTE-028, the study included only patients with PD-L1 combined positive score (CPS) ≥1%. Among 24 patients with relapsed SCLC, 12.5% were treated with pembrolizumab in the second-line setting and 50% in the third-line. ORR was 33%, median PFS was 1.9 months, one-year PFS was 23.8%, median OS was 9.7 months, and the one-year OS was 37.7% [44]. In the KEYNOTE-158 trial, 79% of 107 patients with relapsed SCLC were treated with pembrolizumab in the second-line or third-line setting. A total of 47% of patients were PD-L1-negative, with an ORR of 18.7% (35.7% in the PD-L1-positive subgroup and 6.0% PD-L1-negative subgroup). The median PFS was 2 months, and median OS was 9.1 months [45]. This led to the approval of pembrolizumab in metastatic SCLC patients whose disease progresses on or after platinum-based chemotherapy and at least one other line of treatment. Considered together, although immunotherapy appears promising for SCLC patients, its benefits are modest, and there is significant room for further improvement.

4. Targeted Therapy

Unlike in the case of NSCLC, there are currently no targeted therapies available for SCLC. The lack of knowledge of the key genetic mutations and molecular targets that drive SCLC initiation and progress to a more aggressive disease has been a major impediment in developing targeted therapies. However, recent genome-wide studies have identified the universal loss of tumor suppressor genes such as tumor protein 53 (TP53) in 75–90% of patients and retinoblastoma 1 (RB1) and by frequent 3P deletion [46–51]. Consistent with these observations, studies using genetically engineered mouse models have confirmed that the introduction of these two events in pulmonary cells can give rise to high frequency of SCLC development [52]. Nonetheless, more than 120 clinical trials are ongoing that are evaluating new drugs in SCLC targeting various/multiple pathways. Below, we review a few key studies and are depicted in Figure 1.

Aberrant signaling driven by epidermal growth factor receptor (EGFR), stem cell factor receptor tyrosine kinase (c-KIT), PI3K/AKT/mTOR, insulin-like growth factor receptor (IGFR1), and hedgehog signaling pathways have been identified in SCLC. However, inhibitors targeting these pathways have shown minimal efficacy in first-line, maintenance and relapsed SCLC [34,53–70]. Additionally, overexpression and amplification of MET and fibroblast growth factor receptor (FGFR) that are associated with regulating cell proliferation, survival, motility, ability of invasion, and chemoresistance were also observed in SCLC. However, therapies targeting these pathways have not fared well and next generation inhibitors need to be evaluated in combination with either chemotherapy or immunotherapy [71–76].

The apoptotic pathway and the cell cycle checkpoint are some of the other pathways that have been targeted in SCLC. In the former case, B-cell lymphoma 2 (BCL-2) is the favorite therapeutic target. However, BCL-2 antisense oligonucleotide oblimersen and other agents, including obatoclax and navitoclax, have not shown significant activity against SCLC in both phase I and phase II trials [77,78]. Another BCL-2-specific inhibitor venetoclax, demonstrated efficacy in SCLC cell lines expressing high levels of BCL-2 [79] and a phase I trial of venetoclax together with ABBV-075, a bromodomain and extra-terminal domain (BET) inhibitor, is currently under way (NCT02391480). As far as the cell cycle checkpoint is concerned, ataxia telangiectasia and Rad3-related protein (ATR), checkpoint kinase-1 (CHK1), WEE1, and aurora kinase (AURKA), have been the preferred targets among others [80].

In addition to the pathways discussed above, transcription and DNA repair pathways have also been investigated in SCLC. Of these, the MYC pathway stands out since MYC is amplified in a significant (~20%) fraction of SCLC patients and appears to have higher sensitivity to certain newer targeted therapies, such as AURKA and BET inhibitors [81–84]. Other agents that are currently being evaluated are: chiauranib, an aurora B kinase inhibitor for relapsed SCLC (NCT03216343), GSK525762, a BET inhibitor as monotherapy for patients harboring MYC amplification (NCT01587703), and in combination with trametinib for patients carrying RAS mutations (NCT03266159).

Wee-like protein kinase 1 (WEE1) is a key tyrosine kinase involved in halting the G2-to-M phase transition of the cell cycle upon DNA damage [85] that is overexpressed in SCLC [86]. In a preclinical study, the combination of Poly(ADP-Ribose) Polymerase (PARP) inhibitors and WEE1 inhibitors demonstrated a synergistic effect [87]. A phase II, multi-arm trial (BALTIC) is currently evaluating the efficacy of novel therapies in patients with ES-SCLC refractory to platinum-based agents. These novel therapies include PD-L1 inhibitor durvalumab, PARP inhibitor olaparib, and WEE1 kinase inhibitor AZD1775.

Poly (ADP-ribose) polymerase 1 (PARP1) another key player in DNA repair is overexpressed in SCLC [88]. PARP inhibitors prevent cancer cells from repairing DNA damage caused by cytotoxic drugs. Several PARP inhibitors have demonstrated antitumor efficacy in preclinical SCLC models and are currently being studied in several clinical trials. A phase II study investigating veliparib in combination with cisplatin and etoposide in untreated ES-SCLC patients showed improvement in the primary endpoint PFS (6.1 months vs. 5.5 months) although no significant differences in OS were observed [89]. However, Schlafen-11 (SLFN11), which is involved in regulating response to DNA damage and is overexpressed in about 48% of SCLC, has been identified as a potential biomarker for veliparib benefit [90]. Recently, another PARP inhibitor talazoparib also caused higher sensitization to radiotherapy in SCLC cell lines and patient-derived xenografts. Thus, PARP inhibitors have great potential to emerge as a promising therapy for SCLC [91].

Activation of the Notch pathway is oncogenic in some cancer types, but in SCLC, the inhibition of Notch pathway is involved in tumorigenic signaling, progression, and chemoresistance [92]. Consistently, the inhibitory Notch ligand Delta-like protein 3 (DLL3) is upregulated in 85% of SCLCs compared to normal lung [93]. Rovalpituzumab tesirine (Rova-T), a first-in-class DLL3 antibody-drug conjugate, initially exhibited promising results of 18% ORR in heavily pretreated SCLC [94]. Unfortunately, high toxicity rates in the phase II TRINITY trial (NCT02674568) precluded the study from meeting its primary endpoint. In addition, the phase III MERU trial (NCT03033511) evaluating Rova-T in the maintenance setting following first-line chemotherapy, was also terminated early as a result of lack of survival benefit at an interim analysis. Likewise, another phase III (TAHOE) study that assessed Rova-T as a second-line therapy for advanced SCLC compared to topotecan, stopped enrollment due to shorter OS in the Rova-T group compared with the topotecan control group [95,96]. A phase I/II study evaluating the safety of Rova-T administered in combination with nivolumab or nivolumab and ipilimumab for adults with ES-SCLC has been recently completed and could decide the future of Rova-T (NCT03026166).

5. Protein Phosphatase 2A (PP2A)

Protein phosphatase 2A (PP2A), a serine/threonine phosphatase that functions as a tumor suppressor in many cancers [97], is also involved in various cellular processes, such as protein synthesis, cellular signaling, cell cycle, apoptosis, metabolism, and stress responses [98]. Several small-molecule activators of PP2A (SMAPs) have emerged as first-in-class agents for this target [99–102]. Further, a recent study has shown that PP2A suppression leads to resistance to kinase inhibitors in KRAS-driven lung cancer cell lines. In KRAS-driven xenograft mouse models, combination treatment of SMAP and selumetinib (a MEK inhibitor used in clinical trials) led to significant tumor regression compared to either agent alone [103,104]. Although PP2A is generally held to have tumor suppressor function, several lines of evidence suggest that it could also function as an oncogene. Thus, small molecule inhibitors of PP2A such as LB-100 [105], are emerging as novel strategies for SCLC. Furthermore, since PP2A is also associated with immune response by downregulating cytotoxic T-lymphocyte function [106,107], PP2A inhibition combined with immunotherapy appears to be effective in mediating an antitumor response. Indeed, in colon cancer and melanoma cells, a combination of LB-100 and an immune checkpoint inhibitor led to greater T-cell-dependent anti-tumor response, with more effector T-cell and reduced regulatory T-cell infiltration [106]. Carbonic anhydrase IX (CAIX), an enzyme involved in hypoxia inducible factor 1 alpha (HIF-1α) hypoxic signaling, is a promising target for chimeric antigen receptor-T (CAR-T) cells in an intracranial mouse model for glioblastoma [108]. In this mouse model, LB-100 was shown to augment the cytotoxic response of anti-carbonic anhydrase (CAIX) CAR-T cells, underscoring the therapeutic potential of synergistic LB-100 and CAR-T cell therapy in SCLC and other solid tumors [109].

6. Mitochondria

Mitochondria play an essential role in cell survival, apoptosis, adenosine triphosphate (ATP) production, as well as tumorigenesis [110]. Multiple therapeutic strategies have been developed to target mitochondrial functions, such as oxidative phosphorylation, glycolysis, tricarboxylic acid (TCA) cycle, apoptosis, reactive oxygen species (ROS) regulation, permeability transition pore complex, mitochondrial DNA, and dihydroorotate de-hydrogenase (DHODH)-linked pyrimidine synthesis [111]. Drugs that target mitochondrial metabolism through inhibition of pyruvate dehydrogenase (CPI-613, dichloroacetate), isocitrate dehydrogenase (AG-22, AG-120, AG-881) and targeting apoptotic pathways (birinapant, Minnelide, ME-334, Debio 1143, ONC201, LCL161) have been studied in early phase clinical trials [112–117]. These drugs have modest clinical activity as single agents in various tumors including SCLC and are currently being explored as combination therapies with chemotherapy, immunotherapy, and other targeted therapies [118].

7. Stem Cell Therapy

Cancer stem cells (CSCs) are defined as a small population of cells within a heterogeneous tumor that exhibit similar traits of normal stem cells. CSCs can originate from either somatic stem cells or differentiated progenitor cells. They prompt tumorigenic activity by undergoing self-renewal and differentiation, leading to tumor relapse, resistance to therapy, and metastasis [119–121]. Hence, targeting CSCs has become a novel therapeutic strategy for cancer treatment. CSCs often have upregulated signaling involved in development and tissue homeostasis, such as Notch, Hedgehog and wingless type 1 (WNT) pathways, all of which can be found in SCLC [122,123]. Unfortunately, Notch signaling inhibition with Rova-T and tarextumab have failed, but combination therapies studies are ongoing that could potentially yield positive results. Lysine demethylase 1 (LSD1) is implicated in maintaining stemness properties and hence, has emerged as a potential target for inhibiting lung CSCs [124]. A phase II trial (CLEPSIDRA) investigating the LSD1 inhibitor iadademstat in combination with standard-of-care in relapsing SCLC patients showed remarkable response rates (up to 75%). Preclinical studies with another LSD1 inhibitor GSK2879552 using 150 cancer cell lines, showed that SCLC and acute myeloid leukemia (AML) cell lines were sensitive to growth inhibition by the LSD1 inhibitor [125–127]. Furthermore, dual inhibition of LSD1 and PD-1 appear to be more effective than either therapy alone [128]. Another route to target stem cells is through CD47 inhibition by RRx-001, which targets tumor-associated macrophages and CSCs via downregulation of the antiphagocytic CD47/SIRPα checkpoint axis. A phase II trial (QUADRUPLE THREAT) involving 26 previously platinum-treated third-line SCLC patients showed that the OS and PFS for patients treated with RRx-001 and a reintroduced platinum doublet were 8.6 months and 7.5 months, respectively, which is much higher for a third-line treatment reported in literature [129]. Interestingly, biopsies taken from patients have correlated response to CD47 inhibition with a high density of infiltrated tumor-associated macrophages that are abundant in SCLC. Based on these observations, a phase III (REPLATINUM) randomized study of RRx-001 with platinum doublet vs. only platinum doublet in third-line SCLC is currently ongoing (NCT03699956).

8. Improving Outcomes

8.1. Biomarker-Based Therapy

Although immunotherapy has improved median survival for treatment-naïve ES-SCLC patients, the benefits have been limited with improvement in both PFS and OS approximately 1 and 2 months, respectively, with only 12.6% of patients remaining progression-free after one-year [39]. To improve the outcomes, better selection of patients based on predictive biomarkers, given the high mutational load and rapid resistance in SCLC, and therapies targeting multiple pathways with combination strategies need to be developed.

PD-L1 remains the most common immune-based biomarker for several malignancies. PD-L1 staining in SCLC is less intense and infrequent compared to NSCLC [130]. In KEYNOTE-158, a combined score >1 for PD-L1 expression by the Dako 22C3 assay appeared to predict increased response to pembrolizumab and improved survival when compared with patients negative for PD-L1 [44]; however, the PD-L1 positivity based on Dako 28-8 assay as in the CheckMate 032 did not replicate those results [131]. The assays differ in that KEYNOTE-158 used a PD-L1 score based on staining of tumor cells, lymphocytes and macrophages, whereas CheckMate 032 used staining of only tumor cells to determine positivity. The ongoing phase II REACTION (NCT02580994) and the phase III KEYNOTE-604 (NCT03066778) trials will require measurement of PD-L1 at baseline to provide insight into the predictive role of PD-L1 expression. Higher tumor mutation burden (TMB) has been recognized as a likely predictor of response to immunotherapy across disease types [132]. In an exome-sequencing analysis of CheckMate 032, patients with high TMB appeared to have a greater improvement in OS when treated with nivolumab. Patients with high-, medium-, and low-TMB had a median OS of 5.4 months, 3.9 months, and 3.1 months, respectively; the one-year OS rates were 35.2%, 26.0%, and 22.1%, respectively [133]. However, in the IMpower-133, a blood-based TMB failed to predict benefit for atezolizumab, thus requiring further prospective randomized validation TMB studies. Circulating tumor cells (CTCs) can be detected in 85% of SCLC patients and can potentially serve as a biomarker [134]. CTCs have been explored in multiple studies as a biomarker to predict response and resistance to therapy; however, additional studies looking into the genomic, epigenetic, and transcriptomic heterogeneity of CTCs at diagnosis and during relapse need to be done before it can be applied in clinics [135,136]. Cell-free DNA (cfDNA) widely used in NSCLC has also been examined in SCLC. A study with 27 patients showed cfDNA was able to mirror treatment response and even identified disease recurrence before radiological progression [137]. Future work based on tumor or blood-based biomarkers will help a long way in understanding treatment resistance in SCLC.

8.2. Combination Therapy

To overcome treatment resistance, novel combination approaches targeting multiple pathways are being explored in combination with chemotherapy and immunotherapies. Lurbinectedin, a novel cytotoxic drug, is a transcriptional inhibitor that inhibits RNA polymerase II. In a phase II trial for both sensitive and resistant disease, lurbinectedin was active as a single agent in second-line SCLC with an ORR of 35.2% [138]. Based on this study, the FDA has approved lurbinectedin for the treatment of ES-SCLC patients with disease progression after platinum-based chemotherapy. A phase III study (ATLANTIS trial, NCT02566993) of lurbinectedin in combination with doxorubicin vs. chemotherapy has completed recruitment and results are pending. Current trials investigating targeted therapies with or without chemotherapy include WEE1 inhibitor AZD1775 in combination with carboplatin (NCT02937818) and olaparib (NCT02511795), checkpoint kinase 1 (CHK1) inhibitor SRA737 in combination with cisplatin/gemcitabine (NCT027979770), ataxia–telangiectasia and Rad3 related (ATR) inhibitor AZD6738 in combination with olaparib (NCT02937818), another ATR inhibitor VX-970 in combination with topotecan (NCT02487095), Bcl-2 inhibitor navitoclax and mTOR inhibitor vistusertib (NCT03366103), Bcl-2 inhibitor venetoclax and ABBV-075 (NCT02391480), and Aurora B kinase inhibitor (NCT02579226) are all ongoing, which should shed some light on the future of targeted therapy in SCLC. There are numerous early phase trials investigating the combination of immunotherapy and targeted drugs as well. Durvalumab with olaparib (NCT02734004, MENDIOLA), avelumab with utomilumab, which is a humanized monoclonal antibody (mAb) that stimulates signaling through CD137 (NCT02554812), nivolumab plus ipilimumab with dendritic cell-based p53 vaccine 9 (NCT03406715) in relapsed SCLC, atezolizumab with chemotherapy and a CDK 4/6 inhibitor trilaciclib (NCT03041311) in first-line ES-SCLC are some of the novel combinations of immunotherapy with targeted agents.

8.3. Other Modalities

Other modalities of therapies targeting cell surface antigens expressed on tumor cells by monoclonal antibodies or surface-targeting immunotherapies, such as CAR-T cells and bispecific T-cell engagers (BiTEs), are in early stages of development. CD56 is expressed in almost all SCLC tumors, and thus, presents to be an attractive target for treating SCLC [139]. In a preclinical study, promiximab-duocarmycin (DUBA), a CD56 antibody conjugated to a potent DNA alkylating agent with a novel linker, showed promising results. This antibody drug conjugate (ADC) demonstrated high efficacy in SCLC xenograft models [140], suggesting that further clinical evaluation of this compound may be beneficial. Another ADC sacituzumab govitecan is comprised of a humanized mAb targeting Trop-2 (trophoblastic antigen-2), which is highly expressed in several epithelial cancers [141], fused to SN-38 (the active metabolite of irinotecan), which induces double- and single-strand DNA breaks by inhibiting topoisomerase I [142]. Sacituzumab govitecan is currently being investigated in several trials, including a phase I/II trial where it is being evaluated as a single agent in patients with previously treated, advanced SCLC (NCT01631552). CAR-T cells targeting DLL3 have entered a phase I clinical trial (NCT03392064). AMG 757, a BiTE, is also being evaluated in a phase I trial that includes ES-SCLC patients requiring first-line maintenance therapy and those with SCLC recurrence (NCT03319940). In patients with metastatic solid tumors including relapsed SCLC, targeting other immune checkpoints, such as PD-1 and CTLA-4, with immunotherapies, including TIM3 and LAG3, are being evaluated in clinical trials in combination with anti-PD-1 or anti-PD-L1 antibodies (NCT03708328, NCT03365791). Finally, radiation therapy is assumed to modulate immune response, as it can increase tumor antigen production and presentation and also enhance cytotoxic T-lymphocyte activity [143]. Potential synergy of radiotherapy in combination with immunotherapy in patients with ES-SCLC is being evaluated in innovative ongoing trials, and results are expected in the near future. Altogether, advancement in biomarkers, targeting multiple critical pathways, and enhancing immunotherapy efficacy in SCLC will hopefully improve the survival outcomes for SCLC patients, which has been elusive for many years.

9. Community Network-City of Hope Experience

City of Hope is a National Cancer Institute (NCI)-designated Comprehensive Cancer Center and a member of the National Comprehensive Cancer Network (NCCN). In addition, all clinical sites accept the Via Oncology Pathways (modified by City of Hope) for evaluation, antitumor treatment and surveillance after treatments have concluded. City of Hope is composed of a central academic site in Duarte and several satellite sites within Southern California. At the academic center, preclinical work is performed, and clinical trials on that translational research can be rapidly deployed across the entire enterprise, making bench-to-bedside research feasible and fascicle. The collaboration between basic research done on the main campus and clinical research done at both the main and satellite campuses, furthers the discovery of disease biomarkers and novel drug targets. This results in more rational drug design, improved therapeutic efficacy, and quicker optimization of high priority drugs for clinical use (Figure 2).

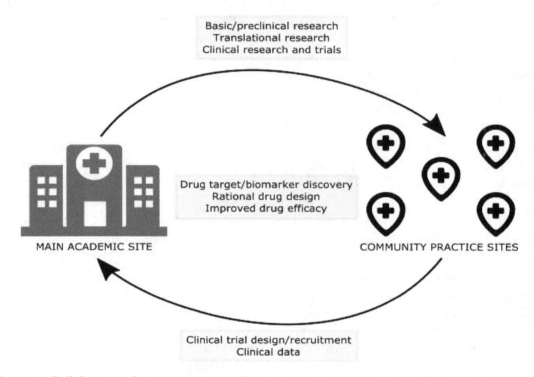

Figure 2. Collaboration between main academic site and community sites for clinical research.

Clinical trials are initiated at the academic campus in Duarte and at one or more of our 27 affiliated network community cancer center offices that are staffed with 43 medical oncologists, 40 radiation oncologists, seven advanced practice providers (APPs) and a clinical trials coordinator. As directed by the Recalcitrant Cancer Research Congressional Act of 2012 (H.R.733), the National Cancer Institute (NCI) allocates resources for research and treatment of recalcitrant cancers having five-year relative survival rates of <20% and estimated to cause at least 30,000 deaths in the US per year. SCLC is considered a recalcitrant cancer having a dismal five-year survival rate of less than 7%. One of the major limitations to ongoing research in SCLC is tumor tissue availability, as the disease is rarely treated surgically. Another issue is many clinical trials in SCLC cannot be completed due to lack of accrual. Using the academic collaboration model with the academic center along with 27 community sites, enrollment becomes more feasible. The rapid progression of disease in SCLC relapse also places research on an urgent timeline to test new agents with a small window to observe treatment efficacy. Given single Institutional Review Board (IRB) approval in our institution, clinical trials can be opened at multiple sites in a rapid fashion. At the academic site, preclinical investigations are done, and clinical trials based on translational research data can be rapidly designed and disseminated across the entire enterprise, facilitating bench-to-bedside SCLC research in a more feasible manner. The collective knowledge gained from the interaction between the academic and community sites will provide insight into how to overcome challenges that continuously hinder therapeutic advancements in SCLC.

10. Future Directions

Traditionally, SCLC has been regarded as a homogenous disease, which led to most SCLC patients being treated with essentially one standard regimen. Recent studies from molecular analysis of patient tissues and genetically defined models indicate that there is notable heterogeneity among SCLCs in terms of histology, growth characteristics, expression of neuroendocrine cell differentiation markers, MYC activation, Notch pathway inactivation, and role of neuronal lineage-specific transcription factors in this disease (ASCL1, achaete-scute homologue 1; NeuroD1, neurogenic differentiation factor 1; POU2F3, POU class 2 homeobox 3; YAP1, yes-associated protein 1) [144–148]. Currently, SCLC is classified into four subtypes based on increased expression of different markers: ASCL1 high (SCLC-A), NEUROD1 high (SCLC-N), POU2F3 high (SCLC-P), and YAP1 high (SCLC-Y) [79]. SCLC-A and SCLC-N are neuroendocrine subtypes, whereas SCLC-P and SCLC-Y are non-neuroendocrine subtypes. These subtypes can be associated with specific biomarkers that are either drug-specific targets or predictors of drug response (e.g., DLL3 in SCLC-A, AURKA in SCLC-N, CDK4/6 in SCLC-Y and IGF1R in SCLC-P). These distinct gene expression profiles will guide us in designing new clinical trials. Recent advances in using patient-derived xenograft (PDX) models based on biopsy/resected tumors, CTCs, genetically engineered mouse models (GEMM), as well as omics profiling will drastically enhance our capacity to identify and test novel drugs and discover biomarkers for treatment and prognostication [93,149].

In conclusion, we recommend: (i) setting up a centralized biobank and repository leading to creation of a database incorporating full genomic, proteomic, and microRNA information; (ii) enrolling a higher proportion of SCLC patients into clinical trials with obligatory biomarker analysis; (iii) creating a master protocol which will help reduce duplicative effort and thus ease the eligibility requirements for clinical trials; (iv) create and incentivize academic and community research partnership centers of excellence, since most SCLC patients are treated in community sites; (v) collaborate with bioengineers, cancer biologists, and biophysicists to gather the genetic aberrations discovered and harness the power of computational modeling of genetic information, which will be a powerful tool in understanding SCLC and developing future therapies. Given the academic and community partnership we have established at City of Hope, this should be achievable and pave way for success in treating this challenging disease.

Author Contributions: Conceptualization, S.S., A.N., and R.S.; methodology, S.S., A.N., and N.G.; writing—original draft preparation, S.S. and A.N.; writing—review and editing, S.S., A.N., N.G., A.B., P.K., and R.S.; supervision, R.S.; project administration, P.K.; funding acquisition, R.S. All authors have read and agreed to the published version of the manuscript.

References

1.   Centers for Disease Control and Prevention. National Center for Health Statistics. CDC On-Line Database, Compiled from Compressed Mortality File 1999–2016 Series 20 No. 2V, 2017. Available online: https://www.cdc.gov/nchs/data_access/cmf.htm (accessed on 28 July 2020).

2.   Gazdar, A.F.; Bunn, P.A.; Minna, J.D. Small-cell lung cancer: What we know, what we need to know and the path forward. *Nat. Rev. Cancer* **2017**, *17*, 765. [CrossRef] [PubMed]

3.   Herbst, R.S.; Morgensztern, D.; Boshoff, C. The biology and management of non-small cell lung cancer. *Nature* **2018**, *553*, 446–454. [CrossRef] [PubMed]

4.   Kalemkerian, G.P. Staging and imaging of small cell Lung cancer. *Cancer Imaging* **2012**, *11*, 253–258. [CrossRef] [PubMed]

5.   Navarro, A.; Felip, E. Pembrolizumab in advanced pretreated small cell lung cancer patients with PD-L1 expression: Data from the KEYNOTE-028 trial: A reason for hope? *Transl. Lung Cancer Res.* **2017**, *6* (Suppl. S1), S78–S83. [CrossRef]

6.   U.S. Food & Drug Administration. FDA Grants Nivolumab Accelerated Approval for Third-Line Treatment of Metastatic Small Cell Lung Cancer. Available online: https://www.fda.gov/drugs/resources-information-approved-drugs/fda-grants-nivolumab-accelerated-approval-third-line-treatment-metastatic-small-cell-lung-cancer (accessed on 28 July 2020).

7.   NCCN. *NCCN Clinical Practice Guidelines in Oncology: Small Cell Lung Cancer*; The National Comprehensive Cancer Network (NCCN): Whitemarsh, PA, USA, 2019.

8.   Warde, P.; Payne, D. Does thoracic irradiation improve survival and local control in limited-stage small-cell carcinoma of the lung? A meta-analysis. *J. Clin. Oncol.* **1992**, *10*, 890–895. [CrossRef]

9.   Pignon, J.P.; Arriagada, R.; Ihde, D.C.; Johnsosn, D.H.; Perry, M.C.; Souhami, R.L.; Brodin, O.; Joss, R.A.; Kies, M.S.; Lebeau, B.; et al. A meta-analysis of thoracic radiotherapy for small-cell lung cancer. *N. Engl. J. Med.* **1992**, *327*, 1618–1624. [CrossRef]

10.   Turrisi, A.T., III; Kim, K.; Blum, R.; Sause, W.T.; Livingston, R.B.; Komaki, R.; Wagner, H.; Aisner, S.; Johnson, D.H. Twice-daily compared with once-daily thoracic radiotherapy in limited small-cell lung cancer treated concurrently with cisplatin and etoposide. *N. Engl. J. Med.* **1999**, *340*, 265–271. [CrossRef]

11.   Faivre-Finn, C.; Snee, M.; Ashcroft, L.; Appel, W.; Barlesi, F.; Bhatnagar, A.; Bezjak, A.; Cardenal, F.; Fournel, P.; Harden, S.; et al. Concurrent once-daily versus twice-daily chemoradiotherapy in patients with limited-stage small-cell lung cancer (CONVERT): An open-label, phase 3, randomised, superiority trial. *Lancet Oncol.* **2017**, *18*, 1116–1125. [CrossRef]

12.   Fukuoka, M.; Furuse, K.; Saijo, N.; Nishiwaki, Y.; Ikegami, H.; Tamura, T.; Shimoyama, M.; Suemasu, K. Randomized trial of cyclophosphamide, doxorubicin, and vincristine versus cisplatin and etoposide versus alternation of these regimens in small-cell lung cancer. *J. Natl. Cancer Inst.* **1991**, *83*, 855–861. [CrossRef]

13.   Roth, B.J.; Johnson, D.H.; Einhorn, L.H.; Schacter, L.P.; Cherng, N.C.; Cohen, H.J.; Crawford, J.; Randolph, J.A.; Goodlow, J.L.; Broun, G.O.; et al. Randomized study of cyclophosphamide, doxorubicin, and vincristine versus etoposide and cisplatin versus alternation of these two regimens in extensive small-cell lung cancer: A phase III trial of the Southeastern cancer study group. *J. Clin. Oncol.* **1992**, *10*, 282–291. [CrossRef]

14.   Noda, K.; Nishiwaki, Y.; Kawahara, M.; Negoro, C.; Sugiura, T.; Yokoyama, A.; Fukuoka, M.; Mori, K.; Watanabe, K.; Tamura, T.; et al. Irinotecan plus cisplatin compared with etoposide plus cisplatin for extensive small-cell lung cancer. *N. Engl. J. Med.* **2002**, *346*, 85–91. [CrossRef] [PubMed]

15.   Jackman, D.M.; Johnson, B.E. Small-cell lung cancer. *Lancet* **2005**, *366*, 1385–1396. [CrossRef]

16.   O'Brien, M.E.R.; Ciuleanu, T.E.; Tsekov, H.; Shparyk, Y.; Cuceviá, B.; Juhasz, G.; Thatcher, N.; Ross, G.A.; Dane, G.C.; Crofts, T. Phase III trial comparing supportive care alone with supportive care with oral topotecan in patients with relapsed small-cell lung cancer. *J. Clin. Oncol.* **2006**, *24*, 5441–5447. [CrossRef] [PubMed]

17.   Von Pawel, J.; Schiller, J.H.; Shepherd, F.A.; Fields, S.Z.; Kleisbauer, J.P.; Chrysson, N.G.; Stewart, D.J.; Clark, P.I.; Palmer, M.C.; Depierre, A.; et al. Topotecan versus cyclophosphamide, doxorubicin, and vincristine for the treatment of recurrent small-cell lung cancer. *J. Clin. Oncol.* **1999**, *17*, 658–667. [CrossRef]

18.   Horita, N.; Yamamoto, M.; Sato, T.; Tsukahara, T.; Nagakura, H.; Tashiro, K.; Shinata, Y.; Watanabe, H.; Nagai, K.; Inoue, M.; et al. Topotecan for relapsed small-cell lung cancer: Systematic review and meta-analysis of 1347 patients. *Sci. Rep.* **2015**, *5*, 15437. [CrossRef]

19.   Masters, G.A.; Declerck, L.; Blanke, C.; Sandler, A.; DeVore, R.; Miller, K.; Johnson, D.; Eastern Cooperative Oncology Group. Phase II trial of gemcitabine in refractory or relapsed small-cell lung cancer: Eastern Cooperative Oncology Group Trial 1597. *J. Clin. Oncol.* **2003**, *21*, 1550–1555. [CrossRef]

20.   Smyth, J.F.; Smith, I.E.; Sessa, C.; Schoffski, P.; Wanders, J.; Franklin, H.; Kaye, S.B. Activity of docetaxel (Taxotere) in small cell lung cancer: The Early Clinical Trials Group of the EORTC. *Eur. J. Cancer* **1994**, *30A*, 1058–1060. [CrossRef]

21.   Yamamoto, N.; Tsurutani, J.; Yoshimura, N.; Asai, G.; Moriyama, A.; Nakagawa, K.; Kudoh, S.; Takada, M.; Minato, Y.; Fukuoka, M. Phase II study of weekly paclitaxel for relapsed and refractory small cell lung cancer. *Anticancer Res.* **2006**, *26*, 777–781.

22.	Pietanza, M.C.; Kadota, K.; Huberman, K.; Sima, C.S.; Fiore, J.J.; Sumner, D.K.; Travis, W.D.; Heguy, A.; Ginsberg, M.S.; Holodny, A.I.; et al. Phase II trial of temozolomide in patients with relapsed sensitive or refractory small cell lung cancer, with assessment of methylguanine-DNA methyltransferase as a potential biomarker. *Clin. Cancer Res.* **2012**, *18*, 1138–1145. [CrossRef]

23.	Masuda, N.; Fukuoka, M.; Kusunoki, Y.; Matsui, K.; Takifuji, N.; Kudoh, S.; Negoro, S.; Nishioka, M.; Nakagawa, K.; Takada, M. CPT-11: A new derivative of camptothecin for the treatment of refractory or relapsed small-cell lung cancer. *J. Clin. Oncol.* **1992**, *10*, 1225–1229. [CrossRef]

24.	Jassem, J.; Karnicka-Mlodkowska, H.; van Pottelsberghe, C.; van Glabbeke, M.; Noseda, M.A.; Ardizzoni, A.; Gozzelino, F.; Planting, A.; van Zandwijk, N. Phase II study of vinorelbine (Navelbine) in previously treated small cell lung cancer patients: EORTC Lung Cancer Cooperative Group. *Eur. J. Cancer* **1993**, *29A*, 1720–1722. [CrossRef]

25.	Ding, Q.; Zhan, J. Amrubicin: Potential in combination with cisplatin or carboplatin to treat small-cell lung cancer. *Drug Des. Dev. Ther.* **2013**, *7*, 681–689.

26.	Miller, A.B.; Fox, W.; Tall, R. Five-year follow-up of the Medical Research Council comparative trial of surgery and radiotherapy for the primary treatment of small-celled or oat-celled carcinoma of the bronchus. *Lancet* **1969**, *2*, 501–505. [CrossRef]

27.	Fox, W.; Scadding, J.G. Treatment of oat-celled carcinoma of the bronchus. *Lancet* **1973**, *2*, 616–617. [CrossRef]

28.	Lad, T.; Piantadosi, S.; Thomas, P.; Payne, D.; Ruckdeschel, J.; Giaccone, G. A prospective randomized trial to determine the benefit of surgical resection of residual disease following response of small cell lung cancer to combination chemotherapy. *Chest* **1994**, *106* (Suppl. S6), 320S–323S. [CrossRef]

29.	Rostad, H.; Naalsund, A.; Jacobsen, R.; Strand, T.E.; Scott, H.; Strøm, E.H.; Norstein, J. Small cell lung cancer in Norway. Should more patients have been offered surgical therapy? *Eur. J. Cardiothorac. Surg.* **2004**, *26*, 782–786. [CrossRef]

30.	Brock, M.V.; Hooker, C.M.; Syphard, J.E.; Westra, W.; Xu, L.; Alberg, A.J.; Mason, D.; Baylin, S.B.; Herman, J.G.; Yung, R.C.; et al. Surgical resection of limited disease small cell lung cancer in the new era of platinum chemotherapy: Its time has come. *J. Thorac. Cardiovasc. Surg.* **2005**, *129*, 64–72. [CrossRef]

31.	Lim, E.; Belcher, E.; Yap, Y.K.; Nicholson, A.G.; Goldstraw, P. The role of surgery in the treatment of limited disease small cell lung cancer: Time to reevaluate. *J. Thorac. Oncol.* **2008**, *3*, 1267–1271. [CrossRef]

32.	Schreiber, D.; Rineer, J.; Weedon, J.; Vongtama, D.; Wortham, A.; Kim, A.; Han, P.; Choi, K.; Rotman, M. Survival outcomes with the use of surgery in limited-stage small cell lung cancer: Should its role be re-evaluated? *Cancer* **2010**, *116*, 1350–1357. [CrossRef]

33.	Liu, T.; Chen, Z.; Dang, J.; Li, G. The role of surgery in stage I to III small cell lung cancer: A systematic review and meta-analysis. *PLoS ONE* **2018**, *13*, e0210001. [CrossRef]

34.	Peifer, M.; Fernández-Cuesta, L.; Sos, M.L.; George, J.; Seidel, D.; Kasper, L.H.; Plenker, D.; Leenders, F.; Sun, R.; Zander, T.; et al. Integrative genome analyses identify key somatic driver mutations of small-cell lung cancer. *Nat. Genet.* **2012**, *44*, 1104–1110. [CrossRef] [PubMed]

35.	Alexandrov, L.B.; Nik-Zainal, S.; Wedge, D.C.; Aparicio, S.A.; Behjati, S.; Biankin, A.V.; Bignell, G.R.; Bolli, N.; Borg, A.; Børrensen-Dale, A.L.; et al. Signatures of mutational processes in human cancer. *Nature* **2013**, *500*, 415–421. [CrossRef] [PubMed]

36.	Horn, L.; Reck, M.; Spigel, D.R. The future of immunotherapy in the treatment of small cell lung cancer. *Oncologist* **2016**, *21*, 910–921. [CrossRef] [PubMed]

37.	Reck, M.; Heigener, D.; Reinmuth, N. Immunotherapy for small-cell lung cancer: Emerging evidence. *Future Oncol.* **2016**, *12*, 931–943. [CrossRef] [PubMed]

38.	Horn, L.; Mansfield, A.S.; Szczęsna, A.; Havel, L.; Krzakowski, M.; Hochmair, M.J.; Huemer, F.; Losonczy, G.; Johnson, M.L.; IMpower133 Study Group; et al. First-line atezolizumab plus chemotherapy in extensive-stage small-cell lung cancer. *N. Engl. J. Med.* **2018**, *379*, 2220–2229. [CrossRef]

39.	Paz-Ares, L.; Dvorkin, M.; Chen, Y.; Reinmuth, N.; Hotta, K.; Trukhin, D.; Statsenko, G.; Hochmair, M.J.; Özgüroğlu, M.; Ji, J.H.; et al. Durvalumab plus platinum–etoposide versus platinum–etoposide in first-line treatment of extensive-stage small-cell lung cancer (CASPIAN): A randomised, controlled, open-label, phase 3 trial. *Lancet* **2019**, *394*, 1929–1939. [CrossRef]

40. Reck, M.; Luft, A.; Szczesna, A.; Havel, L.; Kim, S.-W.; Akerley, W.; Pietanza, M.C.; Wu, Y.-L.; Zielinski, C.; Thomas, M.; et al. Phase III randomized trial of ipilimumab plus etoposide and platinum versus placebo plus etoposide and platinum in extensive-stage small-cell lung cancer. *J. Clin. Oncol.* **2016**, *34*, 3740–3748. [CrossRef]

41. Owonikoko, T.K.; Kim, H.R.; Govindan, R.; Ready, N.; Reck, M.; Peters, S.; Dakhil, S.R.; Navarro, A.; Rodriguez-Cid, J.; Schenker, M.; et al. Nivolumab (nivo) plus ipilimumab (ipi), nivo, or placebo (pbo) as maintenance therapy in patients (pts) with extensive disease small cell lung cancer (ED-SCLC) after first-line (1L) platinum-based chemotherapy (chemo): Results from the double-blind, randomized phase III CheckMate 451 study. *Ann. Oncol.* **2019**, *30* (Suppl. S2), ii77–ii80.

42. Ready, N.E.; Ott, P.A.; Hellmann, M.D.; Zugazagoitia, J.; Hann, C.L.; de Braud, F.; Antonia, S.J.; Ascierto, P.A.; Moreno, V.; Atmaca, A.; et al. Nivolumab Monotherapy and Nivolumab Plus Ipilimumab in Recurrent Small Cell Lung Cancer: Results from the CheckMate 032 Randomized Cohort. *J. Thorac. Oncol.* **2020**, *15*, 426–435. [CrossRef]

43. Ott, P.A.; Elez, E.; Hiret, S.; Kim, D.-W.; Morosky, A.; Saraf, S.; Piperdi, B.; Mehnert, J.M. Pembrolizumab in patients with extensive-stage small-cell lung cancer: Results from the phase Ib KEYNOTE-028 study. *J. Clin. Oncol.* **2017**, *35*, 3823–3829. [CrossRef]

44. Chung, H.C.; Lopez-Martin, J.A.; Kao, S.C.-H.; Miller, W.H.; Ros, W.; Gao, B.; Marabelle, A.; Gottfried, M.; Zer, A.; Delord, J.-P.; et al. Phase 2 study of pembrolizumab in advanced small-cell lung cancer (SCLC): KEYNOTE-158. *J. Clin. Oncol.* **2018**, *15*, 8506. [CrossRef]

45. Rudin, C.M.; Poirier, J.T. Small-cell lung cancer in 2016: Shining light on novel targets and therapies. *Nat. Rev. Clin. Oncol.* **2017**, *14*, 75–76. [CrossRef] [PubMed]

46. Miller, C.W.; Simon, K.; Aslo, A.; Kok, Y.; Yokota, J.; Buys, C.H.; Terada, M.; Koeffler, H.P. p53 mutations in human lung tumors. *Cancer Res.* **1992**, *52*, 1695–1698. [PubMed]

47. Takahashi, T.; Takahashi, T.; Suzuki, H.; Hida, T.; Sekido, Y.; Ariyoshi, Y.; Ueda, R. The p53 gene is very frequently mutated in small-cell lung cancer with a distinct nucleotide substitution pattern. *Oncogene* **1991**, *6*, 1775–1778. [PubMed]

48. Helin, K.; Holm, K.; Niebuhr, A.; Eiberg, H.; Tommerup, N.; Hougaard, S.; Poulsen, H.S.; Spang-Thomsen, M.; Norgaard, P. Loss of the retinoblastoma protein-related p130 protein in small cell lung carcinoma. *Proc. Natl. Acad. Sci. USA* **1997**, *94*, 6933–6938. [CrossRef] [PubMed]

49. Kaye, F.J. RB and cyclin dependent kinase pathways: Defining a distinction between RB and p16 loss in lung cancer. *Oncogene* **2002**, *21*, 6908–6914. [CrossRef]

50. Wistuba, I.I.; Behrens, C.; Virmani, A.K.; Mele, G.; Milchgrub, S.; Girard, L.; Fondon, J.W., 3rd; Garner, H.R.; McKay, B.; Latif, F.; et al. High resolution chromosome 3p allelotyping of human lung cancer and preneoplastic/preinvasive bronchial epithelium reveals multiple, discontinuous sites of 3p allele loss and 3 regions of frequent breakpoints. *Cancer Res.* **2000**, *60*, 1949–1960.

51. Wistuba, I.I.; Berry, J.; Behrens, C.; Maitra, A.; Shivapurkar, N.; Milchgrub, S.; Mackay, B.; Minna, J.D.; Gazdar, A.F. Molecular changes in the bronchial epithelium of patients with small cell lung cancer. *Clin. Cancer Res.* **2000**, *6*, 2604–2610.

52. Bordi, P.; Tiseo, M.; Barbieri, F.; Bavieri, M.; Sartori, G.; Marchetti, A.; Buttitta, F.; Bortesi, B.; Ambrosini-Spaltro, A.; Gnetti, L.; et al. Gene mutations in small-cell lung cancer (SCLC): Results of a panel of 6 genes in a cohort of Italian patients. *Lung Cancer* **2014**, *86*, 324–328. [CrossRef]

53. Ross, J.S.; Wang, K.; Elkadi, O.R.; Tarasen, A.; Foulke, L.; Sheehan, C.E.; Otto, G.A.; Palmer, G.; Yelensky, R.; Lipson, D.; et al. Next-generation sequencing reveals frequent consistent genomic alterations in small cell undifferentiated lung cancer. *J. Clin. Pathol.* **2014**, *67*, 772–776. [CrossRef]

54. Wakuda, K.; Kenmotsu, H.; Serizawa, M.; Koh, Y.; Isaka, M.; Takahashi, S.; Ono, A.; Taira, T.; Naito, T.; Murakami, H.; et al. Molecular profiling of small cell lung cancer in a Japanese cohort. *Lung Cancer* **2014**, *84*, 139–144. [CrossRef] [PubMed]

55. Metro, G.; Duranti, S.; Fischer, M.J.; Cappuzzo, F.; Crinò, L. Emerging drugs for small cell lung cancer—An update. *Expert Opin. Emerg. Drugs* **2012**, *17*, 31–36. [CrossRef] [PubMed]

56. Rudin, C.M.; Durinck, S.; Stawiski, E.W.; Poirier, J.T.; Modrusan, Z.; Shames, D.S.; Bergbower, E.A.; Guan, Y.; Shin, J.; Guillory, J.; et al. Comprehensive genomic analysis identifies SOX2 as a frequently amplified gene in small-cell lung cancer. *Nat. Genet.* **2012**, *44*, 1111–1116. [CrossRef]

57. Umemura, S.; Mimaki, S.; Makinoshima, H.; Tada, S.; Ishii, G.; Ohmatsu, H.; Niho, S.; Yoh, K.; Matsumoto, S.; Takahashi, A.; et al. Therapeutic priority of the PI3K/AKT/mTOR pathway in small cell lung cancers as revealed by a comprehensive genomic analysis. *J. Thorac. Oncol.* **2014**, *9*, 1324–1331. [CrossRef] [PubMed]

58. Umemura, S.; Tsuchihara, K.; Goto, K. Genomic profiling of small-cell lung cancer: The era of targeted therapies. *Jpn. J. Clin. Oncol.* **2015**, *45*, 513–519. [CrossRef] [PubMed]

59. Badzio, A.; Wynes, M.W.; Dziadziuszko, R.; Merrick, D.T.; Pardo, M.; Rzyman, W.; Kowalczyk, A.; Singh, S.; Ranger-Moore, J.; Manriquez, G.; et al. Increased insulin-like growth factor 1 receptor protein expression and gene copy number in small cell lung cancer. *J. Thorac. Oncol.* **2010**, *5*, 1905–1911. [CrossRef] [PubMed]

60. Potti, A.; Moazzam, N.; Ramar, K.; Hanekom, D.S.; Kargas, S.; Koch, M. CD117 (c-KIT) overexpression in patients with extensive-stage small-cell lung carcinoma. *Ann. Oncol.* **2003**, *14*, 894–897. [CrossRef]

61. Park, K.S.; Martelotto, L.G.; Peifer, M.; Sos, M.L.; Karnezis, A.N.; Mahjoub, M.R.; Bernard, K.; Conklin, J.F.; Szczepny, A.; Yuan, J.; et al. A crucial requirement for Hedgehog signaling in small cell lung cancer. *Nat. Med.* **2011**, *17*, 1504–1508. [CrossRef]

62. Belani, C.P.; Dahlberg, S.E.; Rudin, C.M.; Fleisher, M.; Chen, H.X.; Takebe, N.; Ramalingam, S.S.; Schiller, J.H. Three-arm randomized phase II study of cisplatin and etoposide (CE) versus CE with either vismodegib (V) or cixutumumab (Cx) for patients with extensive stage-small cell lung cancer (ES-SCLC) (ECOG 1508). *J. Clin. Oncol.* **2013**, *31*, 7508. [CrossRef]

63. Johnson, B.E.; Fischer, T.; Fischer, B.; Dunlop, D.; Rischin, D.; Silberman, S.; Kowalski, M.O.; Sayles, D.; Dimitrijevic, S.; Fletcher, C.; et al. Phase II study of imatinib in patients with small cell lung cancer. *Clin. Cancer Res.* **2003**, *9*, 5880–5887.

64. Pandya, K.J.; Dahlberg, S.; Hidalgo, M.; Cohen, R.B.; Lee, M.W.; Schiller, J.H.; Johnson, D.H.; Eastern Cooperative Oncology Group. A randomized, phase II trial of two dose levels of temsirolimus (CCI-779) in patients with extensive-stage small cell lung cancer who have responding or stable disease after induction chemotherapy: A trial of the Eastern Cooperative Oncology Group (E1500). *J. Thorac. Oncol.* **2007**, *2*, 1036–1041. [CrossRef] [PubMed]

65. Schneider, B.J.; Kalemkerian, G.P.; Ramnath, N.; Kraut, M.J.; Wozniak, A.J.; Worden, F.P.; Ruckdeschel, J.C.; Zhang, X.; Chen, W.; Gadgeel, S.M. Phase II trial of imatinib maintenance therapy after irinotecan and cisplatin in patients with c-Kit-positive, extensive-stage small-cell lung cancer. *Clin. Lung Cancer* **2010**, *11*, 223–227. [CrossRef] [PubMed]

66. Spigel, D.R.; Hainsworth, J.D.; Simons, L.; Meng, C.; Burris, H.A., 3rd; Yardley, D.A.; Grapski, R.; Schreeder, M.; Mallidi, P.V.; Greco, F.A.; et al. Irinotecan, carboplatin, and imatinib in untreated extensive-stage small-cell lung cancer: A phase II trial of the Minnie Pearl Cancer Research Network. *J. Thorac. Oncol.* **2007**, *2*, 854–861. [CrossRef]

67. Krug, L.M.; Crapanzano, J.P.; Azzoli, C.G.; Miller, V.A.; Rizvi, N.; Gomez, J.; Kris, M.G.; Pizzo, B.; Tyson, L.; Dunne, M.; et al. Imatinib mesylate lacks activity in small cell lung carcinoma expressing c-kit protein: A phase II clinical trial. *Cancer* **2005**, *103*, 2128–2131. [CrossRef]

68. Moore, A.M.; Einhorn, L.H.; Estes, D.; Govindan, R.; Axelson, J.; Vinson, J.; Breen, T.E.; Yu, M.; Hanna, N.H. Gefitinib in patients with chemo-sensitive and chemo-refractory relapsed small cell cancers: A Hoosier Oncology Group phase II trial. *Lung Cancer* **2006**, *52*, 93–97. [CrossRef]

69. Tarhini, A.; Kotsakis, A.; Gooding, W.; Shuai, Y.; Petro, D.; Friedland, D.; Belani, C.P.; Dacic, S.; Argiris, A. Phase II study of everolimus (RAD001) in previously treated small cell lung cancer. *Clin. Cancer Res.* **2010**, *16*, 5900–5907. [CrossRef]

70. Sattler, M.; Salgia, R. Molecular and cellular biology of small cell lung cancer. *Semin. Oncol.* **2003**, *30*, 57–71. [CrossRef]

71. Bikfalvi, A.; Klein, S.; Pintucci, G.; Rifkin, D.B. Biological roles of fibroblast growth factor-2. *Endocr. Rev.* **1997**, *18*, 26–45.

72. Ruotsalainen, T.; Joensuu, H.; Mattson, K.; Salven, P. High Pretreatment Serum Concentration of Basic Fibroblast Growth Factor Is a Predictor of Poor Prognosis in Small Cell Lung Cancer. *Cancer Epidemiol. Biomark. Prev.* **2002**, *11*, 1492–1495.

73. Dai, S.; Zhou, Z.; Chen, Z.; Xu, G.; Chen, Y. Fibroblast Growth Factor Receptors (FGFRs): Structures and Small Molecule Inhibitors. *Cells* **2019**, *8*, 614. [CrossRef] [PubMed]

74. Koch, J.P.; Aebersold, D.M.; Zimmer, Y.; Medová, M. MET targeting: Time for a rematch. *Oncogene* **2020**, *39*, 2845–2862. [CrossRef] [PubMed]

75.   Desai, A.; Adjei, A.A. FGFR signaling as a target for lung cancer therapy. *J. Thorac. Oncol.* **2016**, *11*, 9–20. [CrossRef] [PubMed]

76.   Rudin, C.M.; Salgia, R.; Wang, X.; Hodgson, L.D.; Masters, G.A.; Green, M.; Vokes, E.E. Randomized phase II study of carboplatin and etoposide with or without the bcl-2 antisense oligonucleotide oblimersen for extensive-stage small-cell lung cancer: CALGB 30103. *J. Clin. Oncol.* **2008**, *26*, 870–876. [CrossRef] [PubMed]

77.   Rudin, C.M.; Hann, C.L.; Garon, E.B.; de Oliveira, M.R.; Bonomi, P.D.; Camidge, D.R.; Chu, Q.; Giaccone, G.; Khaira, D.; Ramalingam, S.S.; et al. Phase II study of single-agent navitoclax (ABT-263) and biomarker correlates in patients with relapsed small cell lung cancer. *Clin. Cancer Res.* **2012**, *18*, 3163–3169. [CrossRef] [PubMed]

78.   Lochmann, T.L.; Floros, K.V.; Naseri, M.; Powell, K.M.; Cook, W.; March, R.J.; Stein, G.T.; Greninger, P.; Maves, Y.K.; Saunders, L.R.; et al. Venetoclax is effective in small-cell lung cancers with high BCL-2 expression. *Clin. Cancer Res.* **2018**, *24*, 360–369. [CrossRef]

79.   Rudin, C.M.; Poirier, J.T.; Byers, L.A.; Dive, C.; Dowlati, A.; George, J.; Heymach, J.V.; Johnson, J.E.; Lehman, J.M.; MacPherson, D.; et al. Molecular subtypes of small cell lung cancer: A synthesis of human and mouse model data. *Nat. Rev. Cancer* **2019**, *19*, 289–297. [CrossRef]

80.   Simos, D.; Sajjady, G.; Sergi, M.; Liew, M.S.; Califano, R.; Ho, C.; Leighl, N.; White, S.; Summers, Y.; Petrcich, W.; et al. Third-line chemotherapy in small-cell lung cancer: An international analysis. *Clin. Lung Cancer* **2014**, *15*, 110–118. [CrossRef]

81.   Sos, M.L.; Dietlein, F.; Peifer, M.; Schöttle, J.; Balke-Want, H.; Müller, C.; Koker, M.; Richters, A.; Heynck, S.; Malchers, F.; et al. A framework for identification of actionable cancer genome dependencies in small cell lung cancer. *Proc. Natl. Acad. Sci. USA* **2012**, *109*, 17034–17039. [CrossRef]

82.   Mertz, J.A.; Conery, A.R.; Bryant, B.M.; Sandy, P.; Balasubramanian, S.; Mele, D.A.; Bergeron, L.; Sims, R.J., 3rd. Targeting MYC dependence in cancer by inhibiting BET bromodomains. *Proc. Natl. Acad. Sci. USA* **2011**, *108*, 16669–16674. [CrossRef]

83.   Owonikoko, T.; Nackaerts, K.; Csoszi, T.; Ostoros, G.; Baik, C.; Ullmann, C.D.; Zagadailov, E.; Sheldon-Waniga, E.; Huebner, D. OA05.05 randomized phase 2 study: Alisertib (MLN8237) or placebo + paclitaxel as second-line therapy for small-cell lung cancer (SCLC). *J. Thorac. Oncol.* **2017**, *12*, S261–S262. [CrossRef]

84.   Mir, S.E.; De Witt Hamer, P.C.; Krawczyk, P.M.; Balaj, L.; Claes, A.; Niers, J.M.; Van Tilborg, A.A.G.; Zwinderman, A.H.; Geerts, D.; Kaspers, G.J.L.; et al. In silico analysis of kinase expression identifies WEE1 as a gatekeeper against mitotic catastrophe in glioblastoma. *Cancer Cell* **2010**, *18*, 244–257. [CrossRef] [PubMed]

85.   Sen, T.; Tong, P.; Diao, L.; Li, L.; Fan, Y.; Hoff, J.; Heymach, J.V.; Wang, J.; Byers, L.A. Targeting AXL and mTOR pathway overcomes primary and acquired resistance to WEE1 inhibition in small-cell lung cancer. *Clin. Cancer Res.* **2017**, *23*, 6239–6253. [CrossRef] [PubMed]

86.   Fang, Y.; McGrail, D.J.; Sun, C.; Labrie, M.; Chen, X.; Zhang, D.; Ju, Z.; Vellano, C.P.; Lu, Y.; Li, Y.; et al. Sequential therapy with PARP and WEE1 inhibitors minimizes toxicity while maintaining efficacy. *Cancer Cell* **2019**, *35*, 851.e7–867.e7. [CrossRef] [PubMed]

87.   Cardnell, R.J.; Feng, Y.; Mukherjee, S.; Diao, L.; Tong, P.; Stewart, C.A.; Masrorpour, F.; Fan, Y.; Nilsson, M.; Shen, Y.; et al. Activation of the PI3K/mTOR pathway following PARP inhibition in small cell Lung cancer. *PLoS ONE* **2016**, *11*, e0152584. [CrossRef]

88.   Owonikoko, T.K.; Dahlberg, S.E.; Sica, G.L.; Wagner, L.I.; Wade, J.L.; Srkalovic, G.; Lash, B.W.; Leach, J.W.; Leal, T.B.; Aggarwal, C.; et al. Randomized phase II trial of cisplatin and etoposide in combination with veliparib or placebo for extensive-stage small-cell lung cancer: ECOG-ACRIN 2511 study. *J. Clin. Oncol.* **2018**, *3*, 222–229. [CrossRef]

89.   Inno, A.; Stagno, A.; Gori, S. Schlafen-11 (SLFN11): A step forward towards personalized medicine in small-cell lung cancer? *Transl. Lung Cancer Res.* **2018**, *7* (Suppl. S4), S341–S345. [CrossRef]

90.   Laird, J.H.; Lok, B.H.; Ma, J.; Bell, A.; de Stanchina, E.; Poirier, J.T.; Rudin, C.M. Talazoparib is a potent radiosensitizer in small cell lung cancer cell lines and xenografts. *Clin. Cancer Res.* **2018**, *24*, 5143–5152. [CrossRef]

91.   Kunnimalaiyaan, M.; Chen, H. Tumor suppressor role of Notch-1 signaling in neuroendocrine tumors. *Oncologist* **2007**, *12*, 535–542. [CrossRef]

92. Chapman, G.; Sparrow, D.B.; Kremmer, E.; Dunwoodie, S.L. Notch inhibition by the ligand DELTA-LIKE 3 defines the mechanism of abnormal vertebral segmentation in spondylocostal dysostosis. *Hum. Mol. Genet.* **2011**, *20*, 905–916. [CrossRef]

93. Saunders, L.R.; Bankovich, A.J.; Anderson, W.C.; Aujay, M.A.; Bheddah, S.; Black, K.; Desai, R.; Escarpe, P.A.; Hampl, J.; Laysang, A.; et al. A DLL3-targeted antibody-drug conjugate eradicates high-grade pulmonary neuroendocrine tumor initiating cells in vivo. *Sci. Transl. Med.* **2015**, *7*, 302ra136. [CrossRef]

94. Morgensztern, D.; Besse, B.; Greillier, L.; Santana-Davila, R.; Ready, N.; Hann, C.L.; Glisson, B.S.; Farago, A.F.; Dowlati, A.; Rudin, C.M.; et al. Efficacy and safety of rovalpituzumab tesirine in third-line and beyond patients with DLL3-Expressing, relapsed/refractory small-cell lung cancer: Results from the phase II trinity study. *Clin. Cancer Res.* **2019**, *25*, 6958–6966. [CrossRef] [PubMed]

95. Mullard, A. Cancer stem cell candidate Rova-T discontinued. *Nat. Rev. Drug Discov.* **2019**, *18*, 814. [CrossRef] [PubMed]

96. Mumby, M. PP2A: Unveiling a reluctant tumor suppressor. *Cell* **2007**, *130*, 21–24. [CrossRef] [PubMed]

97. Perrotti, D.; Neviani, P. Protein phosphatase 2A: A target for anticancer therapy. *Lancet Oncol.* **2013**, *14*, e229–e238. [CrossRef]

98. Neviani, P.; Perrotti, D. SETting OP449 into the PP2A-activating drug family. *Clin. Cancer Res.* **2014**, *20*, 2026–2028. [CrossRef] [PubMed]

99. Matsuoka, Y.; Nagahara, Y.; Ikekita, M.; Shinomiya, T. A novel immunosuppressive agent FTY720 induced Akt dephosphorylation in leukemia cells. *Br. J. Pharmacol.* **2003**, *138*, 1303–1312. [CrossRef]

100. Cristóbal, I.; Madoz-Gúrpide, J.; Manso, R.; González-Alonso, P.; Rojo, F.; García-Foncillas, J. Potential anti-tumor effects of FTY720 associated with PP2A activation: A brief review. *Curr. Med. Res. Opin.* **2016**, *32*, 1137–1141. [CrossRef]

101. Gutierrez, A.; Pan, L.; Groen, R.W.J.; Baleydier, F.; Kentsis, A.; Marineau, J.; Grebliunaite, R.; Kozakewich, E.; Reed, C.; Pflumio, F.; et al. Phenothiazines induce PP2A-mediated apoptosis in T cell acute lymphoblastic leukemia. *J. Clin. Investig.* **2014**, *124*, 644–655. [CrossRef]

102. Kauko, O.; O'Connor, C.M.; Kulesskiy, E.; Sangodkar, J.; Aakula, A.; Izadmehr, S.; Yetukuri, L.; Yadav, B.; Padzik, A.; Laajala, T.D.; et al. PP2A inhibition is a druggable MEK inhibitor resistance mechanism in KRAS-mutant lung cancer cells. *Sci. Transl. Med.* **2018**, *10*, eaaq1093. [CrossRef]

103. Shimizu, T.; Tolcher, A.W.; Papadopoulos, K.P.; Beeram, M.; Rasco, D.W.; Smith, L.S.; Gunn, S.; Smetzer, L.; Mays, T.A.; Kaiser, B.; et al. The clinical effect of the dual-targeting strategy involving PI3K/AKT/mTOR and RAS/MEK/ERK pathways in patients with advanced cancer. *Clin. Cancer Res.* **2012**, *18*, 2316–2325. [CrossRef]

104. Chung, V.; Mansfield, A.S.; Braiteh, F.; Richards, D.; Durivage, H.; Ungerleider, R.S.; Johnson, F.; Kovach, J.S. Safety, Tolerability, and Preliminary Activity of LB-100, an Inhibitor of Protein Phosphatase 2A, in Patients with Relapsed Solid Tumors: An Open-Label, Dose Escalation, First-in-Human, Phase I Trial. *Clin. Cancer Res.* **2017**, *23*, 3277–3284. [CrossRef] [PubMed]

105. Ho, W.S.; Wang, H.; Maggio, D.; Kovach, J.S.; Zhang, Q.; Song, Q.; Marincola, F.M.; Heiss, J.D.; Gilbert, M.R.; Lu, R.; et al. Pharmacologic inhibition of protein phosphatase-2A achieves durable immune-mediated antitumor activity when combined with PD-1 blockade. *Nat. Commun.* **2018**, *9*, 2126. [CrossRef] [PubMed]

106. Taffs, R.E.; Redegeld, F.A.; Sitkovsky, M.V. Modulation of cytolytic T lymphocyte functions by an inhibitor of serine/threonine phosphatase, okadaic acid. Enhancement of cytolytic T lymphocyte-mediated cytotoxicity. *J. Immunol.* **1991**, *147*, 722–728. [PubMed]

107. Cui, J.; Wang, H.; Medina, R.; Zhang, Q.; Xu, C.; Indig, I.H.; Zhou, J.; Song, Q.; Dmitriev, P.; Sun, M.Y.; et al. Inhibition of PP2A with LB-100 Enhances Efficacy of CAR-T Cell Therapy Against Glioblastoma. *Cancers* **2020**, *12*, 139. [CrossRef] [PubMed]

108. Hong, C.S.; Ho, W.; Zhang, C.; Yang, C.; Elder, J.B.; Zhuang, Z. LB100, a small molecule inhibitor of PP2A with potent chemo- and radio-sensitizing potential. *Cancer Biol. Ther.* **2015**, *16*, 821–833. [CrossRef]

109. Cui, Q.; Wen, S.; Huang, P. Targeting cancer cell mitochondria as a therapeutic approach: Recent updates. *Future Med. Chem.* **2017**, *9*, 929–949. [CrossRef]

110. Kalyanaraman, B.; Cheng, G.; Hardy, M.; Quari, M.; Lopez, M.; Joseph, J.; Zielonka, J.; Dwinell, M.B. A review of the basics of mitochondrial bioenergetics, metabolism, and related signaling pathways in cancer cells: Therapeutic targeting of tumor mitochondria with lipophilic cationic compounds. *Redox Biol.* **2018**, *14*, 316–327. [CrossRef]

111. Hamilton, E.P.; Birrer, M.J.; DiCarlo, B.A.; Gaillard, S.; Martin, L.P.; Nemunaitis, J.J.; Perez, R.P.; Schilder, R.J.; Annunziata, C.M.; Begley, C.G.; et al. A phase 1b, open-label, non-randomized multicenter study of birinapant in combination with conatumumab in subjects with relapsed epithelial ovarian cancer, primary peritoneal cancer, or fallopian tube cancer. *J. Clin. Oncol.* **2015**, *33*, 5571. [CrossRef]

112. Hurwitz, H.I.; Smith, D.C.; Pitot, H.C.; Brill, J.M.; Chugh, R.; Rouits, E.; Rubin, J.; Strickler, J.; Vuagniaux, G.; Sorensen, J.M.; et al. Safety, pharmacokinetics and pharmacodynamics properties of oral DEBIO1143 (AT-406) in patients with advanced cancer: Results of a first-in-man study. *Cancer Chemother. Pharmacol.* **2015**, *75*, 851–859. [CrossRef]

113. Bendell, J.C.; Patel, M.R.; Infante, J.R.; Kurkjian, C.D.; Jones, S.F.; Pant, S.; Burris, H.A., 3rd; Moreno, O.; Esquibel, V.; Levin, W.; et al. Phase 1, open-label, dose escalation, safety, and pharmacokinetics study of ME-344 as a single agent in patients with refractory solid tumors. *Cancer* **2015**, *121*, 1056–1063. [CrossRef]

114. Diamond, J.R.; Goff, B.; Forster, M.D.; Bendell, J.C.; Britten, C.D.; Gordon, M.S.; Gabra, H.; Waterhouse, D.M.; Poole, M.; Camidge, D.R.; et al. Phase Ib study of the mitochondrial inhibitor ME-344 plus topotecan in patients with previously treated, locally advanced or metastatic small cell lung, ovarian and cervical cancers. *Investig. New Drugs* **2017**, *35*, 627–633. [CrossRef] [PubMed]

115. Greeno, E.; Borazanci, E.H.; Gockerman, J.P.; Korn, R.L.; Saluja, A.; VonHoff, D.D. Phase I dose escalation and pharmokinetic study of a modified schedule of 14-ophosphonooxymethyltriptolide. *J. Clin. Oncol.* **2016**, *34*, TPS472. [CrossRef]

116. Stein, M.N.; Bertino, J.R.; Kaufman, H.L.; Mayer, T.; Moss, R.; Silk, A.; Chan, N.; Malhotra, J.; Rodriguez, L.; Aisner, J.; et al. First-in-human clinical trial of oral ONC201 in patients with refractory solid tumors. *Clin. Cancer Res.* **2017**, *23*, 4163–4169. [CrossRef] [PubMed]

117. Roth, K.G.; Mambetsariev, I.; Kulkarni, P.; Salgia, R. The mitochondrion as an emerging therapeutic target in cancer. *Trends Mol. Med.* **2020**, *26*, 119–134. [CrossRef] [PubMed]

118. Lobo, N.A.; Shimono, Y.; Qian, D.; Clarke, M.F. The biology of cancer stem cells. *Annu. Rev. Cell Dev. Biol.* **2007**, *23*, 675–699. [CrossRef]

119. Yang, Y.M.; Chang, J.W. Current status and issues in cancer stem cell study. *Cancer Investig.* **2008**, *26*, 741–755. [CrossRef]

120. Wicha, M.S.; Liu, S.; Dontu, G. Cancer stem cells: An old idea—A paradigm shift. *Cancer Res.* **2006**, *66*, 1883–1896. [CrossRef]

121. Takebe, N.; Miele, L.; Harris, P.J.; Jeong, W.; Bando, H.; Kahn, M.; Yang, S.X.; Ivy, S.P. Targeting Notch, Hedgehog, and Wnt pathways in cancer stem cells: Clinical update. *Nat. Rev. Clin. Oncol.* **2015**, *12*, 445–464. [CrossRef]

122. Codony-Servat, J.; Verlicchi, A.; Rosell, R. Cancer stem cells in small cell lung cancer. *Transl. Lung Cancer Res.* **2016**, *5*, 16–25.

123. Stewart, C.A.; Byers, L.A. Altering the course of small cell lung cancer: Targeting cancer stem cells via LSD1 inhibition. *Cancer Cell* **2015**, *28*, 4–6. [CrossRef]

124. Bauer, T.M.; Besse, B.; Martinez-Marti, A.; Trigo, J.M.; Moreno, V.; Garrido, P.; Ferron-Brady, G.; Wu, Y.; Park, J.; Collingwood, T.; et al. Phase I, Open-Label, Dose-Escalation Study of the Safety, Pharmacokinetics, Pharmacodynamics, and Efficacy of GSK2879552 in Relapsed/Refractory SCLC. *J. Thorac. Oncol.* **2019**, *14*, 1828–1838. [CrossRef] [PubMed]

125. Mohammad, H.P.; Kruger, R.G. Antitumor activity of LSD1 inhibitors in Lung cancer. *Mol. Cell Oncol.* **2016**, *3*, e1117700. [CrossRef] [PubMed]

126. Ropacki, M.; Navarro, A.; Maes, T.; Gutierrez, S.; Bullock, R.; Buesa, C. P2.12-04 CLEPSIDRA: A Phase II Trial Combining Iadademstat with Platinum-Etoposide in Platinum-Sensitive Relapsed SCLC Patients. *J. Thorac. Oncol.* **2019**, *14*, S813. [CrossRef]

127. Sheng, W.; LaFleur, M.W.; Nguyen, T.H.; Chen, S.; Chakravarthy, A.; Conway, J.R.; Li, Y.; Chen, H.; Yang, H.; Hsu, P.-H.; et al. LSD1 ablation stimulates anti-tumor immunity and enables checkpoint blockade. *Cell* **2018**, *174*, 549–563. [CrossRef]

128. Morgensztern, D.; Rose, M.; Waqar, S.N.; Morris, J.; Ma, P.C.; Reid, T.; Brzezniak, C.E.; Zeman, K.G.; Padmanabhan, A.; Hirth, J.; et al. RRx-001 followed by platinum plus etoposide in patients with previously treated small-cell lung cancer. *Br. J. Cancer* **2019**, *121*, 211–217. [CrossRef] [PubMed]

129. Weiskopf, K.; Jahchan, N.S.; Schnorr, P.J.; Cristea, S.; Ring, A.M.; Maute, R.L.; Volkmer, A.K.; Volkmer, J.-P.; Liu, J.; Lim, J.S.; et al. CD47-blocking immunotherapies stimulate macrophage-mediated destruction of small-cell lung cancer. *J. Clin. Investig.* **2016**, *126*, 2610–2620. [CrossRef]

130. Bonanno, L.; Pavan, A.; Dieci, M.V.; Di Liso, E.; Schiavon, M.; Comacchio, G.; Attili, I.; Pasello, G.; Calabrese, F.; Rea, F.; et al. The role of immune microenvironment in small-cell lung cancer: Distribution of PD-L1 expression and prognostic role of FOXP3-positive tumour infiltrating lymphocytes. *Eur. J. Cancer* **2018**, *101*, 191–200. [CrossRef]

131. Antonia, S.J.; López-Martin, J.A.; Bendell, J.; Ott, P.A.; Taylor, M.; Eder, J.P.; Jäger, D.; Pietanza, M.C.; Le, D.T.; de Braud, F.; et al. Nivolumab alone and nivolumab plus ipilimumab in recurrent small-cell lung cancer (CheckMate 032): A multicentre, open-label, phase 1/2 trial. *Lancet Oncol.* **2016**, *17*, 883–895. [CrossRef]

132. Goodman, A.M.; Kato, S.; Bazhenova, L.; Patel, S.P.; Frampton, G.M.; Miller, V.; Stephens, P.J.; Daniels, G.A.; Kurzrock, R. Tumor mutational burden as an independent predictor of response to immunotherapy in diverse cancers. *Mol. Cancer Ther.* **2017**, *16*, 2598–2608. [CrossRef]

133. Hellmann, M.D.; Callahan, M.K.; Awad, M.M.; Calvo, E.; Ascierto, P.A.; Atmaca, A.; Rizvi, N.A.; Hirsch, F.R.; Selvaggi, G.; Szustakowski, J.; et al. Tumor mutational burden and efficacy of Nivolumab monotherapy and in combination with ipilimumab in small-cell lung cancer. *Cancer Cell* **2018**, *33*, 853.e4–861.e4. [CrossRef]

134. Hou, J.M.; Krebs, M.G.; Lancashire, L.; Sloane, R.; Backen, A.; Swain, R.K.; Priest, L.J.; Greystoke, A.; Zhou, C.; Morris, K.; et al. Clinical significance and molecular characteristics of circulating tumor cells and circulating tumor microemboli in patients with small-cell lung cancer. *J. Clin. Oncol.* **2012**, *30*, 525–532. [CrossRef] [PubMed]

135. Belani, C.P.; Dahlberg, S.E.; Rudin, C.M.; Fleisher, M.; Chen, H.X.; Takebe, N.; Velasco, M.R., Jr.; Tester, W.J.; Sturtz, K.; Hann, C.L.; et al. Vismodegib or cixutumumab in combination with standard chemotherapy for patients with extensive-stage small cell lung cancer: A trial of the ECOG-ACRIN Cancer Research Group (E1508). *Cancer* **2016**, *122*, 2371–2378. [CrossRef] [PubMed]

136. Pietanza, M.C.; Litvak, A.M.; Varghese, A.M.; Krug, L.M.; Fleisher, M.; Teitcher, J.B.; Holodny, A.I.; Sima, C.S.; Woo, K.M.; Ng, K.K.; et al. A phase I trial of the Hedgehog inhibitor, sonidegib (LDE225), in combination with etoposide and cisplatin for the initial treatment of extensive stage small cell lung cancer. *Lung Cancer* **2016**, *99*, 23–30. [CrossRef] [PubMed]

137. Almodovar, K.; Iams, W.T.; Meador, C.B.; Zhao, Z.; York, S.; Horn, L.; Yan, Y.; Hernandez, J.; Chen, H.; Shyr, Y.; et al. Longitudinal cell-free DNA analysis in patients with small cell lung cancer reveals dynamic insights into treatment efficacy and disease relapse. *J. Thorac. Oncol.* **2018**, *13*, 112–123. [CrossRef]

138. Paz-Ares, L.G.; Trigo Perez, J.M.; Besse, B.; Moreno, V.; Lopez, R.; Sala, M.A.; Aix, S.P.; Fernandez, C.M.; Siguero, M.; Kahatt, C.M.; et al. Efficacy and safety profile of lurbinectedin in second-line SCLC patients: Results from a phase II single-agent trial. *J. Clin. Oncol.* **2019**, *37*, 8506. [CrossRef]

139. Kontogianni, K.; Nicholson, A.G.; Butcher, D.; Sheppard, M.N. CD56: A useful tool for the diagnosis of small cell lung carcinomas on biopsies with extensive crush artefact. *J. Clin. Pathol.* **2005**, *58*, 978–980. [CrossRef]

140. Yu, L.; Lu, Y.; Yao, Y.; Liu, Y.; Wang, Y.; Lai, Q.; Zhang, R.; Li, W.; Wang, R.; Fu, Y.; et al. Promiximab-duocarmycin, a new CD56 antibody-drug conjugates, is highly efficacious in small cell lung cancer xenograft models. *Oncotarget* **2017**, *9*, 5197–5207. [CrossRef]

141. Zaman, S.; Jadid, H.; Denson, A.C.; Gray, J.E. Targeting Trop-2 in solid tumors: Future prospects. *Onco Targets Ther.* **2019**, *12*, 1781–1790. [CrossRef]

142. Ocean, A.J.; Starodub, A.N.; Bardia, A.; Vahdat, L.T.; Isakoff, S.J.; Guarino, M.; Messersmith, W.A.; Picozzi, V.J.; Mayer, I.A.; Wegener, W.A.; et al. Sacituzumab govitecan (IMMU-132), an Anti-Trop-2-SN-38 antibody-drug conjugate for the treatment of diverse epithelial cancers: Safety and pharmacokinetics. *Cancer* **2017**, *123*, 3843–3854. [CrossRef]

143. Simone, C.B., 2nd; Berman, A.T.; Jabbour, S.K. Harnessing the potential synergy of combining radiation therapy and immunotherapy for thoracic malignancies. *Transl. Lung Cancer Res.* **2017**, *6*, 109–112. [CrossRef]

144. McColl, K.; Wildey, G.; Sakre, N.; Lipka, M.B.; Behtaj, M.; Kresak, A.; Chen, Y.; Yang, M.; Velcheti, V.; Fu, P.; et al. Reciprocal expression of INSM1 and YAP1 defines subgroups in small cell lung cancer. *Oncotarget* **2017**, *8*, 73745–73756. [CrossRef] [PubMed]

145. Huang, Y.H.; Klingbeil, O.; He, X.Y.; Wu, X.S.; Arun, G.; Lu, B.; Somerville, T.; Milazzo, J.P.; Wilkinson, J.E.; Demerdash, O.E.; et al. POU2F3 is a master regulator of a tuft cell-like variant of small cell lung cancer. *Genes Dev.* **2018**, *32*, 915–928. [CrossRef] [PubMed]

146. Polley, E.; Kunkel, M.; Evans, D.; Silvers, T.; Delosh, R.; Laudeman, J.; Ogle, C.; Reinhart, R.; Selby, M.; Connelly, J.; et al. Small cell lung cancer screen of oncology drugs, investigational agents, and gene and microRNA expression. *J. Natl. Cancer Inst.* **2016**, *108*, djw122. [CrossRef] [PubMed]

147. Barretina, J.; Caponigro, G.; Stransky, N.; Venkatesan, K.; Margolin, A.A.; Kim, S.; Wilson, C.J.; Lehár, J.; Kryukov, G.V.; Sonkin, D.; et al. The Cancer Cell Line Encyclopedia enables predictive modelling of anticancer drug sensitivity. *Nature* **2012**, *483*, 603–607. [CrossRef]

148. Mollaoglu, G.; Guthrie, M.R.; Böhm, S.; Brägelmann, J.; Can, I.; Ballieu, P.M.; Marx, A.; George, J.; Heinen, C.; Chalishazar, M.D.; et al. MYC drives progression of small cell lung cancer to a variant neuroendocrine subtype with vulnerability to aurora kinase inhibition. *Cancer Cell* **2017**, *31*, 270–285. [CrossRef]

149. Sonkin, D.; Vural, S.; Thomas, A.; Teicher, B.A. Neuroendocrine negative SCLC is mostly RB1 WT and may be sensitive to CDK4/6 inhibition: Supplemental Tables. *bioRxiv* **2019**. [CrossRef]

8

New Chondrosarcoma Cell Lines with Preserved Stem Cell Properties to Study the Genomic Drift During In Vitro/In Vivo Growth

Veronica Rey [1,2,†], Sofia T. Menendez [1,2,3,†], Oscar Estupiñan [1,2,3], Aida Rodriguez [1], Laura Santos [1], Juan Tornin [1], Lucia Martinez-Cruzado [1], David Castillo [4], Gonzalo R. Ordoñez [4], Serafin Costilla [5], Carlos Alvarez-Fernandez [6], Aurora Astudillo [7], Alejandro Braña [8] and Rene Rodriguez [1,2,3,*]

[1]   University Central Hospital of Asturias—Health and Research Institute of Asturias (ISPA), 33011 Oviedo, Spain; reyvazquezvero@gmail.com (V.R.); sofiatirados@gmail.com (S.T.M.); o_r_e_s_@hotmail.com (O.E.); aidarp.finba@gmail.com (A.R.); laurasd.finba@gmail.com (L.S.); juantornin@gmail.com (J.T.); lucialmc24@gmail.com (L.M.-C.)

[2]   University Institute of Oncology of Asturias, 33011 Oviedo, Spain

[3]   CIBER in Oncology (CIBERONC), 28029 Madrid, Spain

[4]   Disease Research and Medicine (DREAMgenics) S.L., 33011 Oviedo, Spain; david.castillo@dreamgenics.com (D.C.); gonzalo.ordonez@dreamgenics.com (G.R.O.)

[5]   Department of Radiology of the Servicio de Radiología of the University Central Hospital of Asturias, 33011 Oviedo, Spain; costillaserafin@uniovi.es

[6]   Department of Medical Oncology of the Servicio de Radiología of the University Central Hospital of Asturias, 33011 Oviedo, Spain; carlos.alvfer@gmail.com

[7]   Department of Pathology of the Servicio de Radiología of the University Central Hospital of Asturias, 33011 Oviedo, Spain; astudillo@hca.es

[8]   Department of Traumatology of the University Central Hospital of Asturias, 33011 Oviedo, Spain; albravigil@gmail.com

*   Correspondence: renerg.finba@gmail.com

†   These authors contributed equally to the manuscript.

Abstract: For the cancer genomics era, there is a need for clinically annotated close-to-patient cell lines suitable to investigate altered pathways and serve as high-throughput drug-screening platforms. This is particularly important for drug-resistant tumors like chondrosarcoma which has few models available. Here we established and characterized new cell lines derived from two secondary (CDS06 and CDS11) and one dedifferentiated (CDS-17) chondrosarcomas as well as another line derived from a CDS-17-generated xenograft (T-CDS17). These lines displayed cancer stem cell-related and invasive features and were able to initiate subcutaneous and/or orthotopic animal models. Different mutations in Isocitrate Dehydrogenase-1 (*IDH1*), Isocitrate Dehydrogenase-2 (*IDH2*), and Tumor Supressor P53 (*TP53*) and deletion of Cyclin Dependent Kinase Inhibitor 2A (*CDKN2A*) were detected both in cell lines and tumor samples. In addition, other mutations in *TP53* and the amplification of Mouse Double Minute 2 homolog (*MDM2*) arose during cell culture in CDS17 cells. Whole exome sequencing analysis of CDS17, T-CDS17, and matched patient samples confirmed that cell lines kept the most relevant mutations of the tumor, uncovered new mutations and revealed structural variants that emerged during in vitro/in vivo growth. Altogether, this work expanded the panel of clinically and genetically-annotated chondrosarcoma lines amenable for in vivo studies and cancer stem cell (CSC) characterization. Moreover, it provided clues of the genetic drift of chondrosarcoma cells during the adaptation to grow conditions.

Keywords: chondrosarcoma; primary cell lines; cancer stem cells; whole exome sequencing; genomic drift; animal model; cancer preclinical model

1. Introduction

Chondrosarcoma is a malignant cartilage-forming tumor that represents, with approximately 25% of the cases, the second most common bone sarcoma. The most common subtype, representing 80% of the total, is the primary or conventional central chondrosarcoma which is characterized by the pathological formation of hyaline cartilage within the medullar cavity [1]. Other less common subtypes include the periosteal chondrosarcoma, which occurs in the surface of the bone, and secondary chondrosarcoma, which arises in benign lesions such as enchondroma, frequently associated to Ollier disease or Maffucci syndrome, or osteochondroma [1]. The dedifferentiated chondrosarcoma is a distinct variety of chondrosarcoma, accounting for approximately a 10% of the cases. This subtype is characterized by the presence of a low-grade well-differentiated cartilaginous tumor juxtaposed to a high-grade anaplastic sarcoma [1].

Within the complex cytogenetic scenario characteristic of chondrosarcomas, a few chromosomal alterations and gene mutations are frequently found. Thus, mutations in Isocitrate Dehydrogenase-1 (*IDH1*) and -2 (*IDH2*) are found in 87% of enchondromas, up to 70% of conventional central chondrosarcomas and 54% of dedifferentiated chondrosarcomas and may drive sarcomagenic processes [2–4]. In addition, mutations in the major cartilage collagen (*COL2A1*) or Tumor Supressor P53 (*TP53*) genes have been found in approximately 35% and 20% of the chondrosarcomas respectively [5,6]. Other frequent copy number variations, such as the amplification of the 12q13 region, containing Mouse Double Minute 2 homolog (*MDM2*) and the cyclin-dependent kinase 4 genes, and the deletion of the 9p21 region, which includes the Cyclin Dependent Kinase Inhibitor 2A (*CDKN2A*) locus, contribute to the deregulation of the p53 and Retinoblastoma (RB) pathways [5,7].

Wide surgical resection is the mainstay therapeutic option for localized chondrosarcomas. However, these tumors often show high local recurrence and metastatic potential. Furthermore, chondrosarcomas are inherently resistant to conventional chemo and radiotherapy and nowadays there are no effective treatments available for metastatic or inoperable tumors [8–12]. Proposed mechanisms of chemoresistance include the role of the cartilaginous extracellular matrix as a barrier for drug diffusion, the overexpression of members of the adenosine triphosphate (ATP) binding cassette transmembrane family of efflux pumps and antiapoptotic proteins, and the presence of a high percentage of low proliferating/quiescent cells [9,11,12]. Interestingly, some of these features are related to those described for tumor cell subsets presenting stem cell properties (cancer stem cells, CSC). These CSC subpopulations have been characterized in several subtypes of sarcomas and associated to the expression/activity of pluripotency factors, like Sex Determining Region Y-Box 2 (SOX2), stem cell markers, like Aldehyde Dehydrogenase 1 Family Member A1 (ALDH1), or to the ability to grow as floating clonal spheres (tumorspheres) [13,14]. CSC subpopulations have been barely characterized in chondrosarcoma and therefore new models amenable for the study of these subpopulations are needed to find vulnerabilities against these drug-resistant subpopulations.

Despite their failure to completely reproduce the genetic and microenvironmental conditions of tumors, cell lines are still indispensable models to investigate altered mechanisms in cancer, to study CSC subpopulations, and to serve as drug-screening platforms in a high-throughput and logistically simple and rapid way [15–17]. To our knowledge, 14 tumor-derived chondrosarcoma lines, corresponding to seven conventional, five dedifferentiated, and two secondary chondrosarcomas, have been reported so far [18–27]. In this work, we succeeded in establishing three cell lines from two secondary (CDS06 and CDS11) and one dedifferentiated (CDS-17) chondrosarcoma as well as another cell line derived from a CDS-17 xenograft (T-CDS17). We studied their tumorigenic and invasive potential, characterized the present CSC subpopulations, and analyzed the most relevant chondrosarcoma-related genetic alterations both in the cell lines and their original tumors. Furthermore, using a whole exome sequencing (WES) approach in CDS17 and T-CDS17 cells and their matched patient samples we were able to track the genomic adaptation of tumor cells to in vitro and in vivo growth.

2. Experimental Section

2.1. Establishment of Cell Lines

Human samples and data from donors included in this study were provided by the Principado de Asturias BioBank (PT17/0015/0023) integrated in the Spanish National Biobanks Network upon obtaining of written informed consent from patients. All experimental protocols have been performed in accordance with institutional review board guidelines and were approved by the Institutional Ethics Committee of the University Central Hospital of Asturias (approval number: 45/16). This study was performed in accordance with the Declaration of Helsinki.

Tumor samples were subjected to mechanical disaggregation followed by an enzymatic dissociation using MACS® Tissue Dissociation Kit and the GentleMACS Dissociator system (Miltenyi Biotec, Bergisch Gladbach, Germany). At the end of the incubation, culture medium (DMEM-Dulbecco's Modified Eagle Medium supplemented with 10% FBS, 2 mM L-glutamine, 100 U/mL penicillin and 100 μg/mL streptomicin) was added and the cell suspension was filtered to remove clusters. Tumor cells were collected by centrifugation, resuspended in fresh culture medium and seeded in culture flasks. As an alternative protocol to derived cell lines, some fresh tumor specimens were cut into several small fragments, transferred to dry 25 cm^2 culture flasks, covered with a drop of medium and incubated until outgrowth of tumor cells was observed. Cell cultures derived by both methods were subcultured when they reached 80–90% confluence. As a procedure to select tumoral cells and rid of stromal cells, we performed soft agar colony formation assays using the CytoSelect™ 96-Well Cell Transformation Assay Kit (Cell Biolabs Inc, San Francisco, CA, USA). Cells able to form colonies under these anchorage-independent growth conditions are supposed to be transformed. These colonies were recovered, left to attach to plastic substrate and grow in culture medium as normal adherent cultures. Short Tandem Repeat (STR) analyses were performed to compare the identity of cell lines with matched tumor sample (Supplemental Information).

2.2. Tumorsphere Culture

The tumorsphere formation protocol was previously described [28].

2.3. Western Blotting

Whole cell protein extraction and western blotting analysis were performed as previously described [29]. Antibodies used are described in Supplementary Materials.

2.4. Aldefluor Assay and Cell Sorting

Cells with high Aldehyde Dehydrogenase (ALDH) activity was detected and isolated using the Aldefluor™ reagent (Stem Cells Technologies, Grenoble, France) as previously described [13].

2.5. Three-Dimensional Spheroid Invasion Assay

Invasion assays using 3D spheroids in the presence or not of dasatinib or PF-573228 (Selleckchem, Houston, TX, USA) were performed as previously described [30] (see Supplementary Materials information for details).

2.6. In Vivo Tumor Growth

All animal research protocols were carried out in accordance with the institutional guidelines of the University of Oviedo and were approved by the Animal Research Ethical Committee of the University of Oviedo prior to the study (approval code: PROAE 11/2014; date of approval: 9 December 2014). Experiments were done using female NOD.CB17/Prkdcscid/scid/Rj inbreed mice (Janvier Labs,

St. Berthevin, France). For subcutaneous (s.c.) inoculations in the flanks of the mice, 5×10^5 cells mixed 1:1 with BD Matrigel Matrix High Concentration (Becton Dickinson-BD Biosciences, Erembodegem, Belgium) previously diluted 1:1 in culture medium were injected. Tumor volume was determined using a caliper as previously described [31]. One month after inoculation, mice were sacrificed by CO_2 asphyxiation and tumors were extracted and processed for histological analysis. Limited dilution assays (LDA) and calculation of tumor-initiating frequencies (TIF) was performed as described in Supplemental Information. For the intra-bone (i.b.) inoculation, mice were anesthetized with isoflurane and the leg was bent 90° in order to drill the tip of the tibia with a 25G needle before cell inoculation (2×10^5 cells in 5 µl of culture media per mouse) using a 27G needle [32]. In these experiments, tumor growth was evaluated in the preclinical image laboratory of the University of Oviedo using a computed tomography (CT) system (Argus CT, Sedecal, Madrid, Spain) at week 8 after cell inoculation and a µCT system (SkyScan 1174, Bruker, Antwerp, Belgium) following mice sacrifice at week 12 (see Supplementary Materials for analysis conditions).

2.7. Histological Analysis

Human and xenograft samples were fixed in formol, decalcified using solutions with nitric acid (10%) or formic acid (4%)/chlorhydric acid (4%) and embedded in paraffin. Sections of 4-µm were stained with hematoxylin and eosin (H&E) as previously described [29].

2.8. MDM2 and CDKN2A Gene Copy Number Analysis

Genomic DNA was extracted using the QIAmp DNA Mini Kit (Qiagen, Hilden, Germany) and gene amplification was evaluated by real-time PCR. Reactions were carried out using the following primers: for MDM2 gene, Fw 5′-TGGCTGTGTTCAAGTGGTTC-3′ and Rv 5′-GTGGTGACAGGGTGCTCTAAC-3′; for CDKN2A gene, Fw 5′-CACATTCATGTGGGCATTTC-3′ and Rv 5′-TGCTTGTCATGAAGTCGACAG-3′ (Exon 3, recognizing both p14^{ARF} and p16^{INK4} sequences); and for the reference gene RPPH1 (ribonuclease P RNA component H1), Fw 5′-GAGGGAAGCTCATCAGTGG-3′ and Rv 5′-ACATGGGAGTGGAGTGACAG-3′. Dissociation curve analysis of all PCR products showed a single sharp peak and the relative gene copy number was calculated using the $2^{-\Delta\Delta CT}$ method. For each set of samples, DNA from the corresponding healthy tissue was used as a calibrator.

2.9. Mutational Analysis of TP53, IDH1, IDH2, PI3KCA

Genomic DNA were amplified by PCR (Taq PCR Master Mix (2x), EURx Ltd. (Gdańsk, Poland)). The fragments analyzed include: exon 4 of *IDH1* and *IDH2* genes, identified as mutation hot spots in chondrosarcoma; exon 20 of the *PI3KCA* gene; and exons 4 and 6 of the *TP53* gene. Reactions were carried out using the forward and reverse primers detailed in Supplemental Information and the different PCR products were detected by gel electrophoresis in 1.5% agarose, showing a single band. Samples were purified and sequenced by Macrogen Ltd. (Madrid, Spain) and were aligned with the reference sequences of the genes using SnapGene® 4.2.11 (GSL Biotech; available at snapgene.com).

2.10. Library Construction and WES

WES was performed by Macrogen (Seoul, Korea) using 1 µg of genomic DNA from each sample. DNAs were sheared with a Covaris S2 instrument and used for the construction of a paired-end sequencing library as described in the paired-end sequencing sample preparation protocol provided by Illumina. Enrichment of exonic sequences was then performed for each library using the Sure Select All Exon V6 kits following the manufacturer's instructions (Agilent Technologies, Santa Clara, CA, USA). Exon-enriched DNA was pulled down by magnetic beads coated with streptavidin (Invitrogen, Carlsbad, CA, USA), followed by washing, elution, and additional cycles of amplification of the captured library. Enriched libraries were sequenced (2×101 bp) in an Illumina HiSeq4000 sequencer. WES results were processed using the bioinformatics software HD Genome One (DREAMgenics, Oviedo, Spain), certified with IVD/CE-marking (see Supplementary Materials for a comprehensive description of the exome analysis, [33–47]). The datasets generated during the study are available in the European Nucleotide Archive repository [48].

3. Results

3.1. Establishment of Patient-Derived Chondrosarcoma Cell Lines and Analysis of In Vivo Tumorigenic Potential

Surgically resected tumor samples from 11 patients diagnosed of chondrosarcoma at the Hospital Universitario Central de Asturias (Spain) were processed to establish primary cultures. Cultures from two secondary chondrosarcoma, CDS06 (associated with a previous osteochondroma) and CDS11 (presenting Ollier disease), and one from a dedifferentiated chondrosarcoma (CDS-17), were able to growth long term in vitro (Table S1 show an overview of patient and tumor characteristics). These cell lines were able to form colonies in soft agar, an in vitro transformation assay to test the ability of the cells to grow in anchorage independent conditions (Table 1). In order to select the more tumorigenic populations within the cultures, the colonies able to grow in soft agar were recovered and placed back in adherent culture to continue with the corresponding cell line development. Recovered cell lines could be passaged at least 20 times (Table 1) and their identity with the original tumor was confirmed by STR genotyping (Table S2).

Table 1. Functional characterization of chondrosarcoma cell lines.

Cell Line	Chondrosar. Subtype	Anchorage Independ. Growth §	Passage *	Tumorsphere Growth (% Frequency ± SD)		In Vivo Tumor Growth **			Aldefluor Assay (%)	Invasion ‡
						Subcutaneous		Intra-Bone		
				1st Tumorsph. Passage	2nd Tumorsph. Passage	Tumor Growth (Tumors/Mice)	Mean Volume (mm³ ± SD)	Tumor Growth (Tumors/Mice)		
CDS06	Secondary	Yes	20	Yes (0.24 ± 0.10)	Yes (0.10 ± 0.05)	n/a	n/a	n/a	Yes (4.01)	No
CDS11	Secondary	Yes	25	Yes (0.28 ± 0.11)	Yes (0.16 ± 0.06)	Yes (3/3)	77.00 ± 10.91	n/a	Yes (5.05)	Yes
CDS17	Dedifferent.	Yes	<35	Yes (0.20 ± 0.08)	Yes (0.10 ± 0.01)	Yes (3/3)	198.27 ± 5.11	Yes (1/2)	Yes (2.94)	Yes
T-CDS17	Dedifferent.	Yes	<35	Yes (0.26 ± 0.08)	Yes (0.11 ± 0.01)	Yes (3/3)	350.32 ± 39.45 ¶	Yes (2/2)	Yes (14.50)	Yes

(§) Ability to growth forming colonies in embedded in soft agar. (*) number of passages reached so far in adherent cultures. (**) Tumor growth was follow for 1 and 2.5 months in subcutaneous and intra-bone experiments respectively. (‡) Ability of 3D spheroids to invade collagen matrices. (¶) There is a significant difference between the volumes of tumors generated by CDS17 and T-CDS17 cells ($p = 0.043$; two side Student's t-test. SD: Standard Deviation).

Two of the cell lines (CDS11, CDS17) were assayed for their ability to initiate tumor growth in vivo. Both of them were able to form small slow-growing tumors after subcutaneous (s.c.) inoculation in immunodeficient mice after 1 month (Figure 1A and Table 1). Following this, we generated a new cell line derived from a CDS17-xenograft tumor. Subsequent transplantation of this new cell line, T-CDS17, resulted in a more aggressive tumor growth (formation of significantly bigger tumors in similar latency periods), thus indicating that the tumor could be effectively propagated in vivo (Table 1). Histological analysis showed that the original CDS11 tumor was a malignant chondrosarcoma invading intra-trabecular bone matrix and presenting well differentiated and dedifferentiated areas. There was no inflammatory infiltrate and the dedifferentiated subcomponent displayed a mitotic index of 15 mitoses per 10 high power fields (HPF, 40X). The histology of tumors grown from the CDS11 line resembled that of the more undifferentiated/dedifferentiated areas of the original patient.

Tumor, with tumor cells distributed diffusely in a mesenchymal matrix. No well-differentiated component was found in these tumors. Inflammation was also absent and tumors showed 9 mitoses per 10 HPF (Figure 1A). The CDS17 patient sample was a high-grade chondrosarcoma displaying the characteristic chondroid differentiation, with tumor cells presenting pericellular matrix and surrounded by a chondroid extracellular matrix. There was no inflammation present in this tumor and its mitotic index was 18 mitoses per 10 HPF. Tumors derived from CDS17 and T-CDS17 cells lines maintained chondroid differentiation, with tumor cells presenting pericellular halos and embedded in a chondroid basophilic extracellular matrix. There were no inflammatory infiltrates in these tumors and its mitotic index was 17 and 25 mitoses per 10 HPF for CDS17 and T-CDS17 respectively (Figure 1A).

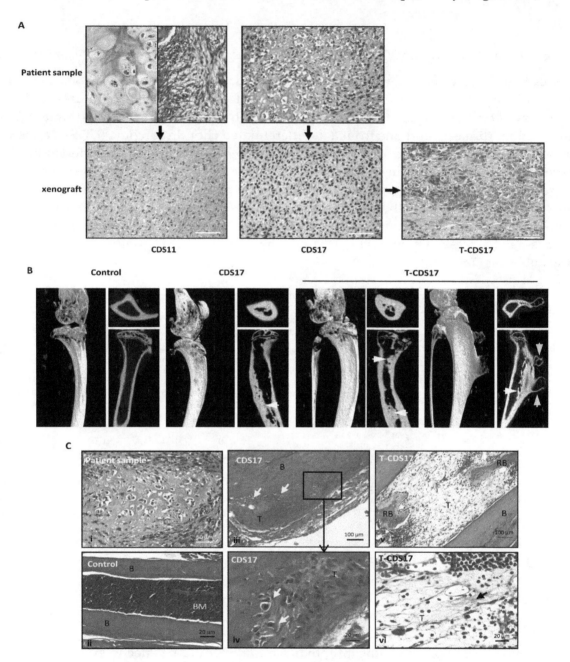

Figure 1. In vivo tumorigenicty of chondrosarcoma cell lines. (**A**) Histological analysis (H&E staining) of original patient tumors and tumors developed 1 month after subcutaneous (s.c.) inoculation of CDS11, CDS17, and T-CDS17 cell lines in immunodeficient mice. Two different areas of the CDS11 patient tumor sample are shown. scale bars = 150 μm. (**B**) Radiologic examination (μCT scan) of tumors developed after intra-bone (i.b.) inoculation of CDS17 and T-CDS17 cells in immunodeficient mice. Coronal, sagittal and axial images are shown. Compared to a control leg, intra-medullar formation of tumor bone/osteoid formation (white arrows) is shown in mice inoculated with both cell lines. In addition, a mouse inoculated with T-CDS17 cells presented an extra-medullar lesion compatible with the radiographic features of osteochondrosarcoma (orange arrows). (**C**) H&E staining of an original patient sample (i), a control leg (ii), and tumors formed after i.b. inoculation of CDS17 (iii and iv) and T-CDS17 (v and vi) cells lines. Chondroid.like cells (yellow arrows) and areas of fibrillar (black arrow) and amorphous (orange arrow) osteo-chondroid matrix are indicated. (B: bone; RB: reactive bone).

In an attempt to create more faithful animal models CDS17 and T-CDS17 cells were inoculated intra-tibia in immunodeficient mice. Both CDS17 (1 out of 2 mice) and T-CDS17 (2 out of 2 mice) cells were able to generate tumor growth in this orthotopic location. Computerized tomography (CT) analysis at day 50 after inoculation (Figure S1) and microCT analysis at the end point of the experiment (day 80) (Figure 1B) revealed the formation of tumors resembling the radiological features of human chondrosarcomas. These tumors showed the presence of a dotted pattern chondroid-like matrix inside the bone marrow cavity. In addition, one of the T-CDS17 generated tumors also displayed extra-medullar tumor growth, forming an osteochondroid exostosis-like lesion (Figure 1B and Figure S1). Histological sections of these orthotopically grown tumors also resembled the main features of the patient sample (Figure 1C(i)), with chondrogenic tumor cells presenting pericellular halos and embedded in cartilaginous matrix (Figure 1C(iii,iv)). In addition, legs inoculated with tumor cells showed bone marrow cavities filled by dedifferentiated mesenchymal cells producing fibrillar and amorphous osteo-chondroid matrix and presenting extensive areas of reactive bone (Figure 1C(v,vi)). None of tumors presented inflammatory component and they showed mitotic indexes between 7 (CDS17) and 10 (T-CDS17) mitoses per 10 HP.

3.2. Genetic Characterization of Chondrosarcoma Cell Lines

Sequencing analysis of common mutations in chondrosarcoma identified point mutations in *IDH1* (p.R132L) in CDS01 cells and *IDH2* (p.R172G) in CDS17 and T-CDS17 cells which were also detected in the corresponding patient tumor samples. Otherwise, CDS06 cells did not show any *IDH1* or *IDH2* mutations. Analysis of *TP53* (exons 4 and 6) revealed the presence of nonsynonymous homozygous in all cell lines. The single nucleotide variants (SNV) p.P72R was found in all cell lines and also in CDS06 and CDS11 patient samples, meanwhile the mutation p.S215R was only found in CDS17 and T-CDS17 cell lines but not in the corresponding patient sample (Figure 2A,C). Additional analysis of hot spot mutations in Phosphatidylinositol-4,5-Bisphosphate 3-Kinase Catalytic Subunit Alpha (*PI3KCA*) showed no alterations in any of the cell lines. Finally, copy number analysis showed a significant gain of *MDM2* in CDS17 and T-CDS17 cells which was not detected in the tumor sample and a homozygous deletion of *CDKN2A* (exon 3) in CDS11 cells and matched patient sample (Figure 2B,C).

3.3. WES of Chondrosarcoma Cell Lines and Clonal Evolution after In Vitro and In Vivo Growth

To better characterize the genomic alterations present in these cells lines, we performed WES in the CDS17 line (passage 14), its xenograft-derived line T-CDS17 (passage 5) and their matched normal (non-tumoral) and tumor patient samples. The average nucleotide coverage in WES studies was approximately 115X, being selected for further analyses only the variants presenting more than 15 reads. Data from WES analysis of tumor the sample were compared to that of normal tissue DNA to exclude germline alterations. Tumor and CDS17 samples showed similar number of somatic mutations (123 and 121 respectively) whereas the T-CDS17 cell line displayed a slightly higher number of mutations (169), corresponding most of them to SNV in the three samples (Figure 3A). All samples displayed a similar profile of SNV transitions and transvertions (Figure 3B and Figure S2A). Similar to other type of tumors, C > T and G > A transitions were the most common mutations found in all samples (Figure 3B). To analyze the genomic evolution of tumor cells after in vitro/in vivo growth adaptation, we used variant allele frequency data of tumors, CDS17 and T-CDS17 samples to delineate the different clonal populations in each sample using the PhyloWGS, and FishPlot software. This analysis retrieves 14 clusters which evolved among samples (Figure 3C,D). The tumor sample contains nine clusters presenting cellular prevalence values higher than 0.05. Among them, cluster 1 is the one including a higher number of SNVs and must be the founder clone since the set of mutations that contain is present in virtually all the tumors cells (cellular prevalence equal to 1) and the other clones seem to derive from it. Notably, the cellular prevalence of cluster 1 is maintained in CDS17 and T-CDS17 samples, thus suggesting that most variants, including driver mutations, are kept by in the cell lines. In addition, cluster 7 remained unchanged in a small proportion of cells in all samples. On the other hand, Clusters

2–4 were positively selected while Clusters 10–14 almost disappeared during the adaptation to in vitro culture, as seen by their variation in cellular prevalence in the CDS17 line. Moreover, Clusters 5 and 6 emerged in the cell line T-CDS17 with a cellular prevalence of 0.25 and 0.15 respectively and were likely acquired during the in vivo growth of tumor cells in immunodeficient mice (Figure 3C,D).

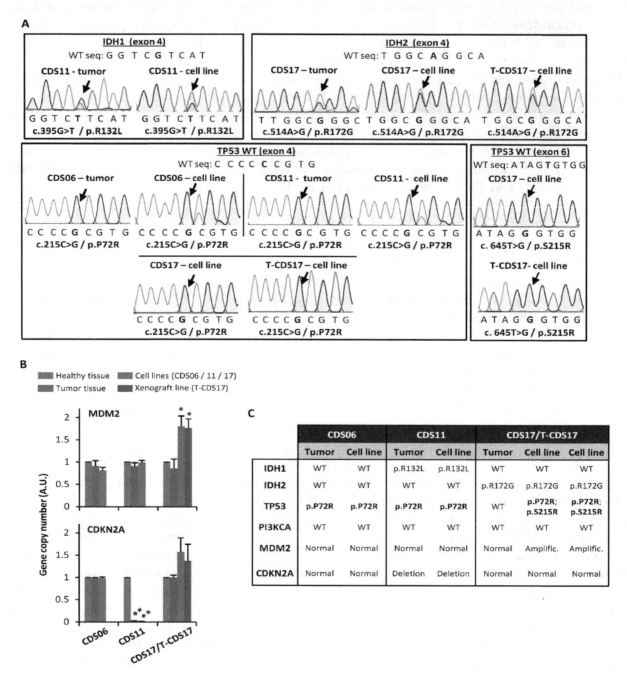

Figure 2. Genetic characterization of chondrosarcoma cell lines. (**A**) Sanger sequencing chromatograms showing mutations (black arrows) in *IDH1*, *IDH2*, and *TP53* genes present in the indicated tumors and cell lines. Reference wild type (WT) sequences are shown. (**B**) Gene copy numbers of the indicated genes were estimated by quantitative PCR on genomic DNA. Results are expressed relative to the corresponding healthy tissue sample and are the mean and standard deviation of three experiments (*: $p < 0.05$; ** $p < 0.005$; two-sided Student's t-test). (**C**) Summary of the genetic characterization of the indicated chondrosarcoma cell lines and tumor samples. Homozygous mutations are highlighted in bold.

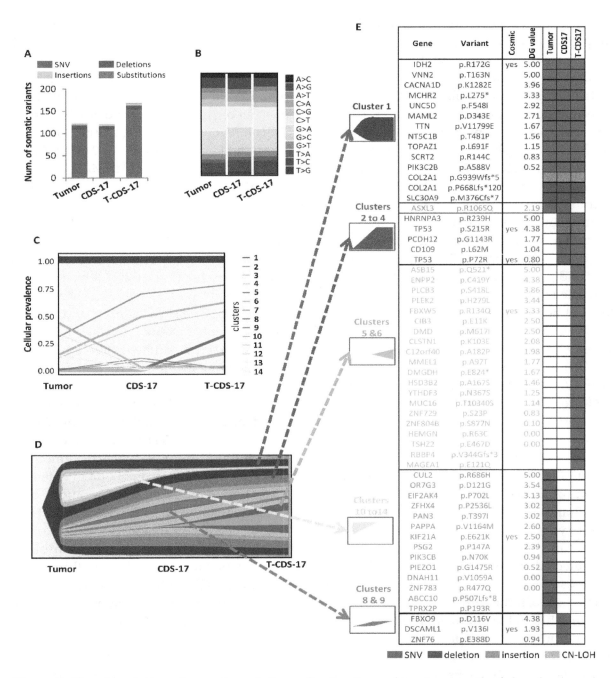

Figure 3. Clonal evolution of somatic mutations after in vitro and in vivo growth of chondrosarcoma cell lines. (**A,B**) Mutational burden data of a tumor patient sample and its derived cell lines CDS-17 and T-CDS17 obtained by whole exome sequencing (WES). The number and type of somatic mutations (**A**) and the profile of SNV transitions and transvertions (**B**) in each sample are shown. (**C,D**) Subclonal reconstruction was performed with PhyloWGS using WES data. The mean cellular prevalence estimates of mutation clusters in originating patient tumor sample and subsequent CDS17 and T-CDS17 cell lines are shown (**C**). Line widths represent the relative abundance of single nucleotide variants (SNVs) in each mutation cluster. Fish-plot representation of the different clusters in each sample is also shown (**D**). (**E**) List of non-synonymous somatic mutations detected in each cluster. Catalogue of Somatic Mutations in Cancer (COSMIC) status, DREAMgenics (DG) algorithm value, and mutation type are indicated.

To select the most relevant somatic mutations included in each group of clusters presenting similar trends we compared tumor versus normal, CDS17 versus tumor and T-CDS17 versus CDS17 samples and filter the results to select variants with non-synonymous effect on coded proteins which presented variant allele frequencies >0.035 in tumor, CDS17 or T-CDS17 samples and maximum allele frequencies <0.01 in population databases (dbSNP, ExAC, ESP, and 1000 Genomes) (Figure 3E). Using this approach, we found a group of 14 mutations included in cluster 1 which were mutated in all the samples. Among these mutations, only the c.514A > G transition (p.R172G) in *IDH2*, previously detected by Sanger sequencing (Figure 2A), was listed in the Catalogue of Somatic Mutations in Cancer (COSMIC). In addition, we also selected two different mutations in the *COL2A1* gene previously found in chondrosarcoma [5,6]. Mutations in the rest of genes were not previously described in cancer. Notably, some of these unreported variants, including SNVs in Vanin2 (*VNN2*), Calcium Voltage-Gated Channel Subunit Alpha1 D (*CACNA1D*), Melanin Concentrating Hormone Receptor 2 (*MCHR2*), Unc-5 Netrin Receptor D (*UNC5D*), or Mastermind Like Transcriptional Coactivator 2 (*MAML2*), showed high values in the 0 to 5 scale assigned by DREAMgenics (DG) value (integrated score of several predictive algorithms [34], see supplemental methods for details) used to predict deleterious mutations and, therefore, they might constitute new driver events in chondrosarcoma (Figures 3E and 4B). Another group of five mutated genes was filtered from variations included in Clusters 2–4, which become enriched in CDS17 and T-CDS17 cells. The most notably alterations in this group was the mutations p.S215R and p.P72R in *TP53*, previously detected by Sanger sequencing (Figure 2A), which was present in both alleles due to a copy-neutral (CN) loss of heterozygosity (LOH) event in chromosome 17 as detailed below. Most relevant variations emerging in T-CDS17 cells (Clusters 5 and 6) included mutations in 20 genes. Among them, a SNV in F-Box and WD Repeat Domain Containing 5 (*FBXW5*) is the only variation previously reported in COSMIC in tumor types different to chondrosarcoma (Figure 3E). Also, the set of variants of the tumor sample that were lost in CDS17 and T-CDS17 cells (Clusters 10–14) included a mutation in Kinesin Family Member 21A (*KIF21A*) previously reported in COSMIC for other types of tumor and other 13 unreported mutations. Finally, three mutations were filtered from variations contained in Clusters 8 and 9, which appear in a small fraction of CDS17 cells and disappeared again in T-CDS17 cells (Figure 3E). Besides the above described changes in somatic mutations, a major consequence of in vitro and in vivo growth of tumor cells was the emergence of structural alterations and copy number variants (CNV) leading to numerous LOH events in many mutations of CDS17 and T-CDS17 cells (Figure 4A,B). Most relevant structural alterations detected in CDS17 and T-CDS17 cells included a CN-LOH affecting chromosome 17, which would explain the homozygous mutations of the *TP53* gene (p.S215R and p.P72R) commented above. Analysis of variant frequencies in this chromosome showed that the CN-LOH affected the whole chromosome and is detected in virtually all cells, as indicated by the disappearance of almost all intermediate frequencies in CDS17 and T-CDS17 cells (Figure 4B,C). Similar CN-LOH events were detected in chromosome 16, although in this case the structural variation affects to only a subset of the cells, as seen by the shift in the intermediate frequencies of variants in CDS17 and T-CDS-17 cells as compared to normal and tumor samples. Noteworthy, the intermediate frequencies shift also indicated that the subpopulation presenting the CN-LOH in chromosome 16 increased in T-CDS17 as compared to CDS-17 cells (Figure 4B,C). Besides these CN variations, other LOH events were due to CNV in several chromosomes. Thus, a copy of chromosome 18 was lost in a subpopulation of CDS-17 cells and in the whole population of non-synonymous mutations undergoing LOH in each sample. COSMIC status, DG algorithm value, and mutation type are indicated.

After filtering LOH events using the criteria described above for somatic variants and including also other LOH variants with a recurrence in the COSMIC database higher than 10, we selected 24 mutations that underwent LOH in CDS17, 17 LOH events which emerged in T-CDS-17 and 5 mutations which were detected as LOH variations in CDS17 but not in T-CDS17 (Figure 4D). Altogether, these data indicate that these cell lines kept the most relevant driver mutations present in the founder clone of the tumor sample. In addition, the adaptation of tumor cells to in vitro cell culture and in vivo growth is accompanied by the gain/loss of additional point mutations and structural variants affecting different subclones of the cell lines.

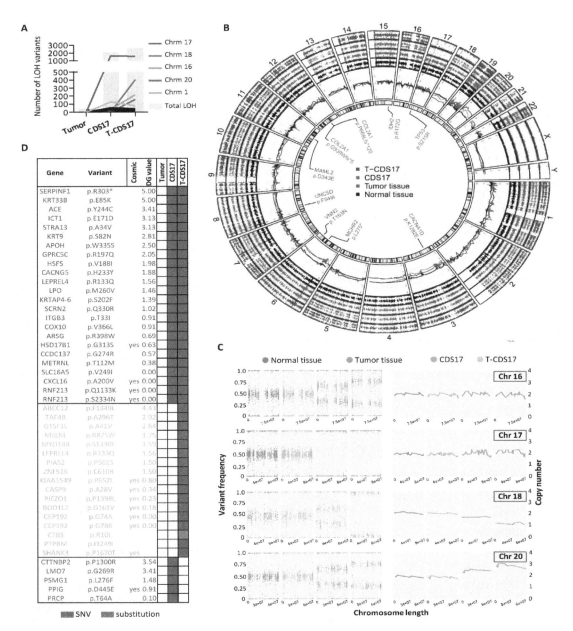

Figure 4. Genomic structural alterations after in vitro and in vivo growth of chondrosarcoma cell lines. (**A**) Number of LOH (total number and distribution between chromosomes) calculated from WES data of tumor, CDS17, and T-CDS17 samples. (**B**) Circular representation of the four samples sequenced through WES. Circles display from the inside outwards: (ring 1) chromosome ideogram, highlighting relevant previously reported (purple) or unreported (grey) somatic variants shared by tumor tissue, CDS17 and T-CDS17, as well as a TP53 homozygous mutation shared by CDS17 and T-CDS17 but not tumor tissue (orange); (ring 2) chromosome copy number (CN) of each sample based on normalized read counts; (rings 3–6) variant frequencies of common polymorphic positions (minimum allele frequency ≥0.01 in at least one major dbSNP population) in each sample. (**C**) Analysis of variant frequencies (left panels) and CN (right panels) extracted from (**B**) in the indicated chromosomes. Similar representations for other chromosomes are show in Figure S3B. (**D**) List of T-CDS17 cells. Conversely, a copy of chromosome 20 was gained in subset of CDS17 cells and in the entire population of T-CDS17 cells (Figure 4B,C). Finally, other copy number variations (CNVs) and/or shifts in variant frequencies affecting subpopulations of CDS-17 and/or T-CDS17 cells, was also detected in other chromosomes like 1, 2, 4, 5, 6, or 7 (Figure 4B and Figure S2B).

3.4. Analysis of CSC Subpopulations in New Chondrosarcoma Cell Lines

All the cell lines (CDS06, CDS11, CDS17, and T-CDS17) could be cultured as tumorspheres for at least two passages showing sphere forming frequencies between 0.20% and 0.28% in the first passage and between 0.1% and 0.16% in the second passage (Figure 5A and Table 1). Regarding the expression of CSC-related factors, CDS17 and T-CDS17 cells displayed high/medium levels of SOX2, while we could not detect SOX2 expression in CDS06 or CDS11 lines (Figure 5B). A similar pattern of expression was detected for ALDH1A1, while all the cell lines expressed ALDH1A3 (Figure 5B). According to the important contribution of these ALDH1A3 isoform to the Aldefluor activity [13], we detected Aldefluor positive cells in all lines in percentages ranging from 2.94% to 14.5% of the cells (Figure 5C). As previously shown in other sarcoma models [13], tumorsphere cultures of the CDS11 cell line are enriched in Aldefluor activity (Figure 5D). Furthermore, to confirm that Aldefluor could be used as a bone fide CSC marker in chondrosarcoma cell lines, we sorted T-CDS17 cells displaying high (ALDH^{high}) and low (ALDH^{low}) Aldefluor activity (Figure 5E) and inoculated several low cellular doses (LDA assays) subcutaneously into immunodeficient mice. We found low incidences of tumor growth after the inoculation of these cellular doses (we detected tumors in 4 out of 30 mice). In any case, ALDH^{low} cells developed only one tumor in the series where the higher number of cells was inoculated, whereas ALDH^{high} cells were able to develop three tumors, one per series. Using ELDA software to calculate the tumor initiation frequency of each population, we found that the ALDH^{high} subpopulation is three times more enriched in CSCs than the ALDH^{low} subpopulation (Figure 5F). Although, due to relatively low tumorigenicity of these cells when injected at low cellular doses, these results do not reach statistical significance, they clearly suggest that ALDH activity could be a suitable stem cell marker in these cells.

3.5. Invasion Ability of Chondrosarcoma Cell Lines

Using live cell time-lapse microscopy we found that spheroids of CDS11, CDS17, and T-CDS17—but not CDS06 cells—were able to invade 3D collagen matrices (Figure 6A,B). In accordance with its enhanced aggressiveness, T-CDS17 also displayed a significantly increased invasive potential when compared to the parental CDS17 cell line.

Deregulated SRC/FAK (Steroid receptor coactivator/Focal adhesion kinase) signaling is related to enhanced migration and invasion in many types of tumors and we previously found that several sarcoma models may invade through a mechanism depending on SRC/FAK signaling [30]. Here, we found that both the SRC inhibitor dasatinib or the FAK inhibitor PF-573228 were able to dose-dependently inhibit cell invasion, thus indicating that this mechanism is also mediating invasion in chondrosarcoma cell lines (Figure 6C–F).

4. Discussion

Chondrosarcomas are inherently resistant to conventional treatments and a range of new therapies aimed to target specific alterations are being currently tested [9,11,12]. Among them, the use of IDH inhibitors have not proved preclinical anti-tumor activity [49] and clinical trials including chondrosarcoma patients have not yet reported positive results [12].

Other therapeutic strategies that are being tested at clinical level include the targeting of signaling pathways controlled by hedgehog, SRC or PI3K/AKT/mTOR, as well as histone deacetylase inhibitors or anti-angiogenic agents, with only a few of them reporting partially encouraging results [12,50,51]. Altogether, there is an urgent need for more research aimed to find and test new therapies for advanced or unresectable chondrosarcomas.

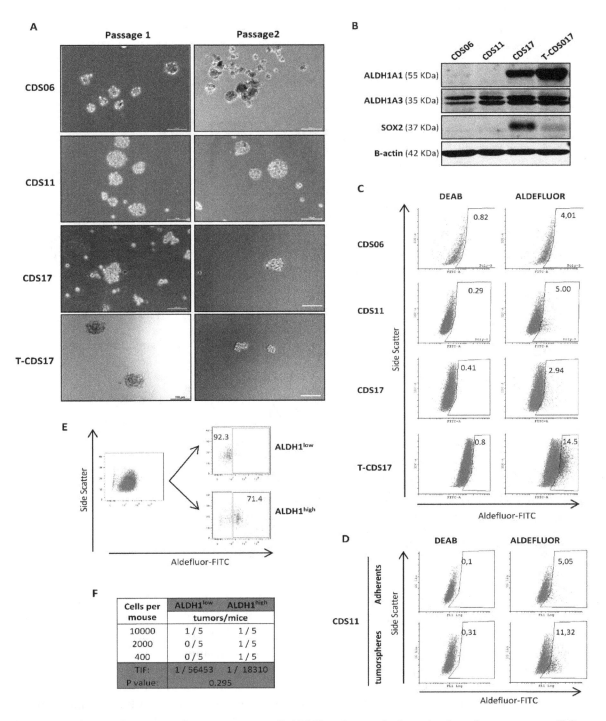

Figure 5. Characterization of cancer stem cell (CSC) subpopulations in chondrosarcoma cell lines. (**A**) Representative images of tumorspheres formed from the indicated cell lines in two successive passages. Scale bar = 100 μm. (**B**) Protein levels of Aldehyde Dehydrogenase 1 Family Member-A1 (ALDH1A1), -A3 (ALDH1A3), and Sex Determining Region Y-Box 2 (SOX2) in the indicated cell lines. β-actin levels were used as a loading control. (**C**) Aldefluor assay showing the activity of ALDH1 in the indicated cell lines. ALDH1 activity was blocked with the specific inhibitor N,N-diethylaminobenzaldehyde (DEAB) to establish the basal levels. (**D**) Comparison of Aldefluor activity in adherent and tumorsphere cultures of CDS11 cells. (**E**) Flow cytometry cell sorting of Aldefluor high (ALDH1^{high}) and low (ALDH1^{low}) populations in T-CDS17 cells. (**F**) Limiting dilution assay to evaluate tumor initiation frequency (TIF) of ALDH1^{high} and ALDH1^{low} T-CDS17 cells. The number of mice that grew tumors after 4 months and the total number of inoculated mice for each condition is indicated. TIF was calculated using ELDA software.

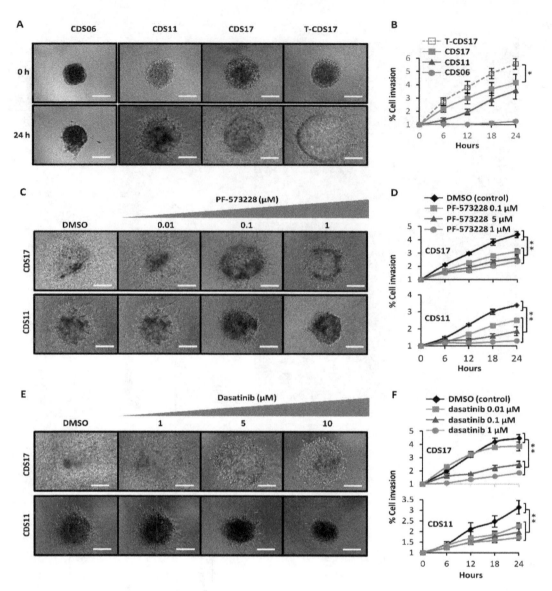

Figure 6. Invasive ability of chondrosarcoma cell lines. (**A,B**) Analysis of the invasive properties of the indicated cell lines using 3D spheroid invasion assays. Representative images of the 3D invading spheroids at the initial and final time points (**A**) and quantification of the invasive area (**B**) are presented. (**C,F**) Effect of increasing concentrations of PF-573228 (**C,D**) or dasatinib (**E,F**) on the invasive ability of CDS11 and CDS17 cells. Representative images of the 3D spheroids treated with the indicated concentrations of PF-573228 (**C**) or dasatinib (**E**) for 24 h and quantification of the invasive area after each treatment (**D,F**) are presented. Scale bars = 200 μm. Error bars represent the SD, and asterisks indicate statistically significant differences between the indicated series (* $p < 0.05$; ** $p < 0.01$; two-sided Student's t-test). (DMSO: Dimethyl sulfoxide).

Cell lines are easy to culture, relatively inexpensive and amenable to high-throughput screening models that have guided advances in cancer research for decades. Despite limitations, such as the accumulation of new mutations after endless in vitro culture [17], international studies reported that large panels of cell lines recapitulated the most relevant alterations of original tumors and, when using a relevant number of well characterized cell lines of a given cancer subtype, they were useful models to predict anti-cancer drug sensitivity and clinical outcomes [15,52–54]. These studies have contributed to retrieve the interest in substituting veteran endless passaged cell lines and replace them with new patient-derived cell lines which should be tagged with clinical information and include genomic characterization of both the cell line and the patient samples. These cell line models would complement more sophisticated models such as organoids or patient-derived xenografts [55].

Here we present four new chondrosarcoma cell lines with related clinical information and genetic characterization of the most common alterations (mutations in *IDH1, IDH2, TP53,* and *PI3KCA* and copy number variants in *MDM2* and *CDKN2*). All the alterations detected were also found in the original tumors with the exception of the *TP53* mutations and *MDM2* amplification found in CDS17 and T-CDS17 cell lines but not in tumor samples. This finding suggests that the loss of functional p53 could be a mechanism of adaptation to in vitro culture in chondrosarcoma cells. Our cell lines expand the panel of available chondrosarcoma cell lines (overviewed in Table S3). Of note, our study provides the first cell line (CDS06) derived from a secondary chondrosarcoma associated to a previous osteochondroma. In addition we add new dedifferentiated cchondrosarcoma cell lines with *IDH2* mutations to only one reported so far. Interestingly, none of previously published dedifferentiated lines described mutations in *IDH1* (Table S3).

Relevant for possible future applications in cancer research, three of the cell lines (CDS11, CDS17, and T-CDS17) were able to initiate tumors in vivo resembling the histology of the patient sample after inoculation in heterotopic and/or orthotopic sites. Some of these cell lines were also able to invade 3D matrices and all of them showed CSC-related features such as the ability to grow as tumorspheres or the presence of subpopulations with ALDH^{high} activity. Related to this, it has been previously shown that sarcoma cells increased their stemness and tumorigenic potential after being grown in mice [13,56]. Therefore cell line/xenograft line tandems, like the one formed by CDS17 and T-CDS17, constitute valuable models for studying/tracking cancer stem cells subpopulations during tumor progression [13]. These studies point ALDH1 as a relevant CSC-associated factor in different types of sarcoma [13,56]. Similarly, we found that the T-CDS17 cell line showed increased ALDH1 expression and activity, enhanced invasive ability and increased in vivo tumorigenic potential than its parental CDS17 cell line. Moreover, our results also suggest a role for ALDH1 as CSC marker in chondrosarcoma.

Our work also includes a WES analysis of CDS17 and T-CDS17 cells lines together with normal and tumor samples from the patient. This is the first time that a chondrosarcoma cell line and matched patient samples include such a level of genomic characterization. This analysis allowed us to know how the cell lines resemble the genomic diversity of the original tumor and also to track the genomic evolution of tumor cells during in vitro and in vivo growth. We found that the putative founder clone, that including a higher number of mutations and is present in all tumor cells, remains unaltered after in vitro cell culture (CDS17 cells) and in vivo growth (T-CDS17 cells). This clone includes previously known mutations, such as that previously found by Sanger sequencing in *IDH2* (R172G) [2,4] or mutations in *COL2A1* (G939Wfs*5 and P668Lfs*120) [5,6], as well as other unreported non-synonymous mutations presenting high scores in impact prediction algorithms, such as *VNN2, CACNA1D, MCHR2, UNC5D,* or *MAML2*, which possibly contribute to chondrosarcoma progression must be studied in detail.

Other mutations affecting different subclones appear or disappear during the adaptation of cells to in vitro/in vivo growth. Although not widely described for sarcomas, this genomic drift is in line with previous studies in other cancer types [57]. An important phenomenon related to the adaptation to growth conditions is the emergence of structural alterations in several chromosomes in CDS17 and T-CDS17 cells. The most relevant change was the CN-LOH affecting the chromosome 17 and responsible for appearance of homozygous mutations in *TP53*. Importantly, alterations in *TP53* were associated with aggressive behavior of chondrosarcomas [58] and similar LOH affecting chromosome 17 was detected in high grade chondrosarcomas [59]. Therefore, despite not being present in the original tumor, the CN-LOH in chromosome 17 detected in CDS17 and T-CDS17 resembles a naturally occurring mechanism for increasing aggressiveness in chondrosarcomas. Other structural variants, such as those detected chromosomes like 16, 18, or 20, affected a sequentially increased cell population in CDS17 and T-CDS17 cells. Given that T-CDS17 cells are more aggressive tan CDS17 cells, some of these structural alterations could be involved in the gain of malignancy in T-CDS17 cells. Whether these alterations occur also in patients during tumor progression or are only due to the adaptation of tumor cells to grow ex-vivo remains to be studied.

Although we could not be completely sure that all the genetic differences observed between CDS17 and T-CDS17 cell lines were due to the in vivo growth in mice and not to the ex-vivo expansion of T-CDS17, the fact that the genomic drift previously observed in patient-derived cell lines were mainly restricted to the first few passages [57] when the adaptation of cells to the in vitro growth conditions occurs, suggests that the new set of genetic alterations detected in T-CDS17 most likely emerged during the in vivo growth phase.

5. Conclusions

In summary, this study provides new patient-derived chondrosarcoma cell lines with clinical and genetic information from patients. These cell lines are suitable for studying CSC subpopulations and to generate in vivo models for this disease. Furthermore, a pioneering genomic analysis using a cell line (CDS17)/xenograft line (T-CDS-17) tandem model confirmed that these cell lines kept the most relevant mutations of the original tumor and described the genetic drift process that tumor cells underwent during the adaptation to in vitro and in vivo growth.

Author Contributions: Conceptualization, R.R.; Methodology, V.R., S.T.M., O.E., A.R., L.S., J.T., L.M.-C. and S.C.; Software, D.C. and G.R.O.; Validation, V.R. and S.T.M.; Formal analysis, V.R., S.T.M., D.C., G.R.O., S.C., and A.A.; Investigation, V.R., S.T.M., O.E., A.R., L.S., J.T., and L.M.-C.; Resources, R.R., A.A., and A.B.; Data curation, D.C. and C.A.-F.; Writing—original draft preparation, R.R.; Writing—review and editing, R.R., V.R., and S.T.M.; Supervision, R.R.; Funding acquisition, R.R.

Acknowledgments: We thank Mario Garcia (Pharmacology laboratory, University of Oviedo) for his help with intra-tibia inoculations. We acknowledge the Spanish Group for Research on Sarcomas (GEIS), co-responsible institution for their support to the study. Finally, we acknowledge the Principado de Asturias BioBank (PT17/0015/0023), financed jointly by Servicio de Salud del Principado de Asturias, Instituto de Salud Carlos III and Fundación Bancaria Cajastur and integrated in the Spanish National Biobanks Network, for its collaboration.

References

1.   Fletcher, C.; Bridge, J.; Hogendoorn, P.; Mertens, F. (Eds.) *WHO Classification of Tumours of Soft Tissue and Bone. Pathology and Genetics of Tumours of Soft Tissue and Bone*, 4th ed.; IARC Press: Lyon, France, 2013.

2.   Amary, M.F.; Bacsi, K.; Maggiani, F.; Damato, S.; Halai, D.; Berisha, F.; Pollock, R.; O'Donnell, P.; Grigoriadis, A.; Diss, T.; et al. IDH1 and IDH2 mutations are frequent events in central chondrosarcoma and central and periosteal chondromas but not in other mesenchymal tumours. *J. Pathol.* **2011**, *224*, 334–343. [CrossRef]

3.   Lu, C.; Venneti, S.; Akalin, A.; Fang, F.; Ward, P.S.; Dematteo, R.G.; Intlekofer, A.M.; Chen, C.; Ye, J.; Hameed, M.; et al. Induction of sarcomas by mutant IDH2. *Genes Dev.* **2013**, *27*, 1986–1998. [CrossRef]

4.   Tinoco, G.; Wilky, B.A.; Paz-Mejia, A.; Rosenberg, A.; Trent, J.C. The biology and management of cartilaginous tumors: A role for targeting isocitrate dehydrogenase. *Am. Soc. Clin. Oncol. Educ. Book* **2015**, e648–e655. [CrossRef]

5.   Tarpey, P.S.; Behjati, S.; Cooke, S.L.; Van Loo, P.; Wedge, D.C.; Pillay, N.; Marshall, J.; O'Meara, S.; Davies, H.; Nik-Zainal, S.; et al. Frequent mutation of the major cartilage collagen gene COL2A1 in chondrosarcoma. *Nat. Genet.* **2013**, *45*, 923–926. [CrossRef]

6.   Totoki, Y.; Yoshida, A.; Hosoda, F.; Nakamura, H.; Hama, N.; Ogura, K.; Fujiwara, T.; Arai, Y.; Toguchida, J.; Tsuda, H.; et al. Unique mutation portraits and frequent COL2A1 gene alteration in chondrosarcoma. *Genome Res.* **2014**, *24*, 1411–1420. [CrossRef] [PubMed]

7.   Schrage, Y.M.; Lam, S.; Jochemsen, A.G.; Cleton-Jansen, A.M.; Taminiau, A.H.; Hogendoorn, P.C.; Bovee, J.V. Central chondrosarcoma progression is associated with pRb pathway alterations: CDK4 down-regulation and p16 overexpression inhibit cell growth in vitro. *J. Cell. Mol. Med.* **2009**, *13*, 2843–2852. [CrossRef] [PubMed]

8.   Boehme, K.A.; Schleicher, S.B.; Traub, F.; Rolauffs, B. Chondrosarcoma: A Rare Misfortune in Aging Human Cartilage? The Role of Stem and Progenitor Cells in Proliferation, Malignant Degeneration and Therapeutic Resistance. *Int. J. Mol. Sci.* **2018**, *19*. [CrossRef] [PubMed]

9.   Bovee, J.V.; Cleton-Jansen, A.M.; Taminiau, A.H.; Hogendoorn, P.C. Emerging pathways in the development of chondrosarcoma of bone and implications for targeted treatment. *Lancet Oncol.* **2005**, *6*, 599–607. [CrossRef]

10. Brown, H.K.; Schiavone, K.; Gouin, F.; Heymann, M.F.; Heymann, D. Biology of Bone Sarcomas and New Therapeutic Developments. *Calcif. Tissue Int.* **2018**, *102*, 174–195. [CrossRef]

11. David, E.; Blanchard, F.; Heymann, M.F.; De Pinieux, G.; Gouin, F.; Redini, F.; Heymann, D. The Bone Niche of Chondrosarcoma: A Sanctuary for Drug Resistance, Tumour Growth and also a Source of New Therapeutic Targets. *Sarcoma* **2011**, *2011*, 932451. [CrossRef]

12. Polychronidou, G.; Karavasilis, V.; Pollack, S.M.; Huang, P.H.; Lee, A.; Jones, R.L. Novel therapeutic approaches in chondrosarcoma. *Future Oncol.* **2017**, *13*, 637–648. [CrossRef]

13. Martinez-Cruzado, L.; Tornin, J.; Santos, L.; Rodriguez, A.; Garcia-Castro, J.; Moris, F.; Rodriguez, R. Aldh1 Expression and Activity Increase During Tumor Evolution in Sarcoma Cancer Stem Cell Populations. *Sci. Rep.* **2016**, *6*, 27878. [CrossRef]

14. Tirino, V.; Desiderio, V.; Paino, F.; De Rosa, A.; Papaccio, F.; Fazioli, F.; Pirozzi, G.; Papaccio, G. Human primary bone sarcomas contain CD133+ cancer stem cells displaying high tumorigenicity in vivo. *FASEB J.* **2011**, *25*, 2022–2030. [CrossRef]

15. Goodspeed, A.; Heiser, L.M.; Gray, J.W.; Costello, J.C. Tumor-Derived Cell Lines as Molecular Models of Cancer Pharmacogenomics. *Mol. Cancer Res.* **2016**, *14*, 3–13. [CrossRef]

16. McDermott, U. Cancer cell lines as patient avatars for drug response prediction. *Nat. Genet.* **2018**, *50*, 1350–1351. [CrossRef]

17. Wilding, J.L.; Bodmer, W.F. Cancer cell lines for drug discovery and development. *Cancer Res.* **2014**, *74*, 2377–2384. [CrossRef]

18. Calabuig-Farinas, S.; Benso, R.G.; Szuhai, K.; Machado, I.; Lopez-Guerrero, J.A.; de Jong, D.; Peydro, A.; San Miguel, T.; Navarro, L.; Pellin, A.; et al. Characterization of a new human cell line (CH-3573) derived from a grade II chondrosarcoma with matrix production. *Pathol. Oncol. Res.* **2012**, *18*, 793–802. [CrossRef]

19. Farges, M.; Mazeau, C.; Gioanni, J.; Ettore, F.; Denovion, H.; Schneider, M. Establishment and characterization of a new cell line derived from a human chondrosarcoma. *Oncol. Rep.* **1997**, *4*, 697–700. [CrossRef]

20. Gil-Benso, R.; Lopez-Gines, C.; Lopez-Guerrero, J.A.; Carda, C.; Callaghan, R.C.; Navarro, S.; Ferrer, J.; Pellin, A.; Llombart-Bosch, A. Establishment and characterization of a continuous human chondrosarcoma cell line, ch-2879: Comparative histologic and genetic studies with its tumor of origin. *Lab. Investig.* **2003**, *83*, 877–887. [CrossRef]

21. Jagasia, A.A.; Block, J.A.; Qureshi, A.; Diaz, M.O.; Nobori, T.; Gitelis, S.; Iyer, A.P. Chromosome 9 related aberrations and deletions of the CDKN2 and MTS2 putative tumor suppressor genes in human chondrosarcomas. *Cancer Lett.* **1996**, *105*, 91–103. [CrossRef]

22. Kalinski, T.; Krueger, S.; Pelz, A.F.; Wieacker, P.; Hartig, R.; Ropke, M.; Schneider-Stock, R.; Dombrowski, F.; Roessner, A. Establishment and characterization of the permanent human cell line C3842 derived from a secondary chondrosarcoma in Ollier's disease. *Virchows Arch.* **2005**, *446*, 287–299. [CrossRef]

23. Kudawara, I.; Araki, N.; Myoui, A.; Kato, Y.; Uchida, A.; Yoshikawa, H. New cell lines with chondrocytic phenotypes from human chondrosarcoma. *Virchows Arch.* **2004**, *444*, 577–586. [CrossRef]

24. Kudo, N.; Ogose, A.; Hotta, T.; Kawashima, H.; Gu, W.; Umezu, H.; Toyama, T.; Endo, N. Establishment of novel human dedifferentiated chondrosarcoma cell line with osteoblastic differentiation. *Virchows Arch.* **2007**, *451*, 691–699. [CrossRef]

25. Kunisada, T.; Miyazaki, M.; Mihara, K.; Gao, C.; Kawai, A.; Inoue, H.; Namba, M. A new human chondrosarcoma cell line (OUMS-27) that maintains chondrocytic differentiation. *Int. J. Cancer* **1998**, *77*, 854–859. [CrossRef]

26. Monderer, D.; Luseau, A.; Bellec, A.; David, E.; Ponsolle, S.; Saiagh, S.; Bercegeay, S.; Piloquet, P.; Denis, M.G.; Lode, L.; et al. New chondrosarcoma cell lines and mouse models to study the link between chondrogenesis and chemoresistance. *Lab. Investig.* **2013**, *93*, 1100–1114. [CrossRef]

27. van Oosterwijk, J.G.; de Jong, D.; van Ruler, M.A.; Hogendoorn, P.C.; Dijkstra, P.D.; van Rijswijk, C.S.; Machado, I.; Llombart-Bosch, A.; Szuhai, K.; Bovee, J.V. Three new chondrosarcoma cell lines: One grade III conventional central chondrosarcoma and two dedifferentiated chondrosarcomas of bone. *BMC Cancer* **2012**, *12*, 375. [CrossRef]

28. Tornin, J.; Martinez-Cruzado, L.; Santos, L.; Rodriguez, A.; Nunez, L.E.; Oro, P.; Hermosilla, M.A.; Allonca, E.; Fernandez-Garcia, M.T.; Astudillo, A.; et al. Inhibition of SP1 by the mithramycin analog EC-8042 efficiently targets tumor initiating cells in sarcoma. *Oncotarget* **2016**, *7*, 30935–30950. [CrossRef]

29. Martinez-Cruzado, L.; Tornin, J.; Rodriguez, A.; Santos, L.; Allonca, E.; Fernandez-Garcia, M.T.; Astudillo, A.; Garcia-Pedrero, J.M.; Rodriguez, R. Trabectedin and Campthotecin Synergistically Eliminate Cancer Stem Cells in Cell-of-Origin Sarcoma Models. *Neoplasia* **2017**, *19*, 460–470. [CrossRef]

30. Tornin, J.; Hermida-Prado, F.; Padda, R.S.; Gonzalez, M.V.; Alvarez-Fernandez, C.; Rey, V.; Martinez-Cruzado, L.; Estupinan, O.; Menendez, S.T.; Fernandez-Nevado, L.; et al. FUS-CHOP Promotes Invasion in Myxoid Liposarcoma through a SRC/FAK/RHO/ROCK-Dependent Pathway. *Neoplasia* **2018**, *20*, 44–56. [CrossRef]

31. Estupinan, O.; Santos, L.; Rodriguez, A.; Fernandez-Nevado, L.; Costales, P.; Perez-Escuredo, J.; Hermosilla, M.A.; Oro, P.; Rey, V.; Tornin, J.; et al. The multikinase inhibitor EC-70124 synergistically increased the antitumor activity of doxorubicin in sarcomas. *Int. J. Cancer* **2018**. [CrossRef]

32. Rubio, R.; Abarrategi, A.; Garcia-Castro, J.; Martinez-Cruzado, L.; Suarez, C.; Tornin, J.; Santos, L.; Astudillo, A.; Colmenero, I.; Mulero, F.; et al. Bone environment is essential for osteosarcoma development from transformed mesenchymal stem cells. *Stem Cells* **2014**, *32*, 1136–1148. [CrossRef]

33. Bolger, A.M.; Lohse, M.; Usadel, B. Trimmomatic: A flexible trimmer for Illumina sequence data. *Bioinformatics* **2014**, *30*, 2114–2120. [CrossRef]

34. Cabanillas, R.; Dineiro, M.; Castillo, D.; Pruneda, P.C.; Penas, C.; Cifuentes, G.A.; de Vicente, A.; Duran, N.S.; Alvarez, R.; Ordonez, G.R.; et al. A novel molecular diagnostics platform for somatic and germline precision oncology. *Mol. Genet. Genomic Med.* **2017**, *5*, 336–359. [CrossRef]

35. Choi, Y.; Sims, G.E.; Murphy, S.; Miller, J.R.; Chan, A.P. Predicting the functional effect of amino acid substitutions and indels. *PLoS ONE* **2012**, *7*, e46688. [CrossRef]

36. Chun, S.; Fay, J.C. Identification of deleterious mutations within three human genomes. *Genome Res.* **2009**, *19*, 1553–1561. [CrossRef]

37. Davydov, E.V.; Goode, D.L.; Sirota, M.; Cooper, G.M.; Sidow, A.; Batzoglou, S. Identifying a high fraction of the human genome to be under selective constraint using GERP++. *PLoS Comput. Biol.* **2010**, *6*, e1001025. [CrossRef]

38. Deshwar, A.G.; Vembu, S.; Yung, C.K.; Jang, G.H.; Stein, L.; Morris, Q. PhyloWGS: Reconstructing subclonal composition and evolution from whole-genome sequencing of tumors. *Genome Biol.* **2015**, *16*, 35. [CrossRef]

39. Dong, C.; Wei, P.; Jian, X.; Gibbs, R.; Boerwinkle, E.; Wang, K.; Liu, X. Comparison and integration of deleteriousness prediction methods for nonsynonymous SNVs in whole exome sequencing studies. *Hum. Mol. Genet.* **2015**, *24*, 2125–2137. [CrossRef]

40. Jagadeesh, K.A.; Wenger, A.M.; Berger, M.J.; Guturu, H.; Stenson, P.D.; Cooper, D.N.; Bernstein, J.A.; Bejerano, G. M-CAP eliminates a majority of variants of uncertain significance in clinical exomes at high sensitivity. *Nat. Genet.* **2016**, *48*, 1581–1586. [CrossRef]

41. Kumar, P.; Henikoff, S.; Ng, P.C. Predicting the effects of coding non-synonymous variants on protein function using the SIFT algorithm. *Nat. Protoc.* **2009**, *4*, 1073–1081. [CrossRef]

42. Li, H.; Handsaker, B.; Wysoker, A.; Fennell, T.; Ruan, J.; Homer, N.; Marth, G.; Abecasis, G.; Durbin, R.; Genome Project Data Processing, S. The Sequence Alignment/Map format and SAMtools. *Bioinformatics* **2009**, *25*, 2078–2079. [CrossRef] [PubMed]

43. Miller, C.A.; McMichael, J.; Dang, H.X.; Maher, C.A.; Ding, L.; Ley, T.J.; Mardis, E.R.; Wilson, R.K. Visualizing tumor evolution with the fishplot package for R. *BMC Genom.* **2016**, *17*, 880. [CrossRef] [PubMed]

44. Puente, X.S.; Pinyol, M.; Quesada, V.; Conde, L.; Ordonez, G.R.; Villamor, N.; Escaramis, G.; Jares, P.; Bea, S.; Gonzalez-Diaz, M.; et al. Whole-genome sequencing identifies recurrent mutations in chronic lymphocytic leukaemia. *Nature* **2011**, *475*, 101–105. [CrossRef]

45. Reva, B.; Antipin, Y.; Sander, C. Predicting the functional impact of protein mutations: Application to cancer genomics. *Nucleic Acids Res.* **2011**, *39*, e118. [CrossRef] [PubMed]

46. Schwarz, J.M.; Cooper, D.N.; Schuelke, M.; Seelow, D. MutationTaster2: Mutation prediction for the deep-sequencing age. *Nat. Methods* **2014**, *11*, 361–362. [CrossRef] [PubMed]

47. Shihab, H.A.; Gough, J.; Mort, M.; Cooper, D.N.; Day, I.N.; Gaunt, T.R. Ranking non-synonymous single nucleotide polymorphisms based on disease concepts. *Hum. Genom.* **2014**, *8*, 11. [CrossRef]

48. European Nucleotide Archive repository. Available online: http://www.ebi.ac.uk/ena/data/view/PRJEB31233 (accessed on 28 February 2019).

49. Suijker, J.; Oosting, J.; Koornneef, A.; Struys, E.A.; Salomons, G.S.; Schaap, F.G.; Waaijer, C.J.; Wijers-Koster, P.M.; Briaire-de Bruijn, I.H.; Haazen, L.; et al. Inhibition of mutant IDH1 decreases D-2-HG levels without affecting tumorigenic properties of chondrosarcoma cell lines. *Oncotarget* **2015**, *6*, 12505–12519. [CrossRef]
50. Campbell, V.T.; Nadesan, P.; Ali, S.A.; Wang, C.Y.; Whetstone, H.; Poon, R.; Wei, Q.; Keilty, J.; Proctor, J.; Wang, L.W.; et al. Hedgehog pathway inhibition in chondrosarcoma using the smoothened inhibitor IPI-926 directly inhibits sarcoma cell growth. *Mol. Cancer Ther.* **2014**, *13*, 1259–1269. [CrossRef]
51. Heymann, D.; Redini, F. Targeted therapies for bone sarcomas. *Bonekey Rep.* **2013**, *2*, 378. [CrossRef]
52. Barretina, J.; Caponigro, G.; Stransky, N.; Venkatesan, K.; Margolin, A.A.; Kim, S.; Wilson, C.J.; Lehar, J.; Kryukov, G.V.; Sonkin, D.; et al. The Cancer Cell Line Encyclopedia enables predictive modelling of anticancer drug sensitivity. *Nature* **2012**, *483*, 603–607. [CrossRef]
53. Iorio, F.; Knijnenburg, T.A.; Vis, D.J.; Bignell, G.R.; Menden, M.P.; Schubert, M.; Aben, N.; Goncalves, E.; Barthorpe, S.; Lightfoot, H.; et al. A Landscape of Pharmacogenomic Interactions in Cancer. *Cell* **2016**, *166*, 740–754. [CrossRef]
54. Lee, J.K.; Liu, Z.; Sa, J.K.; Shin, S.; Wang, J.; Bordyuh, M.; Cho, H.J.; Elliott, O.; Chu, T.; Choi, S.W.; et al. Pharmacogenomic landscape of patient-derived tumor cells informs precision oncology therapy. *Nat. Genet.* **2018**, *50*, 1399–1411. [CrossRef]
55. Ledford, H. US cancer institute to overhaul tumour cell lines. *Nature* **2016**, *530*, 391. [CrossRef]
56. Golan, H.; Shukrun, R.; Caspi, R.; Vax, E.; Pode-Shakked, N.; Goldberg, S.; Pleniceanu, O.; Bar-Lev, D.D.; Mark-Danieli, M.; Pri-Chen, S.; et al. In Vivo Expansion of Cancer Stemness Affords Novel Cancer Stem Cell Targets: Malignant Rhabdoid Tumor as an Example. *Stem Cell Rep.* **2018**, *11*, 795–810. [CrossRef]
57. Ben-David, U.; Ha, G.; Tseng, Y.Y.; Greenwald, N.F.; Oh, C.; Shih, J.; McFarland, J.M.; Wong, B.; Boehm, J.S.; Beroukhim, R.; et al. Patient-derived xenografts undergo mouse-specific tumor evolution. *Nat. Genet.* **2017**, *49*, 1567–1575. [CrossRef]
58. Oshiro, Y.; Chaturvedi, V.; Hayden, D.; Nazeer, T.; Johnson, M.; Johnston, D.A.; Ordonez, N.G.; Ayala, A.G.; Czerniak, B. Altered p53 is associated with aggressive behavior of chondrosarcoma: A long term follow-up study. *Cancer* **1998**, *83*, 2324–2334. [CrossRef]
59. Yamaguchi, T.; Toguchida, J.; Wadayama, B.; Kanoe, H.; Nakayama, T.; Ishizaki, K.; Ikenaga, M.; Kotoura, Y.; Sasaki, M.S. Loss of heterozygosity and tumor suppressor gene mutations in chondrosarcomas. *Anticancer Res.* **1996**, *16*, 2009–2015.

The Community Oncology and Academic Medical Center Alliance in the Age of Precision Medicine: Cancer Genetics and Genomics Considerations

Marilena Melas [1], Shanmuga Subbiah [2], Siamak Saadat [3], Swapnil Rajurkar [4] and Kevin J. McDonnell [5,6,*]

[1] The Steve and Cindy Rasmussen Institute for Genomic Medicine, Nationwide Children's Hospital, Columbus, OH 43205, USA; Marilena.Melas@nationwidechildrens.org

[2] Department of Medical Oncology and Therapeutics Research, City of Hope Comprehensive Cancer Center, Glendora, CA 91741, USA; ssubbiah@coh.org

[3] Department of Medical Oncology and Therapeutics Research, City of Hope Comprehensive Cancer Center, Colton, CA 92324, USA; ssaadat@coh.org

[4] Department of Medical Oncology and Therapeutics Research, City of Hope Comprehensive Cancer Center, Upland, CA 91786, USA; srajurkar@coh.org

[5] Department of Medical Oncology and Therapeutics Research, City of Hope Comprehensive Cancer Center and Beckman Research Institute, Duarte, CA 91010, USA

[6] Center for Precision Medicine, City of Hope Comprehensive Cancer Center, Duarte, CA 91010, USA

* Correspondence: kemcdonnell@coh.org

Abstract: Recent public policy, governmental regulatory and economic trends have motivated the establishment and deepening of community health and academic medical center alliances. Accordingly, community oncology practices now deliver a significant portion of their oncology care in association with academic cancer centers. In the age of precision medicine, this alliance has acquired critical importance; novel advances in nucleic acid sequencing, the generation and analysis of immense data sets, the changing clinical landscape of hereditary cancer predisposition and ongoing discovery of novel, targeted therapies challenge community-based oncologists to deliver molecularly-informed health care. The active engagement of community oncology practices with academic partners helps with meeting these challenges; community/academic alliances result in improved cancer patient care and provider efficacy. Here, we review the community oncology and academic medical center alliance. We examine how practitioners may leverage academic center precision medicine-based cancer genetics and genomics programs to advance their patients' needs. We highlight a number of project initiatives at the City of Hope Comprehensive Cancer Center that seek to optimize community oncology and academic cancer center precision medicine interactions.

Keywords: community oncology; academic cancer center; precision medicine; cancer genetics; cancer genomics

1. Introduction

Historically, the practice and delivery of healthcare in the community contrasted significantly with medical care provided at the academic medical center [1,2]. These differences manifested across specialty practices, including oncology [3,4]. Rapid advances in molecular diagnostics, the advent of targeted therapies and the introduction of precision medicine amplified differences between community and academic oncology practices [5,6]. Reversing this historical divide, however, new financial realities, public policy initiatives and legislative mandateshave forced community oncologists and academic cancer centers to more closely align their healthcare efforts [7]. This forced alliance has lessened the separation between community and academic oncology practices and permitted broader access and utilization of precision medicine-based cancer genetics services and tumor genomic analyses. The alliance between community and academic oncology expands the capabilities and effectiveness of the community practitioner, reinforces the mission of the academic cancer center and, ultimately, secures better oncologic care for the cancer patient.

2. The Emergence and Evolution of the Community Health Care and Academic Medical Center Alliance

A number of key distinctions differentiate the medical care provided at community health centers (CHCs) versus academic health centers (AHCs); these differences result in complementary advantages. The overwhelming majority of patients receive their healthcare through CHCs; the CHC patient population typically exhibits great diversity across economic, racial, ethnic and social spectra [8]. CHCs offer their patients increased accessibility and enhanced client engagement [9]. In contrast, AHCs, characteristically, have focused on specialty medical care, biomedical research, the education and training of health care professionals and the stopgap provision of health care to uninsured and destitute populations [10]. These activities underlie the strengths of AHCs. These strengths include the presence of medical expertise, scientific innovation and clinical trial availability; additionally, AHCs possess unique physical resources such as libraries, computerized database management and informatics infrastructure, research laboratories and emergency room facilities [11,12]. Leveraging these strengths, AHCs have established their reputations and acquired leadership roles in shaping medical care and policy [10].

Until two decades ago, CHCs and AHCs functioned largely in parallel, without administrative or operational intersection. A variety of recent economic, social and regulatory circumstances, however, diminished the independence of AHCs. With the rise of community-based health care markets, particularly managed care plans, many of the operations traditionally carried out at AHCs shifted to CHCs; this shift often undercut the previously reliable revenue streams of AHCs. This situation forced reconsideration of the AHC financial model and provided impetus for the implementation of more efficient, cost-effective health care delivery strategies [13–18]. At the same time, governmental funding agencies, to ensure faithful representation of population diseases, placed a premium on the inclusion of community patients into research protocols. These agencies also issued directives to AHCs to provide comprehensive population care and mandated the formal reporting of AHC involvement with community patient populations [19–25]. Overall, these influences forced AHCs to redefine their core mission with a new emphasis on the integration of the CHC and their patient populations [26–28]. Given their previous work in shaping medical policy, their stewardship of medical education, and their diverse and extensive resources, AHCs readily assumed a leadership role in the restructuring of the CHC/AHC relationship and the creation of integrated partnerships [2,29–35].

The alliance between CHCs and AHCs provides advantages to both partners. CHCs and AHCs enjoy better positioning within the healthcare marketplace. The improved marketplace positioning results primarily from economy of scale pricing that accompanies the integration and expansion of patient services, procedures and therapeutics; the alliance secures for both partners more stable financial footings [36]. The alliance makes possible specific benefits for the CHC. This alliance permits the CHC more direct access to AHC-generated experimental therapeutics, clinical trials, translational research, medical devices and protocols [37]. Further, evidence suggests that affiliation with an AHC often enhances the prestige and attractiveness of the CHC, increases patient and clinical staff retention, fosters more opportunity for continuing professional development, frequently results in greater professional satisfaction and has the potential to enhance the quality and efficacy of the CHC [38–40]. For the AHC, partnerships with a CHC allow for enhanced opportunities to interact more tangibly with the community patient population and expand and diversify patient pools for translational research and clinical trial enrollment; partnerships also increase the ability of AHCs to mitigate outcomes and patient access disparities [41]. Multiple examples of successful CHC/AHC partnerships exist; they serve as models for the feasibility and potential future CHC/AHC partnerships [42–44].

3. Community Oncology and Academic Cancer Center Alliance

The integration of CHCs with AHCs most tangibly manifests as practice changes within specific departments, including, prominently, medical oncology [45–51]. During recent years cancer care has transitioned from primarily private, CHC-based oncology practices to AHC-affiliated and -integrated network cancer centers [51–55]. This transition has advantaged the community cancer patient as the services associated with the academic cancer center provide added value.

At the City of Hope Comprehensive Cancer Center (COHCCC), patients identify a number of key value elements associated with the academic cancer center including access to cancer disease specialists, the availability of clinical, translational and basic science researchers, potential for clinical trial participation and enhanced comprehensive care coordinated through multidisciplinary clinical teams [56].

Across a broad range of cancers, patients experience improved survival when receiving treatment at an academic cancer center or at a community hospital associated with an AHC [57–64]. Academic cancer centers provide additional value to community practices through the discovery and provision of novel drugs, experimental medical devices, treatment protocols and technological advancements [65–71]. Reciprocally, academic cancer centers benefit from their alliance with community oncology practices by expanding clinical trial portfolios [72–74], increasing patient diversity in cancer translational and basic research initiatives [75–79], enhancing cancer center core mission accomplishment through community cancer patient engagement [80] and reducing cancer care costs resulting from increased patient volumes [81].

The introduction of new technologies and scientific techniques underscores the importance and potential of the alliance between community oncology practices and academic cancer centers. Specifically, recent advances in genetics and tumor genomics have provided a foundation for the emergence of precision oncology; the community/academic oncology alliance promises to accelerate significantly the clinical utility of precision oncology for the cancer care of community patients [82–85].

4. The Age of Precision Oncology

Cancers exhibit highly complex genomic and epigenomic alterations; these alterations dictate their overall phenotypic behavior that includes growth characteristics, metastatic potential, interplay between cells and microenvironmental interactions and responses. Over the past several decades, scientific strategies to prevent, diagnose and treat cancer have radically shifted from histology-based to genomically- and immunologically-informed approaches [86].

Since completion of the Human Genome Project in 2003 [87], a series of convergent technological advances resulted from academic-based initiatives. These advances include the introduction and adoption of next generation nucleic acid sequencing (NGS), exponential improvements in computer hardware capabilities, optimization of data processing approaches, evolution of increasingly sophisticated computational biological methods and the discovery and utilization of targeted cancer therapies. Together these advances made possible precision medicine and, more exactly, precision oncology [82,88–90].

NGS arose from innovative DNA sequencing methodologies, most notably massively parallel signature sequencing [91,92]. NGS permits tractable high throughput sequencing of immensely large and complex DNA samples such as whole human exomes and genomes [93,94]. Geneticists first employed NGS to sequence accurately and rapidly the human germline genome [95], allowing insights into the cause of inherited disease [96,97]; investigators then extended the technology to sequence somatic cancer genomes [98]. Scientists further refined the applications of NGS technology. New applications permitted assessment of not only single nucleotide variation and nucleotide insertions and deletions, but also the transcriptome to assess gene expression [99–101], copy number variation [102], complex genomic structural variation [103], protein-DNA interactions [104], targetable epigenetic alterations [105] and epigenetic mechanisms regulating 3D genome structure [106].

In addition to examining tumor genomics, there arose an interest in understanding the immune profiles of the tumor and its microenvironment using NGS; in part, this interest developed from the recognition that tumor genomic changes frequently result in the production of unique, highly immunogenic neoantigens that render the tumor vulnerable to immune surveillance and destruction [107,108]. With the appreciation that the immune system plays an important role in cancer initiation and progression, there has also occurred new interest in targeted therapies aimed at activation of the immune axis [109,110].

NGS generates enormous caches of data; use of these immense data sets for precision oncology requires ever increasing levels of computer hardware performance. Employment of Dennard scaling [111] and multicore architectures [112] have sustained exponential increases in computer chip performance [113–115]. Data processing innovations have included parallel algorithm implementation [116] and parallel data computing [117]; such innovations have force multiplied the efficiency and speed of computation. These approaches allow data analysts to keep pace with the ever increasing information workloads of precision oncology [118].

The realization of precision oncology required adoption of computational biological approaches. The creation of computational biology as an independent academic discipline resulted from the complexity and size of biological data sets. In the case of NGS, the sheer number of nucleotides reads, the task of aligning these reads to reference sequences, predicting functional consequences of genomic variation and the translation of these findings into clinically actionable information necessitated computational biological expertise [119–122]. Computational biological analysis now constitutes an integral element of the data workflow in precision oncology [123–126]; effective clinical translation depends inextricably upon the availability of these computational resources [127–130].

In the early 1970's, Drs. Janet Rowley, Peter Nowell and Alfred Knudson, studying leukemia cell chromosomes under the microscope, suggested that a specific chromosomal translocation that resulted in the formation of the BCR-ABL fusion oncogene caused chronic myelogenous leukemia (CML); this observation established a foundation for clinical cancer genomics [131]. Oncogenic proteins consequently became a focus of therapeutic drug design; targeted therapies aimed to suppress the aberrant functions of these proteins in order to inhibit tumor progression [132,133].

The successful harnessing of precision therapeutics in oncology ultimately relies upon the availability and efficacy of targeted agents. The discovery that imatinib effectively treats CML harboring the BCR-ABL fusion protein [134] led to the drug's FDA approval in 2001 [135], demonstrated the utility of targeted cancer therapy [136,137], kindled enthusiasm for the identification of other genetically vulnerable cancers and their treatments [90,138] and underscored the clinical value and potential of precision oncology [98,139,140]. Since the success of imatinib, the FDA has approved a multitude of additional therapies to target molecularly-altered cancers [141,142].

The clinical provision of precision oncology requires multidisciplinary support [143]; the complexity of this support will become more intense as precision oncology continues to undergo accelerating change [144–146]. AHCs possess the resources and organization to create this support structure; their alliance with CHC oncology practitioners will make precision oncology available to the larger CHC cancer population.

5. The Community Oncology/Academic Cancer Center Alliance in Germline Cancer Genetics

NGS and precision oncology have had a profound effect upon the practice of cancer genetics, including the evaluation and care of community patients with hereditary predisposition to cancer [147–151]. Until recently, genetic testing involved clinical assessment followed by sequential, single gene Sanger sequencing of suspect genes [152–156]. The advent of NGS brought high throughput germline multigene panel [157–161], whole exome [162–167] and whole genome assessment [168–172] to clinical cancer genetics. These platforms provide tremendous benefit to cancer genetics patients both in community oncology practices and at academic cancer centers; these advantages include increased diagnostic yield, increased speed of testing, optimized testing workflows, decreased expense and the discovery of new cancer-causing genes [173–177]. However, together with advantages, challenges and limitations arise; AHCs have the specialized resources to address these issues.

In accordance with the American College of Medical Genetics and the Association for Molecular Pathology guidelines, variants from clinical genetic testing fall along a spectrum ranging from pathogenic/likely pathogenic to benign/likely benign [178]; variants of uncertain significance (VUS) occur when there exists insufficient information for variant assignment to either the pathogenic or benign categories [179,180]. For pathogenic/likely pathogenic and benign/likely benign variants, genetic providers typically have the ability to communicate clear interpretation of results and to provide consensus health recommendations. As their pathogenicity remains uncertain, VUS challenge health care specialists to formulate and relay unambiguous health care instructions [181–185]; furthermore, VUS frequently cause confusion and anxiety for the patient [186–190]. VUS impose a significant clinical burden. More than one third of NGS-based cancer gene panel tests result in identification of a VUS [191]; whole exome and genome testing generate even greater numbers of VUS [192–195]. Moreover, if a patient belongs to a minority group, for whom genome annotations remain less well confirmed, VUS additionally increase [196].

Geneticists classify genes according to their penetrance, that is, how likely will a pathogenic variant of a gene cause disease [197]. For pathogenic variants of high penetrance genes, clinicians more often have firmly established guidelines that inform recommendations for patient screening and surveillance. However, for pathological variants of low penetrance genes, less definitive clinical guidelines exist. NGS-based testing results in increasing detection of pathogenic variants of low penetrance genes; this increased detection adds complexity and uncertainty to patient management [198,199].

Clinicians face another challenge when selecting NGS gene panels for genetic evaluation: they must select the composition of the gene panel that they will employ. This selection requires specialized education and training [200,201]. The cancer genetics expertise required to address this challenge remains scarce [202–205]; the wider use of NGS platforms in clinical oncology and continued technological advances has made this expertise even more scarce [206–208].

AHCs possess the clinical expertise, facilities, support personnel, and administrative structures to meet the burgeoning demands of cancer genetics and to overcome the obstacles associated with the use of NGS in the clinic. Allied community oncology practices and their patients have access to these resources and services through their partnerships with AHCs. Four access models enable community oncology patient engagement with the AHC: (1) patient consultation visits to the academic cancer center, (2) cancer genetics specialist visits to community oncology sites, (3) telemedicine- and web-based remote visits and (4) AHC-sponsored genetic education initiatives that train community oncology practitioners to assess and manage cancer genetic risk and disease (Figure 1).

Conventionally, community oncology patients have received their cancer genetics care by consulting, in person, with a specialist at an AHC [155,209–211]. This model disadvantages community patients who live substantial distances from an AHC as it involves significant travel time and cost commitments [210,212,213]. Alternative cancer genetics delivery models have the potential to mitigate these problems.

In the community satellite clinic model, AHC cancer genetic specialists travel to the CHC clinic on an interval basis to meet the cancer genetic needs of community patients. This approach has proven successful in a variety of circumstances where logistical or economic challenges create barriers to effective cancer genetics care [214–217].

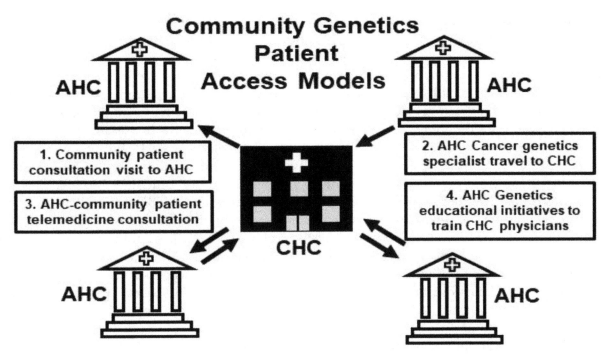

Figure 1. Community health center (CHC) patients requiring genetics care interface with specialists at academic health centers (AHC) through four modes of interaction. (1) The CHC patient may travel to the AHC for assessment. (2) The AHC genetics specialist may travel to a satellite CHC genetics clinic to evaluate the CHC patient. (3) CHC patients and AHC genetic specialists may interact via telemedicine consultation. (4) In order to provide genetics care to their patients, CHC physicians may undergo genetics specialty training sponsored by AHCs.

In our digital era, innovative cancer genetics delivery models have emerged; telemedicine platforms that involve both telephony and video communication platforms represent one such model [218–222]. The Division of Clinical Cancer Genetics (CCG) at COHCCC has assumed a national leadership position in the adoption of digital age technologies to provide academic center cancer genetic services to community oncology practices and their patients.

The CCG formed the Cancer Screening and Program Network (CSPPN), building a bridge to community oncology practices; the CSPPN utilizes innovative videoconferencing, telemedicine and wed-based applications to provide cancer genetics services [223]. Innovation continues at the CCG with the ongoing construction of new software and web-based platforms to permit effective communication between academic cancer genetics providers and community-based patients and practitioners [224].Alongside the use of these digital platforms, the CCG has administered a landmark educational program to provide community oncology healthcare providers with the necessary training that allows them to function as competent cancer risk assessment specialists in their own communities [225]. This program, funded by the National Cancer Institute, has expanded the workforce of qualified germline genetics providers and has helped to alleviate the shortage of cancer genetics expertise in CHC practices.

Educational programs, such as that sponsored by the CCG, have acquired additional practical importance as many healthcare systems now require, prior to genetic testing, assessment by a healthcare provider trained in genetics. These requirements may hinder effective cancer genetics care, particularly in underserved communities [226]; the availability of training will help eliminate this hindrance.

6. The Community Oncology/Academic Cancer Center Alliance in Somatic Tumor Genomics

The use of clinical NGS in oncology has risen exponentially [227]. Hundreds of commercial and academic laboratories now offer NGS-based clinical sequencing of cancer specimens [119,228]. The NGS sequencing formats for somatic tumor sequencing include, among others, whole exome, whole genome, targeted panel, transcriptome and liquid biopsy assessments [229–235]. Various factors have driven the increased clinical application of NGS for somatic tumor assessment. The number of targetable genomic alterations increases substantially each year. Currently, there exist well over one hundred FDA-approved targeted therapies available for the treatment of both solid and hematological cancers [98]; over the past year alone, the FDA granted approval to nearly 20 new drugs or new indications for previously approved drugs [96]. With inclusion of therapy based upon molecular pathway considerations or off-label usage based on tissue-agnostic variant matching, the set of molecular targets and usage indications expands geometrically [236–244]. Purposing NGS-based somatic testing to determine clinical trial eligibility further increases the utility of NGS [245–248]; moreover, the demonstrated efficacy of testing to achieve improved outcomes has also motivated demand [248–252]. The decision by the Centers for Medicare and Medicaid Services to provide insurance coverage for NGS-based sequencing tests removed a financial barrier against the use of NGS, and contributed to the expanded use of this technology [253–255]. All told, currently over three quarters of oncologists use now NGS-base clinical testing to guide treatment decisions [256].

Significant challenges, however, temper enthusiasm for the clinical institution of somatic tumor NGS. A majority of oncologists report difficulty interpreting NGS somatic tumor testing, lack understanding of the clinical indications for testing and have inadequate opportunities to acquire the necessary training to properly use testing. One quarter of oncologists refer patients to other specialists to assist with NGS testing, and approximately 1 in 5 oncologists did not feel they had the proper knowledge to use properly NGS testing [256–258]. Additionally, oncologists report challenges with managing the large data volumes generated from NGS somatic testing. Oncologists also feel that they do not have the ability to distill from these reports actionable information; further, they lack the skill to manage germline variants detected as incidental findings in somatic NGS tumor testing [259–262]. These obstacles may be amplified for the CHC-based oncologist who lacks access to the necessary computational resources, logistical support and expertise in targeted therapeutics [263–266].

The CHC/AHC alliance provides solutions to alleviate these obstacles. Innovative AHC-based web applications make available to community oncologists an analytic framework and the computational tools to aid in the interpretation and clinical implementation of NGS sequencing results (Table 1). CIViC, an open access web resource, serves as a public central repository of NGS data "supporting clinical interpretations related to cancer" [267]. OncoKB, a precision oncology database, aids therapeutic decision-making based upon cancer gene variant status [268]; similarly, the web applications Personalized Cancer Therapy and My Cancer Genome assist both community and academic oncologists in selecting therapeutic options resulting from the somatic NGS of tumor specimens [269,270]. The SMART Cancer Navigator aggregates variant and clinical data from multiple data bases to assist community-based oncologists with the processing of NGS reports and the identification of effective targeted therapies [271]. At the COHCCC, investigators have configured an interactive web interface, HOPE-Genomics, that community patients and oncologists may use to better understand genomic sequencing results and treatment recommendations [224]. The COHCCC also provides to its community practice partners in-house NGS panel testing as part of its HOPESEQ molecular testing panel [272]; HOPESEQ includes genomic test reports designed to assist clinicians with interpreting the genetic testing results and clinical decision making. Furthermore, COHCCC physicians and community partners have access to Via Oncology; this tool provides a web-based clinical pathway system to help match patients with clinical trials and insurance reimbursement for NGS driven treatments [273].

Precision oncology tumor boards (POTBs) represent another solution to the problem of implementing NGS data in the CHC oncology clinic. POTBs arose from the need to assess, process and generate clinical treatment plans from the highly dense and complex data sets that arise from somatic NGS of tumor specimens [274]. POTBs serve two primary functions: targeted therapy drug matching and molecularly-informed clinical trial enrollment [275–280] (Figure 2).

Table 1. Web-based genomics resources available to community oncologists.

WEB-BASED RESOURCE	URL
CIViC	civicdb.org
OncoKB	oncokb.org
Personalized Cancer Therapy	pct.mdanderson.org
My Cancer Genome	mycancergenome.org
SMART Cancer Navigator	smart-cancer-navigator.github.io/home
ASCO Multidisciplinary Molecular Tumor Boards	elearning.asco.org/product-details/multidisciplinary-molecular-tumor/boards-mmtbs
Helio Learn Genomics	healio.com
Know Your Tumor	pancan.org

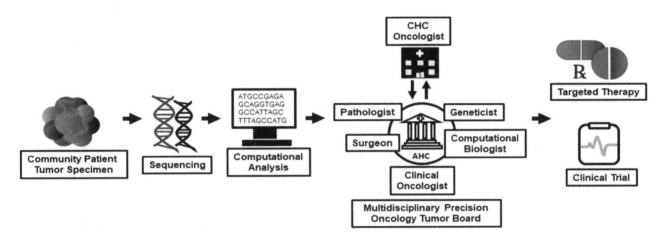

Figure 2. Multidisciplinary precision oncology tumor boards (POTBs) provide expert targeted drug matching and molecularly informed clinical trial enrollment for community oncology patients. Tumor specimens from community patients undergo nucleic acid sequencing with computational analysis to identify molecular alterations; this information provides a basis to discover candidate targeted therapies and determine clinical trial eligibility. An academic health center (AHC) POTB comprising, among others, clinical oncologists, pathologists, surgeons, geneticists and computational biologists, in consultation with community health center (CHC) oncologists, reviews patients' clinical cases and their sequencing results to select appropriate targeted therapies and clinical trials.

POTBs originated within AHCs as these centers possess the multidisciplinary expertise including, among others, clinical oncologists, pathologists, genomics specialists, computational biologists, pharmacologists and clinical geneticists to efficiently identify targeted therapies and clinical trials [281–290]. Targeted therapy drug matching requires comprehensive molecular mutational profiling and downstream pathway analyses of the tumor, combined with the identification of safe and effective therapeutic agents that redress these molecular alterations [291–293]; CHCs typically do not possess the analytic or pharmacologic capabilities to adequately perform these activities. Most clinical trials fail [294–296]; these failures result from a number of factors including deficient clinical trial design, poor proof of concept planning and insufficient administrative support and compliance [297–300]. Such failures have adverse consequences for both the clinical trial sponsors as well as the patients; failure has significant economic cost and results in lost therapeutic opportunity, in addition to potentially exposing the patient to harm from the investigational protocol and drugs [301–303]. These clinical trial-related matters may be more acute at CHCs given their more limited resources and the absence of experienced clinical trialists [304–307]. The POTB provides appropriate, molecularly-informed clinical trial assignment for patients, maximizing both the utility of clinical trial participation and potential patient benefit [308–320].

Given the resource limitations of the CHC oncology clinic, community POTB operation requires innovation and dedicated planning [83,321,322]. One innovation available to community oncologists, the web-based ASCO Multidisciplinary Molecular Tumor Boards, assists oncologists with understanding precision medicine-based tumor testing and the therapy recommendations resulting from these tests [323] (Table 1). Helio Learn Genomics, another web platform, offers a number of educational modules, including POTB cases, to help providers understand the molecular bases of carcinogenesis and precision therapeutics [324]. The Pancreatic Cancer Action Network administers a Know Your Tumor program, a turn-key precision medicine initiative, that allows community oncology practitioners to submit their patients' pancreatic cancer specimens for NGS molecular testing and to receive back a precision medicine-based treatment plan [325].

Another version of the POTB, the virtual POTB, permits the distance participation of community oncologists in an academic POTB. In this model an AHC hosts the POTB and reviews the clinical history and precision oncology testing results of the community oncology patient; subsequently, the POTB discusses with the community oncologist, using a live interactive video teleconferencing link, targeted treatment and clinical trial recommendations [263,311,326–330]. The Translational Genomics Research Institute (TGEN), an academic affiliate of the COHCCC, has successfully built a comprehensive, integrated, high-throughput sequencing and reporting framework that, when combined with remote teleconferencing, has proven tremendously successful in establishing efficient collaborative POTBs [331–335]. Together, these various models of providing clinical somatic NGS demonstrate the feasibility of leveraging precision oncology for the community-based cancer oncologist and their patients.

7. Conclusions

We have entered the age of precision oncology. Precision oncology offers the potential of molecularly informed medicine for the assessment of inherited cancer predisposition, as well as for the diagnosis and treatment of cancers. Realization of this potential depends upon access to specialized expertise and significant analytic and technological resources. While frequently available at AHCs, these resources have previously been limited for CHC oncology practices and their patients. In this paper, we have examined the CHC/AHC alliance and discussed examples illustrating how this alliance provides a structure that allows community cancer patients to benefit from germline and somatic precision oncology advances. Looking forward, multidisciplinary efforts, improved technology and continuing innovation promise to strengthen and facilitate the CHC/AHC alliance in oncology; this alliance offers community oncologists and their patients the prospect of unambiguous interpretation of genetic and genomic test results and optimized precision oncology care.

Author Contributions: Writing-Original Draft Preparation, M.M., S.S. (Shanmuga Subbiah), K.J.M.; Writing-Review and Editing, S.S. (Swapnil Rajurkar). All authors have read and agreed to the published version of the manuscript.

References

1. Wartman, S.A. *The Transformation of Academic Health Centers: Meeting The Challenges Of Healthcare's Changing Landscape*; Academic Press: Fribourg, Switzerland, 2015.
2. Dzau, V.J.; Ackerly, D.C.; Sutton-Wallace, P.; Merson, M.H.; Williams, R.S.; Krishnan, K.R.; Taber, R.C.; Califf, R.M. The role of academic health science systems in the transformation of medicine. *Lancet* **2010**, *375*, 949–953. [CrossRef]
3. Desch, C.E.; Blayney, D.W. Making the choice between academic oncology and community practice: the big picture and details about each career. *J. Oncol. Pract.* **2006**, *2*, 132–136. [CrossRef]
4. Todd, R.F., III. A guide to planning careers in hematology and oncology. *Hematol. Am. Soc. Hemat.* **2001**, *2001*, 499–506. [CrossRef] [PubMed]

5. Levit, L.A.; Kim, E.S.; McAneny, B.L.; Nadauld, L.D.; Levit, K.; Schenkel, C.; Schilsky, R.L. Implementing precision medicine in community-based oncology programs: Three models. *J. Oncol. Pract.* **2019**, *15*, 325–329. [CrossRef] [PubMed]

6. Thompson, M.A.; Godden, J.J.; Weissman, S.M.; Wham, D.; Wilson, A.; Ruggeri, A.; Mullane, M.P.; Weese, J.L. Implementing an oncology precision medicine clinic in a large community health system. *Am. J. Manag. Care* **2017**, *23*, SP425–SP427.

7. Levine, D.M.; Becker, D.M.; Bone, L.R.; Hill, M.N.; Tuggle, M.B., II; Zeger, S.L. Community-academic health center partnerships for underserved minority populations. One solution to a national crisis. *J. Am. Med. Assoc.* **1994**, *272*, 309–311. [CrossRef]

8. Shin, P.; Sharac, J.; Rosenbaum, S. Community health centers and medicaid at 50: An. Enduring relationship essential for health system transformation. *Health Aff. (Millwood)* **2015**, *34*, 1096–1104. [CrossRef]

9. Sharma, A.E.; Huang, B.; Knox, M.; Willard-Grace, R.; Potter, M.B. Patient engagement in community health center leadership: How does it happen? *J. Community Health* **2018**, *43*, 1069–1074. [CrossRef] [PubMed]

10. Blumenthal, D.; Meyer, G.S. Academic health centers in a changing environment. *Health Aff. (Millwood)* **1996**, *15*, 200–215. [CrossRef]

11. Nash, D.B.; Veloski, J.J. Emerging opportunities for educational partnerships between managed care organizations and academic health centers. *West. J. Med.* **1998**, *168*, 319–327. [PubMed]

12. Roper, W.L.; Newton, W.P. The role of academic health centers in improving health. *Ann. Fam. Med.* **2006**, *4*, S55–S57. [CrossRef] [PubMed]

13. Blumenthal, D.; Meyer, G.S. The future of the academic medical center under health care reform. *N. Engl. J. Med.* **1993**, *329*, 1812–1814. [CrossRef]

14. Fox, P.D.; Wasserman, J. Academic medical centers and managed care: Uneasy partners. *Health Aff. (Millwood)* **1993**, *12*, 85–93. [CrossRef]

15. Epstein, A.M. US teaching hospitals in the evolving health care system. *J. Am. Med. Assoc.* **1995**, *273*, 1203–1207. [CrossRef]

16. Iglehart, J.K. Academic medical centers enter the market: The case of Philadelphia. *N. Engl. J. Med.* **1995**, *333*, 1019–1023. [CrossRef] [PubMed]

17. Lofgren, R.; Karpf, M.; Perman, J.; Higdon, C.M. The U.S. health care system is in crisis: Implications for academic medical centers and their missions. *Acad. Med.* **2006**, *81*, 713–720. [CrossRef]

18. Park, B.; Frank, B.; Likumahuwa-Ackman, S.; Brodt, E.; Gibbs, B.K.; Hofkamp, H.; DeVoe, J. Health equity and the tripartite mission: Moving from academic health centers to academic-community health systems. *Acad. Med.* **2019**, *94*, 1276–1282. [CrossRef]

19. Bartlett, S.J.; Barnes, T.; McIvor, R.A. Integrating patients into meaningful real-world research. *Ann. Am. Thorac. Soc.* **2014**, *11*, S112–S117. [CrossRef]

20. Gourevitch, M.N. Population health and the academic medical center: The time is right. *Acad. Med.* **2014**, *89*, 544–549. [CrossRef] [PubMed]

21. Vitale, K.; Newton, G.L.; Abraido-Lanza, A.F.; Aguirre, A.N.; Ahmed, S.; Esmond, S.L.; Evans, J.; Gelmon, S.B.; Hart, C.; Hendricks, D.; et al. Community engagement in academic health centers: A model for capturing and advancing our successes. *J. Commun. Engagem. Scholarsh.* **2018**, *10*, 81–90.

22. Zerhouni, E. Medicine: The NIH roadmap. *Science* **2003**, *302*, 63–72. [CrossRef] [PubMed]

23. Schwenk, T.L.; Green, L.A. The Michigan Clinical Research Collaboratory: Following the NIH Roadmap to the community. *Ann. Fam. Med.* **2006**, *4*, S49–S54. [CrossRef] [PubMed]

24. Zerhouni, E.A. Translational and clinical science—Time for a new vision. *N. Engl. J. Med.* **2005**, *353*, 1621–1623. [CrossRef] [PubMed]

25. Zerhouni, E.A. US biomedical research: Basic, translational, and clinical sciences. *J. Am. Med. Assoc.* **2005**, *294*, 1352–1358. [CrossRef]

26. Kassirer, J.P. Academic medical centers under siege. *N. Engl. J. Med.* **1994**, *331*, 1370–1371. [CrossRef]

27. Iglehart, J.K. Rapid changes for academic medical centers. 2. *N. Engl. J. Med.* **1995**, *332*, 407–411. [CrossRef]

28. Iglehart, J.K. Rapid changes for academic medical centers. 1. *N. Engl. J. Med.* **1994**, *331*, 1391–1395. [CrossRef]

29. Moses, H., III; Matheson, D.H.M.; Poste, G. Serving individuals and populations within integrated health systems: A bridge too far? *J. Am. Med. Assoc.* **2019**, *321*, 1975–1976. [CrossRef]

30. Cutler, D.M.; Morton, F.S. Hospitals, market share, and consolidation. *J. Am. Med. Assoc.* **2013**, *310*, 1964–1970. [CrossRef]

31. Moses, H., III; Matheson, D.H.; Dorsey, E.R.; George, B.P.; Sadoff, D.; Yoshimura, S. The anatomy of health care in the United States. *J. Am. Med. Assoc.* **2013**, *310*, 1947–1963. [CrossRef]

32. Cohen, M.D.; Jennings, G. Mergers involving academic medical institutions: Impact on academic radiology departments. *J. Am. Coll. Radiol.* **2005**, *2*, 174–182. [CrossRef] [PubMed]

33. Denham, A.C.; Hay, S.S.; Steiner, B.D.; Newton, W.P. Academic health centers and community health centers partnering to build a system of care for vulnerable patients: Lessons from Carolina Health Net. *Acad. Med.* **2013**, *88*, 638–643. [CrossRef] [PubMed]

34. Rieselbach, R.E.; Rieselbach, R.E.; Epperly, T.; Friedman, A.; Keahey, D.; McConnell, E.; Nichols, K.; Nycz, G.; Roberts, J.; Schmader, K.; et al. A new community health center/academic medicine partnership for medicaid cost control, powered by the Mega Teaching Health Center. *Acad. Med.* **2018**, *93*, 406–413. [CrossRef]

35. Blumenthal, D.; Campbell, E.G.; Weissman, J.S. The social missions of academic health centers. *N. Engl. J. Med.* **1997**, *337*, 1550–1553. [CrossRef]

36. Fleishon, H.B.; Itri, J.N.; Boland, G.W.; Duszak, R., Jr. Academic medical centers and community hospitals integration: Trends and strategies. *J. Am. Coll. Radiol.* **2017**, *14*, 45–51. [CrossRef]

37. Ellner, A.L.; Stout, S.; Sullivan, E.E.; Griffiths, E.P.; Mountjoy, A.; Phillips, R.S. Health systems innovation at academic health centers: Leading in a new era of health care delivery. *Acad. Med.* **2015**, *90*, 872–880. [CrossRef] [PubMed]

38. Moore, G.T.; Inui, T.S.; Ludden, J.M.; Schoenbaum, S.C. The "teaching HMO": A new academic partner. *Acad. Med.* **1994**, *69*, 595–600. [CrossRef] [PubMed]

39. Poncelet, A.N.; Mazotti, L.A.; Blumberg, B.; Wamsley, M.A.; Grennan, T.; Shore, W.B. Creating a longitudinal integrated clerkship with mutual benefits for an academic medical center and a community health system. *Perm. J.* **2014**, *18*, 50–56. [CrossRef]

40. Berkowitz, S.A.; Brown, P.; Brotman, D.J.; Deutschendorf, A.; Dunbar, L.; Everett, A.; Hickman, D.; Howell, E.; Purnell, L.; Sylvester, C.; et al. Case Study: Johns Hopkins Community Health Partnership: A model for transformation. *Healthc (Amst.)* **2016**, *4*, 264–270. [CrossRef]

41. Institute of Medicine (US) Committee on Understanding and Eliminating Racial and Ethnic Disparities in Health Care. *Unequal Treatment: Confronting Racial and Ethnic Disparities in Health Care*; Smedley, B.D., Stith, A.Y., Nelson, A.R., Eds.; National Academies Press: Washington, DC, USA, 2003.

42. Ahmed, S.M.; Maurana, C.; Nelson, D.; Meister, T.; Young, S.N.; Lucey, P. Opening the black box: Conceptualizing community engagement from 109 community-academic partnership programs. *Prog. Community Health Partnersh.* **2016**, *10*, 51–61. [CrossRef]

43. Croft, C.R.; Dial, R.; Doyle, G.; Schaadt, J.; Merchant, L. Integrating a community hospital-based radiology department with an academic medical center. *J. Am. Coll. Radiol.* **2016**, *13*, 300–302. [CrossRef]

44. Sussman, A.J.; Otten, J.R.; Goldszer, R.C.; Hanson, M.; Trull, D.J.; Paulus, K.; Brown, M.; Dzau, V.; Brennan, T.A. Integration of an academic medical center and a community hospital: The Brigham and Women's/Faulkner hospital experience. *Acad. Med.* **2005**, *80*, 253–260. [CrossRef] [PubMed]

45. Spalluto, L.B.; Thomas, D.; Beard, K.R.; Campbell, T.; Audet, C.M.; McBride Murry, V.; Shrubsole, M.J.; Barajas, C.P.; Joosten, Y.A.; Dittus, R.S.; et al. A community-academic partnership to reduce health care disparities in diagnostic imaging. *J. Am. Coll. Radiol.* **2019**, *16*, 649–656. [CrossRef] [PubMed]

46. Kelley-Quon, L.I.; Thomas, D.; Beard, K.R.; Campbell, T.; Audet, C.M.; McBride Murry, V.; Shrubsole, M.J.; Barajas, C.P.; Joosten, Y.A.; Dittus, R.S.; et al. Academic-community partnerships improve outcomes in pediatric trauma care. *J. Pediatr. Surg.* **2015**, *50*, 1032–1036. [CrossRef] [PubMed]

47. Phillip, C.R.; Mancera-Cuevas, K.; Leatherwood, C.; Chmiel, J.S.; Erickson, D.L.; Freeman, E.; Granville, G.; Dollear, M.; Walker, K.; McNeil, R.; et al. Implementation and dissemination of an African American popular opinion model to improve lupus awareness: An academic-community partnership. *Lupus* **2019**, *28*, 1441–1451. [CrossRef] [PubMed]

48. Rees, T. Academic medical center, community hospital partner to market center of excellence. *Profiles Healthc. Mark.* **1999**, *15*, 40–43.

49. Yaggy, S.D.; Michener, J.L.; Yaggy, D.; Champagne, M.T.; Silberberg, M.; Lyn, M.; Johnson, F.; Yarnall, K.S. Just for Us: An academic medical center-community partnership to maintain the health of a frail low-income senior population. *Gerontologist* **2006**, *46*, 271–276. [CrossRef]

50. Natesan, R.; Yang, W.T.; Tannir, H.; Parikh, J. Strategic expansion models in academic radiology. *J. Am. Coll. Radiol.* **2016**, *13*, 329–334. [CrossRef]

51. Kirkwood, M.K.; Hanley, A.; Bruinooge, S.S.; Garrett-Mayer, E.; Levit, L.A.; Schenkel, C.; Seid, J.E.; Polite, B.N.; Schilsky, R.L. The State of oncology practice in America, 2018: results of the ASCO practice census survey. *J. Oncol. Pract.* **2018**, *14*, e412–e420. [CrossRef]

52. OBR New Perspective Catalyst. *Most Cancer Patients Will Be Treated in Integrated Delivery Networks (IDN) and Cancer Institutions by 2016, Predicts New Report*; OBR New Perspective Catalyst: Sausalito, CA, USA, 2012; Volume 11.

53. Genetech. *The 2018 Genentech Oncology Trend Report*; Genetech: San Francisco, CA, USA, 2018.

54. Genetech. *The 2019 Genentech Oncology Trend Report*; Genetech: San Francisco, CA, USA, 2019.

55. Academic Cancer Centers (NCCC). *Trends Impacting Key Account. Management*; Academic Cancer Centers: Pipersville, PA, USA, 2016.

56. Nardi, E.A.; Wolfson, J.A.; Rosen, S.T.; Diasio, R.B.; Gerson, S.L.; Parker, B.A.; Alvarnas, J.C.; Levine, H.A.; Fong, Y.; Weisenburger, D.D.; et al. Value, access, and cost of cancer care delivery at academic cancer centers. *J. Natl. Compr. Cancer Netw.* **2016**, *14*, 837–847. [CrossRef]

57. Speicher, P.J.; Englum, B.R.; Ganapathi, A.M.; Wang, X.; Hartwig, M.G.; D'Amico, T.A.; Berry, M.F. Traveling to a high-volume center is associated with improved survival for patients with esophageal cancer. *Ann. Surg.* **2017**, *265*, 743–749. [CrossRef] [PubMed]

58. Lidsky, M.E.; Sun, Z.; Nussbaum, D.P.; Adam, M.A.; Speicher, P.J.; Blazer, D.G., III. Going the extra mile: Improved survival for pancreatic cancer patients traveling to high-volume centers. *Ann. Surg.* **2017**, *266*, 333–338. [CrossRef] [PubMed]

59. David, J.M.; Ho, A.S.; Luu, M.; Yoshida, E.J.; Kim, S.; Mita, A.C.; Scher, K.S.; Shiao, S.L.; Tighiouart, M.; Zumsteg, Z.S. Treatment at high-volume facilities and academic centers is independently associated with improved survival in patients with locally advanced head and neck cancer. *Cancer* **2017**, *123*, 3933–3942. [CrossRef]

60. Chen, A.Y.; Fedewa, S.; Pavluck, A.; Ward, E.M. Improved survival is associated with treatment at high-volume teaching facilities for patients with advanced stage laryngeal cancer. *Cancer* **2010**, *116*, 4744–4752. [CrossRef] [PubMed]

61. Pfister, D.G.; Rubin, D.M.; Elkin, E.B.; Neill, U.S.; Duck, E.; Radzyner, M.; Bach, P.B. Risk adjusting survival outcomes in hospitals that treat patients with cancer without information on cancer stage. *JAMA Oncol.* **2015**, *1*, 1303–1310. [CrossRef] [PubMed]

62. Schmitz, R.; Adam, M.A.; Blazer, D.G., III. Overcoming a travel burden to high-volume centers for treatment of retroperitoneal sarcomas is associated with improved survival. *World J. Surg. Oncol.* **2019**, *17*, 180. [CrossRef] [PubMed]

63. Dillman, R.O.; Chico, S.D. Cancer patient survival improvement is correlated with the opening of a community cancer center: Comparisons with intramural and extramural benchmarks. *J. Oncol. Pract.* **2005**, *1*, 84–92. [CrossRef] [PubMed]

64. Ramalingam, S.; Dinan, M.A.; Crawford, J. Survival comparison in patients with stage iv lung cancer in academic versus community centers in the United States. *J. Thorac. Oncol.* **2018**, *13*, 1842–1850. [CrossRef] [PubMed]

65. Carugo, A.; Draetta, G.F. Academic discovery of anticancer drugs: Historic and future perspectives. *Ann. Rev. Cancer Biol.* **2019**, *3*, 385–408. [CrossRef]

66. Everett, J.R. Academic drug discovery: Current status and prospects. *Expert Opin. Drug Discov.* **2015**, *10*, 937–944. [CrossRef] [PubMed]

67. Matter, A. Bridging academic science and clinical research in the search for novel targeted anti-cancer agents. *Cancer Biol. Med.* **2015**, *12*, 316–327. [PubMed]

68. Dorfman, G.S.; Lawrence, T.S.; Matrisian, L.M.; Translational Research Working Group. The Translational Research Working Group developmental pathway for interventive devices. *Clin. Cancer Res.* **2008**, *14*, 5700–5706. [CrossRef] [PubMed]

69. Barrios, C.H.; Reinert, T.; Werutsky, G. Global breast cancer research: Moving forward. *Am. Soc. Clin. Oncol. Educ. Book.* **2018**, *38*, 441–450. [CrossRef] [PubMed]

70. Huber, M.A.; Kraut, N. Key drivers of biomedical innovation in cancer drug discovery. *EMBO Mol. Med.* **2015**, *7*, 12–16. [CrossRef] [PubMed]

71. Grodzinski, P.; Liu, C.H.; Hartshorn, C.M.; Morris, S.A.; Russell, L.M. NCI Alliance for Nanotechnology in Cancer—From academic research to clinical interventions. *Biomed. Microdev.* **2019**, *21*, 32. [CrossRef] [PubMed]

72. Clauser, S.B.; Johnson, M.R.; O'Brien, D.M.; Beveridge, J.M.; Fennell, M.L.; Kaluzny, A.D. Improving clinical research and cancer care delivery in community settings: Evaluating the NCI community cancer centers program. *Implement. Sci.* **2009**, *4*, 63. [CrossRef]

73. Hirsch, B.R.; Locke, S.C.; Abernethy, A.P. Experience of the national cancer institute community cancer centers program on community-based cancer clinical trials activity. *J. Oncol. Pract.* **2016**, *12*, e350-8. [CrossRef]

74. Copur, M.S.; Ramaekers, R.; Gonen, M.; Gulzow, M.; Hadenfeldt, R.; Fuller, C.; Scott, J.; Einspahr, S.; Benzel, H.; Mickey, M.; et al. Impact of the national cancer institute community cancer centers program on clinical trial and related activities at a community cancer center in rural Nebraska. *J. Oncol. Pract.* **2016**, *12*, 67–68. [CrossRef]

75. DH, F. Clinical trials have the best medicine but do not enroll the patients who need it. *Sci. Am.* **2019**, *320*, 61–65.

76. Copur, M.S. Inadequate awareness of and participation in cancer clinical trials in the community oncology setting. *Oncology* **2019**, *33*, 54–57.

77. Green, M.A.; Michaels, M.; Blakeney, N.; Odulana, A.A.; Isler, M.R.; Richmond, A.; Long, D.G.; Robinson, W.S.; Taylor, Y.J.; Corbie-Smith, G. Evaluating a community-partnered cancer clinical trials pilot intervention with African American communities. *J. Cancer Educ.* **2015**, *30*, 158–166. [CrossRef] [PubMed]

78. Best, A.; Hiatt, R.A.; Cameron, R.; Rimer, B.K.; Abrams, D.B. The evolution of cancer control research: An international perspective from Canada and the United States. *Cancer Epidemiol Biomarkers Prev.* **2003**, *12*, 705–712. [PubMed]

79. Greenwald, P.; Cullen, J.W. The new emphasis in cancer control. *J. Natl. Cancer. Inst.* **1985**, *74*, 543–551. [CrossRef]

80. Noel, L.; Phillips, F.; Tossas-Milligan, K.; Spear, K.; Vanderford, N.L.; Winn, R.A.; Vanderpool, R.C.; Eckhardt, S.G. Community-academic partnerships: Approaches to engagement. *Am. Soc. Clin. Oncol. Educ. Book.* **2019**, *39*, 88–95. [CrossRef]

81. Harris, A.; Kumar, P.; Sutaria, S. *Unlocking the Potential of Acdemic and Community Health System Partnerships*; McKinsey and Company: New York, NY, USA, 2015.

82. Johnson, T.M. Perspective on precision medicine in oncology. *Pharmacotherapy* **2017**, *37*, 988–989. [CrossRef] [PubMed]

83. Ersek, J.L.; Black, L.J.; Thompson, M.A.; Kim, E.S. Implementing precision medicine programs and clinical trials in the community-based oncology practice: Barriers and best practices. *Am. Soc. Clin. Oncol. Educ. Book.* **2018**, *38*, 188–196. [CrossRef]

84. Nadauld, L.D.; Ford, J.M.; Pritchard, D.; Brown, T. Strategies for clinical implementation: Precision oncology at three distinct institutions. *Health Aff. (Millwood)* **2018**, *37*, 751–756. [CrossRef]

85. Thompson, M.A.; Godden, J.J.; Wham, D.; Ruggeri, A.; Mullane, M.P.; Wilson, A.; Virani, S.; Weissman, S.M.; Ramczyk, B.; Vanderwall, P.; et al. Coordinating an oncology precision medicine clinic within an integrated health system: lessons learned in year one. *J. Patient Cent. Res. Rev.* **2019**, *6*, 36–45. [CrossRef]

86. Carpten, J.C.; Mardis, E.R. The era of precision oncogenomics. *Cold Spring Harb. Mol. Case Stud.* **2018**, *4*. [CrossRef]

87. International Human Genome Sequencing Consortium. Finishing the euchromatic sequence of the human genome. *Nature* **2004**, *431*, 931–945. [CrossRef]

88. Ashley, E.A. Towards precision medicine. *Nat. Rev. Genet.* **2016**, *17*, 507–522. [CrossRef] [PubMed]

89. Sanchez, N.S.; Mills, G.B.; Mills Shaw, K.R. Precision oncology: Neither a silver bullet nor a dream. *Pharmacogenomics* **2017**, *18*, 1525–1539. [CrossRef] [PubMed]

90. Berger, M.F.; Mardis, E.R. The emerging clinical relevance of genomics in cancer medicine. *Nat. Rev. Clin. Oncol.* **2018**, *15*, 353–365. [CrossRef] [PubMed]

91. Mitra, R.D.; Church, G.M. In situ localized amplification and contact replication of many individual DNA molecules. *Nucleic Acids Res.* **1999**, *27*, e34. [CrossRef]

92. Brenner, S.; Johnson, M.; Bridgham, J.; Golda, G.; Lloyd, D.H.; Johnson, D.; Luo, S.; McCurdy, S.; Foy, M.; Ewan, M.; et al. Gene expression analysis by massively parallel signature sequencing (MPSS) on microbead arrays. *Nat. Biotechnol.* **2000**, *18*, 630–634. [CrossRef]

93. Mardis, E.R. Next-generation DNA sequencing methods. *Annu. Rev. Genomics Hum. Genet.* **2008**, *9*, 387–402. [CrossRef]

94. Shendure, J.; Ji, H. Next-generation DNA sequencing. *Nat. Biotechnol.* **2008**, *26*, 1135–1145. [CrossRef] [PubMed]

95. Bentley, D.R.; Balasubramanian, S.; Swerdlow, H.P.; Smith, G.P.; Milton, J.; Brown, C.G.; Hall, K.P.; Evers, D.J.; Barnes, C.L.; Bignell, H.R.; et al. Accurate whole human genome sequencing using reversible terminator chemistry. *Nature* **2008**, *456*, 53–59. [CrossRef] [PubMed]

96. Mardis, E.R. The impact of next-generation sequencing technology on genetics. *Trends Genet.* **2008**, *24*, 133–141. [CrossRef]

97. Tucker, T.; Marra, M.; Friedman, J.M. Massively parallel sequencing: The next big thing in genetic medicine. *Am. J. Hum. Genet.* **2009**, *85*, 142–154. [CrossRef]

98. Ley, T.J.; Mardis, E.R.; Ding, L.; Fulton, B.; McLellan, M.D.; Chen, K.; Dooling, D.; Dunford-Shore, B.H.; McGrath, S.; Hickenbotham, M.; et al. DNA sequencing of a cytogenetically normal acute myeloid leukaemia genome. *Nature* **2008**, *456*, 66–72. [CrossRef] [PubMed]

99. Reinartz, J.; Bruyns, E.; Lin, J.Z.; Burcham, T.; Brenner, S.; Bowen, B.; Kramer, M.; Woychik, R. Massively parallel signature sequencing (MPSS) as a tool for in-depth quantitative gene expression profiling in all organisms. *Brief. Funct. Genomic. Proteomic.* **2002**, *1*, 95–104. [CrossRef] [PubMed]

100. Torres, T.T.; Metta, M.; Ottenwalder, B.; Schlotterer, C. Gene expression profiling by massively parallel sequencing. *Genome Res.* **2008**, *18*, 172–177. [CrossRef] [PubMed]

101. Cancer Genome Atlas Research, N.; Weinstein, J.N.; Collisson, E.A.; Mills, G.B.; Shaw, K.R.; Ozenberger, B.A.; Ellrott, K.; Shmulevich, I.; Sander, C.; Stuart, J.M. The cancer genome atlas pan-cancer analysis project. *Nat. Genet.* **2013**, *45*, 1113–1120.

102. Wang, H.; Nettleton, D.; Ying, K. Copy number variation detection using next generation sequencing read counts. *BMC Bioinform.* **2014**, *15*, 109. [CrossRef] [PubMed]

103. Medvedev, P.; Stanciu, M.; Brudno, M. Computational methods for discovering structural variation with next-generation sequencing. *Nat. Methods* **2009**, *6*, S13–S20. [CrossRef]

104. Johnson, D.S.; Mortazavi, A.; Myers, R.M.; Wold, B. Genome-wide mapping of in vivo protein-DNA interactions. *Science* **2007**, *316*, 1497–1502. [CrossRef]

105. Morel, D.; Jeffery, D.; Aspeslagh, S.; Almouzni, G.; Postel-Vinay, S. Combining epigenetic drugs with other therapies for solid tumours—Past lessons and future promise. *Nat. Rev. Clin. Oncol.* **2020**, *17*, 91–107. [CrossRef]

106. Lazaris, C.; Aifantis, I.; Tsirigos, A. On epigenetic plasticity and genome topology. *Trends Cancer* **2020**, *6*, 177–180. [CrossRef]

107. Segal, N.H.; Parsons, D.W.; Peggs, K.S.; Velculescu, V.; Kinzler, K.W.; Vogelstein, B.; Allison, J.P. Epitope landscape in breast and colorectal cancer. *Cancer Res.* **2008**, *68*, 889–892. [CrossRef]

108. Alexandrov, L.B.; Nik-Zainal, S.; Wedge, D.C.; Aparicio, S.A.; Behjati, S.; Biankin, A.V.; Bignell, G.R.; Bolli, N.; Borg, A.; Borresen-Dale, A.L.; et al. Signatures of mutational processes in human cancer. *Nature* **2013**, *500*, 415–421. [CrossRef] [PubMed]

109. Sanmamed, M.F.; LChe. A paradigm shift in cancer immunotherapy: From enhancement to normalization. *Cell* **2018**, *175*, 313–326. [CrossRef] [PubMed]

110. Zewde, M.; Kiyotani, K.; Park, J.H.; Fang, H.; Yap, K.L.; Yew, P.Y.; Alachkar, H.; Kato, T.; Mai, T.H.; Ikeda, Y.; et al. The era of immunogenomics/immunopharmacogenomics. *J. Hum. Genet.* **2018**, *63*, 865–875. [CrossRef]

111. Dennard, R.H.; Gaensslen, F.H.; Yu, H.N.; Rideout, V.L.; Bassous, E.; Leblanc, A.R. Design of ion-implanted MOSFET's with very small physical dimensions. *IEEE J. Solid State Circuits* **1974**, *9*, 256–268. [CrossRef]

112. Gorder, P.F. Multicore processors for science and engineering. *Comput. Sci. Eng.* **2007**, *9*, 3–7. [CrossRef]

113. Denning, P.J.; Lewis, T.G. Exponential laws of computing growth. *Commun. Acm* **2017**, *60*, 54–65. [CrossRef]

114. Thackray, A.; Brock, D.C. *Moore's Law: The Life of Gordon Moore, Silicon Valley's Quiet Revolutionary*; Basic Books: New York, NY, USA, 2015.

115. Koomey, J.G.; Berard, S.; Sanchez, M.; Wong, H. Implications of historical trends in the electrical efficiency of computing. *IEEE Comput. Soc.* **2011**, *33*, 46–54. [CrossRef]

116. Hill, M.D.; Marty, M.R. Amdahl's law in the multicore era. *Computer* **2008**, *41*, 33. [CrossRef]

117. Denning, P.J.; Tichy, W.F. Highly parallel computation. *Science* **1990**, *250*, 1217–1222. [CrossRef]

118. Hinkson, I.V.; Davidsen, T.M.; Klemm, J.D.; Kerlavage, A.R.; Kibbe, W.A.; Chandramouliswaran, I. A comprehensive infrastructure for big data in cancer research: Accelerating cancer research and precision medicine. *Front. Cell. Dev. Biol.* **2017**, *5*, 83. [CrossRef]

119. Wing, J.M. Computational thinking. *Commun. Acm* **2006**, *49*, 33–35. [CrossRef]

120. Regev, A.; Shapiro, E. Cellular abstractions: Cells as computation. *Nature* **2002**, *419*, 343-343. [CrossRef] [PubMed]

121. Searls, D.B. The roots of bioinformatics. *PLoS Comput. Biol.* **2010**, *6*. [CrossRef]

122. Moorthie, S.; Hall, A.; Wright, C.F. Informatics and clinical genome sequencing: Opening the black box. *Genet. Med.* **2013**, *15*, 165–171. [CrossRef] [PubMed]

123. Funari, V.; Canosa, S. The importance of bioinformatics in NGS: Breaking the bottleneck in data interpretation. *Science* **2014**, *344*, 653-653. [CrossRef]

124. Oliver, G.R.; Hart, S.N.; Klee, E.W. Bioinformatics for clinical next generation sequencing. *Clin. Chem.* **2015**, *61*, 124–135. [CrossRef] [PubMed]

125. Gullapalli, R.R.; Lyons-Weiler, M.; Petrosko, P.; Dhir, R.; Becich, M.J.; LaFramboise, W.A. Clinical integration of next-generation sequencing technology. *Clin. Lab. Med.* **2012**, *32*, 585–599. [CrossRef]

126. Hundal, J.; Miller, C.A.; Griffith, M.; Griffith, O.L.; Walker, J.; Kiwala, S.; Graubert, A.; McMichael, J.; Coffman, A.; Mardis, E.R. Cancer immunogenomics: computational neoantigen identification and vaccine design. *Cold Spring Harb. Symp. Quant. Biol.* **2016**, *81*, 105–111. [CrossRef]

127. Tenenbaum, J.D. Translational bioinformatics: Past, present, and future. *Genom. Proteomics Bioinform.* **2016**, *14*, 31–41. [CrossRef]

128. Weissenbach, J. The rise of genomics. *C R Biol.* **2016**, *339*, 231–239. [CrossRef]

129. Morganti, S.; Tarantino, P.; Ferraro, E.; D'Amico, P.; Viale, G.; Trapani, D.; Duso, B.A.; Curigliano, G. Complexity of genome sequencing and reporting: Next generation sequencing (NGS) technologies and implementation of precision medicine in real life. *Crit. Rev. Oncol. Hematol.* **2019**, *133*, 171–182. [CrossRef] [PubMed]

130. Koboldt, D.C.; Steinberg, K.M.; Larson, D.E.; Wilson, R.K.; Mardis, E.R. The next-generation sequencing revolution and its impact on genomics. *Cell* **2013**, *155*, 27–38. [CrossRef] [PubMed]

131. Nowell, P.C.; Rowley, J.D.; Knudson, A.G., Jr. Cancer genetics, cytogenetics—Defining the enemy within. *Nat. Med.* **1998**, *4*, 1107–1111. [CrossRef]

132. Druker, B.J.; Lydon, N.B. Lessons learned from the development of an abl tyrosine kinase inhibitor for chronic myelogenous leukemia. *J. Clin. Invest.* **2000**, *105*, 3–7. [CrossRef] [PubMed]

133. Rossari, F.; Minutolo, F.; Orciuolo, E. Past, present, and future of Bcr-Abl inhibitors: From chemical development to clinical efficacy. *J. Hematol. Oncol.* **2018**, *11*, 84. [CrossRef]

134. Druker, B.J.; Talpaz, M.; Resta, D.J.; Peng, B.; Buchdunger, E.; Ford, J.M.; Lydon, N.B.; Kantarjian, H.; Capdeville, R.; Ohno-Jones, S.; et al. Efficacy and safety of a specific inhibitor of the BCR-ABL tyrosine kinase in chronic myeloid leukemia. *N. Engl. J. Med.* **2001**, *344*, 1031–1037. [CrossRef]

135. Savage, D.G.; Antman, K.H. Imatinib mesylate—A new oral targeted therapy. *N. Engl. J. Med.* **2002**, *346*, 683–693. [CrossRef]

136. Lee, Y.T.; Tan, Y.J.; Oon, C.E. Molecular targeted therapy: Treating cancer with specificity. *Eur. J. Pharmacol.* **2018**, *834*, 188–196. [CrossRef]

137. Scholl, C.; Frohling, S. Exploiting rare driver mutations for precision cancer medicine. *Curr. Opin. Genet. Dev.* **2019**, *54*, 1–6. [CrossRef]

138. Jackson, S.E.; Chester, J.D. Personalised cancer medicine. *Int. J. Cancer* **2015**, *137*, 262–266. [CrossRef]

139. Neal, J.W.; Sledge, G.W. Decade in review-targeted therapy: Successes, toxicities and challenges in solid tumours. *Nat. Rev. Clin. Oncol.* **2014**, *11*, 627–628. [CrossRef] [PubMed]

140. Prasad, V.; Fojo, T.; MBrad. Precision oncology: Origins, optimism, and potential. *Lancet Oncol.* **2016**, *17*, e81–e86. [CrossRef]

141. El-Deiry, W.S.; Goldberg, R.M.; Lenz, H.J.; Shields, A.F.; Gibney, G.T.; Tan, A.R.; Brown, J.; Eisenberg, B.; Heath, E.I.; Phuphanich, S.; et al. The current state of molecular testing in the treatment of patients with solid tumors, 2019. *Cancer J. Clin.* **2019**, *69*, 305–343. [CrossRef] [PubMed]

142. National Cancer Institute. Targeted Cancer Therapies. Available online: https://www.cancer.gov/about-cancer/treatment/types/targeted-therapies/targeted-therapies-fact-sheet (accessed on 2 July 2020).

143. Khotskaya, Y.B.; Mills, G.B.; Mills Shaw, K.R. Next-Generation Sequencing and Result Interpretation in Clinical Oncology: Challenges of Personalized Cancer Therapy. *Annu. Rev. Med.* **2017**, *68*, 113–125. [CrossRef]

144. Buchanan, M. The law of accelerating returns. *Nat. Phys.* **2008**, *4*, 507-507. [CrossRef]

145. Kurzweil, R. The Law of Accelerating Returns. 2001. Available online: https://www.kurzweilai.net/the-law-of-accelerating-returns (accessed on 12 April 2020).

146. Blazer, K.R.; Nehoray, B.; Solomon, I.; Niell-Swiller, M.; Culver, J.O.; Uman, G.C.; Weitzel, J.N. Next-generation testing for cancer risk: Perceptions, experiences, and needs among early adopters in community healthcare settings. *Genet. Test. Mol. Biomarkers* **2015**, *19*, 657–665. [CrossRef]

147. Mauer, C.B.; Pirzadeh-Miller, S.M.; Robinson, L.D.; Euhus, D.M. The integration of next-generation sequencing panels in the clinical cancer genetics practice: An. institutional experience. *Genet. Med.* **2014**, *16*, 407–412. [CrossRef]

148. Sabour, L.; Sabour, M.; Ghorbian, S. Clinical applications of next-generation sequencing in cancer diagnosis. *Pathol. Oncol. Res.* **2017**, *23*, 225–234. [CrossRef]

149. Sylvester, D.E.; Chen, Y.; Jamieson, R.V.; Dalla-Pozza, L.; Byrne, J.A. Investigation of clinically relevant germline variants detected by next-generation sequencing in patients with childhood cancer: A review of the literature. *J. Med. Genet.* **2018**, *55*, 785–793. [CrossRef]

150. Obrochta, E.; Godley, L.A. Identifying patients with genetic predisposition to acute myeloid leukemia. *Best Pract. Res. Clin. Haematol.* **2018**, *31*, 373–378. [CrossRef]

151. Gomy, I.; Mdel, P.D. Hereditary cancer risk assessment: Insights and perspectives for the next-generation sequencing era. *Genet. Mol. Biol.* **2016**, *39*, 184–188. [CrossRef] [PubMed]

152. Pensabene, M.; Spagnoletti, I.; Capuano, I.; Condello, C.; Pepe, S.; Contegiacomo, A.; Lombardi, G.; Bevilacqua, G.; Caligo, M.A. Two mutations of BRCA2 gene at exon and splicing site in a woman who underwent oncogenetic counseling. *Ann. Oncol.* **2009**, *20*, 874–878. [CrossRef] [PubMed]

153. Kamps, R.; Brandao, R.D.; Bosch, B.J.; Paulussen, A.D.; Xanthoulea, S.; Blok, M.J.; Romano, A. Next-generation sequencing in oncology: Genetic diagnosis, risk prediction and cancer classification. *Int. J. Mol. Sci.* **2017**, *18*, 308. [CrossRef] [PubMed]

154. Domchek, S.M.; Bradbury, A.; Garber, J.E.; Offit, K.; Robson, M.E. Multiplex genetic testing for cancer susceptibility: Out on the high wire without a net? *J. Clin. Oncol.* **2013**, *31*, 1267–1270. [CrossRef]

155. Weitzel, J.N.; Blazer, K.R.; MacDonald, D.J.; Culver, J.O.; Offit, K. Genetics, genomics, and cancer risk assessment: State of the Art and future directions in the era of personalized medicine. *Cancer J. Clin.* **2011**, *61*, 327–359. [CrossRef] [PubMed]

156. Lynce, F.; Isaacs, C. How far do we go with genetic evaluation. *Am. Soc. Clin. Oncol. Educ. Book.* **2016**, *35*, e72–e78. [CrossRef]

157. Lui, S.T.; Shuch, B. Genetic testing in kidney cancer patients: Who, when, and how? *Eur. Urol. Focus* **2019**, *5*, 973–976. [CrossRef]

158. Piccinin, C.; Panchal, S.; Watkins, N.; Kim, R.H. An update on genetic risk assessment and prevention: The role of genetic testing panels in breast cancer. *Expert Rev. Anticancer Ther.* **2019**, *19*, 787–801. [CrossRef]

159. Plichta, J.K.; Sebastian, M.L.; Smith, L.A.; Menendez, C.S.; Johnson, A.T.; Bays, S.M.; Euhus, D.M.; Clifford, E.J.; Jalali, M.; Kurtzman, S.H.; et al. Germline genetic testing: What the breast surgeon needs to know. *Ann. Surg. Oncol.* **2019**, *26*, 2184–2190. [CrossRef]

160. Valle, L.; Vilar, E.; Tavtigian, S.V.; Stoffel, E.M. Genetic predisposition to colorectal cancer: Syndromes, genes, classification of genetic variants and implications for precision medicine. *J. Pathol.* **2019**, *247*, 574–588. [CrossRef]

161. Suszynska, M.; Klonowska, K.; Jasinska, A.J.; Kozlowski, P. Large-scale meta-analysis of mutations identified in panels of breast/ovarian cancer-related genes—Providing evidence of cancer predisposition genes. *Gynecol. Oncol.* **2019**, *153*, 452–462. [CrossRef] [PubMed]

162. Muskens, I.S.; de Smith, A.J.; Zhang, C.; Hansen, H.M.; Morimoto, L.; Metayer, C.; Ma, X.; Walsh, K.M.; Wiemels, J.L. Germline cancer predisposition variants and pediatric glioma: A population-based study in California. *Neuro. Oncol.* **2020**, *22*, 864–874. [CrossRef] [PubMed]

163. Abdel-Rahman, M.H.; Sample, K.M.; Pilarski, R.; Walsh, T.; Grosel, T.; Kinnamon, D.; Boru, G.; Massengill, J.B.; Schoenfield, L.; Kelly, B.; et al. Whole exome sequencing identifies candidate genes associated with hereditary predisposition to uveal melanoma. *Ophthalmology* **2020**, *127*, 668–678. [CrossRef] [PubMed]

164. Johansson, P.A.; Nathan, V.; Bourke, L.M.; Palmer, J.M.; Zhang, T.; Symmons, J.; Howlie, M.; Patch, A.M.; Read, J.; Holland, E.A.; et al. Evaluation of the contribution of germline variants in BRCA1 and BRCA2 to uveal and cutaneous melanoma. *Melanoma Res.* **2019**, *29*, 483–490. [CrossRef] [PubMed]

165. Shivakumar, M.; Miller, J.E.; Dasari, V.R.; Gogoi, R.; Kim, D. Exome-wide rare variant analysis from the discovEHR study identifies novel candidate predisposition genes for endometrial cancer. *Front. Oncol.* **2019**, *9*, 574. [CrossRef]

166. Bertelsen, B.; Tuxen, I.V.; Yde, C.W.; Gabrielaite, M.; Torp, M.H.; Kinalis, S.; Oestrup, O.; Rohrberg, K.; Spangaard, I.; Santoni-Rugiu, E.; et al. High. frequency of pathogenic germline variants within homologous recombination repair in patients with advanced cancer. *NPJ Genom. Med.* **2019**, *4*, 13. [CrossRef]

167. Akhavanfard, S.; Padmanabhan, R.; Yehia, L.; Cheng, F.; Eng, C. Comprehensive germline genomic profiles of children, adolescents and young adults with solid tumors. *Nat. Commun.* **2020**, *11*, 2206. [CrossRef]

168. Jin, Z.B.; Li, Z.; Liu, Z.; Jiang, Y.; Cai, X.B.; Wu, J. Identification of de novo germline mutations and causal genes for sporadic diseases using trio-based whole-exome/genome sequencing. *Biol. Rev. Camb. Philos. Soc.* **2018**, *93*, 1014–1031. [CrossRef]

169. Johnson, L.M.; Hamilton, K.V.; Valdez, J.M.; Knapp, E.; Baker, J.N.; Nichols, K.E. Ethical considerations surrounding germline next-generation sequencing of children with cancer. *Expert Rev. Mol. Diagn.* **2017**, *17*, 523–534. [CrossRef]

170. Stadler, Z.K.; Schrader, K.A.; Vijai, J.; Robson, M.E.; Offit, K. Cancer genomics and inherited risk. *J. Clin. Oncol.* **2014**, *32*, 687–698. [CrossRef]

171. Backman, S.; Bajic, D.; Crona, J.; Hellman, P.; Skogseid, B.; Stalberg, P. Whole genome sequencing of apparently mutation-negative MEN1 patients. *Eur. J. Endocrinol.* **2020**, *182*, 35–45. [CrossRef] [PubMed]

172. Nissim, S.; Leshchiner, I.; Mancias, J.D.; Greenblatt, M.B.; Maertens, O.; Cassa, C.A.; Rosenfeld, J.A.; Cox, A.G.; Hedgepeth, J.; Wucherpfennig, J.I.; et al. Mutations in RABL3 alter KRAS prenylation and are associated with hereditary pancreatic cancer. *Nat. Genet.* **2019**, *51*, 1308–1314. [CrossRef] [PubMed]

173. Okur, V.; Chung, W.K. The impact of hereditary cancer gene panels on clinical care and lessons learned. *Cold Spring Harb. Mol. Case Stud.* **2017**, *3*. [CrossRef] [PubMed]

174. Lumish, H.S.; Steinfeld, H.; Koval, C.; Russo, D.; Levinson, E.; Wynn, J.; Duong, J.; Chung, W.K. Impact of panel gene testing for hereditary breast and ovarian cancer on patients. *J. Genet. Couns.* **2017**, *26*, 1116–1129. [CrossRef] [PubMed]

175. Rosenthal, E.T.; Bernhisel, R.; Brown, K.; Kidd, J.; Manley, S. Clinical testing with a panel of 25 genes associated with increased cancer risk results in a significant increase in clinically significant findings across a broad range of cancer histories. *Cancer Genet.* **2017**, *218–219*, 58–68. [CrossRef]

176. Foley, S.B.; Rios, J.J.; Mgbemena, V.E.; Robinson, L.S.; Hampel, H.L.; Toland, A.E.; Durham, L.; Ross, T.S. Use of whole genome sequencing for diagnosis and discovery in the cancer genetics clinic. *Ebiomedicine* **2015**, *2*, 74–81. [CrossRef]

177. Fewings, E.; Larionov, A.; Redman, J.; Goldgraben, M.A.; Scarth, J.; Richardson, S.; Brewer, C.; Davidson, R.; Ellis, I.; Evans, D.G.; et al. Germline pathogenic variants in PALB2 and other cancer-predisposing genes in families with hereditary diffuse gastric cancer without CDH1 mutation: A whole-exome sequencing study. *Lancet Gastroenterol. Hepatol.* **2018**, *3*, 489–498. [CrossRef]

178. Richards, S.; Aziz, N.; Bale, S.; Bick, D.; Das, S.; Gastier-Foster, J.; Grody, W.W.; Hegde, M.; Lyon, E.; Spector, E.; et al. Standards and guidelines for the interpretation of sequence variants: A joint consensus recommendation of the American College of Medical Genetics and Genomics and the Association for Molecular Pathology. *Genet. Med.* **2015**, *17*, 405–424. [CrossRef]

179. Eccles, D.M.; Mitchell, G.; Monteiro, A.N.; Schmutzler, R.; Couch, F.J.; Spurdle, A.B.; Gomez-Garcia, E.B.; ENIGMA Clinical Working Group. BRCA1 and BRCA2 genetic testing-pitfalls and recommendations for managing variants of uncertain clinical significance. *Ann. Oncol.* **2015**, *26*, 2057–2065. [CrossRef]

180. Li, M.M.; Datto, M.; Duncavage, E.J.; Kulkarni, S.; Lindeman, N.I.; Roy, S.; Tsimberidou, A.M.; Vnencak-Jones, C.L.; Wolff, D.J.; Younes, A.; et al. Standards and guidelines for the interpretation and reporting of sequence variants in cancer: A joint consensus recommendation of the Association for Molecular Pathology, American Society of Clinical Oncology, and College of American Pathologists. *J. Mol. Diagn.* **2017**, *19*, 4–23. [CrossRef]

181. Hoffman-Andrews, L. The known unknown: The challenges of genetic variants of uncertain significance in clinical practice. *J. Law Biosci.* **2017**, *4*, 648–657. [CrossRef] [PubMed]

182. Cheon, J.Y.; Mozersky, J.; Cook-Deegan, R. Variants of uncertain significance in BRCA: A harbinger of ethical and policy issues to come? *Genome. Med.* **2014**, *6*, 121. [CrossRef] [PubMed]

183. Welsh, J.L.; Hoskin, T.L.; Day, C.N.; Thomas, A.S.; Cogswell, J.A.; Couch, F.J.; Boughey, J.C. Clinical decision-making in patients with variant of uncertain significance in BRCA1 or BRCA2 Genes. *Ann. Surg. Oncol.* **2017**, *24*, 3067–3072. [CrossRef] [PubMed]

184. Voelker, R. Quick uptakes: Taking the uncertainty out of interpreting BRCA variants. *J. Am. Med. Assoc.* **2019**, *321*, 1340–1341. [CrossRef]

185. Domchek, S.; Weber, B.L. Genetic variants of uncertain significance: Flies in the ointment. *J. Clin. Oncol.* **2008**, *26*, 16–17. [PubMed]

186. Medendorp, N.M.; Hillen, M.A.; Murugesu, L.; Aalfs, C.M.; Stiggelbout, A.M.; Smets, E.M.A. Uncertainty related to multigene panel testing for cancer: A qualitative study on counsellors' and counselees' views. *J. Community Genet.* **2019**, *10*, 303–312. [CrossRef]

187. Medendorp, N.M.; Hillen, M.A.; van Maarschalkerweerd, P.E.A.; Aalfs, C.M.; Ausems, M.; Verhoef, S.; van der Kolk, L.E.; Berger, L.P.V.; Wevers, M.R.; Wagner, A.; et al. "We don't know for sure": Discussion of uncertainty concerning multigene panel testing during initial cancer genetic consultations. *Fam. Cancer* **2020**, *19*, 65–76. [CrossRef]

188. Hamilton, J.G.; Robson, M.E. Psychosocial effects of multigene panel testing in the context of cancer genomics. *Hastings Cent. Rep.* **2019**, *49*, S44–S52. [CrossRef]

189. Afghahi, A.; AWKuria. The changing landscape of genetic testing for inherited breast cancer predisposition. *Curr. Treat Option Oncol.* **2017**, *18*, 27. [CrossRef]

190. Richter, S.; Haroun, I.; Graham, T.C.; Eisen, A.; Kiss, A.; Warner, E. Variants of unknown significance in BRCA testing: Impact on risk perception, worry, prevention and counseling. *Ann. Oncol.* **2013**, *24*, viii69–viii74. [CrossRef]

191. Idos, G.E.; Kurian, A.W.; Ricker, C.; Sturgeon, D.; Culver, J.O.; Kingham, K.E.; Koff, R.; Chun, N.M.; Rowe-Teeter, C.; Lebensohn, A.P.; et al. Multicenter prospective cohort study of the diagnostic yield and patient experience of multiplex gene panel testing for hereditary cancer risk. *JCO Precis. Oncol.* **2019**. [CrossRef]

192. Federici, G.; Soddu, S. Variants of uncertain significance in the era of high-throughput genome sequencing: A lesson from breast and ovary cancers. *J. Exp. Clin. Cancer Res.* **2020**, *39*, 46. [CrossRef] [PubMed]

193. Valencia, C.A.; Husami, A.; Holle, J.; Johnson, J.A.; Qian, Y.; Mathur, A.; Wei, C.; Indugula, S.R.; Zou, F.; Meng, H.; et al. Clinical impact and cost-effectiveness of whole exome sequencing as a diagnostic tool: A pediatric center's experience. *Front. Pediatr.* **2015**, *3*, 67. [CrossRef] [PubMed]

194. Gieldon, L.; Mackenroth, L.; Kahlert, A.K.; Lemke, J.R.; Porrmann, J.; Schallner, J.; von der Hagen, M.; Markus, S.; Weidensee, S.; Novotna, B.; et al. Diagnostic value of partial exome sequencing in developmental disorders. *PLoS ONE* **2018**, *13*, e0201041. [CrossRef] [PubMed]

195. Maxwell, K.N.; Hart, S.N.; Vijai, J.; Schrader, K.A.; Slavin, T.P.; Thomas, T.; Wubbenhorst, B.; Ravichandran, V.; Moore, R.M.; Hu, C.; et al. Evaluation of ACMG-guideline-based variant classification of cancer susceptibility and non-cancer-associated genes in families affected by breast cancer. *Am. J. Hum. Genet.* **2016**, *98*, 801–817. [CrossRef]

196. Eggington, J.M.; Bowles, K.R.; Moyes, K.; Manley, S.; Esterling, L.; Sizemore, S.; Rosenthal, E.; Theisen, A.; Saam, J.; Arnell, C.; et al. A comprehensive laboratory-based program for classification of variants of uncertain significance in hereditary cancer genes. *Clin. Genet.* **2014**, *86*, 229–237. [CrossRef]

197. Sud, A.; Kinnersley, B.; Houlston, R.S. Genome-wide association studies of cancer: Current insights and future perspectives. *Nat. Rev. Cancer* **2017**, *17*, 692–704. [CrossRef]

198. Turnbull, C.; Sud, A.; Houlston, R.S. Cancer genetics, precision prevention and a call to action. *Nat. Genet.* **2018**, *50*, 1212–1218. [CrossRef]

199. Kurian, A.W.; Hare, E.E.; Mills, M.A.; Kingham, K.E.; McPherson, L.; Whittemore, A.S.; McGuire, V.; Ladabaum, U.; Kobayashi, Y.; Lincoln, S.E.; et al. Clinical evaluation of a multiple-gene sequencing panel for hereditary cancer risk assessment. *J. Clin. Oncol.* **2014**, *32*, 2001–2009. [CrossRef]

200. Grissom, A.A.; Friend, P.J. Multigene panel testing for hereditary cancer risk. *J. Adv. Pract. Oncol.* **2016**, *7*, 394–407.

201. Kurian, A.W.; Ford, J.M. Multigene panel testing in oncology practice: How should we respond? *JAMA Oncol.* **2015**, *1*, 277–278. [CrossRef] [PubMed]

202. Secretary's Advisory Committee on Genetics, Health and Society. *Genetics Education and Training*; The Honorable Kathleen Sebelius Secretary of Health and Human Services: Washington, DC, USA, 2011.

203. Campion, M.; Goldgar, C.; Hopkin, R.J.; Prows, C.A.; Dasgupta, S. Genomic education for the next generation of health-care providers. *Genet. Med.* **2019**, *21*, 2422–2430. [CrossRef] [PubMed]

204. Guttmacher, A.E.; Porteous, M.E.; McInerney, J.D. Educating health-care professionals about genetics and genomics. *Nat. Rev. Genet.* **2007**, *8*, 151–157. [CrossRef] [PubMed]

205. Douma, K.F.; Smets, E.M.; Allain, D.C. Non-genetic health professionals' attitude towards, knowledge of and skills in discussing and ordering genetic testing for hereditary cancer. *Fam. Cancer* **2016**, *15*, 341–350. [CrossRef] [PubMed]

206. Maiese, D.R.; Keehn, A.; Lyon, M.; Flannery, D.; Watson, M.; Working Groups of the National Coordinating Center for Seven Regional Genetics Service Collaboratives. Current conditions in medical genetics practice. *Genet. Med.* **2019**, *21*, 1874–1877. [CrossRef] [PubMed]

207. Salari, K. The dawning era of personalized medicine exposes a gap in medical education. *PLoS Med.* **2009**, *6*, e1000138. [CrossRef]

208. Stoll, K.; Kubendran, S.; Cohen, S.A. The past, present and future of service delivery in genetic counseling: Keeping up in the era of precision medicine. *Am. J. Med. Genet. C Semin. Med. Genet.* **2018**, *178*, 24–37. [CrossRef]

209. Daly, M.B.; Stearman, B.; Masny, A.; Sein, E.; Mazzoni, S. How to establish a high-risk cancer genetics clinic: Limitations and successes. *Curr. Oncol. Rep.* **2005**, *7*, 469–474. [CrossRef]

210. Cohen, S.A.; Bradbury, A.; Henderson, V.; Hoskins, K.; Bednar, E.; Arun, B.K. Genetic counseling and testing in a community setting: Quality, access, and efficiency. *Am. Soc. Clin. Oncol. Educ. Book.* **2019**, *39*, e34–e44. [CrossRef]

211. Stopfer, J.E. Genetic counseling and clinical cancer genetics services. *Semin. Surg. Oncol.* **2000**, *18*, 347–357. [CrossRef]

212. Anderson, B.; McLosky, J.; Wasilevich, E.; Lyon-Callo, S.; Duquette, D.; Copeland, G. Barriers and facilitators for utilization of genetic counseling and risk assessment services in young female breast cancer survivors. *J. Cancer Epidemiol.* **2012**, *2012*, 298745. [CrossRef] [PubMed]

213. Cohen, S.A.; Marvin, M.L.; Riley, B.D.; Vig, H.S.; Rousseau, J.A.; Gustafson, S.L. Identification of genetic counseling service delivery models in practice: A report from the NSGC service delivery model task force. *J. Genet. Couns.* **2013**, *22*, 411–421. [CrossRef] [PubMed]

214. Ricker, C.; Lagos, V.; Feldman, N.; Hiyama, S.; Fuentes, S.; Kumar, V.; Farwell Hagman, K.; Palomares, M.; Blazer, K.; Lowstuter, K.; et al. If we build it . . . will they come?—Establishing a cancer genetics services clinic for an underserved predominantly Latina cohort. *J. Genet. Couns.* **2007**, *15*, 505–514. [CrossRef]

215. Epstein, C.J.; Erickson, R.P.; Hall, B.D.; Golbus, M.S. The center-satellite system for the wide-scale distribution of genetic counseling services. *Am. J. Hum. Genet.* **1975**, *27*, 322–332. [PubMed]

216. Reid, K.J.; Sakati, N.; Prichard, L.L.; Schneiderman, L.J.; Jones, O.W.; Dixson, B.K. Genetic counseling: An evaluation of public health genetic clinics. *West. J. Med.* **1976**, *124*, 6–12. [PubMed]

217. Riccardi, V.M. Health care and disease prevention through genetic counseling: A regional approach. *Am. J. Public Health* **1976**, *66*, 268–272. [CrossRef]

218. Weissman, S.M.; Zellmer, K.; Gill, N.; Wham, D. Implementing a virtual health telemedicine program. in a community setting. *J. Genet. Couns.* **2018**, *27*, 323–325. [CrossRef]

219. Brown, J.; Athens, A.; Tait, D.L.; Crane, E.K.; Higgins, R.V.; Naumann, R.W.; Gusic, L.H.; Amacker-North, L. A comprehensive program: Enabling effective delivery of regional genetic counseling. *Int. J. Gynecol. Cancer* **2018**, *28*, 996–1002. [CrossRef]

220. Fournier, D.M.; Bazzell, A.F.; Dains, J.E. Comparing outcomes of genetic counseling options in breast and ovarian cancer: An integrative review. *Oncol. Nurs. Forum* **2018**, *45*, 96–105. [CrossRef]

221. Buchanan, A.H.; Rahm, A.K.; Williams, J.L. Alternate service delivery models in cancer genetic counseling: A mini-review. *Front. Oncol.* **2016**, *6*, 120. [CrossRef]

222. McDonald, E.; Lamb, A.; Grillo, B.; Lucas, L.; Miesfeldt, S. Acceptability of telemedicine and other cancer genetic counseling models of service delivery in geographically remote settings. *J. Genet. Couns.* **2014**, *23*, 221–228. [CrossRef] [PubMed]

223. MacDonald, D.J.; KRBlazer; JNWeitze. Extending comprehensive cancer center expertise in clinical cancer genetics and genomics to diverse communities: The power of partnership. *J. Natl. Compr. Canc. Netw.* **2010**, *8*, 615–624. [CrossRef] [PubMed]

224. Solomon, I.B.; McGraw, S.; Shen, J.; Albayrak, A.; Alterovitz, G.; Davies, M.; Fitz, C.D.V.; Freedman, R.A.; Lopez, L.N.; Sholl, L.M. Engaging patients in precision oncology: development and usability of a web-based patient-facing genomic sequencing report. *JCO Precis. Oncol.* **2020**, *4*, 307–318. [CrossRef]

225. Blazer, K.R.; Macdonald, D.J.; Culver, J.O.; Huizenga, C.R.; Morgan, R.J.; Uman, G.C.; Weitzel, J.N. Personalized cancer genetics training for personalized medicine: Improving community-based healthcare through a genetically literate workforce. *Genet. Med.* **2011**, *13*, 832–840. [CrossRef] [PubMed]

226. Whitworth, P.; Beitsch, P.; Arnell, C.; Cox, H.C.; Brown, K.; Kidd, J.; Lancaster, J.M. Impact of payer constraints on access to genetic testing. *J. Oncol. Pract.* **2017**, *13*, e47–e56. [CrossRef] [PubMed]

227. Karlovich, C.A.; Williams, P.M. Clinical applications of next-generation sequencing in precision oncology. *Cancer J.* **2019**, *25*, 264–271. [CrossRef]

228. Wadapurkar, R.; Vyas, R. Computational analysis of next generation sequencing data and its applications in clinical oncology. *Inform. Med. Unlocked* **2018**, *11*, 75–82. [CrossRef]

229. Hyman, D.M.; Taylor, B.S.; Baselga, J. Implementing genome-driven oncology. *Cell* **2017**, *168*, 584–599. [CrossRef]

230. Nangalia, J.; Campbell, P.J. Genome sequencing during a patient's journey through cancer. *N. Engl. J. Med.* **2019**, *381*, 2145–2156. [CrossRef]

231. Pleasance, E.D.; Cheetham, R.K.; Stephens, P.J.; McBride, D.J.; Humphray, S.J.; Greenman, C.D.; Varela, I.; Lin, M.L.; Ordonez, G.R.; Bignell, G.R.; et al. A comprehensive catalogue of somatic mutations from a human cancer genome. *Nature* **2010**, *463*, 191–196. [CrossRef]

232. Campbell, P.J.; Getz, G.; Korbel, J.O.; Stuart, J.M.; Jennings, J.L.; Stein, L.D.; Perry, M.D.; Nahal-Bose, H.K.; Ouellette, B.F.F.; Li, C.H.; et al. Pan-cancer analysis of whole genomes. *Nature* **2020**, *578*, 82–93.

233. Demircioglu, D.; Cukuroglu, E.; Kindermans, M.; Nandi, T.; Calabrese, C.; Fonseca, N.A.; Kahles, A.; Lehmann, K.V.; Stegle, O.; Brazma, A.; et al. A pan-cancer transcriptome analysis reveals pervasive regulation through alternative promoters. *Cell* **2019**, *178*, 1465–1477. [CrossRef] [PubMed]

234. Nagahashi, M.; Shimada, Y.; Ichikawa, H.; Kameyama, H.; Takabe, K.; Okuda, S.; Wakai, T. Next generation sequencing-based gene panel tests for the management of solid tumors. *Cancer Sci.* **2019**, *110*, 6–15. [CrossRef] [PubMed]

235. El Achi, H.; Khoury, J.D.; Loghavi, S. Liquid biopsy by next-generation sequencing: A multimodality test for management of cancer. *Curr. Hematol. Malig. Rep.* **2019**, *14*, 358–367. [CrossRef] [PubMed]

236. Kancherla, J.; Rao, S.; Bhuvaneshwar, K.; Riggins, R.B.; Beckman, R.A.; Madhavan, S.; Bravo, H.C.; Boca, S.M. Evidence-based network approach to recommending targeted cancer therapies. *JCO Clin. Cancer Inform.* **2020**, *4*, 71–88. [CrossRef]

237. Zhang, W.; Chien, J.; Yong, J.; Kuang, R. Network-based machine learning and graph theory algorithms for precision oncology. *NPJ Precis. Oncol.* **2017**, *1*, 25. [CrossRef]

238. Jiang, X.L.; Martinez-Ledesma, E.; Morcos, F. Revealing protein networks and gene-drug connectivity in cancer from direct information. *Sci. Rep.* **2017**, *7*, 3739. [CrossRef]

239. Zhang, Y.; Tao, C. Network analysis of cancer-focused association network reveals distinct network association patterns. *Cancer Inform.* **2014**, *13*, 45–51.

240. Cheng, F.; Liu, C.; Jiang, J.; Lu, W.; Li, W.; Liu, G.; Zhou, W.; Huang, J.; Tang, Y. Prediction of drug-target interactions and drug repositioning via network-based inference. *PLoS Comput. Biol.* **2012**, *8*, e1002503. [CrossRef]

241. Garber, K. In a major shift, cancer drugs go "tissue-agnostic". *Science* **2017**, *356*, 1111–1112. [CrossRef]

242. Luoh, S.W.; Flaherty, K.T. When tissue is no longer the issue: tissue-agnostic cancer therapy comes of age. *Ann. Intern. Med.* **2018**, *169*, 233–239. [CrossRef] [PubMed]

243. Mullard, A. FDA approves landmark tissue-agnostic cancer drug. *Nat. Rev. Drug Discov.* **2018**, *1*, 87. [CrossRef] [PubMed]

244. Torres-Ayuso, P.; Sahoo, S.; Ashton, G.; An, E.; Simms, N.; Galvin, M.; Leong, H.S.; Frese, K.K.; Simpson, K.; Cook, N.; et al. Signaling pathway screening platforms are an efficient approach to identify therapeutic targets in cancers that lack known driver mutations: A case report for a cancer of unknown primary origin. *NPJ Genom. Med.* **2018**, *3*, 15. [CrossRef] [PubMed]

245. Siu, L.L.; Conley, B.A.; Boerner, S.; LoRusso, P.M. Next-generation sequencing to guide clinical trials. *Clin. Cancer Res.* **2015**, *21*, 4536–4544. [CrossRef] [PubMed]
246. Beaubier, N.; Bontrager, M.; Huether, R.; Igartua, C.; Lau, D.; Tell, R.; Bobe, A.M.; Bush, S.; Chang, A.L.; Hoskinson, D.C.; et al. Integrated genomic profiling expands clinical options for patients with cancer. *Nat. Biotechnol.* **2019**, *37*, 1351–1360. [CrossRef]
247. Lih, C.J.; Harrington, R.D.; Sims, D.J.; Harper, K.N.; Bouk, C.H.; Datta, V.; Yau, J.; Singh, R.R.; Routbort, M.J.; Luthra, R.; et al. Analytical validation of the next-generation sequencing assay for a nationwide signal—Finding clinical trial: Molecular analysis for therapy choice clinical trial. *J. Mol. Diagn.* **2017**, *19*, 313–327. [CrossRef]
248. Bitzer, M.; Ostermann, L.; Horger, M.; Biskup, S.; Schulze, M.; Ruhm, K.; Hilke, F.; Öner, Ö.; Nikolaou, K.; Schroeder, C.; et al. Next-generation sequencing of advanced gi tumors reveals individual treatment options. *JCO Precis. Oncol.* **2020**, *4*, 258–271. [CrossRef]
249. Sicklick, J.K.; Kato, S.; Okamura, R.; Schwaederle, M.; Hahn, M.E.; Williams, C.B.; De, P.; Krie, A.; Piccioni, D.E.; Miller, V.A.; et al. Molecular profiling of cancer patients enables personalized combination therapy: The I-PREDICT study. *Nat. Med.* **2019**, *25*, 744–750. [CrossRef]
250. Rodon, J.; Soria, J.C.; Berger, R.; Miller, W.H.; Rubin, E.; Kugel, A.; Tsimberidou, A.; Saintigny, P.; Ackerstein, A.; Brana, I.; et al. Genomic and transcriptomic profiling expands precision cancer medicine: The WINTHER trial. *Nat. Med.* **2019**, *25*, 751–758. [CrossRef]
251. Rothwell, D.G.; Ayub, M.; Cook, N.; Thistlethwaite, F.; Carter, L.; Dean, E.; Smith, N.; Villa, S.; Dransfield, J.; Clipson, A.; et al. Utility of ctDNA to support patient selection for early phase clinical trials: The TARGET study. *Nat. Med.* **2019**, *25*, 738–743. [CrossRef]
252. Reitsma, M.; Fox, J.; Vanden Borre, P.; Cavanaugh, M.; Chudnovsky, Y.; Erlich, R.L.; Gribbin, T.E.; Anhorn, R. Effect of a collaboration between a health plan, oncology practice, and comprehensive genomic profiling company from the payer perspective. *J. Manag. Care Spec. Pharm.* **2019**, *25*, 601–611. [CrossRef] [PubMed]
253. Luh, F.; Yen, Y. Benefits and harms of the centers for medicare & medicaid services ruling on next-generation sequencing. *JAMA Oncol.* **2018**, *4*, 1171–1172. [PubMed]
254. Phillips, K.A.; Trosman, J.R.; Deverka, P.A.; Quinn, B.; Tunis, S.; Neumann, P.J.; Chambers, J.D.; Garrison, L.P., Jr.; Douglas, M.P.; Weldon, C.B. Insurance coverage for genomic tests. *Science* **2018**, *360*, 278–279.
255. Trosman, J.R.; Weldon, C.B.; Gradishar, W.J.; Benson, A.; Cristofanilli, M.; Kurian, A.W.; Ford, J.M.; Balch, A.; Watkins, J.; Phillips, K.A. From the past to the present: Insurer coverage frameworks for next-generation tumor sequencing. *Value Health* **2018**, *21*, 1062–1068. [CrossRef] [PubMed]
256. Freedman, A.N.; Klabunde, C.N.; Wiant, K.; Enewold, L.; Gray, S.W.; Filipski, K.K.; Keating, N.L.; Leonard, D.G.B.; Lively, T.; McNeel, T.S.; et al. Use of next-generation sequencing tests to guide cancer treatment: Results from a nationally representative survey of oncologists in the United States. *JCO Precision Oncol.* **2018**, *13*, 1–13. [CrossRef]
257. Miller, F.A.; Krueger, P.; Christensen, R.J.; Ahern, C.; Carter, R.F.; Kamel-Reid, S. Postal survey of physicians and laboratories: Practices and perceptions of molecular oncology testing. *BMC Health Serv. Res.* **2009**, *9*, 131. [CrossRef]
258. Gray, S.W.; Hicks-Courant, K.; Cronin, A.; Rollins, B.J.; Weeks, J.C. Physicians' attitudes about multiplex tumor genomic testing. *J. Clin. Oncol.* **2014**, *32*, 1317–1323. [CrossRef]
259. Gray, S.W.; Park, E.R.; Najita, J.; Martins, Y.; Traeger, L.; Bair, E.; Gagne, J.; Garber, J.; Janne, P.A.; Lindeman, N.; et al. Oncologists' and cancer patients' views on whole-exome sequencing and incidental findings: Results from the CanSeq study. *Genet. Med.* **2016**, *18*, 1011–1019. [CrossRef]
260. Malone, E.R.; Oliva, M.; Sabatini, P.J.B.; Stockley, T.L.; Siu, L.L. Molecular profiling for precision cancer therapies. *Genome Med.* **2020**, *12*, 8. [CrossRef]
261. Bieg-Bourne, C.C.; Millis, S.Z.; Piccioni, D.E.; Fanta, P.T.; Goldberg, M.E.; Chmielecki, J.; Parker, B.A.; Kurzrock, R. Next-generation sequencing in the clinical setting clarifies patient characteristics and potential actionability. *Cancer Res.* **2017**, *77*, 6313–6320. [CrossRef]
262. Clark, D.F.; Maxwell, K.N.; Powers, J.; Lieberman, D.B.; Ebrahimzadeh, J.; Long, J.M.; McKenna, D.; Shah, P.; Bradbury, A.; Morrissette, J.J.D.; et al. Identification and confirmation of potentially actionable germline mutations in tumor-only genomic sequencing. *JCO Precis. Oncol.* **2019**, *3*. [CrossRef]

263. Madhavan, S.; Subramaniam, S.; Brown, T.D.; Chen, J.L. Art and challenges of precision medicine: Interpreting and integrating genomic data into clinical practice. *Am. Soc. Clin. Oncol. Educ. Book. Educ. Book.* **2018**, *38*, 546–553. [CrossRef] [PubMed]

264. Gutierrez, M.E.; Choi, K.; Lanman, R.B.; Licitra, E.J.; Skrzypczak, S.M.; Pe Benito, R.; Wu, T.; Arunajadai, S.; Kaur, S.; Harper, H.; et al. Genomic profiling of advanced non-small cell lung cancer in community settings: Gaps and opportunities. *Clin. Lung. Cancer* **2017**, *18*, 651–659. [CrossRef]

265. Trosman, J.R.; Weldon, C.B.; Kelley, R.K.; Phillips, K.A. Challenges of coverage policy development for next-generation tumor sequencing panels: Experts and payers weigh in. *J. Natl. Compr. Canc. Netw.* **2015**, *13*, 311–318. [CrossRef] [PubMed]

266. Hughes, K.S.; Ambinder, E.P.; Hess, G.P.; Yu, P.P.; Bernstam, E.V.; Routbort, M.J.; Clemenceau, J.R.; Hamm, J.T.; Febbo, P.G.; Domchek, S.M.; et al. Identifying health information technology needs of oncologists to facilitate the adoption of genomic medicine: Recommendations from the 2016 American Society of Clinical Oncology Omics and Precision Oncology Workshop. *J. Clin. Oncol.* **2017**, *35*, 3153–3159. [CrossRef]

267. Griffith, M.; Spies, N.C.; Krysiak, K.; McMichael, J.F.; Coffman, A.C.; Danos, A.M.; Ainscough, B.J.; Ramirez, C.A.; Rieke, D.T.; Kujan, L.; et al. CIViC is a community knowledgebase for expert crowdsourcing the clinical interpretation of variants in cancer. *Nat. Genet.* **2017**, *49*, 170–174. [CrossRef] [PubMed]

268. Chakravarty, D.; Phillips, S.; Kundra, R.; Zhang, H.; Wang, J.; Rudolph, J.E.; Yaeger, R.; Soumerai, T.; Nissan, M.H.; Chang, M.T.; et al. OncoKB: A precision oncology knowledge base. *JCO Precis. Oncol.* **2017**. [CrossRef] [PubMed]

269. Kurnit, K.C.; Bailey, A.M.; Zeng, J.; Johnson, A.M.; Shufean, M.A.; Brusco, L.; Litzenburger, B.C.; Sanchez, N.S.; Khotskaya, Y.B.; Holla, V.; et al. "Personalized cancer therapy": A publicly available precision oncology resource. *Cancer Res.* **2017**, *77*, e123–e126. [CrossRef]

270. My Cancer Genome: Genetically Informed Cancer Medicine. Available online: https://www.mycancergenome.org/ (accessed on 25 April 2020).

271. Warner, J.L.; Prasad, I.; Bennett, M.; Arniella, M.; Beeghly-Fadiel, A.; Mandl, K.D.; Alterovitz, G. SMART cancer navigator: A framework for implementing ASCO workshop recommendations to enable precision cancer medicine. *JCO Precis. Oncol.* **2018**. [CrossRef]

272. City of Hope. Molecular Oncology. Available online: https://www.cityofhope.org/clinical-molecular-diagnostic-laboratory/list-of-cmdl-tests/molecular-oncology (accessed on 3 June 2020).

273. Ellis, P.G. Development and implementation of oncology care pathways in an integrated care network: The via oncology pathways experience. *J. Oncol. Pract.* **2013**, *9*, 171–173. [CrossRef]

274. Luchini, C.; Lawlor, R.T.; Milella, M.; Scarpa, A. Molecular tumor boards in clinical practice. *Trends Cancer* **2020**. [CrossRef]

275. Rolfo, C.; Manca, P.; Salgado, R.; Van Dam, P.; Dendooven, A.; Machado Coelho, A.; Ferri Gandia, J.; Rutten, A.; Lybaert, W.; Vermeij, J.; et al. Multidisciplinary molecular tumour board: A tool to improve clinical practice and selection accrual for clinical trials in patients with cancer. *ESMO Open.* **2018**, *3*, e000398. [CrossRef] [PubMed]

276. Remon, J.; Dienstmann, R. Precision oncology: Separating the wheat from the chaff. *ESMO Open* **2018**, *3*, e000446. [CrossRef] [PubMed]

277. Romero, D. Optimizing access to matched therapies. *Nat. Rev. Clin. Oncol.* **2019**, *16*, 401. [CrossRef] [PubMed]

278. Andre, F.; Mardis, E.; Salm, M.; Soria, J.C.; Siu, L.L.; Swanton, C. Prioritizing targets for precision cancer medicine. *Ann. Oncol.* **2014**, *25*, 2295–2303. [CrossRef] [PubMed]

279. Dalton, W.S.; Sullivan, D.; Ecsedy, J.; Caligiuri, M.A. Patient enrichment for precision-based cancer clinical trials: Using prospective cohort surveillance as an approach to improve clinical trials. *Clin. Pharmacol. Ther.* **2018**, *104*, 23–26. [CrossRef] [PubMed]

280. Chakradhar, S. Matching up. *Nat. Med.* **2018**, *24*, 882–884. [CrossRef]

281. Roychowdhury, S.; Iyer, M.K.; Robinson, D.R.; Lonigro, R.J.; Wu, Y.M.; Cao, X.; Kalyana-Sundaram, S.; Sam, L.; Balbin, O.A.; Quist, M.J.; et al. Personalized oncology through integrative high-throughput sequencing: A pilot study. *Sci. Transl. Med.* **2011**, *3*, 111ra121. [CrossRef]

282. Kurnit, K.C.; Dumbrava, E.E.I.; Litzenburger, B.; Khotskaya, Y.B.; Johnson, A.M.; Yap, T.A.; Rodon, J.; Zeng, J.; Shufean, M.A.; Bailey, A.M.; et al. Precision oncology decision support: Current approaches and strategies for the future. *Clin. Cancer Res.* **2018**, *24*, 2719–2731. [CrossRef]

283. Dalton, W.B.; Forde, P.M.; Kang, H.; Connolly, R.M.; Stearns, V.; Gocke, C.D.; Eshleman, J.R.; Axilbund, J.; Petry, D.; Geoghegan, C.; et al. Personalized medicine in the oncology clinic: Implementation and outcomes of the Johns Hopkins Molecular Tumor Board. *JCO Precis. Oncol.* **2017**. [CrossRef]

284. Meric-Bernstam, F.; Johnson, A.; Holla, V.; Bailey, A.M.; Brusco, L.; Chen, K.; Routbort, M.; Patel, K.P.; Zeng, J.; Kopetz, S.; et al. A decision support framework for genomically informed investigational cancer therapy. *J. Natl. Cancer Inst.* **2015**, *107*. [CrossRef]

285. Hyman, D.M.; Solit, D.B.; Arcila, M.E.; Cheng, D.T.; Sabbatini, P.; Baselga, J.; Berger, M.F.; Ladanyi, M. Precision medicine at Memorial Sloan Kettering Cancer Center: Clinical next-generation sequencing enabling next-generation targeted therapy trials. *Drug Discov. Today* **2015**, *20*, 1422–1428. [CrossRef] [PubMed]

286. Huang, L.D.; Fernandes, H.; Zia, H.; Tavassoli, P.; Rennert, H.; Pisapia, D.; Imielinski, M.; Sboner, A.; Rubin, M.A.; Kluk, M.; et al. The cancer precision medicine knowledge base for structured clinical-grade mutations and interpretations. *J. Am. Med. Inform. Assoc.* **2017**, *24*, 513–519. [CrossRef] [PubMed]

287. Beltran, H.; Eng, K.; Mosquera, J.M.; Sigaras, A.; Romanel, A.; Rennert, H.; Kossai, M.; Pauli, C.; Faltas, B.; Fontugne, J.; et al. Whole-exome sequencing of metastatic cancer and biomarkers of treatment response. *JAMA Oncol.* **2015**, *1*, 466–474. [CrossRef] [PubMed]

288. Schwaederle, M.; Parker, B.A.; Schwab, R.B.; Daniels, G.A.; Piccioni, D.E.; Kesari, S.; Helsten, T.L.; Bazhenova, L.A.; Romero, J.; Fanta, P.T.; et al. Precision oncology: The UC San Diego Moores Cancer Center PREDICT Experience. *Mol. Cancer Ther.* **2016**, *15*, 743–752. [CrossRef] [PubMed]

289. Said, R.; Tsimberidou, A.M. Basket trials and the MD Anderson Precision Medicine Clinical trials platform. *Cancer J.* **2019**, *25*, 282–286. [CrossRef] [PubMed]

290. Trivedi, H.; Acharya, D.; Chamarthy, U.; Meunier, J.; Ali-Ahmad, H.; Hamdan, M.; Herman, J.; Srkalovic, G. Implementation and outcomes of a molecular tumor board at Herbert-Herman Cancer Center, Sparrow Hospital. *Acta Med. Acad.* **2019**, *48*, 105–115.

291. Grandori, C.; Kemp, C.J. Personalized cancer models for target. discovery and precision medicine. *Trends Cancer* **2018**, *4*, 634–642. [CrossRef]

292. Pauli, C.; Hopkins, B.D.; Prandi, D.; Shaw, R.; Fedrizzi, T.; Sboner, A.; Sailer, V.; Augello, M.; Puca, L.; Rosati, R.; et al. Personalized in vitro and in vivo cancer models to guide precision medicine. *Cancer Discov.* **2017**, *7*, 462–477. [CrossRef]

293. Chen, H.Z.; Bonneville, R.; Roychowdhury, S. Implementing precision cancer medicine in the genomic era. *Semin. Cancer Biol.* **2019**, *55*, 16–27. [CrossRef]

294. Wong, C.H.; Siah, K.W.; Lo, A.W. Estimation of clinical trial success rates and related parameters. *Biostatistics* **2019**, *20*, 273–286. [CrossRef] [PubMed]

295. Sacks, L.V.; Shamsuddin, H.H.; Yasinskaya, Y.I.; Bouri, K.; Lanthier, M.L.; Sherman, R.E. Scientific and regulatory reasons for delay and denial of FDA approval of initial applications for new drugs, 2000–2012. *J. Am. Med. Assoc.* **2014**, *311*, 378–384. [CrossRef] [PubMed]

296. Hay, M.; Thomas, D.W.; Craighead, J.L.; Economides, C.; Rosenthal, J. Clinical development success rates for investigational drugs. *Nat. Biotechnol.* **2014**, *32*, 40–51. [CrossRef] [PubMed]

297. Fogel, D.B. Factors associated with clinical trials that fail and opportunities for improving the likelihood of success: A review. *Contemp. Clin. Trials Commun.* **2018**, *11*, 156–164. [CrossRef] [PubMed]

298. Khozin, S.; Liu, K.; Jarow, J.P.; Pazdur, R. Regulatory watch: Why do oncology drugs fail to gain US regulatory approval? *Nat. Rev. Drug. Discov.* **2015**, *14*, 450–451. [CrossRef]

299. Heneghan, C.; Goldacre, B.; Mahtani, K.R. Why clinical trial outcomes fail to translate into benefits for patients. *Trials* **2017**, *18*, 122. [CrossRef]

300. Seruga, B.; Ocana, A.; Amir, E.; Tannock, I.F. Failures in phase III: Causes and consequences. *Clin. Cancer Res.* **2015**, *21*, 4552–4560. [CrossRef]

301. Schmidt, C. The struggle to do no harm. *Nature* **2017**, *552*, S74–S75. [CrossRef]

302. Mullard, A. How much do phase III trials cost? *Nat. Rev. Drug Discov.* **2018**, *1*, 7777-7777. [CrossRef]

303. Vincent Rajkumar, S. The high cost of prescription drugs: Causes and solutions. *Blood Cancer J.* **2020**, *10*, 71. [CrossRef]

304. Sanders, A.B.; Fulginiti, J.V.; Witzke, D.B.; Bangs, K.A. Characteristics influencing career decisions of academic and nonacademic emergency physicians. *Ann. Emerg. Med.* **1994**, *23*, 81–87. [CrossRef]

305. Tsang, J.L.Y.; Ross, K. It's time to increase community hospital-based health research. *Acad. Med.* **2017**, *92*, 727. [CrossRef]

306. Dimond, E.P.; St Germain, D.; Nacpil, L.M.; Zaren, H.A.; Swanson, S.M.; Minnick, C.; Carrigan, A.; Denicoff, A.M.; Igo, K.E.; Acoba, J.D.; et al. Creating a "culture of research" in a community hospital: Strategies and tools from the National Cancer Institute Community Cancer Centers Program. *Clin. Trials* **2015**, *12*, 246–256. [CrossRef]

307. Boaz, A.; Hanney, S.; Jones, T.; Soper, B. Does the engagement of clinicians and organisations in research improve healthcare performance: A three-stage review. *BMJ Open* **2015**, *5*, e009415. [CrossRef]

308. Knepper, T.C.; Bell, G.C.; Hicks, J.K.; Padron, E.; Teer, J.K.; Vo, T.T.; Gillis, N.K.; Mason, N.T.; McLeod, H.L.; Walko, C.M. Key lessons learned from moffitt's molecular tumor board: The clinical genomics action committee experience. *Oncologist* **2017**, *22*, 144–151. [CrossRef] [PubMed]

309. Overman, M.J.; Morris, V.; Kee, B.; Fogelman, D.; Xiao, L.; Eng, C.; Dasari, A.; Shroff, R.; Mazard, T.; Shaw, K.; et al. Utility of a molecular prescreening program in advanced colorectal cancer for enrollment on biomarker-selected clinical trials. *Ann. Oncol.* **2016**, *27*, 1068–1074. [CrossRef] [PubMed]

310. Dienstmann, R.; Garralda, E.; Aguilar, S.; Sala, G.; Viaplana, C.; Ruiz-Pace, F.; González-Zorelle, J.; LoGiacco, D.G.; Ogbah, Z.; Masdeu, L.R.; et al. Evolving landscape of molecular prescreening strategies for oncology early clinical trials. *JCO Precis. Oncol.* **2020**, *4*, 505–513. [CrossRef]

311. Pishvaian, M.J.; Blais, E.M.; Bender, R.J.; Rao, S.; Boca, S.M.; Chung, V.; Hendifar, A.E.; Mikhail, S.; Sohal, D.P.S.; Pohlmann, P.R.; et al. A virtual molecular tumor board to improve efficiency and scalability of delivering precision oncology to physicians and their patients. *JAMIA Open* **2019**, *2*, 505–515. [CrossRef]

312. Schwaederle, M.; Zhao, M.; Lee, J.J.; Lazar, V.; Leyland-Jones, B.; Schilsky, R.L.; Mendelsohn, J.; Kurzrock, R. Association of biomarker-based treatment strategies with response rates and progression-free survival in refractory malignant neoplasms: A meta-analysis. *JAMA Oncol.* **2016**, *2*, 1452–1459. [CrossRef]

313. Schwaederle, M.; Zhao, M.; Lee, J.J.; Eggermont, A.M.; Schilsky, R.L.; Mendelsohn, J.; Lazar, V.; Kurzrock, R. Impact of precision medicine in diverse cancers: A meta-analysis of phase II clinical trials. *J. Clin. Oncol.* **2015**, *33*, 3817–3825. [CrossRef]

314. Stockley, T.L.; Oza, A.M.; Berman, H.K.; Leighl, N.B.; Knox, J.J.; Shepherd, F.A.; Chen, E.X.; Krzyzanowska, M.K.; Dhani, N.; Joshua, A.M.; et al. Molecular profiling of advanced solid tumors and patient outcomes with genotype-matched clinical trials: The Princess Margaret IMPACT/COMPACT trial. *Genome Med.* **2016**, *8*, 109. [CrossRef] [PubMed]

315. Haslem, D.S.; Van Norman, S.B.; Fulde, G.; Knighton, A.J.; Belnap, T.; Butler, A.M.; Rhagunath, S.; Newman, D.; Gilbert, H.; Tudor, B.P.; et al. A retrospective analysis of precision medicine outcomes in patients with advanced cancer reveals improved progression-free survival without increased health care costs. *J. Oncol. Pract.* **2017**, *13*, e108–e119. [CrossRef] [PubMed]

316. Radovich, M.; Kiel, P.J.; Nance, S.M.; Niland, E.E.; Parsley, M.E.; Ferguson, M.E.; Jiang, G.; Ammakkanavar, N.R.; Einhorn, L.H.; Cheng, L.; et al. Clinical benefit of a precision medicine based approach for guiding treatment of refractory cancers. *Oncotarget* **2016**, *7*, 56491–56500. [CrossRef]

317. Aust, S.; Schwameis, R.; Gagic, T.; Mullauer, L.; Langthaler, E.; Prager, G.; Grech, C.; Reinthaller, A.; Krainer, M.; Pils, D.; et al. Precision medicine tumor boards: Clinical applicability of personalized treatment concepts in ovarian cancer. *Cancers* **2020**, *12*, 548. [CrossRef] [PubMed]

318. Tafe, L.J.; Gorlov, I.P.; de Abreu, F.B.; Lefferts, J.A.; Liu, X.; Pettus, J.R.; Marotti, J.D.; Bloch, K.J.; Memoli, V.A.; Suriawinata, A.A.; et al. Implementation of a molecular tumor board: The impact on treatment decisions for 35 patients evaluated at Dartmouth-Hitchcock Medical Center. *Oncologist* **2015**, *20*, 1011–1018. [CrossRef]

319. Lamping, M.; Benary, M.; Leyvraz, S.; Messerschmidt, C.; Blanc, E.; Kessler, T.; Schutte, M.; Lenze, D.; Johrens, K.; Burock, S.; et al. Support of a molecular tumour board by an evidence-based decision management system for precision oncology. *Eur. J. Cancer* **2020**, *127*, 41–51. [CrossRef]

320. Boddu, S.; Walko, C.M.; Bienasz, S.; Bui, M.M.; Henderson-Jackson, E.; Naghavi, A.O.; Mullinax, J.E.; Joyce, D.M.; Binitie, O.; Letson, G.D.; et al. Clinical utility of genomic profiling in the treatment of advanced sarcomas: A single-center experience. *JCO Precis. Oncol.* **2018**, 1–8. [CrossRef]

321. Lane, B.R.; Bissonnette, J.; Waldherr, T.; Ritz-Holland, D.; Chesla, D.; Cottingham, S.L.; Alberta, S.; Liu, C.; Thompson, A.B.; Graveel, C.; et al. Development of a center for personalized cancer care at a regional cancer center: Feasibility trial of an institutional tumor sequencing advisory board. *J. Mol. Diagn.* **2015**, *17*, 695–704. [CrossRef]

322. Overton, L.C.; Corless, C.L.; Agrawal, M.; Assikis, V.J.; Beegle, N.L.; Blau, S.; Chernoff, M.; Divers, S.G.; Henry, D.H.; Nikolinakos, P.; et al. Impact of next-generation sequencing (NGS) on treatment decisions in the community oncology setting. *J. Clin. Oncol.* **2014**, *32*, 11028-11028. [CrossRef]

323. ASCO eLearning. Multidisciplinary Molecular Tumor Boards (MMTBs). Available online: https://elearning. asco.org/product-details/multidisciplinary-molecular-tumor-boards-mmtbs (accessed on 1 May 2020).

324. Healio Learn Genomics. Available online: https://www.healio.com/hematology-oncology/learn-genomics (accessed on 1 May 2020).

325. Pishvaian, M.J.; Bender, R.J.; Halverson, D.; Rahib, L.; Hendifar, A.E.; Mikhail, S.; Chung, V.; Picozzi, V.J.; Sohal, D.; Blais, E.M.; et al. Molecular profiling of patients with pancreatic cancer: Initial results from the know your tumor initiative. *Clin. Cancer Res.* **2018**, *24*, 5018–5027. [CrossRef]

326. Burkard, M.E.; Deming, D.A.; Parsons, B.M.; Kenny, P.A.; Schuh, M.R.; Leal, T.; Uboha, N.; Lang, J.M.; Thompson, M.A.; Warren, R.; et al. Implementation and clinical utility of an integrated academic-community regional molecular tumor board. *JCO Precis. Oncol.* **2017**, 1–10. [CrossRef]

327. Heifetz, L.J.; Christensen, S.D.; Devere-White, R.W.; Meyers, F.J. A model for rural oncology. *J. Oncol. Pract.* **2011**, *7*, 168–171. [CrossRef] [PubMed]

328. Shea, C.M.; Teal, R.; Haynes-Maslow, L.; McIntyre, M.; Weiner, B.J.; Wheeler, S.B.; Jacobs, S.R.; Mayer, D.K.; Young, M.; Shea, T.C. Assessing the feasibility of a virtual tumor board program: A case study. *J. Healthc. Manag.* **2014**, *59*, 177–193. [CrossRef] [PubMed]

329. Farhangfar, C. Utilization of consultative molecular tumor board in community setting. *J. Clin. Oncol.* **2017**, *35*, 6508. [CrossRef]

330. Marshall, C.L.; Petersen, N.J.; Naik, A.D.; Vander Velde, N.; Artinyan, A.; Albo, D.; Berger, D.H.; Anaya, D.A. Implementation of a regional virtual tumor board: A prospective study evaluating feasibility and provider acceptance. *Telemed. J. E Health* **2014**, *20*, 705–711. [CrossRef]

331. Nasser, S.; Kurdolgu, A.A.; Izatt, T.; Aldrich, J.; Russell, M.L.; Christoforides, A.; Tembe, W.; Keifer, J.A.; Corneveaux, J.J.; Byron, S.A.; et al. An Integrated framework for reporting clinically relevant biomarkers from paired tumor/normal genomic and transcriptomic sequencing data in support of clinical trials in personalized medicine. *Pac. Symp. Biocomput.* **2015**, *2015*, 56–67.

332. Von Hoff, D.; Han, H. *Precision Medicine in Cancer Therapy*; Springer International Publishing: New York, NY, USA, 2019.

333. Weiss, G.J.; Byron, S.A.; Aldrich, J.; Sangal, A.; Barilla, H.; Kiefer, J.A.; Carpten, J.D.; Craig, D.W.; Whitsett, T.G. A prospective pilot study of genome-wide exome and transcriptome profiling in patients with small cell lung cancer progressing after first-line therapy. *PLoS ONE* **2017**, *12*, e0179170. [CrossRef]

334. Byron, S.A.; Tran, N.L.; Halperin, R.F.; Phillips, J.J.; Kuhn, J.G.; de Groot, J.F.; Colman, H.; Ligon, K.L.; Wen, P.Y.; Cloughesy, T.F.; et al. Prospective feasibility trial for genomics-informed treatment in recurrent and progressive glioblastoma. *Clin. Cancer Res.* **2018**, *24*, 295–305. [CrossRef]

335. Mueller, S.; Jain, P.; Liang, W.S.; Kilburn, L.; Kline, C.; Gupta, N.; Panditharatna, E.; Magge, S.N.; Zhang, B.; Zhu, Y.; et al. A pilot precision medicine trial for children with diffuse intrinsic pontine glioma-PNOC003: A report from the Pacific Pediatric Neuro-Oncology Consortium. *Int. J. Cancer* **2019**, *145*, 1889–1901. [CrossRef]

10

Use of HER2-Directed Therapy in Metastatic Breast Cancer and How Community Physicians Collaborate to Improve Care

Joanne E. Mortimer [1,*], Laura Kruper [2], Mary Cianfrocca [1], Sayeh Lavasani [1], Sariah Liu [1], Niki Tank-Patel [1], Mina Sedrak [1], Wade Smith [1], Daphne Stewart [1], James Waisman [1], Christina Yeon [1], Tina Wang [1] and Yuan Yuan [1]

[1] Department of Medical Oncology and Therapeutics Research, City of Hope Comprehensive Cancer Center, Duarte, CA 91010, USA; mcianfrocca@coh.org (M.C.); slavasani@coh.org (S.L.); sarliu@coh.org (S.L.); nikpatel@coh.org (N.T.-P.); msedrak@coh.org (M.S.); wsmith@coh.org (W.S.); dapstewart@coh.org (D.S.); jwaisman@coh.org (J.W.); cyeon@coh.org (C.Y.); tinawang@coh.org (T.W.); yuyuan@coh.org (Y.Y.)
[2] Department of Surgery, Division of Breast Surgery, City of Hope Comprehensive Cancer Center, Duarte, CA 91010, USA; lkruper@coh.org
* Correspondence: jmortimer@coh.org

Abstract: The development of new HER2-directed therapies has resulted in a significant prolongation of survival for women with metastatic HER2-positive breast cancer. Discoveries in the laboratory inform clinical trials which are the basis for improving the standard of care and are also the backbone for quality improvement. Clinical trials can be completed more rapidly by expanding trial enrollment to community sites. In this article we review some of the challenges in treating metastatic breast cancer with HER2-directed therapies and our strategies for incorporating our community partners into the research network.

Keywords: breast cancer; community; research; HER2-directed therapy

1. Introduction

Although breast cancers arise from a single organ, the biology and natural history of the disease can be extremely variable. Gene expression profiling allows us to subcategorize breast cancer into four "intrinsic subtypes", each with a unique natural history and response to therapy—Luminal A, Luminal B, Basal-like, and HER2 (human epidermal growth factor receptor 2) "enriched" [1,2]. However, until uniform genomic profiling becomes feasible, clinical decision making is based on tumor histology, stage, hormone receptor status, and HER2 status. This paper focuses on the use of HER2-targeted therapies in metastatic breast cancer and the importance of clinical trials and community practice collaboration in understanding the biology of this disease and advancing therapy.

2. HER2 and Breast Cancer

Four membrane tyrosine kinase receptors constitute the HER family. HER1 (also known as EGFR; epidermal growth factor receptor), HER3, and HER4 bind to almost a dozen different ligands, while HER2 has no known ligands. Rather, HER2 is activated through homo- and heterodimerization with other HER family members, and these complexes activate intracellular signaling pathways such as MAPK (mitogen-activated protein kinase) and PI3K (phosphoinositide 3-kinase) that results in tumor growth, invasion, migration, and survival [3]. The different receptors, ligands, and intracellular signaling pathways provide opportunities for drug development with agents used alone, in combination with each other, and with chemotherapy. The gene that encodes HER2 is amplified in 15–20% of all breast cancers and defines a uniquely aggressive natural history with high grade histologies, greater likelihood to metastasize to visceral sites, and shortened survivals [4,5]. Gene amplification or protein over expression identifies patients who are candidates for HER2-directed therapies.

The humanized IgG monoclonal antibody, trastuzumab, targets the extracellular domain of HER2 effectively preventing intracellular signaling. While trastuzumab has minimal activity as a single agent, when combined with chemotherapy there is a prolongation in survival for women with metastatic breast cancer [6–8]. Trastuzumab has been shown to improve disease outcomes in all stages of HER2-amplified breast cancer [9]. The development of HER2-directed therapies, and trastuzumab in particular, is one of the greatest success stories in the treatment of breast cancer and is as important as hormone receptor status in its clinical impact.

3. Assessment of HER2 Status

Candidacy for HER2-directed therapies is based on a pathologic determination from the primary tumor or metastatic focus of disease. It is generally agreed that HER2 positivity is defined as 3+ staining by immunohistochemical staining (IHC) of the protein or gene amplification of HER2 by fluorescence in situ hybridization (FISH). Recently, companion studies described using in situ hybridization to report gene copy number per cell. This resulted in a HER2 "equivocal" status and required modification of the ASCO/CAP (American Society of Clinical Oncology/College of American Pathologists) guidelines for HER2 assessment [10].

The standard of care dictates that a tumor biopsy be performed on all patients suspected of having recurrent or metastatic breast cancer in order to document the disease as well as to determine the hormone receptor and HER2 status, which guide the choice of systemic therapy. The estrogen receptor (ER), progesterone receptor (PR), or HER2 status on a recurrence may differ from the original primary in 20–30% of instances. Furthermore, although it is not feasible to biopsy all sites of metastatic disease, discordance of receptors within an individual patient occurs in 15–20% of lesions [11–13]. Ultimately, the choice of systemic therapy is determined on a small sample of tumor obtained on a larger site of disease and thus may not reflect the tumor status at all sites.

HER2-directed therapies are effective only in patients whose cancers are HER2-positive. The NSABP B47 randomized over 3000 women with early stage breast cancer whose HER2 status was negative (1+, and 2+ by IHC of FISH< 2.0) to receive conventional adjuvant chemotherapy with or without 12 months of trastuzumab. No benefit was seen with the addition of trastuzumab and cardiac toxicity was observed in 2.3% receiving trastuzumab [14]. It is probably not realistic to assume that all HER2-positive patients benefit from HER2-directed therapies. Given a predictable incidence of cardiac toxicity, it would be ideal to treat only women who are likely to benefit from these treatments. The goal of precision medicine is to identify which patients benefit from HER2-directed therapies.

4. Functional Imaging to Predict Response to HER2 Therapies

We have developed ^{64}Cu-labeled trastuzumab as a PET imaging agent to study women with recurrent/metastatic breast cancer. In our experience uptake on ^{64}Cu-trastuzumab PET/CT correlates with the qualitative assessment of HER2 by IHC. Higher uptake of ^{64}Cu-trastuzumab is seen in women with IHC levels of 3+ compared to 1+ [15,16]. Functional imaging with ^{64}Cu-trastuzumab PET/CT does not assess HER2 status, but demonstrates that trastuzumab is effectively delivered to the cancer. This pharmacodynamics data is clinically more relevant than knowing the intensity of uptake by IHC or degree of gene amplification. The current standard of care for patients with newly diagnosed metastatic HER2-positive cancer utilizes a combination of chemotherapy, trastuzumab, and pertuzumab. It is, therefore, not possible for functional imaging with radiolabeled trastuzumab to predict impact of trastuzumab on treatment efficacy when response to therapy is confounded by the concurrent administration of chemotherapy.

Ado-trastuzumab emtansine (TDM1) binds to the extracellular domain of HER2 and undergoes receptor-mediated internalization inhibiting intracellular signaling pathways [17]. Because its activity is dependent upon trastuzumab binding to the HER2 protein, it is the ideal drug to test whether functional imaging with ^{64}Cu-trastuzumab PET/CT is able to predict for response to therapy. In our experience, pretreatment ^{64}Cu-trastuzumab PET/CT in women with recurrent/metastatic disease is able to identify which individuals are unlikely to benefit from TDM1. Additionally, ^{64}Cu-trastuzumab PET/CT has identified disease within the CNS and has also demonstrated that uptake of ^{64}Cu-trastuzumab can be heterogeneous within a single patient. If that uptake in individual sites falls below a certain level, TDM1 is not effective in those areas and the response is mixed [18].

5. Current Treatment for Metastatic HER2-Positive Breast Cancer

Like trastuzumab, pertuzumab is also a monoclonal antibody that binds to the extracellular domain of HER2, but at a different epitope from that bound by trastuzumab. Pertuzumab prevents dimerization with other HER family members (HER1, HER3, and HER4) [19]. Neither trastuzumab or pertuzumab are very active as single agents, but the combination is synergistic. In women with metastatic HER2-positive breast cancer that has progressed on a trastuzumab-containing regimen, the combination of pertuzumab with trastuzumab produces clinical benefit in more than half of patients [20]. The CLEOPATRA study demonstrated that the addition of pertuzumab to trastuzumab and docetaxel improved overall survival and established this three-drug combination as first-line therapy in metastatic disease. With more than 8 years of follow up, 37% of women who started treatment with pertuzumab, trastuzumab, and docetaxel are still alive. The study was designed to administer at least 6 cycles of docetaxel or until toxicity, and the duration of docetaxel was left to the discretion of the treating oncologist. Pertuzumab and trastuzumab were continued until disease progression. The median number of treatment cycles containing docetaxel was 8 (range 6–10) and the median total cycles was 24 with a maximum of 167 [21,22]. The prolonged survival in this population is also related to the efficacy of subsequent treatment.

Two antibody drug conjugates (ADC) have utilized trastuzumab to deliver a cytotoxic payload. Ado-trastuzumab emtansine (TDM1) utilizes maytansine as the cytotoxic component and has been found to be superior to other regimens containing chemotherapy and HER2-directed agents. It is currently considered second or third line therapy [17,23]. Fam-trastuzumab-deruxtecan uses the topoisomerase I inhibitor, deruxtecan as its payload. In the DESTINY 01 trial, 184 women with HER2-positive metastatic breast cancer who had received a median of six prior therapies were treated with fam-trastuzumab-deruxtecan. Objective responses were observed in 112 (60.9%) women with a median duration of response of 14.8 months [24]. Fam-trastuzumab-deruxtecan is used as third-line therapy.

The two ADCs differ in other ways. Fam-trastuzumab-deruxtecan has a higher drug-to-antibody ratio than TDM1 (DAR = 8 vs. DAR = 3.4, respectively) and fam-trastuzumab-deruxtecan is selectively cleaved by cathepsins that are up regulated in tumor cells. Deruxtecan is also highly cell-membrane permeable and is readily released across cell membranes. A potential benefit for this mechanism is that release of the cytotoxic component may have cytotoxic effects on adjacent tumor cells regardless of the tumor's HER2 dependency [25]. Since the majority of breast cancers (~60%) express HER2 to some degree, fam-trastuzumab-deruxtecan has the potential to benefit many patients [26,27]. Currently the drug is considered for 3rd line and beyond [28].

The oral tyrosine kinase inhibitor, tucatinib, is a selective inhibitor of HER2. In combination with capecitabine and trastuzumab, objective tumor responses have been demonstrated in heavily pretreated patients with metastatic HER2-positive breast cancer including women with brain metastases. The HER2CLIMB study randomized women with metastatic HER2-positive breast cancer who had received prior trastuzumab, pertuzumab, and TDM1 to receive trastuzumab and capecitabine with or without tucatinib. Progression-free survival (PFS) favored the addition of tucatinib (7.8 months compared with 5.4 months). The overall survival also favored the tucatinib arm with a survival prolongation of 4.5 months; 21.9 months vs. 17.4 months. For the 291 women with brain metastases, the median PFS was 7.6 months in the tucatinib arm and 5.4 months in the control arm ($p < 0.001$) [29].

Tucatinib was recently approved by the FDA. Tucatinib + trastuzumab + capecitabine is currently considered as a treatment for advanced unresectable or metastatic HER2-positive breast cancer, including patients with brain metastases, who have received one or more lines of prior HER2-targeted therapy in the metastatic setting [30]. In the HER2CLIMB study, 291 patients were enrolled who had brain metastases—48% in the tucatinib arm and 46% in the control arm. The CNS (central nervous system) progression-free survival and median overall survival favored the tucatinib arm making this an important therapy in patients with HER2+ breast cancer metastatic to brain [31].

There are additional active agents that also deserve mention. Lapatinib was the first dual inhibitor of HER2 and HER1. Until the development of TDM1, lapatinib and capecitabine were considered to be second-line therapy [32]. Currently, lapatinib is combined with trastuzumab as a "next-line" of therapy [33]. The NALA trial randomized patients who had received at least two prior treatments for metastatic disease to receive either neratinib or lapatinib in combination with capecitabine. At 6 and 12 months, the progression-free survival was significantly longer with neratinib as well as a significant increase in the time to intervention for symptomatic CNS. Neratinib provides another treatment option for treating metastatic disease [34]. Even after disease progression on trastuzumab, additional chemotherapy with trastuzumab has been shown to be more effective than chemotherapy alone [35].

The explosion in new and highly effective therapies has transformed metastatic HER2-positive breast cancer into a chronic disease. Conventional chemotherapy still has a role as salvage treatment and is more effective when combined with trastuzumab [35]. New drug development and combining the currently available HER2-directed agents with drugs that modulate intracellular signaling are currently on-going in the clinic.

6. HER2 Activating Mutations—A Unique Clinical Entity

Bose used DNA sequencing on samples obtained from ACOSOG (American College of Surgeons Oncology Groupz) 1031 and data from other sequencing studies to identify somatic mutations in tumors that were pathologically determined to be HER2-negative. Seven of the 13 mutations were classified as activating mutations. Cell line studies showed a unique dependence on EGFR phosphorylation and led to an assessment of the therapeutic efficacy of the dual kinase inhibitors of HER2 and EGFR, lapatinib and neratinib. Neratinib demonstrated a stronger inhibition of cell growth than lapatinib and was effective in all activating mutations [36]. It is estimated that HER2-activating mutations occur in 1.6–2.5% of invasive ductal carcinomas and 7.5% of invasive lobular cancers [36,37]. Clinical trials of neratinib in this population have demonstrated efficacy and have identified another way of targeting HER2 [38,39]. This unique genotype demonstrates the potential use of next generation sequencing in breast cancer.

7. Engaging the Community in Clinical Research

City of Hope recently acquired 30 community practice sites and in doing so dramatically expanded the number of colleagues in surgical, medical, and radiation oncology and almost tripled the number of new breast patients. With such a rapid expansion, our goal was to develop a common culture of research and quality clinical care that is at the heart of City of Hope's values. This initiative was led by a steering committee of interdisciplinary subspecialty physicians and business leaders who met regularly. This team identified the individual community physicians who had an interest in treating breast cancer and in conducting clinical research and worked with all the stakeholders to define quality of care. We convened a meeting of all clinical faculty with an interest in breast cancer, compiled a brief resource inventory (systematic identification and access to any potential contributions to this program), and identified barriers to achieving our predefined quality of care. The sharing of our unique differences in practice and the challenges that each individual experienced, resulted in a respect for what each partner brought to the program and how we could work together to solve these problems. Through a culture of respect and trust we were able to define quality metrics for the clinical care of patients with breast cancer and created treatment guidelines which included eligibility for clinical trial participation (see Table 1). Clinical research requires physicians who are interested in conducting clinical trials and a practice site that has a patient population interested in study participation. It is also critical to have competent clinical research coordinators, a research pharmacy, and radiologists who support serial radiologic interpretation of x-rays using RECIST and PERCIST.

Table 1. City of Hope Institutional guidelines HER2+ metastatic disease.

HR− and HER2+ Breast Cancer	HR+ and HER2+ Breast Cancer
FIRST: Biopsy confirmation of Diagnosis and Receptor Status ALL Pt should have BRCA tested	
1st line #19339 NRG Trial pertuzumab, trastuzumab, taxane +/− atezolizumab	**1st line #19339 NRG Trial** pertuzumab, trastuzumab, taxane +/− atezolizumab
1st Line* pertuzumab, trastuzumab and taxane	**1st Line*** pertuzumab, trastuzumab and taxane
* #20048 Alpelisib in maintenance alpelisib combination in PIK3CA mutation	*** #20048 Alpelisib in maintenance** alpelisib combination in PIK3CA mutation
2nd Line #19599 (HER2CLIMB-02) tucatinib or placebo in combination with TDM1 for unresectable locally-advanced or metastatic disease	**2nd Line #19599 (HER2CLIMB-02)** tucatinib or placebo in combination with TDM1 for unresectable locally-advanced or metastatic disease
2nd Line TDM1or tucatinib/capecitabine/trastuzumab	**2nd Line** TDM1 or tucatinib/capecitabine/trastuzumab
3rd Line tucatinib/capecitabine/trastuzumab or fam-trastuzumab-deruxtecan	**3rd Line** tucatinib/capecitabine/trastuzumab or or fam-trastuzumab-deruxtecan
4th or + Line Prior pertuzumab, trastuzumab, TDM1 consider fam-trastuzumab-deruxtecan or neratinib/capecitabine, lapatinib/trastuzumab Chemo + trastuzumab	**4th or + Line** Prior pertuzumab, trastuzumab, TDM1 consider fam-trastuzumab-deruxtecan or neratinib/capecitabine, lapatinib/trastuzumab or Chemo + trastuzumab or an AI or LHRH agonist + Tamoxifen/trastuzumab
Bone Directed Therapy— Zometa q1 month x 9, then q3 months until Hospice or Xgeva q1 month until Hospice (Xgeva is 2x more expensive)	

All research decision-making is made by the breast cancer research team (Breast Disease Team), composed of medical, surgical, and radiation oncologists, basic scientists, statisticians, pharmacists, research nurses, clinical research associates, and the Executive Director for Affiliate sites. Breast Disease Team meetings are available on a remote platform so that our community partners can participate, and meeting minutes are submitted to all. The Breast Disease Team meets on a weekly basis to review proposed study concepts, endorse the written protocols developed from an approved concept, troubleshoot operational problems, and review active patients on study. Our current clinical research portfolio in HER2-positive breast cancer focuses on two main areas: 1. Defining new therapies and new roles for these systemic therapies (an area largely driven by the cooperative groups and Pharma), and 2. Identifying which patients are likely to benefit from HER2-directed therapies using functional imaging, which is a City of Hope research initiative.

The Executive Director for Affiliates oversees research at the community sites and is aware of the physicians' interests, patient population, and clinical trial infrastructure at the individual offices. The full clinical trial portfolio is not activated at every site and phase I clinical trials are generally restricted to the main campus. The most successful clinical trials to conduct in the community are those therapeutic trials that focus on improving disease outcomes through the use of new agents or testing approved agents used in different settings. For example, mutations in PIK3A have been associated with worse outcomes in adjuvant therapy trials and in CLEOPATRA [21,40]. A phase III NRG trial builds on the positive results of CLEOPATRA in women with metastatic HER2-positive disease and tests the benefit of adding the immune checkpoint inhibitor, atezolizumab, as first line therapy. A Novartis sponsored trial randomizes women with metastatic disease and a PIK3A mutation to a placebo controlled double blind trial of alpelisib added during the patients' maintenance of trastuzumab and pertuzumab. We are currently enrolling patients with documented HER2-activating mutations to a phase II trial sponsored by PUMA of neratinib, trastuzumab, (and fulvestrant if also ER-positive).

Our radiolabeled trastuzumab imaging studies require a radiopharmacy and expertise by a committed team of radiologists and physicist who interpret the images. Our community oncologists play an important role in these studies by referring patients, thereby allowing us to complete accrual expeditiously. They are authors on our publications and are recognized by their local communities as true experts who participate in innovative research.

8. Optimizing Partnerships

The Breast Disease Team has a number of initiatives to ensure inclusion of our community partners in research, and the weekly Breast Disease Team meeting is at the heart of these collaborations. Discussions at weekly Tumor Boards and a bi-weekly treatment planning meeting frequently highlight on-going studies and identify study candidates. City of Hope is a founding member of the NCCN (national comprehensive cancer network) and has a long history of participating in guideline panels. While some of the guidelines for treating breast cancer are definitive, others offer acceptable treatment options. The breast cancer team on the main campus meets on an annual basis to compile our guideline preferences for treatment, including, not only standard of care but the open studies for clinical trial participation as well (see Table 1).

9. Future Directions

We continue to activate investigator-initiated, cooperative group, and Pharma trials in the community that focus on improving the outcomes for women with metastatic HER2-positive disease. Our imaging research will utilize radiolabeled trastuzumab to predict for response to new agents such as fam-trastuzumab-deruxtecan and tucatinib [24,29]. These studies will rely on our community partners to refer interested patients for study participation.

National Cancer Institute-designated Comprehensive Cancer Centers (NCI-CCC) such as City of Hope strive to provide expert interdisciplinary clinical care and cutting-edge treatments and technologies. Between 1998 and 2008, 6.4% of adults between 22 and 65 years of age who were diagnosed with cancer in Los Angeles County received treatment at an NCI-CCC. For all primary tumor sites, the survival of patients treated at an NCI-CCC was superior to patients treated at a non-NCI-CCC. In this study, 6.5% of the 31,764 breast cancer patients included in the analysis were treated at an NCI-CCC and their survival was superior to those treated at non NCI-CCC sites [41]. Realistically, the majority of cancer patients will receive their care in community sites, and it is an important part of the mission of a Comprehensive Cancer Center to ensure that the standard of care in the community is comparable to the care that is delivered in these large research centers. Clinical research is at the heart of improving quality care.

Author Contributions: Conceptualization and writing, J.E.M., L.K. and Y.Y.; writing, review and editing, M.C., S.L. (Sayeh Lavasani), S.L. (Sariah Liu), N.T.-P., M.S., W.S., D.S., J.W., C.Y. and T.W. All authors have read and agreed to the published version of the manuscript.

Acknowledgments: The authors thank Nicola Welch, CMPP for editorial assistance and critical review of the manuscript.

References

1.   Prat, A.; Pineda, E.; Adamo, B.; Galván, P.; Fernández, A.; Gaba, L.; Díez, M.; Viladot, M.; Arance, A.; Muñoz, M. Clinical implications of the intrinsic molecular subtypes of breast cancer. *Breast* **2015**, *24*, S26–S35. [CrossRef]

2.   Prat, A.; Pascual, T.; Adamo, B. Intrinsic molecular subtypes of HER2+ breast cancer. *Oncotarget* **2017**, *8*, 73362–73363. [CrossRef]

3.   Hayes, D.F. HER2 and Breast Cancer—A Phenomenal Success Story. *N. Engl. J. Med.* **2019**, *381*, 1284–1286. [CrossRef]

4.   Slamon, D.; Clark, G.; Wong, S.; Levin, W.; Ullrich, A.; McGuire, W. Human breast cancer: Correlation of relapse and survival with amplification of the HER-2/neu oncogene. *Science* **1987**, *235*, 177–182. [CrossRef]

5.   Press, M.F.; Pike, M.C.; Chazin, V.R.; Hung, G.; Udove, J.A.; Markowicz, M.; Danyluk, J.; Godolphin, W.; Sliwkowski, M.; Akita, R.; et al. Her-2/*neu* Expression in Node-negative Breast Cancer: Direct Tissue Quantitation by Computerized Image Analysis and Association of Overexpression with Increased Risk of Recurrent Disease. *Cancer Res.* **1993**, *53*, 4960–4970.

6.   Cobleigh, M.A.; Vogel, C.L.; Tripathy, D.; Robert, N.J.; Scholl, S.; Fehrenbacher, L.; Wolter, J.M.; Paton, V.; Shak, S.; Lieberman, G.; et al. Multinational Study of the Efficacy and Safety of Humanized Anti-HER2 Monoclonal Antibody in Women Who Have HER2-Overexpressing Metastatic Breast Cancer That Has Progressed After Chemotherapy for Metastatic Disease. *J. Clin. Oncol.* **1999**, *17*, 2639. [CrossRef]

7.   Vogel, C.; Cobleigh, M.; Tripathy, D.; Harris, L.; Fehrenbacher, L.; Slamon, D.; Ash, M.; Novotny, W.; Stewart, S.; Shak, S. First-line, non-hormonal, treatment of women with HER2 overexpressing metastatic breast cancer with herceptin (trastuzumab, humanised anti-HER2 antibody) [abstract 275]. *Proc. Am. Soc. Clin. Oncol.* **2001**, *20*, 71a.

8.   Slamon, D.J.; Leyland-Jones, B.; Shak, S.; Fuchs, H.; Paton, V.; Bajamonde, A.; Fleming, T.; Eiermann, W.; Wolter, J.; Pegram, M.; et al. Use of Chemotherapy plus a Monoclonal Antibody against HER2 for Metastatic Breast Cancer That Overexpresses HER2. *N. Engl. J. Med.* **2001**, *344*, 783–792. [CrossRef]

9.   Giordano, S.H.; Temin, S.; Chandarlapaty, S.; Crews, J.R.; Esteva, F.J.; Kirshner, J.J.; Krop, I.E.; Levinson, J.; Lin, N.U.; Modi, S.; et al. Systemic Therapy for Patients With Advanced Human Epidermal Growth Factor Receptor 2–Positive Breast Cancer: ASCO Clinical Practice Guideline Update. *J. Clin. Oncol.* **2018**, *36*, 2736–2740. [CrossRef]

10. Wolff, A.C.; Hammond, M.E.H.; Allison, K.H.; Harvey, B.E.; Mangu, P.B.; Bartlett, J.M.S.; Bilous, M.; Ellis, I.O.; Fitzgibbons, P.; Hanna, W.; et al. Human Epidermal Growth Factor Receptor 2 Testing in Breast Cancer: American Society of Clinical Oncology/College of American Pathologists Clinical Practice Guideline Focused Update. *J. Clin. Oncol.* **2018**, *36*, 2105–2122. [CrossRef]

11. Niehans, G.A.; Singleton, T.P.; Dykoski, D.; Kiang, D.T. Stability of HER-2/neu Expression Over Time and at Multiple Metastatic Sites. *J. Natl. Cancer Inst.* **1993**, *85*, 1230–1235. [CrossRef] [PubMed]

12. Bergh, J. Quo Vadis With Targeted Drugs in the 21st Century? *J. Clin. Oncol.* **2009**, *27*, 2–5. [CrossRef] [PubMed]

13. Blancas, I.; Muñoz-Serrano, A.J.; Legerén, M.; Ruiz-Ávila, I.; Jurado, J.M.; Delgado, M.T.; Garrido, J.M.; González Bayo, B.; Rodríguez-Serrano, F. Immunophenotypic Conversion between Primary and Relapse Breast Cancer and its Effects on Survival. *Gynecol. Obstet. Investig.* **2020**, in press. [CrossRef] [PubMed]

14. Fehrenbacher, L.; Cecchini, R.S.; Jr, C.E.G.; Rastogi, P.; Costantino, J.P.; Atkins, J.N.; Crown, J.P.; Polikoff, J.; Boileau, J.-F.; Provencher, L.; et al. NSABP B-47/NRG Oncology Phase III Randomized Trial Comparing Adjuvant Chemotherapy With or Without Trastuzumab in High-Risk Invasive Breast Cancer Negative for HER2 by FISH and With IHC 1+ or 2+. *J. Clin. Oncol.* **2020**, *38*, 444–453. [CrossRef] [PubMed]

15. Mortimer, J.; Conti, P.; Shan, T.; Carroll, M.; Kofi, P.; Colcher, D.; Raubitschek, A.; Bading, J. 64Cu-DOTA-trastuzumab positron emission tomography imaging of HER2 in women with advanced breast cancer. *Cancer Res.* **2012**, *72*, 229s.

16. Mortimer, J.E.; Bading, J.R.; Colcher, D.M.; Conti, P.S.; Frankel, P.H.; Carroll, M.I.; Tong, S.; Poku, E.; Miles, J.K.; Shively, J.E.; et al. Functional Imaging of Human Epidermal Growth Factor Receptor 2–Positive Metastatic Breast Cancer Using 64Cu-DOTA-Trastuzumab PET. *J. Nucl. Med.* **2014**, *55*, 23–29. [CrossRef]

17. Burris, H.A.; Rugo, H.S.; Vukelja, S.J.; Vogel, C.L.; Borson, R.A.; Limentani, S.; Tan-Chiu, E.; Krop, I.E.; Michaelson, R.A. Girish, S.; et al. Phase II Study of the Antibody Drug Conjugate Trastuzumab-DM1 for the Treatment of Human Epidermal Growth Factor Receptor 2 (HER2)–Positive Breast Cancer After Prior HER2-Directed Therapy. *J. Clin. Oncol.* **2011**, *29*, 398–405. [CrossRef]

18. Mortimer, J.E.; Shively, J.E. Functional Imaging of Human Epidermal Growth Factor Receptor 2–Positive Breast Cancers and a Note about NOTA. *J. Nucl. Med.* **2019**, *60*, 23–25. [CrossRef]

19. Barthélémy, P.; Leblanc, J.; Goldbarg, V.; Wendling, F.; Kurtz, J.-E. Pertuzumab: Development Beyond Breast Cancer. *Anticancer Res.* **2014**, *34*, 1483–1491.

20. Baselga, J.; Gelmon, K.A.; Verma, S.; Wardley, A.; Conte, P.; Miles, D.; Bianchi, G.; Cortes, J.; McNally, V.A.; Ross, G.A.; et al. Phase II Trial of Pertuzumab and Trastuzumab in Patients With Human Epidermal Growth Factor Receptor 2–Positive Metastatic Breast Cancer That Progressed During Prior Trastuzumab Therapy. *J. Clin. Oncol.* **2010**, *28*, 1138–1144. [CrossRef]

21. Swain, S.M.; Miles, D.; Kim, S.-B.; Im, Y.-H.; Im, S.-A.; Semiglazov, V.; Ciruelos, E.; Schneeweiss, A.; Loi, S.; Monturus, E.; et al. Pertuzumab, trastuzumab, and docetaxel for HER2-positive metastatic breast cancer (CLEOPATRA): End-of-study results from a double-blind, randomised, placebo-controlled, phase 3 study. *Lancet Oncol.* **2020**, *21*, 519–530. [CrossRef]

22. Swain, S.M.; Baselga, J.; Kim, S.-B.; Ro, J.; Semiglazov, V.; Campone, M.; Ciruelos, E.; Ferrero, J.-M.; Schneeweiss, A.; Heeson, S.; et al. Pertuzumab, Trastuzumab, and Docetaxel in HER2-Positive Metastatic Breast Cancer. *N. Engl. J. Med.* **2015**, *372*, 724–734. [CrossRef]

23. Yan, H.; Yu, K.; Zhang, K.; Liu, L.; Li, Y. Efficacy and safety of trastuzumab emtansine (T-DM1) in the treatment of HER2-positive metastatic breast cancer (MBC): A meta-analysis of randomized controlled trial. *Oncotarget.* **2017**, *8*, 102458. [CrossRef] [PubMed]

24. Modi, S.; Saura, C.; Yamashita, T.; Park, Y.H.; Kim, S.-B.; Tamura, K.; Andre, F.; Iwata, H.; Ito, Y.; Tsurutani, J.; et al. Trastuzumab Deruxtecan in Previously Treated HER2-Positive Breast Cancer. *N. Engl. J. Med.* **2020**, *382*, 610–621. [CrossRef] [PubMed]

25. Ogitani, Y.; Aida, T.; Hagihara, K.; Yamaguchi, J.; Ishii, C.; Harada, N.; Soma, M.; Okamoto, H.; Oitate, M.; Arakawa, S.; et al. DS-8201a, A Novel HER2-Targeting ADC with a Novel DNA Topoisomerase I Inhibitor, Demonstrates a Promising Antitumor Efficacy with Differentiation from T-DM1. *Clin. Cancer Res.* **2016**, *22*, 5097–5108. [CrossRef] [PubMed]

26. Cuadros, M.; Villegas, R. Systematic Review of HER2 Breast Cancer Testing. *Appl. Immunohistochem. Mol. Morphol.* **2009**, *17*, 1–7. [CrossRef] [PubMed]

27. Yau, T.K.; Sze, H.; Soong, I.S.; Hioe, F.; Khoo, U.S.; Lee, A.W.M. HER2 overexpression of breast cancers in Hong Kong: Prevalence and concordance between immunohistochemistry and in-situ hybridisation assays. *Hong Kong Med. J.* **2008**, *14*, 130–135. [PubMed]

28. NCCN. Clinical Practice Guidelines in Oncology: Prostate Cancer (v.3.2011). Available online: http: //www.nccn.org (accessed on 9 June 2011).

29. Murthy, R.K.; Loi, S.; Okines, A.; Paplomata, E.; Hamilton, E.; Hurvitz, S.A.; Lin, N.U.; Borges, V.; Abramson, V.; Anders, C.; et al. Tucatinib, Trastuzumab, and Capecitabine for HER2-Positive Metastatic Breast Cancer. *N. Engl. J. Med.* **2019**, *382*, 597–609. [CrossRef]

30. Network, N.C.C. Breast Version 4. 2020. Available online: https://www.nccn.org/professionals/physician_gls/ pdf/breast.pdf (accessed on 28 April 2020).

31. Lin, N.U.; Borges, V.; Anders, C.; Murthy, R.K.; Paplomata, E.; Hamilton, E.; Hurvitz, S.; Loi, S.; Okines, A.; Abramson, V.; et al. Intracranial Efficacy and Survival With Tucatinib Plus Trastuzumab and Capecitabine for Previously Treated HER2-Positive Breast Cancer With Brain Metastases in the HER2CLIMB Trial. *J. Clin. Oncol.* **2020**, in press. [CrossRef]

32. Geyer, C.E.; Forster, J.; Lindquist, D.; Chan, S.; Romieu, C.G.; Pienkowski, T.; Jagiello-Gruszfeld, A.; Crown, J.; Chan, A.; Kaufman, B.; et al. Lapatinib plus Capecitabine for HER2-Positive Advanced Breast Cancer. *N. Engl. J. Med.* **2006**, *355*, 2733–2743. [CrossRef]

33. Blackwell, K.L.; Burstein, H.J.; Storniolo, A.M.; Rugo, H.S.; Sledge, G.; Aktan, G.; Ellis, C.; Florance, A.; Vukelja, S.; Bischoff, J.; et al. Overall Survival Benefit With Lapatinib in Combination With Trastuzumab for Patients With Human Epidermal Growth Factor Receptor 2–Positive Metastatic Breast Cancer: Final Results From the EGF104900 Study. *J. Clin. Oncol.* **2012**, *30*, 2585–2592. [CrossRef] [PubMed]

34. Nasrazadani, A.; Brufsky, A. Neratinib: The emergence of a new player in the management of HER2+ breast cancer brain metastasis. *Future Oncol.* **2020**, *16*, 247–254. [CrossRef] [PubMed]

35. Tripathy, D.; Slamon, D.J.; Cobleigh, M.; Arnold, A.; Saleh, M.; Mortimer, J.E. Safety of treatment of metastatic breast cancer with trastuzumab beyond disease progression. *J. Clin. Oncol.* **2004**, *22*, 1063–1070. [CrossRef]

36. Bose, R.; Kavuri, S.M.; Searleman, A.C.; Shen, W.; Shen, D.; Koboldt, D.C.; Monsey, J.; Goel, N.; Aronson, A.B.; Li, S.; et al. Activating HER2 Mutations in HER2 Gene Amplification Negative Breast Cancer. *Cancer Discov.* **2013**, *3*, 224–237. [CrossRef]

37. Ma, C.X.; Bose, R.; Gao, F.; Freedman, R.A.; Telli, M.L.; Kimmick, G.; Winer, E.; Naughton, M.; Goetz, M.P.; Russell, C.; et al. Neratinib Efficacy and Circulating Tumor DNA Detection of *HER2* Mutations in *HER2* Nonamplified Metastatic Breast Cancer. *Clin. Cancer Res.* **2017**, *23*, 5687–5695. [CrossRef]

38. Ben-Baruch, N.E.; Bose, R.; Kavuri, S.M.; Ma, C.X.; Ellis, M.J. HER2-Mutated Breast Cancer Responds to Treatment With Single-Agent Neratinib, a Second-Generation HER2/EGFR Tyrosine Kinase Inhibitor. *J. Natl. Compr. Cancer Netw.* **2015**, *13*, 1061–1064. [CrossRef]

39. Hyman, D.M.; Piha-Paul, S.A.; Won, H.; Rodon, J.; Saura, C.; Shapiro, G.I.; Juric, D.; Quinn, D.I.; Moreno, V.; Doger, B.; et al. HER kinase inhibition in patients with HER2- and HER3-mutant cancers. *Nature* **2018**, *554*, 189–194. [CrossRef] [PubMed]

40. Pogue-Geile, K.L.; Kim, C.; Jeong, J.-H.; Tanaka, N.; Bandos, H.; Gavin, P.G.; Fumagalli, D.; Goldstein, L.C.; Sneige, N.; Burandt, E.; et al. Predicting Degree of Benefit From Adjuvant Trastuzumab in NSABP Trial B-31. *J. Natl. Cancer Inst.* **2013**, *105*, 1782–1788. [CrossRef]

41. Wolfson, J.A.; Sun, C.-L.; Wyatt, L.P.; Hurria, A.; Bhatia, S. Impact of care at comprehensive cancer centers on outcome: Results from a population-based study. *Cancer* **2015**, *121*, 3885–3893. [CrossRef] [PubMed]

11

Bioengineered Skin Substitutes: The Role of Extracellular Matrix and Vascularization in the Healing of Deep Wounds

Francesco Urciuolo [1,2,*, Costantino Casale [1], Giorgia Imparato [3] and Paolo A. Netti [1,2,3]**

[1]   Department of Chemical, Materials and Industrial Production Engineering (DICMAPI) University of Naples Federico II, P.le Tecchio 80, 80125 Naples, Italy; costantino.casale@unina.it (C.C.); nettipa@unina.it (P.A.N.)
[2]   Interdisciplinary Research Centre on Biomaterials (CRIB), University of Naples Federico II P.le Tecchio 80, 80125 Naples, Italy
[3]   Center for Advanced Biomaterials for HealthCare@CRIB, Istituto Italiano di Tecnologia, Largo Barsanti e Matteucci 53, 80125 Naples, Italy; giorgia.imparato@iit.it
*   Correspondence: urciuolo@unina.it

Abstract: The formation of severe scars still represents the result of the closure process of extended and deep skin wounds. To address this issue, different bioengineered skin substitutes have been developed but a general consensus regarding their effectiveness has not been achieved yet. It will be shown that bioengineered skin substitutes, although representing a valid alternative to autografting, induce skin cells in repairing the wound rather than guiding a regeneration process. Repaired skin differs from regenerated skin, showing high contracture, loss of sensitivity, impaired pigmentation and absence of cutaneous adnexa (i.e., hair follicles and sweat glands). This leads to significant mobility and aesthetic concerns, making the development of more effective bioengineered skin models a current need. The objective of this review is to determine the limitations of either commercially available or investigational bioengineered skin substitutes and how advanced skin tissue engineering strategies can be improved in order to completely restore skin functions after severe wounds.

Keywords: skin substitutes; tissue engineering; wound healing; extracellular matrix; bottom-up tissue engineering; vascularization; bioreactors; dermal substitutes; scar tissue

---

1. Introduction

The skin is the largest organ of the body, accounting for about 15% of the total adult body weight. It is made up of three layers: the epidermis, dermis, and the hypodermis (Figure 1, [1]). Bioengineered skin substitutes, in the form of either cellularized engineered skin grafts or acellular dermal regeneration templates (DRT), have been developed to address two main issues still affecting the repair of extended deep wounds [2–10]: firstly, limiting the amount of healthy skin removed from the patient needed for closure; and secondly, acting as promoter for the restoration of the physiologic conditions of the skin avoiding the formation of severe scars. Skin acts not only as a barrier between the organism and the environment preventing invasion of pathogens and fending off chemical and physical assaults [11], it also plays a crucial role in the regulation of body temperature, moisture, and trafficking of water and solutes [12]. In addition, the sensory system of the skin allows the sensing of pain, temperature, light touch, discriminative touch, vibration and pressure. Finally, other important adnexal structures, such as sweat glands and hair follicles, contribute to the functionality of the healthy skin. In addition to the epidermis, severe damage due to burns, chronic ulcers and reconstructive surgeries, induce the destruction of the dermis. Unlike the epidermis, the dermis is characterized by an impaired healing process in which the final assembly of the extracellular matrix (ECM) is far from physiologic conditions.

This mismatch compromises the reestablishment of the aforementioned regulatory functions of the whole organ [13–15]. The components of the ECM of the dermis (collagen elastin, hyaluronic acid, fibronectin, perlacan, water and other molecules), possess specific three-dimensional arrangements of sequences orchestrating the cross-talk among the different cell populations comprising the skin. Ultimately, such cross-talk affects the attachment, migration, differentiation and morphogenetic phenomena. For instance, the ECM promotes 'appropriate' communications between keratinocytes and the fibroblasts, and it is responsible for the formation and maintenance of the adnexal structures such as hair follicles, sweat glands and innervations [16–18]. Furthermore, when such adnexal structures become compromised, the self-regeneration of the epidermis cannot occur, and the wound becomes hard to heal. The repair of a deep wound can be divided into four subsequent phases [19,20]: (i) the coagulation and homeostasis phase (immediately after injury); (ii) the inflammatory phase (shortly after injury to tissue), during which swelling takes place; (iii) the proliferation period, where new tissues and blood vessels are formed; and (iv) the maturation phase, in which remodeling of new tissues takes place. How the maturation phase takes place determines the difference between repair and regeneration. The former is a "mere" closure process where fibroblasts bridge the wound gap by organizing their ECM differently from the healthy status. The latter restores the organization of the ECM that will appear indistinguishable from the healthy status [21]. The impaired ECM organization featuring the repair process depresses the regulatory and repository role of the extracellular space that ultimately forms an extended scar characterized by the loss of biological functionalities, inducing the insurgence of severe aesthetics and mobility-associated concerns. A classical approach to skin grafting and repairing is depicted in Figure 2. After debridement of the wound bed, a DRT is applied. Fibroblasts and endothelial cells from the recipient take at least one month to invade the DRT. After this time, it is possible to apply a split thickness skin graft (STSG): an epidermis with a layer of dermis removed from healthy sites of the patient. Both vascularization and fibroblast-secreted ECM molecules affect the take of the STSG that serves to trigger the regeneration of the epidermis due to the lack of adnexa and basal lamina [22–26]. As shown in Figure 2, with a period of two years, the remodeling of the neodermis occurs. To date, even though progress in biomaterials science and tissue engineering has led to the realization of different classes of skin substitutes (either cellularized or not), their healing potential is still limited in triggering a repair process instead of regeneration. In addition to economics, safety and regulatory (in case of allogenic or xenogeneic materials) concerns, in this work the currently available skin substitutes will be reviewed in the light of the composition of the dermis compartment and how this can affect the regeneration process. DRT can be fabricated starting from connective tissues of either allogenic or xenogeneic origin after removal of the cellular component [27,28]. The decellularization processes remove the associated risk of transmission of pathogens, preserving the composition of the ECM. On the other hand, the functionality of molecules of the ECM resulting from the decellularization processes compromise the correct signal presentation to the cells [16–18]. Pre-cellularization with endothelial cells, fibroblasts and keratinocytes seems to improve the biological performance of reconstructed three-dimensional matrices of both natural or synthetic origins [2,27,29–31], by speeding up the vascularization, the synthesis of neodermis, the take of the STSG and the closure of the wounds [32–34]. Nevertheless, the reconstructed three-dimensional matrices used to accommodate living cells prior to the implant are composed of exogenous biomatrices that possess composition, stiffness and three-dimensional arrangements that are quite different from the native dermis. For this reason, some doubts on their effectiveness in triggering a regeneration process have been raised [17]. Finally, a tissue engineering strategy that use patients' own cells to build up in vitro a human-like vascularized ECM featured by the absence of any exogenous material, is presented as an alternative to guide the wound toward a physiological regeneration process [35–37].

2. Tissue Engineering Strategies for Skin Regeneration

Tissue engineering aims at developing strategies to allow tissue and organ regeneration [32] by two approaches: (i) In in vitro tissue engineering the patient's human skin is re-built in a laboratory using either endogenous or allogenic cell lines (keratinocytes and fibroblasts); after a period of cultivation in three-dimensional matrices [24] and bioreactors [10,38], the engineered skin is then implanted [32]; (ii) in in vivo tissue engineering a three-dimensional matrix is introduced in the wound bed; such matrices are bio-functionalized in order to attract both cells and growth factors supporting skin regeneration [38]. The use of de novo fabricated skin becomes necessary when skin self-regeneration is hindered by adverse conditions [10]; in particular, when severe burns (second-, third-, and fourth-degree burns), chronic ulcers, surgery or trauma lead to the destruction of the dermis and underlying tissues (fat, muscle or bone) are exposed [39,40]. Bioengineered skin substitutes can be classified according to the following categories.

- Cellularized epithelial tissues: used for superficial wounds, when the dermis is not (or is partially) damaged; autologous, allogenic or xenogeneic epithelial tissues are cultured in vitro and then implanted. In this case, the application of an STSG is not required. Engineered epithelial tissues are in general formed by cell sheets two or three cell layers thick [41,42].
- Cellularized dermis: when the dermis is damaged, autologous or allogenic fibroblasts are embedded in a three-dimensional matrix and then implanted in the wound bed. This procedure implies a second surgical step for the application of an epithelial layer using an STSG as shown in Figure 2 [41,42].
- Cellularized composite skin (or full thickness): engineered tissues containing both epithelial and dermal tissues. They are composed of epithelial tissue grown on a dermis surrogate composed of fibroblasts entrapped in a biomaterial [4,41–43]. Due to the presence of an epidermis layer, the application of an STSG can be avoided.
- Acellular dermal substitutes: or derma regeneration templates (DRT) that are porous 3D biomaterials (non-containing cells) applied in the missing dermis after wound debridement. This procedure implies a second surgical step for the application of an epithelial layer coming from an STSG, as shown in Figure 2 [4,41–43].

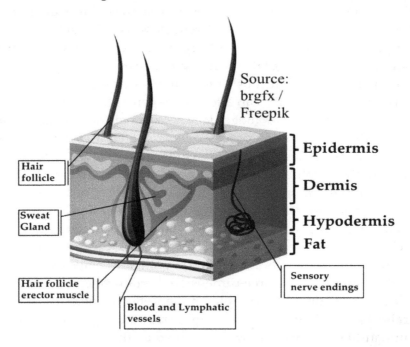

Figure 1. Main components of the human skin. (Image source: brgfx/Freepik).

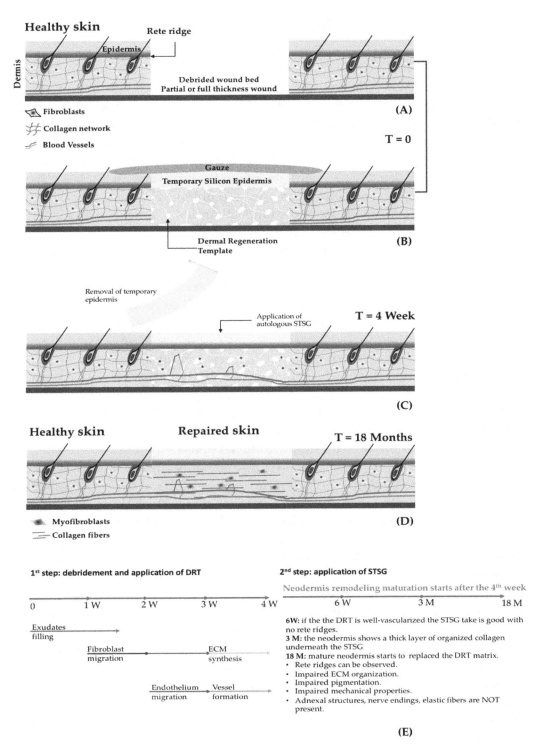

Figure 2. The main steps of a two-step procedure to treat deep and partial wounds with the application of a DRT. (**A**) Healthy skin and wound bed after debridement. (**B**) Application of a DRT possessing an artificial silicone epidermis and covered with gauze. (**C**) Removal of the silicone epidermis and application of the STSG. (**D**) Long-term appearance of the repaired dermis. (**E**) Cellular end extracellular dynamics occurring during the wound healing process after the application of a DRT. W = week; M = month. DRT, dermal regeneration templates; STSG, split thickness skin graft; ECM, extracellular matrix.

2.1. Dermal Regeneration Templates (DRT): Materials and Fabrication Techniques

Porous and fibrous materials. Regardless of the tissue engineering strategy used (in vitro vs. in vivo approaches), a 3D scaffold supporting cell growth is required [42]. Scaffolds are biomaterials acting as temporary porous structures mimicking the 3D architecture of human tissue. In the case of skin tissue engineering, the tissue that one would like to mimic is the dermis. The scaffolds mimicking the dermis can be made by either natural or synthetic polymers (or a combination of both) and, regardless of their origin, they must have different characteristics: non-immunogenic; biocompatible; be able to resist the activity of proteolytic enzymes; stiff and flexible in order to withstand surgical procedures; be able to control the wound contracture; and to possess a degradation rate synchronous with the neo-dermis ingrowth and assembling. Furthermore, the scaffold should support epidermis attachment, maintenance and stratification, and it should promote the blood vessels' influx when implanted [23,34,42]. Three-dimensional porous structures can be obtained by different fabrication techniques allowing the production of different 3D architectures. Starting from melt polymers or polymer solutions, the use of porogen agents, or phase separation techniques, allows the production of sponge-like structures with interconnected pores and porosity ranging from 50 to 500 μm [44]. When porogens are used, the final mechanical properties of the scaffold can be modulated by varying the polymer concentration, the volume fraction and the dimension of the porogens. Phase separation technique exploits the thermodynamic instability of either polymeric solutions or blends [42]. The instability can be induced physically (i.e., temperature) or chemically (i.e., introduction of a solvent/non-solvent agent). The thermodynamic instability induces a segregation process with the formation of a dispersed and a continuum phase. The dispersed phase forms globular structures and after its removal porosity is created. The parameters affecting the final properties of the scaffold (mechanical properties, porosity, pore diameter and pore interconnection) are the initial composition of the polymer solution and, in the case of thermally induced phase separation, the cooling/heating rate is used to induce the thermodynamic instability. Woven and non-woven assembly of nano-fibers using electrospinning allows the production of porous structures categorized as fibrillar scaffolds [30,45,46]. Nanofibrous materials can be also produced by means of different techniques such as self-assembly, phase separation, fiber bonding and electrospinning. This kind of structure is able to mimic better the fibrous nature of the natural extracellular matrix. In in vitro tissue engineering, such preformed structures (either porous or fibrous) are colonized by the cells after the preparation, since their fabrication techniques represent severe conditions for cell viability. This could represent a limitation because a homogenous cell seeding through the thickness of the scaffolds is difficult to achieve and sophisticated bioreactors need to be used [38,47–49]. Hydrogels represent another class of fibrous scaffolds. These are highly hydrated 3D structures obtained by physical, ionic or covalent cross-linking of different polymers of both natural or synthetic origins [49–52]. Three-dimensional hydrogels can be obtained by the assembly and crosslinking of a liquid monomeric phase. This represents an advantage because the monomeric solution can be mixed with the cell suspension. At the end of the gelling process, cells remain entrapped in the 3D structures obtaining a homogenous cellularization of the final 3D scaffold. Although the final properties can be modulated by different parameters (monomer concentration, temperature, pH, UV radiation, ionic strength) the presence of cells poses the same constraints on the control of the final mechanical properties. For instance, UV radiation, pH, temperature and other methods used to induce cross-link of polymeric networks may affect cell viability. Hydrogel are, in general, considered soft materials. Hydrogels composed of gelatin–chitosan hydrogels [53], fibronectin–hyaluronan, or dextran-based hydrogels, in combination with nano-fibrous poly lactic-co-glycolic acid (PLGA) scaffolds have been extensively used for wound healing and regeneration applications [54–56]. In particular, dextran-based hydrogels demonstrated efficient vascularization. Composite hydrogels formed by glycosaminoglycan (GAG)–collagen showed good wound healing in rabbit models [56]. Self-assembling peptide-based hydrogel scaffolds have been reported to reduce burn wound healing time and skin cell proliferation [56].

Protein-based naturals biomaterials. Biomaterials of protein nature can be realized using (but not limited to) collagen, gelatin, silk and fibrinogen. Collagen is the most abundant structural protein of the human dermis secreted by fibroblasts, and is responsible for tensile stiffness. Collagen in skin tissue engineering is used as both acellular scaffold or cell-populated scaffold [56]. Collagen for tissue engineering application is extracted from animals: bovine, ovine and avian are the mostly exploited sources. Examples of acellular/porous scaffolds are the commercially available dermis substitutes Alloderm® or Integra®, while examples of cell-populated collagen hydrogels are represented by Apligraft® and Transcyte®. In addition, collagen-based biomaterials have been processed in the form of membranes, sponges, composite sponges and electrospun biomaterials with nanometric features [56]. Gelatin is a protein obtained by collagen denaturation possessing higher advantages in terms of cell adhesion and inducing a reduced immunogenic response. In the treatment of wounds and burns, gelatin has been used as electrospun nanofibers [57], membranes [58] and gelatin sponges loaded with growth factors [59]. Silk fibroin in the form of sponges, nanofibers and porous films have shown decreased inflammatory response, and promising results in wound healing and skin regeneration has been reported [60].

Polysaccharide-based biomaterials. Polysaccharide-based biomaterials are mainly used in the form of hydrogels. Those mostly used in skin regeneration and wound healing are dextran [54], cellulose [26], chitosan [61], alginate [62] and hyaluronic acid (HA) [63–65]. Among these, HA has been extensively used in skin regeneration leading to the commercialization of different skin substitutes, such as Hyaff®, Laserskin® and Hyalograft®.

Synthetic and composite biomaterials. Synthetic biomaterials comprise [30] the class of aliphatic polyesters, such as polylactic acid (PLA), polyglycolic (PGA) and polycaprolactone (PCL). They possess controllable mechanical stiffness and high process flexibility and are biocompatible and nontoxic. Moreover, PLA, PGA, PCL, and their blends and copolymers are FDA approved. An example of a commercially available skin substitute made using such materials is Dermagraft®.

Decellularized matrices. To date, no biomaterials yet exist that are able to mimic the composition of the native extracellular matrix as a whole [16–18]. Decellularized matrices of allogenic or xenogeneic origin should bridge such a gap. This is very important in skin regeneration because the lack of a functional extracellular matrix is the main cause affecting the impaired wound healing process. Currently available decellularized biomaterials comprise decellularized mesothelium, intestine, amniotic membrane, dermis and skin flaps [9]. Allogenic dermis can be obtained by treating fresh dermis from a cadaver with Dispase–Triton X-100 or NaCl–sodium dodecyl sulfate (SDS). In this way, collagen bundles and basement membranes retain their structure. The abstained biomaterial is further lyophilized. An FDA-approved decellularized dermis obtained with such a technique is Alloderm® [9]. Its use in combination with split-thickness autologous skin grafts allows complete cellularization of skin defects after 12 weeks post application when applied to full-thickness or partial-thickness burn wounds, thereby reducing subsequent scarring [65]. Other acellular dermal matrices are of porcine origin (e.g., Permacol®) and the decellularization process is similar to that of Alloderm®. Different techniques use a foaming process in order to destroy the cellular component, as well as any immunogenic agent. On the other hand, foaming compromises extracellular matrix structure and functions. In general, this kind of decellularized dermis is similar to porous scaffolds and is used for hemostatic applications. Other kinds of decellularized matrices are derived from the mesothelium, including peritoneum, pleura and pericardium [27,66,67]. Decellularized peritoneum is obtained using detergent agents and the processes are designed to maximize the preservation of the extracellular matrix architecture and composition. Because growth factors have a limited shelf life, such biomaterials are often combined with fibroblast growth factor (FGF) and epidermal growth factor (EGF) to promote wound repair. Decellularized mesothelium of porcine origin is used, for instance, in breast reconstruction. Bovine sources are another font of decellularized mesothelium showing a faster healing process than that observed for other decellularized dermis substitutes such as Alloderm® [27]. The intestine is another source to obtain decellularized extracellular matrices.

Interestingly, many cytokines and growth factors (FGF and TGF-β families) are retained after the decellularization process. Different applications have been reported comprising the reconstruction of cornea, urethra, vagina, and lung. In the case of dermis reconstruction, decellularized intestine and, in particular, the decellularized small intestine submucosa, is a very promising scaffold due to its capability in promoting angiogenesis. OaSIS® and SurgySIS® (Cook Surgical, Bloomington, IN, USA) are two decellularized matrices from small intestine submucosa [9,68]. The human amniotic membrane is rich in basement membrane and avascular stromal matrix. Decellularization can be obtained using ethylenediaminetetraacetic acid (EDTA) and aprotinin, SDS, DNAase and RNAase. Nevertheless, such a process induces the reduction of anti-inflammatory and anti-scarring components by reducing their superiority compared to other matrices. Clinical applications can be found in the reconstruction of the ocular surface, while different studies have been performed on skin reconstruction in nude mice models [27].

2.2. Tissue Engineering Strategies

2.2.1. Traditional Tissue Engineering

Tissue engineering aims at producing functional and living human tissue in vitro that can be implanted to restore and to replace damaged tissues and organs [32], or can be used in vitro as living testing platforms [68]. The classical approach involves the extraction of cells from humans (primary cells or stem cells), their expansion and seeding in a biomaterial [32], followed by a dynamic culture to promote the neo tissue growth [10,38,47,49]. After cell expansion, the skin tissue engineering process involves at least three steps. (i) Fibroblasts are seeded in a biomaterial; this cellular construct acts as a dermis surrogate where the scaffold represents the temporary extracellular matrix of the fibroblast. (ii) After a variable culture period (two weeks–one month), to allow fibroblast attachment and production of endogenous extracellular matrix components, keratinocytes are seeded on the top of the engineered dermis and kept in submerged culture. (iii) After approximately two weeks, the culture conditions are switched from submerged to air liquid interface (ALI) in order to promote the stratification of the epidermis with the formation of the stratum corneum [2,69]. Such full-thickness engineered skin can be eventually implanted, but different requirements need to be satisfied [70]. The engineered skin must be safe for the patient because any cultured cell material possesses an associated risk of contamination, and viral or bacterial infection. Moreover, in the case of allogenic or xenogeneic cells and materials, there is also an associated risk of rejection. The tissue engineered skin should be effective in providing real benefit for the patient: it should attach correctly to the wound area, it should undergo normal healing limiting or discouraging the formation of a scar, and it should restore the correct pigmentation and barrier functions. Then, it should support the vascular network ingrowth [2,24] with subsequent development of other structures useful for the normal life of the patient: innervation should be promoted in order to restore the sensing properties [71] and the growth of both hair follicles and sweat glands [72]. Finally, tissue engineered skin should be cost-effective in order to achieve a concrete clinical uptake. One of the strengths of the tissue engineering approach is the possibility to have fine control over the properties of the final tissue. Indeed, by modulating the initial properties of the scaffold used to accommodate human fibroblasts and optimizing the culture conditions (culture media composition, mechanical stimulation, hydrodynamic stimulation) it is possible to obtain engineered skin with desired properties [10,38,47–49,70]. It has been demonstrated that uniaxial and biaxial stretch can induce the alignment of the de novo synthesized collagen network [73]. Furthermore, by engineering either the stiffness or the porosity of the scaffold, it is possible to control the assembly of the de novo synthesized extracellular matrix [74]. This allows, for instance, to match the final properties of the engineered skin with the properties of the patient's skin in order to lower the structural and functional differences between the restored zone and the surrounding skin [13,21,43,75–78].

2.2.2. Modular Tissue Engineering: Building a Tissue from the Bottom Up

Modular tissue engineering strategy applies the concept of tissue engineering but at a sub-millimeter scale. Cells are arranged in 3D architectures in the form of micromodules or micro tissues, or building blocks having at least one dimension ranging from 50 to 200 μm. Such micrometric tissues can be either scaffold-free or scaffold-based, and they act as building blocks for the fabrication of larger structures [78]. Scaffold-free microtissues can be obtained by organizing cells in sheets [79] (with a thickness ranging from 50 to 100 μm) or spheres [80,81] (diameters up to 200 μm). Scaffold-based microtissues are obtained by entrapping cells in micrometric scaffolds, such as porous microspheres [81], non-porous microspheres [82–85], non-spherical microparticles [78] or wires of hydrogels [84]. Sheets of human fibroblast are obtained by culturing fibroblasts in flat dishes and promoting the synthesis of the extracellular matrix. When the sheets achieve confluency, they are detached from the culture dishes and, by stacking different sheets of cells, a thicker tissue can be obtained [85]. When placed in close proximity, cell–cell contacts and extracellular matrix–extracellular matrix contacts lead to the formation of continuum structures made by fibroblasts embedded in their own extracellular matrix. One of the limitations of this technique is represented by the high cell density. This induces the formation of a dermis equivalent featuring a cell: ECM ratio higher than that found in the human dermis. The presence of high traction forces exerted by fibroblasts on the immature collagen fibers induces the formation of a highly packed ECM. Moreover, the over-expressed cell density increases the metabolic request. For these reasons, the cell-sheets are often characterized by a very low thickness and by the presence of a necrotic core. The detachment of the cell sheets from the culture plate and the subsequent stacking procedures represent other issues [86–88]. The fabrication of centimeter-sized tissues can be obtained by casting spherical microtissues in molds having any shape and dimensions [83]. Fibroblasts can be entrapped in both spherical and non-spherical hydrogels under continuous conditions using microfluidic devices [89,90]. Dermal microtissues obtained using this approach have been successfully used to build up large pieces of living dermis in vitro. In this direction, fibroblasts laden hydrogel has been used as a building block to fabricate a doll-shaped dermis equivalent [83]. In this study, the possibility of building up a centimeter-sized piece of dermis was demonstrated, but the final tissue underwent sever contracture. Since fibroblasts were imbedded in collagen hydrogel, the lack of a mature cell-synthesized extracellular matrix capable of withstanding the traction force of fibroblasts caused the shrinking of the final tissue. Finally, the presence of an exogenous collagen did not guarantee the complete replication of the native extracellular microenvironment [83]. To reduce the presence of exogenous matrices and promote the synthesis and the assembly of an endogenous dermal microenvironment, human fibroblasts have been seeded in porous gelatin microspheres kept in suspension cultures [89]. Under optimized culture conditions, fibroblasts were able to produce and assemble their extracellular matrix in the inner pores of the microspheres. The microspheres were designed in order to degrade during the extracellular matrix assembly process so the final microtissue was a sort of a sub-millimeter-sized "ball of human dermis", named Dermal-μTissue (Figure 3), composed of fibroblasts and fibroblast-assembled-collagen, elastin and hyaluronic acid [83,91,92]. Dermal-μTissues, having an average diameter of about 200 μm, have been cast in centimeter-sized molds in order to promote biological sintering. The molds containing the Dermal-μTissues have been inserted in bioreactors working under engineered fluid dynamic regimes, which have been developed to improve mass transport during the assembly of the Dermal-μTissue [91,92]. In these works, shear stress and optimized fluid velocity fields were used to guide the correct assembly of the de novo synthetized ECM [92,93]. Moreover, the final dermis equivalent was completely formed by a fibroblast assembled extracellular matrix, leading to the fabrication of skin substitutes with superior functionalities compared to the engineered skin composed of exogenous ECM. For instance, when cultured in vitro in the presence of human keratinocytes and dorsal root ganglion cells, the first spontaneous formation of follicle-like structures in vitro [72] and functional innervation [35] were observed. Finally, tissue wire technology can be used to produce living fibers treated as textile and woven fibers [84]. These modular approaches lead to several advantages, such as fine control over the final architecture, control over the final shape, and control over the spatial organization of engineered biologic structures [79–87,92,93].

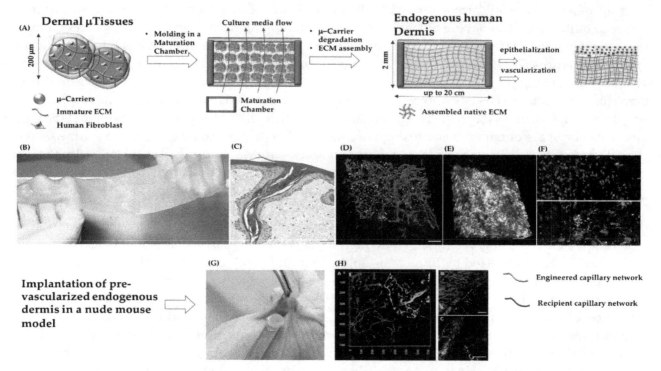

Figure 3. The main steps for the production of a DRT composed of fibroblast-assembled/pre-vascularized human dermis substitutes, and its morphological features before and after implantation in a nude mice model. (**A**) From left to right: production of Dermal-µTissues; their molding and assembly in a maturation chamber that is kept under dynamic culture conditions; formation of a continuum of fibroblasts embedded in their own dermal extracellular matrix; epithelization and vascularization of the endogenous human dermis. (**B**) Fabrication of large pieces of endogenous human dermis (major dimension 20 cm). (**C**) Histology of the endogenous human dermis supporting the differentiation of epidermis with the formation of spontaneous rete ridge profile. (**D**) Vascularized endogenous human dermis: cell nuclei in green and capillary network in red. (**E**) Vascularized endogenous human dermis: fibroblast-assembled collagen bundles observed under label-free multiphoton microscopy in gray; capillary network in red. (**F**) Top: fibroblast-assembled hyaluronic acid in green, cell nuclei in blue; Bottom: fibroblast-assembled elastin network in yellow, cell nuclei in blue. (**G**) Implantation of a piece of the pre-vascularized endogenous human dermis. (**H**) Connection between engineered capillary network (green) and recipient capillary network (red); fibroblast-assembled collagen in gray. Figure 3B, 3D, 3E, 3G, and 3H are from reference [34] "Mazio, C. et al. Pre-vascularized dermis model for fast and functional anastomosis with host vasculature. Biomat. 192, 159–170 (2019)".

Three-Dimensional Bio-Printing

Three-dimensional bio-printing [94] techniques are used to achieve correct positioning of different cell types. The aim is the fabrication of intricate biologic architectures with high spatial resolution in a standardized manner [82,95–97]. Moreover, the obtainment of a full-thickness human skin equivalent takes at least four weeks, representing an issue in the case of production of autologous skin engineering grafts that should be implanted in a shorter time frame. The positioning of different cell strata in their final configuration could reduce the time required for the development of the full-thickness graft. Other advantages of 3D printing techniques are represented by the possibility of printing a vascular network and its insertion in its final configuration in important adnexal structures such as the hair follicle precursors [97–100]. This should represent a plus in the case of deep skin damage where neither innervation nor hair follicle development during the healing process has been observed [20]. Finally, the use of 3D printing techniques aims at reducing the batch-to-batch variability by providing a standardized and controlled process. By precisely locating different matrix materials, growth factors, and different cells in a layer-by-layer assembly, functional living skin tissues would be fabricated possessing designed and personalized structures with neither size nor shape limitations, in a high throughput, and in a highly reproducible manner. In general, the equipment used to print skin tissues consists of independently controlled cell-dispensing channels. Electromechanical valves operate the dispenser, which is positioned on a three-axis robotic stage possessing high spatial resolution (below 50 μm). The dispenser can deliver pre-hydrogel solutions containing cells. Once delivered, the hydrogel solution solidifies via chemical or physical routes. According to this strategy, fibroblasts embedded in rat tail collagen have been printed layer-by-layer, forming a dermis surrogate upon which keratinocytes have been deposited in order to form the epidermal layer [101]. In this study, it was demonstrated that a 3D dermis can be formed in an automated and controlled fashion by printing nanoliter droplets of collagen containing living cells [95,99]. A printed skin equivalent can be obtained using fibrin hydrogels as bio-ink containing cells [95,100]. It was demonstrated that a dermis equivalent as large as 100 cm^2 could be obtained in less than 35 minutes. After this time, a layer of keratinocytes was printed on the top of the dermis equivalent and, after confluency was obtained (24 h), the bilayer engineered skin was implanted in immunodeficient mouse. After implantation, the dermis was able to integrate with the recipient tissue and the epidermis was able to differentiate until forming the stratum corneum. Nevertheless, the dermal–epidermal interface did not present the physiological rete ridge profile. Finally, techniques for the printing of a microvasculature network have been assessed. Endothelial cells can be inserted in fibrinogen solution and printed in a gelling bath according to a prescribed 3D architecture. Together with the vascular network, a hydrogel solution containing fibroblasts can be printed by means of an independent dispenser in order to obtain a more complex dermis formed by a connective tissue equivalent containing a 3D designed microvasculature [102].

3. Commercially Available Skin Substitutes

3.1. Acellular Dermal Substitutes

The most used commercially available acellular dermal substitutes (Table 1) are composed of natural extracellular matrix components and can be divided in two categories: decellularized extracellular matrices and reconstructed extracellular matrices. The first category is formed by natural connective tissues (dermis, mesothelium, intestine) deprived of any cellular components and allergenic/immunogenic agents.

The most used commercially available decellularized matrices (Table 1) for the treatment of deep wounds after burns and trauma, or for reconstruction and treatment of diabetic/venous/pressure ulcers are (but not limited to): Alloderm®, Dermacell®, Dermamatrix®, SureDerm®, OASIS®, Permacoll® and EZ-DERM®. Alloderm®, Dermacell®, Dermamatrix® and SureDerm®, are decellularized cadaveric dermis, non-cross-linked, that can be incorporated into the wound bed [4,6–9,40,42,103,104]. In general, such systems retain the basement membrane after the decellularization process but lack an epidermal layer. The acellular matrix provides a good natural 3D environment for fibroblasts and endothelial cells influx in order to promote the formation of a new extracellular matrix and vascular network. OASIS®, Permacoll® and EZ-DERM® are decellularized matrices of porcine origins. OASIS® is obtained using similar processing methods to those of human derived matrices but start from porcine small intestine submucosa. Permacoll® and EZ-DERM® are decellularized porcine dermis that are further cross-linked. Alloderm® was approved and considered as banked human tissue by the FDA; it has been used to treat burns since 1992 and has also been used to treat severe soft tissue defects [105]. This product has been shown to have good graft take rates and to reduce subsequent scarring of full-thickness wounds, even though the graft take of split-skin grafts in a one-step procedure is low. Alloderm® is considered medically necessary in post-mastectomy breast reconstructive surgery for at least one of the following indications: there is insufficient tissue expander or implant coverage by the pectoralis major muscle and additional coverage is required; there are thin post-mastectomy skin flaps that are at risk of dehiscence or necrosis; or the infra-mammary fold and lateral mammary folds have been undermined during mastectomy and re-establishment of these landmarks is needed [39]. By retrieving information form the websites of Dermacell® and Dermamatrix®, it is possible to note that they are intended for soft tissue reconstruction (face defects, nasal reconstruction, abdomen, etc.) and for breast reconstruction. Moreover, different clinical trials involving Dermacell® and Dermamatrix® can be retrieved by consulting the database of clinicaltrials.gov. SureDerm® is indicated by the manufacturer as suitable for gingival and root reconstruction. EZ-DERM® is a porcine-derived xenograft in which the collagen has been chemically cross-linked with aldehyde in order to provide strength and durability [106]; it has FDA 510(k) approval for the treatment of partial-thickness burns and venous, diabetic, and pressure ulcers. In a randomized study involving 157 patients affected by partial-thickness burns, it was found to have satisfactory results: non-correct positioning = 1.5%, infection = 3.0%, incomplete epithelialization at time of separation = 2.2%, need for additional excision and grafting = 4.5%, and hypertrophic scaring = 3.3% [106]. OASIS® Wound Matrix and OASIS® Ultra Tri-Layer Matrix are considered medically necessary for treatment of chronic, noninfected, partial- or full-thickness lower-extremity vascular ulcers, which have not adequately responded following a one-month period of conventional ulcer therapy. They are regulated by the FDA as a Class II (moderate risk) device and received FDA 510(k) approval (K061711), on 19 July, 2006 [39]. OASIS® Wound Matrix was subjected to a randomized controlled study in 120 patients with chronic venous leg ulcers. Significantly more wounds (55% vs. 34%) were observed to be healed in comparison with conventional therapy [67].

Using other routes, the production of acellular dermis is obtained in vitro using the main constituents of the connective tissues (collagen, elastin, glycosaminoglycan, etc.) which are extracted from animals and then reconstructed. Once extracted and purified, the extracellular matrix components can be eventually combined together and processed to form 3D porous structures according to the techniques discussed in Section 2.1 (e.g., cross-linking, lyophilization and electrospinning). In the class of reconstructed extracellular matrices (Table 1), we find: Integra®, Biobrane®, Matriderm® and Hyalomatrix®. Integra® Dermal Regeneration Template consists of a bi-layered extracellular matrix of fibers of cross-linked bovine collagen and chondroitin-6-sulfate (a component of cartilage) with a silicone membrane as transient epithelium. Once the neodermis is formed, the disposable silicone sheet is removed, and an ultrathin autograft is placed over the neodermis [9,20,26]. Integra® Dermal Regeneration Template is considered medically necessary in the post-excisional treatment of severe burns when autografting is not feasible. It has an FDA PMA for treatment of life-threatening, full-thickness or deep partial-thickness thermal injuries where sufficient autograft is not available at the time of excision or not desirable due to the physiologic condition of the individual [39]. This product also has an FDA PMA for repair scar contractures. An issue affecting this kind of skin substitute is the time required for neovascularization. Indeed, when the dermis bed is not well vascularized, or it takes a long time to achieve vascularization, the take of the STSG is compromised. Matriderm® becomes vascularized faster than Integra®, supporting the take of a split-skin graft in a one-step procedure. This is due to the presence of elastin in the Matriderm® model, which is able to attract more vascular cells than the chondroitin-6-sulphate present in Integra®. Biobrane® is an acellular dermal matrix composed of bovine type 1 collagen, silicone and nylon, and mechanically bonded to a flexible knitted nylon fabric. The semipermeable membrane is comparable to human epidermis and controls the loss of water vapor, allows for drainage of exudates, and provides permeability to topical antibiotics. The nylon/silicone membrane provides a flexible adherent covering for the wound surface [2,6,9,10,31,39,41,57,61,67,76,99,107,108]. Biobrane® holds an FDA 510(k) approval for the treatment of clean partial-thickness burn wounds and donor site wounds. It is considered medically necessary [39] for the treatment of burn wounds when all of the following criteria are met: the treatment is specific to non-infected partial-thickness burn wounds and donor site wounds;

excision of the burn wound is complete (e.g., nonviable tissue are removed) and homeostasis achieved; sufficient autograft tissue is not available at the time of excision; and autograft is not desirable due to the individual's physiologic condition (e.g., individual has multisystem injuries such that creating new wounds may cause undue stress). It has been shown to be as effective as frozen human allografts. Furthermore, when used on excised full-thickness burns, it reduces hospitalization time in the case of pediatric patients with second-degree burn injuries. Nylon present in Biobrane® is not incorporated, making such an acellular matrix a wound dressing rather than a skin substitute. Hyalomatrix® [2,6,9,42,107,109–111] is a bilayer, esterified hyaluronic acid (HYAFF®) matrix with an outer silicone membrane. The connective-mimicking layer HYAFF® is a long-acting derivative of hyaluronic acid providing a microenvironment suitable for optimal tissue repair and accelerated wound healing. Specifically intended for the treatment of deep burns and full-thickness wounds, it also provides a wound preparation support for the implantation of autologous skin grafts.

3.2. Cellularized Dermal Substitutes

Cellularized skin substitutes can be divided into three categories: (1) Epithelial sheets: formed by epithelial cells embedded in or seeded on polymeric membranes. Such engineered epithelial tissues will not be discussed in this review because the scope of the survey is to elucidate the role of dermis regeneration during the closure of deep wounds. (2) Dermis equivalents: composed of 3D porous matrices or hydrogels containing fibroblasts. (3) Full-thickness (or composite) skin equivalents: composed of a dermis equivalent and epidermis.

In the class of cellularized dermis (Table 2) we find (but are not limited to): Dermagraft®, TransCyte®, and Hyalograft3D®. Dermagraft® is classified by the FDA as an interactive wound and burn dressing approved under the PMA process as a class III, high-risk device, and requires clinical data to support their claims for use: treatment of full-thickness diabetic foot ulcers of greater than six weeks duration that extend through the dermis, but without tendon, muscle, joint capsule, or bone exposure. It is a living dermal replacement composed of a bio-absorbable PLGA mesh seeded with cryopreserved neonatal allogeneic foreskin fibroblasts. Dermagraft® is considered medically necessary when used for at least one of the following indications: the treatment of full-thickness diabetic foot ulcers of greater than six weeks duration that have not adequately responded to standard therapy, that extend through the dermis, but without tendon, muscle, joint capsule or bone exposure; or when used on wounds with dystrophic epidermolysis bullosa. It is advised that this material should be used in patients that have adequate blood supply [39]. This dermal substitute appears to produce results as good as allografts with regard to wound infection, wound exudate, wound-healing time, wound closure and graft take, and is more readily removed than allograft, with significantly higher levels of patient satisfaction [111]. The advantages of this skin substitute include good resistance to tearing, ease of handling and lack of rejection [112]. TransCyte® is a nylon mesh coated with bovine collagen and seeded with allogenic neonatal human foreskin fibroblasts which proliferate and synthesize growth factors and extracellular matrix components. It was shown that the presence of a cell-assembled ECM was able to hasten the re-epithelialization process of partial-thickness burns [113]. Furthermore, a multicenter randomized clinical study showed it to be even superior to frozen human cadaver allograft for the temporary closure of excised burn wounds [114].

TransCyte® received an FDA PMA as a temporary wound covering for surgically excised full-thickness and deep partial-thickness burn wounds (detailed reports can be retrieved on the web site of the FDA). It is considered medically necessary for the following uses: temporary wound covering to treat surgically excised full-thickness (third-degree) and deep partial-thickness (second-degree) thermal burn wounds in persons who require such a covering before autograft placement; and the treatment of mid-dermal to indeterminate depth burn wounds that typically require debridement, and that may be expected to heal without autografting [39].

Hyalograft3D (FDA 510(k) approval) comprises esterified hyaluronic acid fibers seeded with autologous fibroblasts and covered by a silicone membrane. Its use in diabetic ulcer therapy has been reported, showing significant improvement of the wound closure compared to other devices [115]. Apligraft® consists of neonatal fibroblasts seeded onto a bovine type I collagen gel and neonatal keratinocytes cultured on top of this dermal layer [116–118]. It gained an FDA PMA based on its efficacy with venous ulcers. Apligraf® also has an FDA PMA for use in the treatment of diabetic foot ulcers.

In the case of venous insufficiency, it is considered medically necessary for at least one of the following indications: chronic, non-infected, partial- or full-thickness ulcers due to venous insufficiency; standard therapeutic compression also in use; and at least one month of conventional ulcer therapy (such as standard dressing changes, and standard therapeutic compression) has been ineffective [39]. In the case of diabetic foot ulcers, it is considered medically necessary for at least one of the following indications: full-thickness neuropathic diabetic foot ulcers that extend through the dermis but without tendon, muscle, joint capsule, or bone exposure; and at least four weeks of conventional ulcer therapy (such as surgical debridement, complete off-loading and standard dressing changes) has been ineffective. It has been reported that adding Apligraf® to compression therapy for chronic venous ulcers doubled the number of healed wounds at six months. Furthermore, in chronic diabetic foot ulcers, 56% of patients in the Apligraf® group had reached complete healing by 12 weeks compared with only 38% in the control group with moist gauze dressing treatment [118]. Use of Apligraft® in other skin defects, such as donor-site wounds and epidermolysis bullosa [119], has been reported. Disadvantages are its uneven pigmentation and contracture, short shelf life of five days, fragility, the risk of disease transfer due to its allogeneic constituents, and the high cost [4]. Tissuetech® is composed of hyaluronic acid-based matrix seeded with fibroblasts with autologous keratinocytes on top. It was shown to be effective in the treatment of the lower limbs. Furthermore, in 401 diabetic ulcers, 70.3% treated with Tissuetech® healed within less than one year [2,42,107]. OrCel® is a bi-layered skin substitute formed by human derma fibroblasts entrapped in a bovine collagen sponge, with human keratinocytes on top.

OrCel® has received an FDA PMA for the treatment of fresh, clean split-thickness donor sites associated with mitten-hand deformities in individuals who have recessive dystrophic epidermolysis bullosa. It is considered medically necessary for the following indications: epidermolysis bullosa in children after reconstructive surgery; and full-thickness (third-degree) or partial-thickness (second-degree burns) [3,39,41,116,120,121]. Once placed in the defect, OrCel® dissolves and is replaced by the patient's own skin.

Table 1. Acellular dermal substitutes.

Product	Composition	Indications	FDA Status
ALLODERM®	Acellular human dermis– non crosslinked	Repair or replacement of damaged or inadequate integument tissue	HCT/P
DERMACELL®	Acellular human dermis– non crosslinked	Chronic non-healing wounds	HCT/P
DERMAMATRIX®	Acellular human dermis– non crosslinked	Soft tissue replacement Breast Reconstruction	Available through the Musculoskeletal Transplant Foundation which meets and exceeds the standards and regulations of the American Association of Tissue Banks (AATB) and the Food and Drug Administration (FDA)
SUREDERM®	Acellular human dermis– non crosslinked	Soft tissue replacement	HCT/P
OASIS®	Porcine acellular lyophilized small intestine submucosa– non crosslinked	Acute, chronic and burns wounds. It delivers growth factors to stimulate and cell migration angiogenesis	510(k)
PERMACOLL®	Porcine acellular diisocyanite -crosslinked	Full-thickness defects such as burns and for soft tissue reconstruction such as hernia repair	510(k)

Table 1. *Cont.*

Product	Composition	Indications	FDA Status
EZ-DERM®	Porcine aldehyde cross-linked reconstituted dermal collagen	Partial-thickness burns	510(k)
INTEGRA®	Acellular Bovine type I collagen and chondroitin-6-sulfate copolymer coated with a thin silicone elastomer-crosslinked	Deep partial thickness and full thickness burns	PMA (1996) 510(k) (2002)
BIOBRANE®	Ultrathin silicone as epidermal analog film and 3D nylon filament as dermal analog with type I collagen peptides	Partial-thickness burns in children; toxic epidermal necrolysis, paraneoplastic pemphigus and chronic wounds	510(k)
MATRIDERM®	Bovine non-crosslinked lyophilized dermis, coated with α-elastin hydrolysate	Full-thickness burns	510(k)
HYALOMATRIX®	Acellular non-woven pad of benzyl ester of hyaluronic acid and a silicone membrane–non crosslinked	Burns, chronic wounds.	510(k)

Adapted from [9,29,39,40]. FDA status (retrieved from FDA website): A preamendment device is one that was in commercial distribution before May 28, 1976, the date the Medical Device Amendments were signed into law. After the Medical Device Amendments became law, the classification of devices was determined by FDA classification panels. Eventually all Class III devices will require a PMA. However, preamendment Class III devices require a PMA only after FDA publishes a regulation calling for PMA submissions. The preamendment devices must have a PMA filed for the device by the effective date published in the regulation in order to continue marketing the device. The CFR will state the date that a PMA is required. Prior to the PMA effective date, the devices must have a cleared Premarket Notification 510(k) prior to marketing. Class III Preamendment devices that require a 510(k) are identified in the CFR as Class III and include the statement "Date premarket approval application (PMA) or notice of completion of product development protocol (PDP) is required. No effective date has been established of the requirement for premarket approval.".

Table 2. Cellularized skin substitutes.

Product	Composition	Indications	Status
DERMAGRAFT® (d)	Human cultured neonatal fibroblasts seeded on polyglactin scaffold	Treatment of diabetic foot ulcers, epidermolysisbullosa	PMA (2001)
TRANSCYTE® (d)	Nylon mesh coated with bovine collagen and seeded with allogenic neonatal human foreskin fibroblasts	Full and partial thickness burns	PMA (1998)
ICX-SKN® (d)	A fibrin matrix seeded with neonatal human fibroblasts	Deep dermal wounds	-
DENOVODERM® (d)	Autologous fibroblasts in collagen hydrogel	Deep defect of the skin	In development, under clinical trials
HYALOGRAFT3D® (d)	Based on estherified hyaluronic acid derivate with cultured fibroblasts and covered by a silicone membrane	Use in diabetic ulcer therapy has been reported	510(k)
APLIGRAFT® (ft)	Bovine collagen matrix seeded with neonatal foreskin fibroblasts and keratinocytes	Treatment of various forms of epidermolysisbullosa Diabetic and venous ulcers	PMA Commercially available in the USA
TISSUETECH® (ft)	Hyaluronic acid with cultured autologous keratinocytes and fibroblasts (Hyalograft 3D® + Laserskin®)	Ulcers	-
PERMADERM® (ft)	Autologous fibroblasts and keratinocytes in culture with bovine collagen and GAG substrates	Sever Burns	-
ORCEL® (ft)	Type I bovine collagen matrix seeded with allogenic neonatal foreskin fibroblasts and keratinocyte	Donor sites in Epidermolysis Bullosa Fresh, clean split thickness donor site wounds in burn patients	PMA (2001)
DENOVOSKIN® (ft)	Autologous fibroblasts in collagen hydrogel and autologous keratinocytes	Deep defect of the skin	In development, under clinical trials

D = composed of one layer (engineered dermis); FT = full-thickness, composed of engineered dermis and engineered epidermis. Adapted from [9,29,39,40]. FDA status: see caption in Table 1.

3.3. Clinical Effectiveness of Skin Substitutes

3.3.1. Effectiveness of Acellular Dermal Regeneration Templates

Dermal substitutes must guarantee correct regeneration of the dermis compartment [13]. After implantation, a dermal substitute has to allow a fast recruitment of endothelial cells in order to guarantee the correct take of a thin STSG. As a long-term aim, the skin substitute should guide a correct regeneration avoiding the formation of scar tissue. It has been recognized that an ideal dermal substitute must satisfy the following requirements [38]:

- avoid the immune response, inflammation and any kind of rejection;
- protect the wounds from infection and loss of fluid;
- easy to handle and flexible, but stiff enough to withstand surgical procedures;
- enable the influx of cells (fibroblasts and endothelial cells) that will build the neodermis;
- stable enough to guarantee the correct neo-synthesis and assembly of immature extracellular matrix; on the other hand, its rate of degradation should be synchronous with the rate of formation of the neo-tissue;
- enable a correct vascularization in less than 14 days post implantation in order to increase the probability of the take of the STSG;
- be able to guide the regeneration avoiding the formation of scar tissue.

To date it is difficult to make a comparison between the efficacy of the different commercially available dermal substitutes because of the lack of long-term follow-up studies in which different dermal substitutes have been studied in parallel. Even where different clinical studies exist for each of the skin substitutes, it is difficult to make an objective comparison due to different factors. Notably, different studies use different methods for the evaluation of the success of the healing. Indeed, different scales exist to evaluate the features of the scar after implantation: Vancouver Scar Scale, Hamilton Burn Scar Rating, Patient and Observer Scar Assessment Scale, Manchester Scar Scale and Visual Analog Scale [121–124]. Moreover, the studies are conducted starting from different type of wounds (burns, ulcers, trauma, etc.). Finally, the experience of the surgeon plays a crucial role in the success of the take of both dermal regeneration template and STSG. This is highlighted by analyzing the results on the take of grafts coming from multicenter and single center studies: the former possesses higher degrees of uncertainty than the latter [124].

Nevertheless, it is possible to extrapolate some general indications showing the benefits and downsides of the different dermal substitutes. By focusing attention on partial- to full-thickness wounds, the gold standard treatment is the application of a partial- or full-thickness STSG. The application of an STSG is an autografting procedure and possesses two main issues: (i) the use of an STSG is an invasive technique because after the removal of large parts of healthy tissues, other damage is induced; and (ii) if the total burn surface is higher than 25% of the total body area, the donor site cannot provide enough tissue to cover the wounded area. For this reason, the majority of the clinical trials have been conducted by comparing the efficacy of a dermis substitute to the efficacy of the gold standard treatment. Among the acellular dermal substitutes, Integra®, Matriderm® and Alloderm® have been subjected to a systematic review [38] thanks to the availability of long-term follow-up studies starting from similar wounds (partial- or full-thickness wounds due to thermal burns). The comparison between the dermal substitutes and the control groups has been performed by analyzing primary outcomes (graft take, wound infection, scar quality) and secondary outcomes (donor site morbidity, convalescence of the patient, need to re-graft). Compared with an STSG, only Integra® showed a significantly lower take ($p < 0.001$). Concerning the infection rate, a value of 85% of infection in patients having a total burn surface of 45% and treated with Integra® has been reported [125,126]. However, other studies reported no difference in infection percentage between Integra® and the control group [26,126,127]. A 6% rate of infection has been detected in a study where Alloderm® was used [127]. Matriderm® did not reveal any difference of infection rate compared with the controls [128]. Concerning scar quality, data only showed better scar quality for Integra® compared to that of an STSG. For all other models, no significant differences were detected in scar quality compared with the control groups. A relevant increase in donor site healing (lower donor site morbidity) has been detected in all studies [38]. This is because by using a dermal substitute to fill the wound bed, the thickness of the STSG can be reduced to 0.006 of an inch, compared to 0.01 of an inch for gold standard treatments.

With the exception of Integra®, few data concerning the mortality and length of stay of patients have been found [38]. No significant differences in rates of re-graft were reported between the dermal substitutes and control groups. Other studies have compared five dermal substitutes (involving Integra®, Matriderm® and Hyalomatrix®) in a preclinical pig model [110]. No difference was found at the end of the survey (six months after implantation) in terms of scar quality and healing properties. A difference was found in the evolution of the healing process. Integra® took more time for fibroblast and blood vessel influx and was still present, as a fragmented matrix, at the end of the survey. Hyalomatrix® showed a lower degradation rate than Matriderm®, but both had completely disappeared at the end of the survey. The quality of the scar assessed with the Vancouver Scar Scale was similar. A long-term follow-up revealed both histological and clinical outcomes in a randomized study using Integra® and Nevelia® [103]. Nevelia® is a porous degradable matrix of about 2 mm thickness made of stabilized native collagen type 1 from calf hides and a silicone sheet of about 200 μm thickness mechanically reinforced with a polyester fabric, and does not contain any chondroitin-6-sulphate GAG. Collagen is purified from calf hides from animals younger than nine months sourced from safe countries. Collagen is then cross-linked with a very low percentage of glutaraldehyde. Clinical results were evaluated through the healing time, Manchester Scar Scale (MSS) and Visual Analog Scale (VAS) up to three years. The differences in healing time between groups, pain and self-estimation was not statistically significant up to a one-year follow-up. Nevelia® showed early regenerative properties in terms of epidermal proliferation and dermal renewal at three weeks, compared with Integra®. Furthermore, Nevelia® showed a more evident angiogenesis vs. Integra®, evaluated as α-SMA immunohistochemistry. Differences in the MSS score were statistically significant at three years follow up in favor of Nevelia® group ($p = 0.001$), together with clinical outcomes. Histological and immunohistochemistry data showed that Nevelia® allows faster neo-angiogenesis and tissue regeneration with neo-formed tissue architecture closer to the physiology of the skin. This data confirms the importance of both vascularization and neodermis influx within the dermal substitute. Indeed, it is well accepted that the faster the vascularization, the higher the take of the STSG. Integra® contains a fraction of chondroitin-6-sulphate GAG that had two side effects: firstly, such a kind of GAG slows the influx of endothelial cells; secondly, the presence of such a high hydrophilic component may retain lesion inflammatory exudates. Furthermore, the high degree of cross-linking in Integra® masks both the adhesion site for fibroblasts and the proteolytic degradation sites, hampering the recipient cells' influx and the degradation of such exogenous ECM. Finally, it seems that rapid vascularization and presence of endogenous dermal cells (fibroblast and vascular network) may play a crucial role in the effectiveness of the dermal substitute.

3.3.2. Effectiveness of Cellularized Skin Substitutes

The introduction of cellularized skin substitutes in the treatment of full-thickness wounds has been necessary in order to overcome some limitations of the acellular dermis. In particular, the presence of dermic cell lines (fibroblast or endothelial cells) serves to reduce the time for neodermis influx after implant. By using acellular dermal substitutes, surgeons have to wait at least four weeks for the implantation of the STSG in order to allow fibroblast and endothelial cells' influx. Without such cellular components, the take of the STSG is not possible. Moreover, the larger the delay before the STSG is implanted, the higher the probability of infection. Thus, the success of the regeneration process is strictly related to both "colonization" time and the quality of the neodermis formed in the porosity of the acellular dermis. A cell populated scaffold introduced in the wound bed aims at reducing such colonization time as a primary task. We can highlight additional requirements that engineered skin substitutes have to possess compared with acellular substitutes:

- Safety concerns: any cultured cell material carries the risk of transmitting viral or bacterial infection, and some support materials (such as bovine collagen and murine feeder cells) may also have a disease risk.
- Clinical efficacy: since the biological risk is higher, the benefits in terms of quality of the healed tissue must be significantly superior, and not only equal, to conventional therapies.
- Convenience: in general, the cost of tissue engineered products is at least ten-fold higher compared to that of non-cellularized materials; in order to achieve clinical uptake, the benefits must include the reduction of hospitalization time, surgical operations after the implants, pain and the associated cost of the treatment.

To date, the use of tissue engineered products for the treatment of burns, although it has received broad scientific success, seems to be not convenient in terms of commercial outcomes. For this reason, many companies have focused their attention on the commercialization of engineered tissues for the treatment of chronic diseases: venous valve insufficiency, arterial diseases, diabetes, vasculitis, skin malignancies and blistering diseases. Regardless of the origin of the wound, the major aim is to reestablish the physiological conditions of the dermis layer. The cells that act to maintain the dermis are the fibroblasts [108], which synthesize and assemble collagen, elastin, and proteoglycans. When inflammation occurs, fibroblasts migrate to the wound site, attracted by bFGF and TGF-β secreted by inflammatory cells and platelets, where the fibroblasts are stimulated to replicate, migrate into the wound, and secrete IGF-1, bFGF, TGF-β, platelet-derived growth factor, and KGF, enabling fibroblast–keratinocyte interaction. When the wound is chronic, the continuous inflammation state induces a premature and stress-induced cellular senescence of the fibroblasts. Moreover, a decreased proliferative potential, impaired capacity to react to growth factors and abnormal protein production is observed. When the percentage of senescent cells in the defect is greater than 15%, wounds are described as hard to heal [14,15,129,130]. The use of Dermagraft® for the treatment of non-healing ulcers has been demonstrated in different clinical studies [130–132]. Summarizing the results, it is possible to establish that the percentage of healing using Dermagraft® ranged from 50% to 71.4%. The complete closure of the wound can be obtained only for ulcers with 12 months of duration or less.

The most popular bi-layered skin substitute (containing fibroblasts and keratinocytes) is Apligraf®, which has been studied since 1999. It has been demonstrated that use of such a bi-layered engineered skin is an effective treatment for ulcers of greater than one-year duration, with a percentage of wound closure of about 50%. Moreover, the number of osteomyelitis and lower-limb amputations were less frequent in the Apligraf® group. The advantage of dermal–epidermal substitutes is the presence of the living epidermal layer that avoids the use of gauzes and two-step procedures. This reduces the risk of infections and improves the healing process due to the presence of fibroblast–keratinocyte cross-talk, which plays a crucial role in the healing process of deep wounds. One of the limitations of the aforementioned categories of skin grafts is the presence of allogenic cell lines, which contain an associated biological risk. This limitation is being overcame by developing models containing autologous cell lines. Two models that use autologous fibroblasts and keratinocytes are denovoDerm® and denovoSkin®, which are under clinical trials at University Children's Hospital of Zurich [71,133–135]. Finally, to deeply investigate on both FDA status and the effectiveness of current skin substitutes the reader can refer to "FDA" and "clinicaltrial" databases by searching for the desired skin model [136,137].

4. Advanced Bioengineered Skin Equivalents: A Future Perspective

4.1. Pre–Vascularization of Dermis Substitutes

The treatment and the evolution of deep wounds due to thermal burns is schematized in Figure 2A-D. After the debridement of the wound, the bed is filled with a DRT supporting an artificial layer of silicone-based epidermis. After a period of four weeks, the epidermal layer is detached and an autologous STSG is applied. In a clinical study that used Integra® as the DRT, 20 patients presenting deep wounds were treated using the procedure described in Figure 2A-D. The evolution of the wound was analyzed by means of histology, immunocytochemistry and the Vancouver Scar Scale [20]. It was observed that the vascularization of the DRT played a crucial role in the take of the STSG. For instance, if the STSG was applied after two or three weeks, the take rate was very low. On the contrary, if the STSG was applied after the fourth week, the take increased up to 95%. Histological and immunostaining analyses demonstrated that at two weeks the vascularization of DRT was poor but increased four weeks after implantation. These data suggest that vascularization of the DRT and the take of the STSG are strictly related [20].

Other relevant findings concern the evolution of the dermis compartment over the time. Weekly histological investigation revealed that influx of exudates and host fibroblasts occurred during weeks one–two. At three weeks, the influx of endothelial cells and the synthesis of immature extracellular matrix components by fibroblasts began. During week four, the formation of a capillary network (Figure 2E) was observed. After the application of the STSG, the wound continued its evolution: at week six a well-organized capillary network was observed, but the dermis–epidermis interface presented no rete ridge profile; at month three, a layer of endogenous collagen network was observed underneath the STSG; after two months, the wound was completely repaired but the neo-tissue was different from the healthy skin. Finally, the complete substitution of the initial DRT with the neodermis occurred at two years post implantation. Even though the patients recovered partial mobility of the damaged parts, it was observed that the repaired zone showed an impaired pigmentation, the mechanical properties between healthy and repaired sites were different, and the organization of the collagen network of the neodermis was different than that of the collagen in the healthy dermis. Finally, neither elastin nor adnexa were present, and differentiation of fibroblasts in myofibroblasts was observed. On the basis of such findings two main issues affecting the DRT emerge: (i) the lack of vascularization [22,23]; and (ii) the limited capability in inducing regeneration instead of repairing processes [135]. The take of the STSG has huge implications related to the repairing process, patient mortality, and morbidity and healthcare costs. Indeed, a low take percentage increases the number of re-grafts and the risk of infection by causing either the death of the patient or an increase of hospitalization time in case of morbidity. To increase the take of STSGs, new emerging strategies involve the use of pre-vascularized DRTs [22,23,33,34,36]. By seeding a DRT with adipose tissue-derived microvasculature fragments, a faster vascularization after implants was observed [138]. Complete reperfusion of the DRT occurred at day six. The percentage of the take was high if the STSG was applied just after day six, indicating that reperfusion rather than simple vascularization played a crucial role in the take. These data suggest that pre-vascularization of the DRT can contribute to shortening the timeframe needed for the application of an STSG. On the other hand, a one-step surgery, which may decrease the number of surgical operations, cannot be performed yet. To do this, not only vascularization, but also fast reperfusion should be promoted.

4.2. Engineered Skin Composed of Fibroblast-Assembled Extracellular Matrix

The lack of vascularization at the moment of implantation has been recognized as the main issue affecting the take of the STSG. No studies have been performed yet on the role that the extracellular matrix comprising the DRT may play on both vascularization and longtime dermal remodeling [17]. The dermis compartment of the totality of the skin substitutes (either cellularized or acellular) are composed by exogenous extracellular materials, i.e., not assembled by the fibroblasts of the patient. This should represent the limitation of the currently available tissue engineering skins. Indeed, exogenous matrices, even though of natural origins, cannot fully replicate the complexity of the living dermis. This may ultimately compromise the repository and regulatory role that the native cell-assembled extracellular matrix plays [16–18]. Such a mismatch between an exogenous material and the living dermis may be responsible for the impaired repair process at both cellular and extracellular levels. Firstly, because the repository and regulatory role of the native ECM is depressed, the growth factors secreted by fibroblasts are not correctly presented to other cell types (e.g., keratinocytes and endothelial cells) neither in space nor time, generating a possible "mistake" in cell–cell signaling [16,17]. This could explain both the delay in the vascularization time and the delayed formation of the rete ridge profile at dermal epidermal interfaces [20,26,72]. As confirmation of this, in vitro tissue engineered skin made by exogenous natural hydrogels (i.e., collagen, fibrin, etc.) presents a flat dermal–epidermal interface. On the contrary, if epithelial cells are grown on a fibroblast-assembled ECM, it is possible to observe a rete ridge profile with spontaneous formation of epithelial invagination and follicular-like structures (Figure 3C) [72], which are typical of the physiologic dermal–epidermal cross-talk mediated by the extracellular matrix [72]. The lack of endogenous ECM-mediated signaling may also explain the absence of both cutaneous adnexa and nerve endings in repaired deep wounds [20,26,129]. Secondly, when fibroblasts colonize the inner porosity of the DRT, they produce an immature extracellular matrix with a degree of assembly much lower than the degree of assembly of the surrounding healthy dermis. Such an immature protein network is not able to withstand the traction forces of the fibroblasts [74,110], generating a different architecture of the collagen fibers in the wound compared to the healthy dermis [15,19,21,77]. Macroscopically, these phenomena generate a portion of the cutis possessing different mechanical properties, different pigmentation, absence of sensing properties and high contracture, provoking both severe functional and aesthetic concerns.

To overcome such limitations, a tissue engineering strategy to produce a human dermis substitute composed of a fibroblast-assembled extracellular matrix has been developed [73,75]. The innovative idea of such strategy is to let human fibroblasts producing their own ECM in vitro. This process provides the possibility of modulating the properties of the cell-synthesized ECM, in order to obtain a final dermis having both composition and assembly degree of the collagen network relatively similar to those present in vivo. Moreover, no exogenous materials are present. This bottom-up tissue engineering strategy starts with the fabrication of dermal building blocks obtained [81] by seeding human fibroblasts in porous gelatin microspheres (Figure 3A). It has been demonstrated that by optimizing the culture conditions, the fibroblasts can produce their own extracellular matrix. Such building blocks, named Dermal-µTissues, were subsequently molded and packed in maturation chambers where both cell–cell and ECM–ECM interactions took place, leading to the formation of a continuum, up to 2 mm thick, made of an endogenous dermis containing fibroblasts and gelatin microspheres. By modulating the stiffness and the degradation rate of the gelatin microspheres and by engineering the dynamic culture conditions (Figure 3), it was possible to obtain fine control over the maturation status and assembly of both collagen and elastin networks [74,91]. During the duration of the process (approximately five weeks), gelatin microspheres were degraded by protease digestion and the final tissue, named EndoDermis, was completely made up of fibroblasts embedded in their own extracellular matrix (Figure 3A). Interestingly, the collagen network was characterized by a stiffness and degree of assembly similar to that featuring the human skin. In the ECM elastin, hyaluronic acid, fibronectin and elastin were also present (Figure 3B-F). In order to produce a pre-vascularized endogenous human dermis model, human umbilical vein endothelial cells (HUVECs) were seeded on the EndoDermis and it was allowed to form an interconnected capillary network [34] that occurred within three weeks (Figure 3D, E). At the best of our knowledge, other than a capillary network, such an engineered DRT is the first model completely formed by a fibroblast-assembled extracellular matrix [34]. After subcutaneous implant in a nude mouse model, fibroblasts and their own ECM (the neodermis) were already present and well-assembled. Thus, no additional time is required for fibroblast influx and neodermis formation. The only phenomenon required is the anastomosis and perfusion of the engineered capillary network. This was shown to occur within seven days of implantation (Figure 3H). Although further investigations are currently being conducted of a more representative wound model, such data are encouraging. In addition to vascularization, which has been recognized as a critical issue [22,23,25,33,34] affecting the effectiveness of a DRT, the described tissue engineered strategy allows the fabrication of a DRT composed of a native extracellular matrix starting from a small number of fibroblasts derived from the patient. In this way, the risks associated with the allogenic nature of the cells and the impaired ECM assembly during wound closure, can be drastically reduced. According to this idea, the formation of severe scars can be reduced.

5. Discussion and Conclusions

Dermal regeneration templates and tissue engineered skin [40] has been reviewed in the light of their effectiveness in guiding the closure of deep wounds toward a regeneration process rather than a repair process [38]. By analyzing the literature, no strategies are currently available that are able to completely restore the whole functionality of the reconstructed part, including pigmentation, mechanical properties, adnexal structures and sensing properties. In other words, the formation of severe scarring still represents a concern in the field of skin reconstruction. Many advances have been made to limit the use of thick STSGs. Indeed, using a last generation DRT, the thickness of STSGs can be reduced to 0.006 of an inch, compared to 0.01 of an inch for gold standard treatments. Furthermore, the take of STSGs has been improved by promoting the vascularization of the DRT [22,23,25]. It has been observed that a DRT composed of non-cross-linked matrices promotes the invasion of fibroblasts and endothelial cells, increasing the take of the STSG compared to the case of cross-linked matrices [9]. On the other hand, cross-linked matrices are able to better withstand contracture during the neodermis remodeling process, due to their superior stiffness. To hasten neodermis growth after implantation, tissue engineering strategies aim at cellularizing the dermis compartment prior to implantation with either fibroblasts or endothelial cells. Pre-vascularization has been shown to improve the take of the STSG and the reperfusion of the dermal bed. This aids the oxygenation of the zone and the removal of waste. The presence of fibroblasts serves to shorten the migration time of fibroblasts from the recipient and to also promote the synthesis of the neo-ECM in the wound bed [26]. Nevertheless, once assembled, the final ECM is still far from its physiologic condition. By analyzing the composition of the bioengineered skin models, it is possible to highlight that they are characterized by a common denominator: cells are always embedded in exogenous matrices (i.e., not synthesized by fibroblasts). This can represent an issue, since native ECMs possess a specific arrangement of moieties, which regulates the cross-talk between fibroblasts and keratinocytes that ultimately leads to the formation of skin adnexa and skin appendages [16–18]. The in vitro fabrication of human bioengineered dermis composed of a fibroblast-assembled ECM incorporating a vascularized network may provide a means of overcoming the scarring process. In this regard, it has been shown that a tissue engineering strategy allows the control of the assembly of the ECM produced by fibroblasts. By modulating the process variables, it is possible to produce an engineered dermis possessing composition, organization, and signal presentation capabilities relatively similar to the native dermis [19,34,35,72,74,81]. This may led to different benefits in the scenario of skin regeneration: (i) To date, the neodermis takes at least two years to form; by introducing the reconstructed patients' dermis in the wound bed, possessing the final architecture and composition at the moment of the implant, no further time will be required for neodermis formation; (ii) by controlling in vitro the degree of assembly of the ECM, it will possible to decrease the differences between repaired and healthy tissues; and (iii) the spatial organization and the functionality of ECM components is not compromised by external factors (e.g., chemicals or physical treatments) and communications among all cell types (e.g., fibroblasts, keratinocytes, nerve endings and macrophages) are correctly orchestrated.

Author Contributions: F.U. collected the majority of the data from the literature, performed a critical analysis of data retrieved from both literature and FDA-CRINICAL TRIAL database, then it wrote the manuscript with inputs from all authors (C.C., G.I. and P.A.N.). C.C. collected data from bottom up tissue engineering skin models and produced histological images and bioengineered skin samples described in the in the Figure 3. He participated to critical discussions during the editing phase. G.I. worked on the arrangement of paragraphs togheter with F.U. and contributed to the development of figures and participated to critical discussions. P.A.N. was the supervisor of the project; he gave inputs about the organization of the manuscript, he gave a crucial contribution concerning the arrangement of discussion in the scientific framework.

Acknowledgments: The authors would like to acknowledge Alessia Larocca, for her contribution in the preparation of the Graphical Abstract.

References

1.   Kanitakis, J. Anatomy, histology and immunohistochemistry of normal human skin. *Eur. J. Dermatol.* **2002**, *12*, 390–401.

2.   Vig, K.; Atul, C.; Shweta, T.; Saurabh, D.; Rajnish, S.; Shreekumar, P.; Vida, A.D.; Shree, R.S. Advances in Skin Regeneration Using Tissue Engineering. *Int. J. Mol. Sci.* **2017**, *18*, 789. [CrossRef] [PubMed]

3.   Zhang, Z.; Michniak-kohn, B.B. Tissue Engineered Human Skin Equivalents. *Pharmaceutics* **2012**, *4*, 26–41. [CrossRef] [PubMed]

4.   Matrices, D.; Skin, B. Dermal Matrices and Bioengineered Skin Substitutes: A Critical Review of Current Options. *Plast. Reconstr. Surg. Glob. Open* **2015**, *3*, e284.

5.   Heimbach, D.; Luterman, A.; Burke, J.; Cram, A.; Herndon, D.; Hunt, J.; Jordan, M.; McManus, W.; Solem, L.; Warden, G.L. Artificial Dermis for Major Burns. *Ann. Surg.* **1988**, *208*, 313–320. [CrossRef] [PubMed]

6.   Shahrokhi, S.; Arno, A.; Jeschke, M.G. The use of dermal substitutes in burn surgery: Acute phase. *Wound Repair Regen.* **2014**, *22*, 14–22. [CrossRef]

7.   Sun, B.K.; Siprashvili, Z.; Khavari, P.A. Advances in skin grafting and treatment of cutaneous wounds. *Science* **2014**, *346*, 941–946. [CrossRef]

8.   Dhivya, S.; Vijaya, V.; Santhini, E. Review article Wound dressings—A review. *BioMedicine* **2015**, *5*, 24–28. [CrossRef]

9.   Van der Veen, V.C.; van der Wal, M.B.; van Leeuwen, M.C.; Ulrich, M.M.; Middelkoop, E. Biological background of dermal substitutes. *Burns* **2010**, *36*, 305–321. [CrossRef]

10.   Bloemen, M.C.; van Leeuwen, M.C.; van Vucht, N.E.; van Zuijlen, P.P.; Middelkoop, E. Dermal Substitution in Acute Burns and Reconstructive Surgery: A 12-Year Follow-Up. *Plast. Reconstr. Surg.* **2010**, *125*, 1450–1459. [CrossRef]

11.   Proksch, E.; Brandner, J.M.; Jensen, J. The skin: An indispensable barrier. *Exp. Dermatol.* **2008**, *17*, 1063–1072. [CrossRef] [PubMed]

12.   Schlader, Z.J.; Vargas, N.T. Regulation of Body Temperature by Autonomic and Behavioral Thermoeffectors. *Exerc. Sport Sci. Rev.* **2019**, *47*, 116–126. [CrossRef] [PubMed]

13.   Enoch, S.; Leaper, D.J. Basic science of wound healing. *Surgery* **2008**, *26*, 31–37.

14.   Tarnuzzer, R.W.; Gregory, S. Biochemical analysis of acute and chronic wound environments. *Wound Repair Regen.* **1996**, *4*, 321–325. [CrossRef]

15.   Velnar, T.; Bailey, T.; Smrkolj, V. The wound healing process: An overview of the cellular and molecular mechanisms. *J. Int. Med. Res.* **2009**, *37*, 1528–1542. [CrossRef]

16.   Bowers, S.L.; Banerjee, I.; Baudino, T.A. The extracellular matrix: At the center of it all. *J. Mol. Cell Cardiol.* **2010**, *48*, 474–482. [CrossRef]

17.   Rozario, T.; DeSimone, D.W. The extracellular matrix in development and morphogenesis: A dynamic view. *Dev. Biol.* **2010**, *341*, 126. [CrossRef]

18.   Watt, F.M.; Fujiwara, H. Cell-Extracellular Matrix Interactions in Normal and Diseased Skin. *Cold Spring Harb. Perspect. Biol.* **2011**, *3*, a005124. [CrossRef]

19.   Lombardi, B.; Casale, C.; Imparato, G.; Urciuolo, F.; Netti, P.A. Spatiotemporal Evolution of the Wound Repairing Process in a 3D Human Dermis Equivalent. *Adv. Healthc. Mater.* **2017**, *6*, 1–11. [CrossRef]

20.   Moiemen, N.S.; Vlachou, E.; Staiano, J.J.; Thawy, Y.; Frame, J.D. Reconstructive Surgery with Integra Dermal Regeneration Template: Histologic Study, Clinical Evaluation, and Current Practice. *Plast. Reconstr. Surg.* **2006**, *117*, 160S–174S. [CrossRef]

21.   Clark, J.A.; Leung, K.S. Mechanical properties of normal skin and hypetrophic scars. *Burns* **1996**, *22*, 443–446. [CrossRef]

22.   Frueh, F.S.; Sanchez-Macedo, N.; Calcagni, M.; Giovanoli, P.; Lindenblatt, N. The crucial role of vascularization and lymphangiogenesis in skin reconstruction. *Eur. Surg. Res.* **2018**, *59*, 242–254. [CrossRef] [PubMed]

23.   Laschke, M.W.; Menger, M.D. Vascularization in tissue engineering: Angiogenesis versus inosculation. *Eur. Surg. Res.* **2012**, *48*, 85–92. [CrossRef] [PubMed]

24. Chaudhari, A.A.; Vig, K.; Baganizi, D.R.; Sahu, R.; Dixit, S.; Dennis, V.; Singh, S.R.; Pillai, S.R. Future Prospects for Scaffolding Methods and Biomaterials in Skin Tissue Engineering: A Review. *Int. J. Mol. Sci.* **2016**, *17*, 1974. [CrossRef]

25. Hendrickx, B.; Verdonck, K.; Van den Berge, S.; Dickens, S.; Eriksson, E.; Vranckx, J.J.; Luttun, A. Integration of blood outgrowth endothelial cells in dermal fibroblast sheets promotes full thickness wound healing. *Stem Cells* **2010**, *28*, 1165–1177. [CrossRef]

26. Lagus, H.; Sarlomo-Rikala, M.; Böhling, T.; Vuola, J. Prospective study on burns treated with Integra®, a cellulose sponge and split thickness skin graft: Comparative clinical and histological study—Randomized controlled trial. *Burns* **2013**, *39*, 1577–1587. [CrossRef]

27. Cui, H.; Chai, Y.; Yu, Y. Review Article Progress in developing decellularized bioscaffolds for enhancing skin construction. *J. Biomed. Mater. Res. Part A* **2019**, *107*, 1849–1859.

28. Moore, M.A.; Samsell, B.; Wallis, G.; Triplett, S.; Chen, S.; Jones, A.L.; Qin, X. Decellularization of human dermis using non-denaturing anionic detergent and endonuclease: A review. *Cell Tissue Bank.* **2015**, *16*, 249–259. [CrossRef]

29. Macneil, S. Progress and opportunities for tissue-engineered skin. *Nature* **2007**, *445*, 874–880. [CrossRef]

30. Cheung, H.; Lau, K.; Lu, T.; Hui, D. A critical review on polymer-based bio-engineered materials for scaffold development. *Compos. Part B* **2007**, *38*, 291–300. [CrossRef]

31. Zhong, S.P.; Zhang, Y.Z.; Lim, C.T. Tissue scaffolds for skin wound healing and dermal reconstruction. *Nanomed. Nanobiotechnol.* **2010**, *2*, 510–525. [CrossRef] [PubMed]

32. Vacanti, C.A. The history of tissue engineering. *J. Cell. Mol. Med.* **2006**, *10*, 569–576. [CrossRef] [PubMed]

33. Domaszewska-Szostek, A.; Krzyżanowska, M.; Siemionow, M. Cell-Based Therapies for Chronic Wounds Tested in Clinical Studies. *Ann. Plast. Surg.* **2019**, *83*, e96–e109. [CrossRef] [PubMed]

34. Mazio, C.; Casale, C.; Imparato, G.; Urciuolo, F.; Attanasio, C.; De Gregorio, M.; Rescigno, F.; Netti, P.A. Pre-vascularized dermis model for fast and functional anastomosis with host vasculature. *Biomaterials* **2019**, *192*, 159–170. [CrossRef] [PubMed]

35. Martorina, F.; Casale, C.; Urciuolo, F.; Netti, P.A.; Imparato, G. In vitro activation of the neuro-transduction mechanism in sensitive organotypic human skin model. *Biomaterials* **2017**, *113*, 217–229. [CrossRef]

36. Martin, I.; Wendt, D.; Heberer, M. The role of bioreactors in tissue engineering. *TRENDS Biotechnol.* **2004**, *22*, 80–86. [CrossRef]

37. Ratcliffe, A.; Niklason, L.E.E. Bioreactors and Bioprocessing for Tiosue Engineering. *Ann. N. Y. Acad. Sci.* **2002**, *961*, 210–215. [CrossRef]

38. Widjaja, W.; Tan, J.; Maitz, P.K.M.M. Efficacy of dermal substitute on deep dermal to full thickness burn injury: A systematic review. *ANZ J. Surg.* **2017**, *87*, 446–452. [CrossRef]

39. Ucare. *Bioengineering Skin Substitutes—Medical Policy 2016*; Ucare Medical Policy-Policy Number: 2016M0011B; Ucare: Minneapolis, MN, USA, 2016.

40. Mohebichamkhorami, F.; Alizadeh, A. Skin Substitutes: An Updated Review of Products from Year 1980 to 2017. *J. Appl. Biotechnol. Reports* **2017**, *4*, 615–623.

41. Boyce, S.T.; Lalley, A.L. Tissue engineering of skin and regenerative medicine for wound care. *Burns Trauma* **2018**, *6*, 1–10. [CrossRef]

42. Ma, P.X. Scaffolds for tissue fabrication. *Mater. Today* **2004**, *7*, 30–40. [CrossRef]

43. Gibot, L.; Galbraith, T.; Huot, J.; Auger, F.A. A preexisting microvascular network benefits in vivo revascularization of a microvascularized tissue-engineered skin substitute. *Tissue Eng. Part A* **2010**, *16*, 3199–3206. [CrossRef] [PubMed]

44. Hou, Q.; Grijpma, D.W.; Feijen, J. Porous polymeric structures for tissue engineering prepared by a coagulation, compression moulding and salt leaching technique. *Biomaterials* **2003**, *24*, 1937–1947. [CrossRef]

45. Braghirolli, D.I.; Steffens, D.; Pranke, P. Electrospinning for regenerative medicine: A review of the main topics. *Drug Discov. Today* **2014**, *19*, 743–753. [CrossRef]

46. Pörtner, R.; Nagel-Heyer, S.; Goepfert, C.; Adamietz, P.; Meenen, N.M. Bioreactor Design for Tissue Engineering. *J. Biosci. Bioeng.* **2005**, *100*, 235–245. [CrossRef]

47. Helmedag, M.; Weinandy, S.; Marquardt, Y.; Baron, J.M.; Pallua, N. The Effects of Constant Flow Bioreactor Cultivation and Keratinocyte Seeding Densities on Organotypic Skin Grafts Based on a Fibrin Scaffold Corresponding Author. *Tissue Eng. Part A* **2013**, *21*, 1–31.

48. Lei, X.H.; Ning, L.N.; Cao, Y.J.; Liu, S.; Zhang, S.B.; Qiu, Z.F.; Hu, H.M.; Zhang, H.S.; Liu, S.; Duan, E.K. NASA-Approved Rotary Bioreactor Enhances Proliferation of Human Epidermal Stem Cells and Supports Formation of 3D Epidermis-Like Structure. *PLoS ONE* **2011**, *6*, 1–8. [CrossRef]

49. Drury, J.L.; Mooney, D.J. Hydrogels for tissue engineering: Scaffold design variables and applications. *Biomaterials* **2003**, *24*, 4337–4351. [CrossRef]

50. Slaughter, B.B.V.; Khurshid, S.S.; Fisher, O.Z.; Khademhosseini, A.; Peppas, N.A. Hydrogels in Regenerative Medicine. *Adv. Mater.* **2009**, *21*, 3307–3329. [CrossRef]

51. Lee, K.Y.; Mooney, D.J. Hydrogels for Tissue Engineering. *Chem. Rev.* **2001**, *101*, 1869–1880. [CrossRef]

52. Hoffman, A.S. Hydrogels for biomedical applications. *Adv. Drug Deliv. Rev.* **2012**, *64*, 18–23. [CrossRef]

53. Yang, C.; Xu, L.; Zhou, Y.; Zhang, X.; Huang, X.; Wang, M.; Han, Y.; Zhai, M.; Wei, S.; Li, J. A green fabrication approach of gelatin/CM-chitosan hybrid hydrogel for wound healing. *Carbohydr. Polym.* **2010**, *82*, 1297–1305. [CrossRef]

54. Sun, G.; Zhang, X.; Shen, Y.I.; Sebastian, R.; Dickinson, L.E.; Fox-Talbot, K.; Reinblatt, M.; Steenbergen, C.; Harmon, J.W.; Gerecht, S. Dextran hydrogel scaffolds enhance angiogenic responses and promote complete skin regeneration during burn wound healing. *PNAS* **2011**, *108*, 20976–20981. [CrossRef] [PubMed]

55. Ribeiro, M.P.; Morgado, P.I.; Miguel, S.P.; Coutinho, P.; Correia, I.J. Dextran-based hydrogel containing chitosan microparticles loaded with growth factors to be used in wound healing. *Mater. Sci. Eng. C* **2013**, *33*, 2958–2966. [CrossRef] [PubMed]

56. Chattopadhyay, S.; Raines, R.T. Review Collagen-Based Biomaterials for Wound Healing. *Biopolymers* **2014**, *101*, 821–833. [CrossRef]

57. Heo, D.N.; Yang, D.H.; Lee, J.B.; Bae, M.S.; Kim, J.H.; Moon, S.H.; Chun, H.J.; Kim, C.H.; Lim, H.N.; Kwon, I.K. Burn-Wound Healing Effect of Gelatin/Polyurethane Nanofiber Scaffold Containing Silver-Sulfadiazine. *J. Biomed. Nanotechnol.* **2013**, *9*, 511–515. [CrossRef]

58. Nunes, P.S.; Rabelo, A.S.; de Souza, J.C.; Santana, B.V.; da Silva, T.M.; Serafini, M.R.; dos Passos Menezes, P.; dos Santos Lima, B.; Cardoso, J.C.; Alves, J.C.; et al. Gelatin-based membrane containing usnic acid-loaded liposome improves dermal burn healing in a porcine model. *Int. J. Pharm.* **2016**, *513*, 473–482. [CrossRef]

59. Ulubayram, K.; Cakar, A.N.; Korkusuz, P.; Ertan, C.; Hasirci, N. EGF containing gelatin-based wound dressings. *Biomaterials* **2001**, *22*, 1345–1356. [CrossRef]

60. Farokhi, M.; Mottaghitalab, F.; Fatahi, Y.; Khademhosseini, A.; Kaplan, D.L. Overview of Silk Fibroin Use in Wound Dressings. *Trends Biotechnol.* **2018**, *36*, 907–922. [CrossRef]

61. Boucard, N.; Viton, C.; Agay, D.; Mari, E.; Roger, T.; Chancerelle, Y.; Domard, A. The use of physical hydrogels of chitosan for skin regeneration following third-degree burns. *Biomaterials* **2007**, *28*, 3478–3488. [CrossRef]

62. Opasanon, S.; Muangman, P.; Namviriyachote, N. Clinical effectiveness of alginate silver dressing in outpatient management of partial-thickness burns. *Int. Wound J.* **2010**, *7*, 467–471. [CrossRef] [PubMed]

63. Voigt, J.; Driver, V.R. Hyaluronic acid derivatives and their healing effect on burns, epithelial surgical wounds, and chronic wounds: A systematic review and meta-analysis of randomized controlled trials. *Wound Repair Regen.* **2012**, *20*, 317–331. [CrossRef] [PubMed]

64. Harris, P.A.; Di Francesco, F.; Barisoni, D.; Leigh, I.M.; Navsaria, H.A. Use of hyaluronic acid and cultured autologous keratinocytes and fibroblasts in extensive burns. *Lancet* **1999**, *353*, 35–36. [CrossRef]

65. Sood, R.; Roggy, D.; Zieger, M.; Balledux, J.; Chaudhari, S.; Koumanis, D.J.; Mir, H.S.; Cohen, A.; Knipe, C.; Gabehart, K.; et al. Cultured Epithelial Autografts for Coverage of Large Burn Wounds in Eighty-Eight Patients: The Indiana University Experience. *J. Burn Care Res.* **1990**, *31*, 559–568. [CrossRef] [PubMed]

66. Alexandra, P.M.; Rogeério, P.P.; Mariana, T.C.; Rui, L.R. *Skin Tissue Models*, 1st ed.; Mica Haley: Amsterdam, The Netherlands, 2018; pp. 1–451.

67. Mostow, E.N.; Haraway, G.D.; Dalsing, M.; Hodde, J.P.; King, D.; OASIS Venus Ulcer Study Group. Effectiveness of an extracellular matrix graft (OASIS Wound Matrix) in the treatment of chronic leg ulcers: A randomized clinical trial. *J. Vasc.* **2005**, *41*, 837–843. [CrossRef] [PubMed]

68. Groeber, F.; Engelhardt, L.; Lange, J.; Kurdyn, S.; Schmid, F.F.; Rücker, C.; Mielke, S.; Walles, H.; Hansmann, J. A first vascularized skin equivalent as an alternative to animal experimentation. *ALTEX-Altern. Anim. Exp.* **2016**, *33*, 415–422. [CrossRef] [PubMed]

69. Sun, T.; Norton, D.; Haycock, J.W.; Ryan, A.J.; MacNeil, S. Development of a Closed Bioreactor System for Culture of Tissue-Engineered Skin at an Air—Liquid Interface. *Tissue Eng.* **2005**, *11*, 1824–1831. [CrossRef]

70. Hartmann-Fritsch, F. About ATMPs, SOPs and GMP: The Hurdles to Produce novel skin grafts for clinical use. *Transfus. Med. Hemother.* **2016**, *43*, 344–352. [CrossRef]

71. Griffin, J.W.; Mcarthur, J.C.; Polydefkis, M. Assessment of cutaneous innervation by skin biopsies. *Curr. Opin. Neurol.* **2001**, *14*, 655–659. [CrossRef]

72. Casale, C.; Imparato, G.; Urciuolo, F.; Netti, P. Endogenous human skin equivalent promotes in vitro morphogenesis of follicle-like structures. *Biomaterials* **2016**, *101*, 86–95. [CrossRef]

73. Vader, D.; Kabla, A.; Weitz, D.; Mahadevan, L. Strain-Induced Alignment in Collagen Gels. *PLoS ONE* **2009**, *4*, e5902. [CrossRef]

74. Imparato, G.; Urciuolo, F.; Casale, C.; Netti, P.A.; Imparato, G.; Urciuolo, F.; Casale, C.; Netti, P.A. The role of microscaffold properties in controlling the collagen assembly in 3D dermis equivalent using modular tissue engineering. *Biomaterials* **2013**, *34*, 7851–7861. [CrossRef] [PubMed]

75. Varkey, M.; Ding, J.; Tredget, E.E. Advances in Skin Substitutes—Potential of Tissue Engineered Skin for Facilitating Anti-Fibrotic Healing. *J. Funct. Biomater.* **2015**, *6*, 547–563. [CrossRef] [PubMed]

76. van Zuijlen, P.P.; Ruurda, J.J.; van Veen, H.A.; van Marle, J.; van Trier, A.J.; Groenevelt, F.; Kreis, R.W.; Middelkoop, E. Collagen morphology in human skin and scar tissue: No adaptations in response to mechanical loading at joints. *Burns* **2003**, *29*, 423–431. [CrossRef]

77. Sidgwick, G.P.; McGeorge, D.; Bayat, A. A comprehensive evidence-based review on the role of topicals and dressings in the management of skin scarring. *Arch. Dermatol. Res.* **2015**, *307*, 461–477. [CrossRef] [PubMed]

78. Nichol, J.W.; Khademhosseini, A.; Nichol, J.W. Modular tissue engineering: Engineering biological tissues from the bottom up. *Soft Matter* **2009**, *5*, 1312–1319. [CrossRef] [PubMed]

79. Yang, J.; Yamato, M.; Kohno, C.; Nishimoto, A. Cell sheet engineering: Recreating tissues without biodegradable scaffolds $. *Biomaterials* **2005**, *26*, 6415–6422. [CrossRef]

80. Mironov, V.; Visconti, R.P.; Kasyanov, V.; Forgacs, G.; Drake, C.J.; Markwald, R.R. Organ printing: Tissue spheroids as building blocks. *Biomaterials* **2009**, *30*, 2164–2174. [CrossRef]

81. Urciuolo, F.; Garziano, A.; Imparato, G.; Panzetta, V.; Fusco, S.; Casale, C.; Netti, P.A. Biophysical properties of dermal building-blocks affect extra cellular matrix assembly in 3D endogenous macrotissue. *Biofabrication* **2016**, *8*, 015010. [CrossRef]

82. Leong, W.; Wang, D. Cell-laden Polymeric Microspheres for Biomedical Applications. *Trends Biotechnol.* **2015**, *33*, 653–666. [CrossRef]

83. Matsunaga, Y.T.; Morimoto, Y.; Takeuchi, S. Molding Cell Beads for Rapid Construction of Macroscopic 3D Tissue Architecture. *Adv. Healthc. Mater.* **2011**, *23*, 90–94. [CrossRef] [PubMed]

84. Onoe, H.; Okitsu, T.; Itou, A.; Kato-Negishi, M.; Gojo, R.; Kiriya, D.; Sato, K.; Miura, S.; Iwanaga, S.; Kuribayashi-Shigetomi, K.; et al. Metre-long cell-laden microfibres exhibit tissue morphologies and functions. *Nat. Mater.* **2013**, *12*, 584–590. [CrossRef] [PubMed]

85. Larouche, D.; Cantin-warren, L.; Moulin, J.; Germain, L. Improved Methods to Produce Tissue-Engineered Skin Substitutes Suitable for the Permanent Closure of Full-Thickness Skin Injuries. *Biores. Open Access* **2016**, *5*, 320–329. [CrossRef] [PubMed]

86. Kim, M.S.; Lee, B.; Kim, H.N.; Bang, S.; Yang, H.S.; Kang, S.M.; Suh, K.Y.; Park, S.H. 3D tissue formation by stacking detachable cell sheets formed on nanofiber mesh tissues and organs. *Biofabrication* **2017**, *9*, 15029. [CrossRef]

87. Toma, C.C.; Corato, R.; Di Rinaldi, R. Microfluidics and BIO-encapsulation for drug-and cell-therapy. In Proceedings of the Organic Sensors and Bioelectronics X—International Society for Optics and Photonics 2017, San Diego, CA, USA, 6–7 August 2017.

88. Jiang, W.; Li, M.; Chen, Z.; Leong, K.W. Cell-laden microfluidic microgels for tissue regeneration. *Lab Chip* **2016**, *16*, 4482–4506. [CrossRef]

89. Palmiero, C.; Imparato, G.; Urciuolo, F.; Netti, P.A. Engineered dermal equivalent tissue in vitro by assembly of microtissue precursors. *Acta Biomater.* **2010**, *6*, 2548–2553. [CrossRef]

90. Urciuolo, F.; Imparato, G.; Totaro, A.; Netti, P.A. Building a Tissue In Vitro from the Bottom Up: Implications in Regenerative Medicine. *DeBakey Cardiovasc. J.* **2013**, *9*, 213–217. [CrossRef]

91. Urciuolo, F.; Imparato, G.; Palmiero, C.; Trilli, A.; Netti, P.A. Effect of Process Conditions on the Growth of Three-Dimensional Dermal-Equivalent Tissue Obtained by Microtissue Precursor Assembly. *Tissue Eng. Part C* **2011**, *17*, 155–164. [CrossRef]

92. Urciuolo, F. Lab on a Chip A micro-perfusion bioreactor for on line hydrodynamic and biochemical stimulation. *Lab Chip* **2016**, *16*, 855–867.

93. Jakab, K.; Norotte, C.; Damon, B.; Marga, F.; Neagu, A.; Besch-Williford, C.L.; Kachurin, A.; Church, K.H.; Park, H.; Mironov, V.; et al. Tissue Engineering by Self-Assembly of Cells Printed into Topologically Defined Structures. *Tissue Eng. Part A* **2008**, *14*, 413–421. [CrossRef]

94. Moroni, L.; Boland, T.; Burdick, J.A.; De Maria, C.; Derby, B.; Forgacs, G.; Mota, C. Biofabrication: A guide to technology and terminology. *Trends Biotechnol.* **2018**, *36*, 384–402. [CrossRef] [PubMed]

95. Cui, X.; Boland, T. Human microvasculature fabrication using thermal inkjet printing technology. *Biomaterials* **2009**, *30*, 6221–6227. [CrossRef] [PubMed]

96. Patra, S.; Young, V. A Review of 3D Printing Techniques and the Future in Biofabrication of Bioprinted Tissue. *Cell Biochem. Biophys.* **2016**, *74*, 93–98. [CrossRef] [PubMed]

97. Fetah, K.; Tebon, P.; Goudie, M.J.; Eichenbaum, J.; Ren, L.; Barros, N.; Nasiri, R.; Ahadian, S.; Ashammakhi, N.; Dokmeci, M.R.; et al. The emergence of 3D bioprinting in organ-on-chip systems. *Reports Prog. Biomed. Eng.* **2019**, *1*, 012001. [CrossRef]

98. Pourchet, L.J.; Thepot, A.; Albouy, M.; Courtial, E.J.; Boher, A.; Blum, L.J.; Marquette, C.A. Human Skin 3D Bioprinting Using Scaffold-Free Approach. *Adv. Healthc. Mater.* **2017**, *6*, 1–8. [CrossRef]

99. Tarassoli, S.P.; Jessop, Z.M.; Al-Sabah, A.; Gao, N.; Whitaker, S.; Doak, S.; Whitaker, I.S. Skin tissue engineering using 3D bioprinting: An evolving research field. *J. Plast. Reconstr. Aesthetic Surg.* **2018**, *71*, 615–623. [CrossRef]

100. Cubo, N.; Garcia, M.; Cañizo, J.F.; Velasco, D.; Jorcano, J.L. 3D bioprinting of functional human skin: Production and in vivo analysis 3D bioprinting of functional human skin: Production and in vivo analysis. *Biofabrication* **2017**, *9*, 1–12.

101. Lee, W.; Debasitis, J.C.; Lee, V.K.; Lee, J.H.; Fischer, K.; Edminster, K.; Park, J.K.; Yoo, S.S. Multi-layered culture of human skin fibroblasts and keratinocytes through three-dimensional freeform fabrication. *Biomaterials* **2009**, *30*, 1587–1595. [CrossRef]

102. Yanez, M.; Rincon, J.; Dones, A.; De Maria, C.; Gonzales, R.; Boland, T. In Vivo Assessment of Printed Microvasculature in a Bilayer Skin Graft to Treat Full-Thickness Wounds. *Tissue Eng. Part A* **2015**, *21*, 224–233. [CrossRef]

103. De Angelis, B.; Orlandi, F.; Fernandes Lopes Morais D'Autilio, M.; Scioli, M.G.; Orlandi, A.; Cervelli, V.; Gentile, P. Long-term follow-up comparison of two different bi-layer dermal substitutes in tissue regeneration: Clinical outcomes and histological findings. *Int. Wound J.* **2018**, *15*, 695–706. [CrossRef]

104. Shukla, A.; Dey, N.; Nandi, P. Acellular Dermis as a Dermal Matrix of Tissue Engineered Skin Substitute for Burns Treatment. *Ann. Public Heal. Res.* **2015**, *2*, 1023.

105. Wainwright, D.J. Use of an acellular allograft dermal matrix in the management of full-thickness burns. *Burns* **1995**, *21*, 243–248. [CrossRef]

106. Troy, J.; Karlnoski, R.; Downes, K. The Use of EZ Derm R in Partial-Thickness Burns: An Institutional Review of 157 Patients. *Eplasty* **2013**, *13*, 108–119.

107. Baus, A.; Combes, F.; Lakhel, A.; Pradier, J.P.; Brachet, M.; Duhoux, A.; Duhamel, P.; Fossat, S.; Bey, E. Chirurgia delle ustioni gravi in fase acuta. *EMC-Tec. Chir.-Chir. Plast. Ricostr. Estet.* **2017**, *15*, 1–25. [CrossRef]

108. Costa-almeida, R.; Soares, R.; Granja, P.L. Fibroblasts as maestros orchestrating tissue regeneration. *J. Tissue Eng. Regen. Med.* **2018**, *12*, 240–251. [CrossRef] [PubMed]

109. Kamel, R.A.; Ong, J.F.; Junker, J.P.E. Tissue Engineering of Skin. *J. Am. Coll. Surg.* **2013**, *217*, 533–555. [CrossRef]

110. Philandrianos, C.; Andrac-Meyer, L.; Mordon, S.; Feuerstein, J.M.; Sabatier, F.; Veran, J.; Magalon, G.; Casanova, D. Comparison of five dermal substitutes in full-thickness skin wound healing in a porcine model. *Burns* **2012**, *38*, 820–829. [CrossRef]

111. Hansbrough, J.F.; Mozingo, D.W.; Kealey, G.P.; Davis, M.; Gidner, A.; Gentzkow, G.D. Clinical trials of a biosynthetic temporary skin replacement DermagraftTC compared with cryoperserved human cadaver skin for temporary coverage of excised burn. *J. Burn Care Rehabil.* **1997**, *18*, 43–51. [CrossRef]

112. Hart, C.E.; Loewen-rodriguez, A.; Lessem, J. Wound care products dermagraft: Use in the Treatment of Chronic Wounds. *Adv. Wound Care* **2012**, *1*, 6–18. [CrossRef]

113. Demling, R.H.; Desanti, L. Management of partial thickness facial burns (comparison of topical antibiotics and bio-engineered skin substitutes) p. *Burns* **1999**, *25*, 256–261. [CrossRef]

114. Kumar, R.J.; Kimble, R.M.; Boots, R.; Pegg, S.P. Treatment of partial thicness burns: A prospective, randomized trial using TranscyteTM. *ANZ J. Surg.* **2004**, *74*, 622–626. [CrossRef] [PubMed]

115. Santema, T.B.K.; Poyck, P.P.C.; Ubbink, D.T. Systematic review and meta-analysis of skin substitutes in the treatment of diabetic foot ulcers: Highlights of a Cochrane systematic review. *Wound Repair Regen.* **2016**, *24*, 737–744. [CrossRef] [PubMed]

116. Falanga, V.; Sabolinski, M. A bilayered living skin construct (APLIGRAF ®) accelerates complete closure of hard-to-heal venous ulcers. *Wound Repair Regen.* **1999**, *7*, 201–207. [CrossRef] [PubMed]

117. Griffiths, M.; Ojeh, N.; Res, M.; Livingstone, R.; Price, R. Survival of Apligraf in Acute Human Wounds. *Tissue Eng.* **2004**, *10*, 1180–1195. [CrossRef] [PubMed]

118. Kirsner, R.S.; Sabolinski, M.L.; Parsons, N.B.; Skornicki, M.; Marston, W.A. Comparative effectiveness of a bioengineered living cellular construct vs. a dehydrated human amniotic membrane allograft for the treatment of diabetic foot ulcers in a real world setting. *Wound Repair Regen.* **2015**, *23*, 737–744. [CrossRef] [PubMed]

119. Falabella, A.F.; Valencia, I.C.; Eaglstein, W.H.; Schachner, L.A. Tissue-Engineered Skin (Apligraf) in the Healing of Patients with Epidermolysis Bullosa Wounds. *Arch. Dermatol.* **2000**, *136*, 1225–1230. [CrossRef]

120. Efanov, J.I.; Tchiloemba, B.; Duong, A.; Bélisle, A.; Izadpanah, A.; Coeugniet, E.; Danino, M.A. Use of bilaminar grafts as life-saving interventions for severe burns: A single-center experience. *Burns* **2018**, *44*, 1336–1345. [CrossRef]

121. Forbes-Duchart, L.; Marshall, S.; Strock, A.; Cooper, J.E. Determination of Inter-Rater Reliability in Pediatric Burn Scar Assessment Using a Modified Version of the Vancouver Scar Scale. *J. Burn Care Res.* **2007**, *28*, 460–467. [CrossRef]

122. Fearmonti, R.; Bond, J.; Erdmann, D. A Review of Scar Scales and Scar Measuring. *Eplasty* **2010**, *10*, 354–363.

123. Draaijers, L.J.; Tempelman, F.R.; Botman, Y.A.; Tuinebreijer, W.E.; Middelkoop, E.; Kreis, R.W.; van Zuijlen, P.P. The Patient and Observer Scar Assessment Scale: A Reliable and Feasible Tool for Scar Evaluation. *Plast. Reconstr. Surg.* **2003**, *113*, 1960–1965. [CrossRef]

124. Tyack, Z.; Simons, M.; Spinks, A.; Wasiak, J. A systematic review of the quality of burn scar rating scales for clinical and research use. *Burns* **2011**, *38*, 6–18. [CrossRef] [PubMed]

125. Peck, M.D.; Kessler, M.; Meyer, A.A.; Bonham Morris, P.A. A Trial of the Effectiveness of Artificial Dermis in the Treatment of Patients with Burns Greater Than 45% Total Body Surface Area. *J. Trauma* **1988**, *39*, 313–319. [CrossRef] [PubMed]

126. Heimbach, D.A.; Luterman, A.R.; Burke, J.O.; Cram, A.L.; Herndon, D.A.; Hunt, J.O.; Jordan, M.A.; McMANUS, W.I.; Solem, L.Y.; Warden, G.L. Artificial dermis for major burns. A multi-center randomized clinical trial. *Ann. Surg.* **1988**, *208*, 313–320. [CrossRef] [PubMed]

127. Rennekampff, H.O.; Pfau, M.; Schaller, H.E. Acellular allograft dermal matrix: Immediate or delayed epidermal coverage? *Burns* **2001**, *27*, 150–153. [CrossRef]

128. Bloemen, M.C.; van der Wal, M.B.; Verhaegen, P.D.; Nieuwenhuis, M.K.; van Baar, M.E.; van Zuijlen, P.P.; Middelkoop, E. Clinical effectiveness of dermal substitution in burns by topical negative pressure: A multicenter randomized controlled trial. *Wound Repair Regen.* **2012**, *20*, 797–805. [CrossRef]

129. Wall, I.B.; Moseley, R.; Baird, D.M.; Kipling, D.; Giles, P.; Laffafian, I.; Price, P.E.; Thomas, D.W.; Stephens, P. Fibroblast dysfunction is a key factor in the non-healing of chronic venous leg ulcers. *J. Investig. Dermatol.* **2008**, *128*, 2526–2540. [CrossRef]

130. Harding, K.; Sumner, M.; Cardinal, M. A prospective, multicentre, randomised controlled study of human fibroblast-derived dermal substitute (Dermagraft) in patients with venous leg ulcers. *Int. Wound J.* **2013**, *10*, 132–137. [CrossRef]

131. Hanft, J.R.; Surprenant, M.S. Healing of chronic foot ulcers in diabetic patients treated with a human fibroblast-derived dermis. *J. Foot Ankle Surg.* **2002**, *41*, 291–299. [CrossRef]

132. Omar, A.A.; Mavor, A.I.D.; Jones, A.M.; Homer-Vanniasinkam, S. Treatment of venous leg ulcers with Dermagraft. *Eur. J. Vasc. Endovasc. Surg.* **2004**, *27*, 666–672. [CrossRef]

133. ClinicalTraials. Phase I Study for Autologous Dermal Substitutes and Dermo-epidermal Skin Substitutes for Treatment of Skin Defects. 2014. Available online: https://clinicaltrials.gov/ct2/show/NCT02145130 (accessed on 10 September 2019).

134. Braziulis, E.; Diezi, M.; Biedermann, T.; Pontiggia, L.; Schmucki, M.; Hartmann-Fritsch, F.; Luginbühl, J.; Schiestl, C.; Meuli, M.; Reichmann, E. Modified plastic compression of collagen hydrogels provides an ideal matrix for clinically applicable skin substitutes. *Tissue Eng. Part C Methods* **2012**, *18*, 464–474. [CrossRef]

135. Suzuki, M.; Yakushiji, N.; Nakada, Y.; Satoh, A. Limb Regeneration in Xenopus laevis Froglet. *Sci. World J.* **2006**, *6*, 26–37. [CrossRef] [PubMed]
136. Clinical Trials. Available online: https://clinicaltrials.gov/ (accessed on 10 September 2019).
137. FDA. Available online: https://www.accessdata.fda.gov/scripts/cder/daf/ (accessed on 10 September 2019).
138. Frueh, F.S.; Später, T.; Körbel, C.; Scheuer, C.; Simson, A.C.; Lindenblatt, N.; Giovanoli, P.; Menger, M.D.; Laschke, M.W. Prevascularization of dermal substitutes with adipose tissue-derived microvascular fragments enhances early skin grafting. *Sci. Rep.* **2018**, *8*, 1–9. [CrossRef] [PubMed]

Permissions

The contributors of this book come from diverse backgrounds, making this book a truly international effort. This book will bring forth new frontiers with its revolutionizing research information and detailed analysis of the nascent developments around the world.

We would like to thank all the contributing authors for lending their expertise to make the book truly unique. They have played a crucial role in the development of this book. Without their invaluable contributions this book wouldn't have been possible. They have made vital efforts to compile up to date information on the varied aspects of this subject to make this book a valuable addition to the collection of many professionals and students.

This book was conceptualized with the vision of imparting up-to-date information and advanced data in this field. To ensure the same, a matchless editorial board was set up. Every individual on the board went through rigorous rounds of assessment to prove their worth. After which they invested a large part of their time researching and compiling the most relevant data for our readers.

The editorial board has been involved in producing this book since its inception. They have spent rigorous hours researching and exploring the diverse topics which have resulted in the successful publishing of this book. They have passed on their knowledge of decades through this book. To expedite this challenging task, the publisher supported the team at every step. A small team of assistant editors was also appointed to further simplify the editing procedure and attain best results for the readers.

Apart from the editorial board, the designing team has also invested a significant amount of their time in understanding the subject and creating the most relevant covers. They scrutinized every image to scout for the most suitable representation of the subject and create an appropriate cover for the book.

The publishing team has been an ardent support to the editorial, designing and production team. Their endless efforts to recruit the best for this project, has resulted in the accomplishment of this book. They are a veteran in the field of academics and their pool of knowledge is as vast as their experience in printing. Their expertise and guidance has proved useful at every step. Their uncompromising quality standards have made this book an exceptional effort. Their encouragement from time to time has been an inspiration for everyone.

The publisher and the editorial board hope that this book will prove to be a valuable piece of knowledge for researchers, students, practitioners and scholars across the globe.

List of Contributors

Shen Li, Derek J. Erstad, Bryan C. Fuchs and Kenneth K. Tanabe
Division of Surgical Oncology, Massachusetts General Hospital Cancer Center and Harvard Medical School, Boston, MA 02114, USA

Antonio Saviano and Thomas Baumert
Inserm, U1110, Institut de Recherche sur les Maladies Virales et Hépatiques, Université de Strasbourg, 67000 Strasbourg, France

Yujin Hoshida
Simmons Comprehensive Cancer Center, UT Southwestern Medical Center, Department of Internal Medicine, Dallas, TX 75390, USA

Edward Wenge Wang, Sariah Liu, Siamak Saadat, James Shen, Mihaela Cristea and Daphne Stewart
Department of Medical Oncology and Therapeutics Research, City of Hope National Medical Center, Duarte, CA 91010, USA

Christina Hsiao Wei and Sharon Wilczynski
Department of Pathology, City of Hope National Medical Center, Duarte, CA 91010, USA

Stephen Jae-Jin Lee, Thanh Dellinger, Ernest Soyoung Han and Lorna Rodriguez-Rodriguez
Department of Surgical Oncology, City of Hope National Medical Center, Duarte, CA 91010, USA

Susan Shehayeb
Department of Population Sciences, City of Hope National Medical Center, Duarte, CA 91010, USA

Scott Glaser and Richard Li
Department of Radiation Oncology, City of Hope National Medical Center, Duarte, CA 91010, USA

Shanmuga Subbiah, Arin Nam, Natasha Garg, Amita Behal, Prakash Kulkarni and Ravi Salgia
Department of Medical Oncology and Therapeutics Research, City of Hope National Medical Center, Duarte, CA 91010, USA

Isa Mambetsariev, Rebecca Pharaon, Benjamin Leach, TingTing Tan, Prakash Kulkarni and Ravi Salgia
Department of Medical Oncology and Therapeutics Research, City of Hope, Duarte, CA 91010, USA

Marilena Melas
The Steve and Cindy Rasmussen Institute for Genomic Medicine, Nationwide Children's Hospital, Columbus, OH 43205, USA

Shanmuga Subbiah
Department of Medical Oncology and Therapeutics Research, City of Hope Comprehensive Cancer Center, Glendora, CA 91741, USA

Siamak Saadat
Department of Medical Oncology and Therapeutics Research, City of Hope Comprehensive Cancer Center, Colton, CA 92324, USA

Swapnil Rajurkar
Department of Medical Oncology and Therapeutics Research, City of Hope Comprehensive Cancer Center, Upland, CA 91786, USA
Department of Medical Oncology and Therapeutics Research, City of Hope, Duarte, CA 91010, USA

Kevin J. McDonnell
Department of Medical Oncology and Therapeutics Research, City of Hope Comprehensive Cancer Center and Beckman Research Institute, Duarte, CA 91010, USA
Center for Precision Medicine, City of Hope Comprehensive Cancer Center, Duarte, CA 91010, USA

Joanne E. Mortimer, Mary Cianfrocca, Sayeh Lavasani, Niki Tank-Patel, Mina Sedrak, Wade Smith, Daphne Stewart, James Waisman, Christina Yeon, Tina Wang and Yuan Yuan
Department of Medical Oncology and Therapeutics Research, City of Hope Comprehensive Cancer Center, Duarte, CA 91010, USA

Laura Kruper
Department of Surgery, Division of Breast Surgery, City of Hope Comprehensive Cancer Center, Duarte, CA 91010, USA

Federico Salaris and Alessandro Rosa
Center for Life Nano Science, Istituto Italiano di Tecnologia, Viale Regina Elena 291, 00161 Rome, Italy
Department of Biology and Biotechnology Charles Darwin, Sapienza University of Rome, P.le A. Moro 5, 00185 Rome, Italy

Cristina Colosi, Carlo Brighi, Alessandro Soloperto, Valeria de Turris, Silvia Ghirga and Maria Rosito
Center for Life Nano Science, Istituto Italiano di Tecnologia, Viale Regina Elena 291, 00161 Rome, Italy

Maria Cristina Benedetti
Department of Biology and Biotechnology Charles Darwin, Sapienza University of Rome, P.le A. Moro 5,00185 Rome, Italy

Silvia Di Angelantonio
Center for Life Nano Science, Istituto Italiano di Tecnologia, Viale Regina Elena 291, 00161 Rome, Italy
Department of Physiology and Pharmacology, Sapienza University of Rome, P.le A. Moro 5, 00185 Rome, Italy

Aida Rodriguez, Laura Santos, Juan Tornin and Lucia Martinez-Cruzado
University Central Hospital of Asturias – Health and Research Institute of Asturias (ISPA), 33011 Oviedo, Spain

Veronica Rey
University Central Hospital of Asturias – Health and Research Institute of Asturias (ISPA), 33011 Oviedo, Spain
University Institute of Oncology of Asturias, 33011 Oviedo, Spain

Rene Rodriguez, Sofia T. Menendez and Oscar Estupiñan
University Central Hospital of Asturias – Health and Research Institute of Asturias (ISPA), 33011 Oviedo, Spain
University Institute of Oncology of Asturias, 33011 Oviedo, Spain
CIBER in Oncology (CIBERONC), 28029 Madrid, Spain

David Castillo and Gonzalo R. Ordoñez
Disease Research and Medicine (DREAMgenics) S.L., 33011 Oviedo, Spain

Serafin Costilla
Department of Radiology of the Servicio de Radiología of the University Central Hospital of Asturias, 33011 Oviedo, Spain

Carlos Alvarez-Fernandez
Department of Medical Oncology of the Servicio de Radiología of the University Central Hospital of Asturias, 33011 Oviedo, Spain

Aurora Astudillo
Department of Pathology of the Servicio de Radiología of the University Central Hospital of Asturias, 33011 Oviedo, Spain

Alejandro Braña
Department of Traumatology of the University Central Hospital of Asturias, 33011 Oviedo, Spain

Giuseppe Cesarelli and Parisa Pedram
Center for Advanced Biomaterials for Healthcare, Istituto Italiano di Tecnologia (IIT@CRIB), 80125 Naples, Italy
Department of Chemical, Materials and Industrial Production Engineering, University of Naples Federico II, 80125 Naples, Italy

Aurelio Salerno
Center for Advanced Biomaterials for Healthcare, Istituto Italiano di Tecnologia (IIT@CRIB), 80125 Naples, Italy

Paolo Antonio Netti
Center for Advanced Biomaterials for Healthcare, Istituto Italiano di Tecnologia (IIT@CRIB), 80125 Naples, Italy
Department of Chemical, Materials and Industrial Production Engineering, University of Naples Federico II, 80125 Naples, Italy
Interdisciplinary Research Center on Biomaterials (CRIB), University of Naples Federico II, 80125 Naples, Italy

Laura Lossi, Claudia Castagna and Adalberto Merighi
Department of Veterinary Sciences, University of Turin, I-10095 Grugliasco (TO), Italy

Alberto Granato
Department of Psychology, Catholic University of the Sacred Heart, I-20123 Milano (MI), Italy

Costantino Casale
Department of Chemical, Materials and Industrial Production Engineering (DICMAPI) University of Naples Federico II, P.le Tecchio 80, 80125 Naples, Italy

Francesco Urciuolo
Department of Chemical, Materials and Industrial Production Engineering (DICMAPI) University of Naples Federico II, P.le Tecchio 80, 80125 Naples, Italy
Interdisciplinary Research Centre on Biomaterials (CRIB), University of Naples Federico II P.le Tecchio 80, 80125 Naples, Italy

Giorgia Imparato
Center for Advanced Biomaterials for HealthCare@ CRIB, Istituto Italiano di Tecnologia, Largo Barsanti e Matteucci 53, 80125 Naples, Italy

Paolo A. Netti
Department of Chemical, Materials and Industrial
Production Engineering (DICMAPI) University of
Naples Federico II, P.le Tecchio 80, 80125 Naples, Italy

Interdisciplinary Research Centre on Biomaterials
(CRIB), University of Naples Federico II P.le Tecchio
80, 80125 Naples, Italy
Center for Advanced Biomaterials for HealthCare@
CRIB, Istituto Italiano di Tecnologia, Largo Barsanti e
Matteucci 53, 80125 Naples, Italy

Index

Printed in the USA
CPSIA information can be obtained
at www.ICGtesting.com
JSHW052311231023
50683JS00006BA/65

9 781646 466252